Integrating Conventional and Chinese Medicine in Cancer Care

A Clinical Guide

Tai Lahans was voted Faculty of the Year at Bastyr University in 1998.

She was also voted a Seattle Magazine Top Doc in 2003; this is a position voted on by other doctors and providers within the Seattle area health delivery system. Tai Lahans also sits on several boards serving cancer patients, and is extensively published. She founded the only residency program in integrated oncology with Chinese medicine in the United States.

Dedicated to Philip Duncan

For Elsevier:

Commissioning Editor: Karen Morley
Development Editor: Louise Allsop
Project Manager: Morven Dean
Design Direction: Jayne Jones

Integrating Conventional and Chinese Medicine in Cancer Care

A Clinical Guide

Tai Lahans L.AC., M.TCM, M.Ed.

Diplomate Chinese Herbal Medicine, NCCAOM

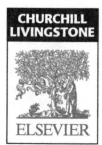

CHURCHILL LIVINGSTONE

ELSEVIER

CHURCHILL
LIVINGSTONE
ELSEVIER

An imprint of Elsevier Limited

First published 2007

ISBN-10; 0443100632
ISBN-13; 9780443100635

British Library Cataloguing in Publication Data
A catalogue record for this book is available from the British Library

Library of Congress Cataloging in Publication Data
A catalogue record for this book is available from the Library of Congress

---

Notice

Knowledge and best practice in this field are constantly changing. As new research and experience broaden our knowledge, changes in practice, treatment and drug therapy may become necessary or appropriate. Readers are advised to check the most current information provided (i) on procedures featured or (ii) by the manufacturer of each product to be administered, to verify the recommended dose or formula, the method and duration of administration, and contraindications. It is the responsibility of the practitioner, relying on their own experience and knowledge of the patient, to make diagnoses, to determine dosages and the best treatment for each individual patient, and to take all appropriate safety precautions. To the fullest extent of the law, neither the Publisher nor the Author assumes any liability for any injury and/or damage to persons or property arising out or related to any use of the material contained in this book.

ELSEVIER   your source for books,
journals and multimedia
in the health sciences

www.elsevierhealth.com

Printed in China

The publisher's
policy is to use
paper manufactured
from sustainable forests

Endorsements

In *Integrating Conventional and Chinese Medicine,* Tai Lahans takes the clear thinking, extensive research, hard-won personal experience and compassion that has marked her courses at our school and puts it in written form. This will be an extremely useful book for any practitioner of Oriental medicine who has the opportunity to treat people with cancer.

Dan Bensky, DO
Director, Seattle Institute of Oriental Medicine, USA

Tai Lahans has done a remarkable job putting together a text on cancer specifically for practitioners of Chinese medicine. She takes the key aspects of western allopathic medicine, making an understanding accessible and clinically valuable. In addition to giving us the most complete discussion of causative factors I have yet to read. She also guides us through the stages of cancer treatment. This is bound to be a well used book in my clinic.

Sharon Weizenbaum, Chinese Medicine Practitioner, MA, USA

As the practice of conventional Western medicine becomes more integrated with other modalities, physicians and other healthcare providers need new reference resources. An expanded understanding of the clinical and scientific paradigms of Chinese medicine and how they can be incorporated into current care will benefit providers and patients alike. This comprehensive text will be an essential additional to the libraries of practitioners and medical schools worldwide.

Patricia L. Dawson MD PhD FACS
Medical Director, Swedish Cancer Institute, Providence Campus; Comprehensive Breast Center Associate; Medical Director, Swedish Cancer Institute Breast Program

Contents

Preface   ix
Introduction   xiii
Disclaimer   xvii

1. General pathophysiology and treatment: conventional and Chinese medicine 1

2. Lung cancer 35

3. Colorectal cancer 61

4. Breast cancer 89

5. Prostate cancer 155

6. Cervical and uterine cancers 177

7. Ovarian cancer 195

8. Bladder and renal cancer 215

9. Pancreatic and hepatic cancers 229

10. Lymphomas 253

11. Leukemia 283

12. Concurrent issues 301

13. Death and dying 331

14. Prevention 341

Appendix   363
Index   365

Preface

Traditional Navajo rug weavers always include a line that runs out of the pattern and into the field of the rug ending at the edge. It looks like a mistake, as though the weaver lost control or fell asleep at a critical moment. But it is, in fact, intentional. This line is called the 'spirit line' and it connects the creative spirit of the weaver of the rug with the creative spirit of the universe. In this way, the rug is a living entity that stays alive forever through its connection to the universe. It is also a way for the creative spirit of the Navajo nation to remain alive throughout the manifestations of its culture. The spirit line is a continual healing.

The weft of Chinese medicine also carries a spirit line. It has evolved through history with a reference line connecting backwards to historic Chinese medicine texts and forward to the future. This ongoing reference back to the classics is one of the remarkable things about Chinese medicine; and, as one of my teachers, Ma Shoucun, has said, 'Chinese medicine has yet to reach its fulfillment'. We are the current carriers of the spirit line of Chinese medicine.

This spirit line has always been open to the creative manifestations of other traditions. For example, the connections between Ayurvedic and Chinese medicine are historic and obvious. The Chinese have imported herbs from all over the world and incorporated them into their own pharmacopoeia. In modern times, Western science has also influenced the ways in which we who practice Chinese medicine understand and treat human illnesses. The TCM system of modern Chinese medicine is very much a composite of the classical science and theory of many ages of Chinese medicine and the science of the West. In herbal medicine the classical usage of herbs is sometimes combined with the pharmacological analysis of those herbs. In oncology this is especially true. For example, e zhu (Curcumae Rhizoma; *Curcuma zedoaria*; zedoary) is a blood-cracking herb and, from the pharmacological perspective, we know that it can extend the life of certain white blood cells. Therefore, we add it to formulas where this newly discovered function is valuable in treating myelosuppression caused by chemotherapy. The Chinese have also implemented new ways of delivering herbal formulas by integrating preparation techniques from western science allowing for intravenous delivery. The list grows by the day.

So the spirit line of Chinese medicine continues to draw from various traditions. No matter what your opinion regarding the mixing and hybridising of paradigms of medicine in relation to classical Chinese medicine, nowhere does the line become more blurred than in cancer treatment. This eclecticism is partially driven by patients. Even in China today patients are drawing from any information they can find about an intervention that might help save their life. Chinese patients use many of the same nutritional supplements as their Western counterparts. The Internet has made for a smaller global community. When someone is fighting for their life, dedication to the purity of classical practice can be one of the first things to go. It is not to say that classical medicine and theory has less to offer the cancer question but rather that, in the scramble to find answers, patients and practitioners, perhaps driven by fear, often tend to become more eclectic. At the same time, a whole new medicine has evolved that is an initiation into the world of global medicine. The fact that this initiation began mainly in the realm of Chinese medicine makes me intensely proud, supportive, and persistent in efforts to share this newer window through which to view healing. It is in this amazingly creative environment that patients and practitioners alike have become aware that cancer is the modern epidemic, the epidemic to a large extent of the developed world.

In 1900 in the United States, cancer caused less than 4% of all deaths; in 1976 cancer accounted for 20% of all deaths; and in the year 2000 cancer accounted for 30% of all deaths in the United States. The rates for solid tumor cancers, including breast, colon, prostate, testis, urinary bladder, kidney, skin, malignant melanoma, and lymphatic and hematopoietic malignancies (leukemias) have all risen dramatically. Since 1970 the rates for testicular cancer have risen by 150% and for non-Hodgkin's lymphoma by 200%. Breast cancer occurred in 1 in 30 women in the 1940s; the breast cancer rate in the year 2000 was 1 in 8 women. Cancer is now the only major killing disease in the developed world the incidence of which is on the rise. All of these statistics are from the United States governmental reports through the National Cancer Institute and from Cancer Statistics published by the American Cancer Society. What is happening? Are human beings somehow more vulnerable to cancers now? Is an extended age range to blame? Is it stress and the modern lifestyle? The governmental statistics have all been adjusted to account for increased age and a greater population.

The primary rationale in conventional medicine is that cancers are predominantly caused by immunodeficiency, chronic viral infection, genetic predisposition, and environmental carcinogens. In this last category, environmental carcinogens used to include naturally occurring radiation exposures (sun flares most commonly) and exposures to heavy metals that have always occurred in the environment. Arsenic and lead and many other known carcinogens occur naturally. It is now believed that animals or humans exposed to a carcinogen may be influenced by a variety of other factors: endocrine, immunological, viral, biochemical, and possibly psychological factors. Therefore, a range of factors can increase one's sensitivity to a carcinogen. Diet is a major external factor; other combined carcinogens may be another; and promoting agents such as alcoholism, lack of exercise, chronic depression, obesity, hyperinsulinemia, diabetes, chronic disease, poor sleep and ageing may be others.

The rate of increase in the production and dissemination of new chemicals since the 1940s has been immense. The number of organic solvents introduced to the marketplace between 1945 and 1970 rose by 750%. The number of nitrogen fertilisers rose by 1050%. In fact, over 85 000 new chemicals were developed during the 20th century. Of these, 33 000 are in common use, and of these only about 1500 have been studied for any human health effects.

The intricate biochemical defenses that living beings have developed to cope with their environment are now being violated constantly by foreign materials introduced into the environment, in petroleum products, petroleum-based synthetic organochlorine chemicals, and pesticides. Many of these products, and especially organochlorine pesticides and other agricultural inputs, drift from their original place of application via the movement of air and water. They accumulate, often far from the locale of their original application, and sometimes up to one million times the original amount. Many have a very long half-life and some never break down in the environment. Many are fat-soluble, which means that fat tissue in living animals, including humans, becomes a repository for these molecules. The higher an animal is placed on the food chain, the greater the possible exposure. Since the food chain in the ocean is longer and more complex than on land, fish tend to be more highly contaminated than land-based animals.

For example, some organochlorine pesticides are xenoestrogenic and carcinogenic. They increase the number of estrogen receptors in the body, vastly increasing the body's exposure to estrogen. The Environmental Working Group sampled tap water in 29 major American cities. They found that the tap water in 28 of the 29 cities studied contained atrazine. According to the EWG, the number of chemical contaminants now found in the average adult human body is between 70 and 90. It is odd that the pharmaceutical industry must spend vast amounts of time and money before a drug is deemed safe for use in treatment of human diseases but, at the same time, the chemical industry, a very close relative, produces new chemicals that appear to have no constraints put upon them regarding safety, and yet these chemicals also end up in the human body, and more and more are causing disease.

There may appear to be an emphasis on cause in this book, particularly from the environmental point of view. This emphasis stems from my deep belief that an ounce of prevention is worth a pound of cure. Considering the quote from the *Art of War* by Sun Tzu about the family of physicians from ancient times in China, then our role becomes more clear. A brother was asked who was the best doctor in his family. He replied, 'My eldest brother sees the spirit of sickness and removes it before it takes shape, so his name does not get out of the house. My elder brother cures sickness when it is still extremely minute, so his name does not get out of the neighborhood. As for me, I puncture veins, prescribe potions, and massage skin, so from time to time my name gets out and is heard among the lords'. The concept of prevention runs deeply in Chinese medicine. If this philosophy was applied to the modern cancer epidemic, we would be seeing and hearing much more information about how we can help ourselves to avoid ever being diagnosed with a cancer. Prevention begins at home and in our neighborhoods.

Cancer is often a long-term evolutionary process that may take several years to detect. When we add the complexity of new exposures it becomes clear that prevention may begin in utero. And so constant vigilance is necessary on the part of the practitioner to teach our patients what we do know in any given moment about causes of cancer. This vigilance includes learning classical Chinese medicine as deeply as we can and learning the new information that becomes available from biomedical research about cancer causation and about environmental contamination. All latent pathogenic factors begin as external exposures, and it may be that the external exposures of modern life are, in fact, latent pathogenic factors that contribute to cancer pathogenesis. We know that yin deficiency and spleen deficiency act as

magnets for latent pathogenic factors and help them to sink more deeply into the body. Perhaps this is a classical explanation of the carcinogenic exposures and the idea of promoting factors in cancer causation. Given this, the role of the modern doctor of Oriental medicine may be that of sage, counselor, physician, environmentalist, and community-oriented political activist.

In conventional medicine most theory and research relating to cancer pathology is aimed at treatment. Most 'prevention' is aimed at early detection. The odd or somewhat obscure resources sometimes given in this book are necessary because conventional research about promoting factors, environmental causation, and prevention of cancer is scarce. Information resulting from research in these realms is often hidden or overlooked because acting upon this information would necessitate dramatic changes in how we live. This is especially true in the arena of environmental contamination. Information about prevention is hard to find, and is rarely given out by oncologists because of a lack of time, because of the politics involved, and because prevention is not taught in medical schools.

Citations have become easier to obtain in the realm of treatment in conventional science and medicine, but not in Chinese medicine. This is unfortunate, since this is one of the problems given for the lack of trust in Chinese herbal medicine. Certainly citing the Shang han za bing lun for references regarding the concept of latent pathogenic factors is a perfectly legitimate approach for the practitioner of herbal medicine. But these citations to classical literature are meaningless to modern science. I have done my best to provide accurate citations of legitimate and well-designed studies of Chinese herbal medicine that would meet the rigorous standards applied in the West. Single-herb studies abound, but not as many studies for formulas. Many references are not available in English. When necessary I have referred to a Chinese or Korean or Japanese language reference. At other times, I have referred to notes taken during my studies in China or Korea with integrative oncologists at various hospitals. All of my teachers have been doctors of Chinese medicine, equally trained in conventional and Chinese medicine, and specialists in integrated oncology. I cannot say how grateful I am for their amazing dedication, persistence, skill and compassion in treating and supporting patients who suffer in all the same ways that our patients suffer here in the West and for the same reasons. If it weren't for these immensely intelligent and courageous doctors, we here would know so much less than we do to care for our patients.

Let us all take up the spirit line of modern Chinese medicine and find strategies for the modern epidemic of cancer. It is emblematic of the tension in modern life between natural living within the land and the developing world and the frenetic constant movement of urban high-density constructed life without room and quiet space for the mind and soul. We are the people we have been waiting for.

Tai Lahans
Seattle, USA 2004

Introduction

It was in the 1950s that the Chinese began to integrate the best of the old (classical Chinese medicine) and the best of the new (modern biomedicine). This integration has been very successful in many areas of medicine, including oncology. Chinese medicine has followed the evolution of biomedicine with regards to the pathophysiology and biology of cancers, and then interpreted these physiological concepts within the framework of classical Chinese medicine. Valuable and compelling information has been developed about many herbs pertaining to their ability to treat myelosuppression, increase many oncologically important components of the immune system, treat hypercoaguability syndrome, enhance the effectiveness of cytotoxic treatments, protect organ function and so on, all within the context of classical theory and its modern analysis within the parameters of biomedicine.

At the same time, Chinese medicine has evolved its own analysis, part classically oriented and part biomedically oriented, of how cancers come about and how they can be more effectively treated and prevented. The integration of the two systems of medicine, Chinese and conventional, within the minds of individual practitioners of Chinese medicine in China and Korea lends to them an ability to synthesise these two systems in ways that directly benefit their patients. For example, not all neutropenic fevers are caused by infection and yet, in the United States, they are often treated prophylactically with antibiotic therapy. The use of antibiotics, although some-times valuable and necessary, is not always the correct treatment especially when laboratory screens show no presence of pathogens. Antibiotic therapies frequently undermine the ability of the middle burner to metabolise fluids and absorb nutrients. This function is very important in cancer treatment because many cancer patients are malnourished due to the cancer itself and due to chemotherapeutic regimens and their side effects. Therefore, adding insult to injury by treating prophylactically for infection that is not present becomes preventable in an integrated approach.

Apparent neutropenic fevers can also be due to yin or qi deficiency, both of which are common in patients who are undergoing chemotherapy or radiotherapy for cancer. Antibiotic use can actually contribute to qi or yin deficiency and undermine normal health. The middle jiao injury from antibiotic treatment leads to a damp accumulation, which causes qi deficiency and leads to stasis, which in turn leads to heat constraint and then to yin deficiency. The ability to differentiate between these two types of fevers, by combining the analysis of Chinese medicine with that of conventional medicine, is a valuable skill that directly contributes to the overall health of cancer patients.

THE BOOK

The chapters of this book are an attempt to organise and present this integration. The understanding and treatment of cancer is an ongoing and evolving specialty. This information changes almost on a daily basis. Certainly the conventional approach changes as new research becomes available and there is a growing change in orientation in conventional medicine away from what would be called in Chinese medicine 'attack' therapy, one of the eight battle arrays. This is welcome on everyone's part. And means that the Chinese medicine approach must change as well since the adjunctive intervention must interface with a deep understanding of the conventional mechanisms. The change in orientation is also evolving from the point of view of Chinese medicine wherein new research from China, Korea, and Japan adds to the overall means by which practitioners view cancer pathogenesis and treatment. For example, newer research is looking at blood-regulating herbs and their ability to prevent metastatic spread, thus buying time for other approaches to act cytotoxically by confining tumors to their local area (unpublished research). Patients usually die of cancer because of complications from metastatic disease. Preventing metastasis is a major accomplishment.

The integration of Chinese herbal medicine into the standard of care for cancer treatment is a highly valuable contribution to our patients, and this integration is full of the basic tenets of both classical Chinese medicine and biomedicine. For example, both systems share the tenet to 'first do no harm'. Upholding this ethic in conventional medical treatment for cancer is much more difficult. On the one hand, our conventional medical colleagues deserve great respect; and we cannot say that we have an alternative for cure given the constraints placed on us in the West. We cannot utilise intravenous herbal medicine nor other delivery methods of traditional medicine that might be as cytotoxic as chemotherapy or radiation. There are some other modalities and techniques, like ultraviolet exposure and others, that are not necessarily cytotoxic but are curative, but those are also outside our scope of practice in the United States. On the other hand, we have a great deal to offer the gap of limiting harm caused by conventional treatment and, in modern China and Korea, higher dose chemotherapy is used because of the supportive care offered by combining treatment with Chinese herbal medicine.

The hope is that the evolving exploration of this integration can be carried on no matter what new information is added by either system. There is a vast number of highly sophisticated and well-designed studies from China, Korea, and Japan that show significant efficacy for the combined medicine approach. At the same time it is necessary to keep up with the mechanism and action of new treatments in cancer in order to better understand the integration. And this means that we must be constantly studying both approaches. The spirit line of Chinese medicine in oncology is not an easy one. This is especially true given that the integration is a hard won effort on the part of Chinese medicine practitioners here in the West who must stop their lives here and travel to China or Korea for extended periods of time in order to learn the medicine. Also, the theory of Chinese medicine is not sought in research settings here in the United States. The contribution from the Chinese medicine side of the integration is disregarded and grossly misunderstood. Treating cancer patients with integrated care can be a lonely path.

Cancer is not one disease but rather over 100 different diseases with commonalities between them all. Therefore, each type of cancer is treated differently. Chinese medicine follows conventional medicine in this regard, but also retains much of the classical approach regarding pathogenesis, particularly pertaining to phlegm and blood stasis and the many ways that toxins are spoken of in the classical literature. The book is organised, therefore, by chapter and by type of cancer. Where possible the conventional medical approach is integrated into the Chinese medicine approach and vice versa. It has been very difficult to write this integration and, at times, it feels awkward. For this I apologise. It has been difficult to find a straightforward way to give voice to the mechanics and the flexibility of the integration except in the cases. It is my hope that the cases make the integration a real and living entity that grounds finally all of the theory from both sides.

The purpose in writing this book has always been to offer information that would encourage practitioners of Chinese medicine to enter the realm of treating serious chronic illness and that place where we are often forced to work alongside our conventional medical colleagues. My intent is to support the Western Chinese medicine practitioners to practice as do the Chinese and Koreans whenever appropriate. Even when we have failed to change the internal and external environment of life to the extent that we have prevented serious disease we still have tremendous skill and value to offer the patient with life-threatening illness or terminal disease. Much of Chinese medicine has evolved out of treating epidemics. The Shang Han Za Bing Lun and the strategies it proposes was written by Zhang Zhong Jing after 80% of his family had died of epidemic disease in the first half of the 3rd century ACE. Cancer is a modern epidemic and we must carry the spirit line of the medicine into this modern epidemic.

At the same time, this book is not meant to be an encyclopedia for the standard of care in a linear approach to integrating Chinese and conventional treatment for cancer patients. Every patient diagnosed with cancer that has the same type, stage, and markers is not the same disease within the parameters of Chinese medicine. So all of these formulas are meant to be modified to meet the individual needs of any given patient in time. This is the art of Chinese medicine. Therefore, the information contained here is meant for the more advanced practitioner who has skill in discerning layers of diagnostic patterns and also skill in interpreting conventional medicine through the lens of Chinese medicine. What is needed more than anything now in the practice of Chinese medicine in the West is the addition of clinical supervised specialty training. In my opinion, nowhere is this more needed than in oncology and chronic viral diseases. Patients come to us with a potentially life-threatening diagnosis and we owe them the highest skill level possible. This can come only from supervised clinical training from specialists. Treating patients from a textbook is not adequate. Treating patients without any training in classical

Chinese herbalism would be unethical. So I ask that you do not lift formulas from this book without modifying them to specifically fit your patient.

You will note that this book does not include acupuncture techniques in the therapeutics. This is because Chinese medicine traditionally has looked upon herbal medicine as the primary interface in the treatment of serious illness. Material medicine is considered crucial. This is especially true in oncology. When there is material disease, like a mass, then material medicine is needed. Acupuncture is used all over the world to treat cancers in adjunctive care. However, there are many forms or systems of acupuncture being used today, and this is another reason for not including the variety of acupuncture therapeutics available. Japanese, Chinese, Korean, and European schools of practice and many others make it impossible to cover the terrain within this context. Acupuncture is immensely valuable in treating cancers, the side effects of conventional treatments, and the spirit of the patient. This book, however, covers only the herbal medicine aspect of the interface.

Chinese medicine has not reached its full potential. As carriers of the spirit line of Chinese medicine, it is our path to meet the challenge of modern illness. That path is complex in that it includes understanding the multiple pathogenic influences of modern life and also finding a way, sometimes in a world that does not care, of bridging the gap between modern biomedicine and classical natural medicine. Is it possible that in bridging the gap, it is not only Chinese medicine that is transformed but also conventional medicine? The time is now; we are the people for whom we have been waiting.

Disclaimer

Materia medica are referred to throughout the book by their pharmaceutical name in Latin. Readers should be aware of the legal status of certain herbs included in this book. Although they are all available in China, a few herbs are subject to export restrictions and others are considered too toxic for use in some Western countries. The situation regarding restrictions and bans tends to change over time and from country to country.

Materia medica that are included in the Appendix of the Convention on International Trade in Endangered Species of Wild Fauna and Flora (CITES) are marked with an asterisk (*), as are other materia medica subject to restrictions or bans in certain countries as a result of their toxicity. Also marked with an asterisk are other animal and mineral materia medica which cannot be sold in unlicensed medical preparations as herbs.

Readers should consult the appropriate authorities in their own countries for the latest developments. Inclusion of materia medica in this book does not imply that their use is permitted in all countries and in all circumstances.

To the extent permissible under applicable laws, no responsibility is assumed by the Publisher, its distributors or licensees for any injury and/or damage to persons or property as a result of any alleged libellous statements, infringement of intellectual property or privacy rights, or products liability, whether resulting from negligence, herbal dosage or otherwise, or from any use or operation of any ideas, instructions, procedures, products or methods contained in the material herein.

Chapter 1

General Pathophysiology and Treatment: Conventional and Chinese Medicine

CHAPTER CONTENTS

Conventional medical approach   1
    Biology   1
    Apparent causal factors   4
    Common modes of presentation   6
    Physiological abnormalities   6
    Diagnosis   8
    Principles of treatment   11
    Integration of care   15

Chinese medicine approach   15
    Pathogenesis   17
    Therapeutic principles   22
    Treatment   25
    Prevention   32

> We are the people we have been waiting for
>
> Hopi saying

CONVENTIONAL MEDICAL APPROACH

BIOLOGY

Neoplastic disorders are now the most common cause of death in the United States. In their lifetime, one-quarter of all women in the United States and one-third of men will be diagnosed with cancer. Of these, approximately 50–60% will die of the disease.[1]

Generally, a neoplastic disease consists of an altered cell population that has become unresponsive to normal controls and to the organising influences of adjacent tissues. Plasma means 'thing formed'; neo means new. Therefore, neoplasms are new and abnormal formations of tissue without useful function and growing at the expense of a healthy organism. There are many types, including benign, histoid, and malignant. Malignancies have the capacity to spread locally and to distant sites, a capacity not shared with benign tumors.[2] It is often the complications of spread that are the cause of death in cancers. There are over 100 different kinds of cancer, each of which has its own specific characteristics and, therefore, treatment.

Neoplastic disorders are defined by their biological characteristics. Certain histologic abnormalities are predictive of neoplastic biologic behavior. Histology is the study of the microscopic structure of tissues. Among the histologic abnormalities of neoplasms is a high frequency of mitotic figures, meaning that many cell nuclei are reproducing. Also there are derangements of the nucleus, the vital body in the protoplasm of the cell and the essential agent in growth, metabolism, reproduction, and the transmission of characteristics of a cell. At the same time that these abnormalities are taking place in the cell, an alteration is taking place in the normal tissue architecture, and evidence begins to accumulate that there is an invasion of adjacent structures and possibly even distant metastatic spread.[2]

Malignant neoplasms commonly arise in tissues with self-renewing cell systems. Self-renewing cell systems include skin, mucosal linings, blood cells, immune cells, and hormonally-responsive cells. Normal cellular replication and maturation takes place at a fairly high frequency in these types of cells. For example, the mucosal lining of the digestive tract replaces itself approximately every 24 hours. Breast tissue cells respond usually on a monthly basis to hormonal influences as part of the menstrual cycle. Cancers can be seen as caricatures of normal cellular replication and maturation. It is thought that the diversity that develops in tumor cell populations probably arises from imperfect attempts at maturation. Maturation refers to a cell changing and growing towards a climax of that type of cell within a given system. Once the cell has fulfilled its life work, it enters apoptosis, or programmed cell death. It is often the lack of controls on replication and growth and the loss of apoptosis that are the underlying causative factors in the cancerisation process.[2]

The main biologic properties displayed by tumor cells are common to many normal cells within the body. For example, lymphocytes, granulocytes, and macrophages are all immune cells that move to distant sites in the body and 'invade' tissues as part of their normal functioning. During embryogenesis various cells move to distant sites, implant, and develop within new organs and tissues. Many of the phenotypic markers found on cancer cells are also present in immature normal cells. These include carcinoembryonic antigen or CEA, α-fetoprotein, fetal isozymes, and others.[3] One could say that normal cells contain genetic

information for cancer-like traits, and that cancerous cells are cells that have been affected in such a way that a mutation occurred, and that the cells have been trying to get back to normal ever since by trying, unsuccessfully, to go through a cellular process.

There are also chromosomal changes that are associated with cancer,[4] and because of this many neoplastic disorders are characterised by specific karyotypic abnormalities. A karyotype refers to the systematic array of the chromosomes of a given cell in the metaphase stage. The chromosome is a microscopic body that develops from the nuclear material of a cell and is especially conspicuous during mitosis or cell division. Chromosomes contain the genes, the hereditary determiners. The numbers of these are stable for a species; the number for humans is 46, or 23 in somatic cells; the ova and sperm each contain 23 chromosomes, one each of the 23 pairs.

When a diagnosis of acute leukemia, for example, is given, very often a genetic abnormality is found at the monosomy 5 and 7 gene sites. An abnormality is often found at the 3p site in small cell cancer of the lung. Chromosome 8 is translocated in Burkitt's lymphoma, and so on. In fact, locating these abnormalities is often part of the histological diagnosis for a cancer.

These chromosomal markers are also used as targets in modern gene therapy for some kinds of cancers. This is important because an understanding of the mechanism of conventional treatment is an important part of integrative care. Some of these same markers are used in monitoring and, therefore, can be used to monitor the impact of Chinese medicine in integrated treatment. If we as practitioners of Chinese medicine can construct formulas that enhance the mechanism of the conventional treatment and change the marker being monitored more significantly, then we have contributed to the outcome in a beneficial way.

Genes that have been frequently found to be associated with cancer pathogenesis are called oncogenes.[4] Cells expressing mutated forms of these genes have a high probability of progressing to malignancy. The normal genes before being 'switched on' are called proto-oncogenes. The mutated forms are called oncogenes, and are said to be activated. These genes are denoted by three-letter names, such as *sis*, *ras*, and *myc*. Since many of the oncogenes were first discovered as mutated cellular genes incorporated into the nucleic acid of RNA tumor viruses, the activated forms are denoted v-onc, as in v-*sis*, and the proto-oncogenes are c-onc, as in c-*sis*.

Arguments have been put forward that support qualitative and quantitative abnormalities of oncogene expression as key to the process of tumorigenesis. Cellular DNA sequences have a high degree of similarity in structure and in origin to the known transforming sequences of retroviruses. There is currently a great deal of study in this realm because these genes are highly conserved in nature and are found in a large number of animal species. It is possible that they play a role in normal growth and development, and when injured in some way contribute to abnormal growth processes. To date, approximately 25 oncogenes have been identified. Gene therapy is one of the driving forces in cancer treatment and is also used in vaccine therapies to prevent a cancer from forming.

Proto-oncogenes code for proteins involved in the receptor-activated proliferation/differentiation pathways. Proto-oncogenes are classified into four groups:

1. Growth factors that stimulate cell signaling, such as platelet-derived growth factors. These are important because platelet aggregation is a key in tumorogenesis. There are herbs in the blood-regulating category that affect platelet aggregation.[5]
2. Growth-factor receptors receive oncogenic information.[5] Many growth-factor receptors contain tyrosine kinase activity, e.g. erbB-2 protein, which is found in more aggressive forms of breast cancer. There are herbs in the toxin-clearing category that affect these receptors by clearing the toxin.
3. Signal transducers that are components of the intracellular signaling pathways. Signals are transmitted from cell-membrane receptors to the nucleus by second messengers. Cascades of protein kinases are involved in mediating these signals by way of proto-oncogenes. The *ras* gene plays a role here. Cyclin-dependent kinases (CDKs) are involved in many cancers. CDK-1 plays a role in cell division and has a role in 90% of all breast cancers. Its

presence facilitates the proliferation of vascular endothelial cells. These cells form the basis for the creation of new blood vessels, which feed tumors (angiogenesis). Many supplement therapies and probably many Chinese herbs interact with growth factors and growth-factor receptors to limit tyrosine kinase activity and stop cell proliferation.

4. Nuclear transcription factors bind DNA and activate gene expression. The proto-oncogene c-*sis* is the gene for one form of platelet-derived growth factor. The oncogene, v-*sis*, causes fibroblasts to proliferate because, whereas the normal cellular *sis* gene, c-*sis*, is repressed in fibroblasts, the viral copy, v-*sis*, is under the control of the active viral regulatory region and is highly expressed. Thus, the cell makes its own growth factor and grows continuously. Many categories of Chinese herbs can be thought of as regulators, detoxifiers, and harmonisers in relation to nuclear transcription factors.

One growth factor gene is c-*erbB*. Normal receptor activation triggers the extensive network of reactions that culminate in mitosis. The mutated gene, v-*erbB*, activates this cascade without the normally present EGF, a polypeptide growth factor, and a cell with this mutated receptor is continuously stimulated to grow. The *erbB-2* (which is probably a hormone receptor) is a gene expression that is frequently amplified in breast cancer. The *erbB-2* is an example of a proto-oncogene with a point mutation or translocation. The *her-2neu* oncogene is related to *erbB-2*, and a newer form of chemotherapy for *her-2neu*-positive breast tumors, trastuzumab (Herceptin®), is an example of the utilisation of the concept of oncogene expression in antineoplastic therapy.

Another proto-oncogene is the c-*myc* one, which is probably involved with regulatory rates in cell growth. Mutations in the v-*myc* gene cause increased expression and, therefore, persistent proliferation. In cancers, it is important to note that proliferation per se is not necessarily abnormal, but the differentiation to terminal or mature cells is abnormal, delayed or absent in the malignant clone of the original normal cell.

What likely turns on these mutations is what would be considered 'toxin' in Chinese medicine.

Toxins come in many forms and the utilisation of heat and toxin-clearing herbs acts to release these toxins and flush them from the environment. This action potentiates the cytotoxic therapy used in conventional medicine.

Tumor-suppressor genes are active genes that suppress the formation of tumors.[6] They are a normal part of the body's immune system. Tumor-suppressor genes can be 'knocked out' through inheritance, giving the individual a predisposition to develop cancer. They can also be knocked out by other, as yet unknown, means. It seems probable that exposures to toxic chemicals may have a negative effect on the functioning of tumor-suppressor genes. For example, the *p53* tumor suppressor gene is frequently knocked out in lung cancer. The end products of carcinogenic chemicals made by heating tobacco are toxic and affect the *p53* gene as it relates to the lung tissue.

Tumor-suppressor genes are regulators that control the expression of other genes. The most common gene mutation is in the tumor-suppressor gene *p53*. Many cancers are the result of a defect in the *p53* gene. For example, 70% of all colorectal cancers, 30% of all breast cancers, 50% of all ovarian cancers, and all small-cell lung cancers have defects in the *p53* tumor-suppressor genes. The flavone quercitin, found in brassicas (broccoli, cauliflower, kale, Brussels sprouts) helps to prevent a defect in this gene. It is not known whether there are Chinese herbs that have this effect but several formulas have been tested over time in the prevention of the recurrence of lung cancer. It seems safe to say that the efficacy of these formulas (like Fei liu ping) is partially based on re-establishing the *p53* tumor suppressor gene activity.

Oncoviruses are a cause of insertional mutagenesis that occurs when cells are infected by viral genes.[7] This causes mutation to already existing DNA. Epstein–Barr virus (EBV) is linked to esophageal cancer and one type of lymphoma. Herpes simplex virus (HSV) and human papilloma virus (HPV) are linked to cervical cancer. Hepatitis B and C (HBV and HCV, respectively) are linked to hepato-cellular cancer.

There are 63 trillion cells in the body, each of which undergoes mutations each day. It is amazing that more malignancies do not occur when viewed from this perspective. Mutation occurs when there is a build-up of oxidative damage whereby the gene itself is altered and then initiates the process of malignancy. The protective mechanisms within the body to prevent malignancy from occurring as a result of mutation include:

- inhibition of mutation by reducing the overall number of mutational changes
- repair of mutations that do occur
- inhibition of an occurrence by turning off a damaged cell so that it cannot proliferate.

APPARENT CAUSAL FACTORS

Epidemiological studies have identified environmental hazards, social practices, and heritable factors that seem to be responsible for many cancers. Because there is often a prolonged period of development into a cancer, the precise etiological agents responsible are sometimes difficult to ascertain. Many cancers are multifactorial. This is one of the reasons given why cancer prevention is not really a possibility and, therefore, is one reason why research focuses on treatment rather than prevention of cancers. This is an area of great frustration among families who have lost loved ones to cancer and among those who treat cancers on a daily basis. It is also an area of frustration for cancer patients and survivors who often realise too late that there are specific things that can be done to prevent or at least lower risk for cancer. Each chapter in this book includes a section on risk factors. This provides a means by which practitioners can advise patients about how to survive their cancer and prevent recurrence.

There do seem to be clearly increased incidences of neoplastic diseases within certain families, but a clearly defined pattern of inheritance is established only rarely. Retinoblastoma, lipomatosis, and colonic polyposis may present in families with a pattern of dominant inheritance. Also, multiple endocrine neoplasm syndromes involving the pituitary, thyroid, and pancreatic islet cells follow a dominant inheritance pattern in some cases. However, for the most part, the chromosomal instability syndromes and immunodeficiency disorders are transmitted as autosomal recessive characteristics, making patterns difficult to identify. However, identifying families at higher risk allows the practitioner of Chinese medicine to begin advising and treating to prevent an occurence of cancer.

The relative incidence of various cancers to age, gender, and other constitutional factors indicates that other determinants do exist. For example, acute lymphocytic leukemia is essentially a disease of childhood. Protecting children from exposure to causative factors is primary. Malignant melanoma is a post-pubertal phenomenon. Testicular tumors and Hodgkin's disease are most frequently diseases of young adults. Breast cancer is far more common in women than in men. The rates for breast cancer are now so high in the US that it would seem that every woman is at risk. Therefore, advising and treating women on how to prevent a primary occurrence is important. Other kinds of cancer like chronic leukemia, myeloma, and many solid tumors, have increasing rates of incidence with age. These cancers appear to be connected not with aging and immunodeficiency, but rather with a growing load of toxins that eventually overwhelm the whole system. More research needs to be done in this realm. One good resource in this regard is the Environmental Working Group website (www.ewg.org).

Acquired clinical disorders that are not neoplastic are often associated with increased incidence of malignant tumors. Usually these tumors arise from tissue that has been undergoing prolonged regenerative activity. Perhaps the increased rate of cellular proliferation enhances the possibility for and development of a neoplasia. For example, Bowen's disease of the skin tends to evolve into a squamous cell cancer. Non-familial polyps of a certain type are regarded as precursors for malignant lesions. Human papilloma virus of certain types is considered causative for cervical cancer.

The number of chemicals introduced for the first time has climbed astronomically since the 1940s. Of the approximately 85 000 new chemicals introduced since that time, only about 1500 have been tested for carcinogenicity or any other human health effects. Neither have combinations of various new chemicals been tested. New, more sophisticated, techniques for measuring the levels of 150 chemicals stored in human body tissue show that most people, by the age of 60, are carrying at least 80 chemicals in various body tissues. The carcinogenicity of these chemicals is untested, as is their contribution to other diseases.

Petroleum-based chemicals, especially the organochlorines used in the monoculture agribusiness industry, are especially problematic. Organochlorines are used to make pesticides and certain chemical fertilisers. Organochlorines persist in the environment, some for thousands of years. They accumulate downstream or downwind from their original application area, in concentrations sometimes a million-fold that of the original application.[8,9] They are fat-soluble, and when ingested accumulate and can act xenoestrogenically in many ways to cause and promote cancers.[10,11] Israel eliminated three organochlorine pesticides from agricultural use and in 10 years breast cancer rates in Israel dropped by 30%.[12–14] This is only one example of how a chemical used ubiquitously in agriculture can affect human health.

Viruses have been shown to be oncogenic in several animal species.[15] At least 12 strains of human adenoviruses are capable of inducing tumors in newborn laboratory animals. HPV is linked to papillomas; EBV is linked to Burkitt's lymphoma and esophageal cancer; HSVII has been associated, along with HPV, with cervical cancer; a retrovirus has been associated with aggressive T-cell leukemia-lymphoma; HCV has been linked to liver cancer, and so on.

Serologic studies have identified tumor-related antigens in patients with leukemia, osteogenic sarcoma, melanoma, and other soft-tissue sarcomas. Similar antibodies have been found in family members. This implies a possible link with a virus or other infectious agent and tumor pathogenesis. It also implies that unrecognised infections in normal individuals may be responsible for some cancers. Hepatitis C and HPV are the most obvious examples.

Antigens are substances that induce the formation of antibodies; antibodies are protein substances developed by the body, usually in response to the presence of an antigen. Antibodies are present in the circulation, and may be transferred to an infant in utero by the mother, or may be developed during life by subclinical contact with the disease-producing agent, thereby providing immunity to the disease. For example, there is distinct antigenicity associated with Burkitt's lymphoma, nasopharyngeal cancer, melanoma, and neuroblastoma, among others. Fetal antigens have been demonstrated in cancer of the colon, pancreas, and lung (CEA). α-Fetoprotein is associated with hepatoma and embryonal carcinoma and testicular cancer. CEA is also present in the blood of pregnant women, heavy smokers, and in some patients with hepatic cirrhosis, pulmonary emphysema, and ulcerative colitis.

There is a defined humoral and cell-mediated response to tumor-related antigens. Sensitised lymphocytes can be prevented from acting against tumor cells by the presence of blocking or enhancing antibodies. Immunologic responsiveness to tumor antigens may be thwarted by the presence of suppressor T cells, large amounts of tumor (immune paralysis), or tolerance due to the introduction of tumor antigen very early in life. The role of immunologic surveillance and tumorogenesis is an area requiring much investigation.

Table 1.1 shows environmental agents known to be associated with neoplasms,[16] and Box 1.1 lists some known and suspected carcinogens.[17]

One of the primary health problems that we now face is how to decontaminate the human and general environment of these carcinogens.

COMMON MODES OF PRESENTATION

Neoplastic diseases present themselves in various and inconsistent ways. The onset of a neoplasm is difficult to date. Even when there is a known exposure to a carcinogen, a prolonged latent or induction period is common before clinically-detectable disease evolves. For example, in a ductal carcinoma of the breast it generally takes seven to ten years for a neoplastic tumor to develop into a 1 cm tumor (several billion cells), which is just barely palpable.

Carcinoma-in-situ is considered a premalignant lesion. The most common site for this earliest stage of a cancer is the uterine cervix. Many non-invasive lesions like this do not develop into cancer. Often the biopsy procedure will remove the entire carcinoma in situ; thus the diagnostic technique is also the treatment technique. Ductal carcinoma in situ (DCIS) in breast cancer is also in this realm, and the lumpectomy surgical biopsy procedure can be curative, although radiation to the site is often performed as added insurance against local spread.

Malignant neoplastic diseases may exist in a human for months and even years and remain asymptomatic. Often their presence is found through routine screening, either for cancer or for general health. Prostate cancer can fall into this realm as well as cervical and breast cancers. Prostate cancer is sometimes so indolent that it is only on autopsy that it is found. Another example is chronic lymphocytic leukemia, which may exist for long periods without symptoms.

Usually in non-leukemic neoplasms the presentation of the patient relates to problems arising from physical alterations in adjacent organ systems. Findings often include the presence of an obvious tumor mass; the presence of an ulcerative lesion that will not heal; chronic bleeding and the results of blood loss; bone destruction; involvement of the central or peripheral nervous system with resultant seizures, paralysis, and pain; acute or chronic obstruction of a hollow organ, e.g. the lungs, colon, stomach, gallbladder, urinary bladder; and obstruction of mediastinal structures. When mass lesions are present the initial presentation may be in relation to a distant site from the origin of the cancer, as in metastatic disease. Common sites for metastatic spread are the lymph nodes, lungs, liver, bones, and brain. Box 1.2 shows metastatic sites and the most probable primary source of the tumor.

PHYSIOLOGICAL ABNORMALITIES

Tumor growth necessarily causes many functional abnormalities. As tumor masses enlarge they cease to grow exponentially. The cells themselves cease to proliferate and the internal cells in the tumor begin to die. One function of a tumor is to produce a blood supply for itself. Cells most distant from the blood supply begin to lose access and then die, in a sense, of malnutrition. Therefore, most tumors will have areas of necrosis. This will often set up an inflammatory response and local and possibly systemic fever. Hormonal-like substances are secreted by the tumor to induce angiogenesis.

Table 1.1   Etiological agents in cancer – environmental carcinogens[16]

Causal factor	Neoplasm	Evidence of exposure	Occupation/exposure
Chemical agents			
Aromatic amines	Papilloma, cancer of the bladder and urinary tract	Compounds in urine	Chemical workers
Benzol	Leukemia, lymphoma	Anemia, bone marrow aplasia	Coal tar, solvents, painters
Coal tar, pitch, creosote, anthracene	Cancer of skin, larynx, bronchus	Chronic dermatitis, warts, photosensitivity	Chemical industries, lumber
Petroleum, paraffin oils, waxes, tars	Cancer of the skin	Chronic dermatitis, boils, warts	Oil refinery, asphalt, mechanics
Isopropyl oil	Cancer of sinus, larynx, bronchus		Isopropyl alcohol producers
Asbestos	Cancer of bronchus, mesothelioma	Pulmonary asbestosis, asbestos warts on hands	Asbestos miners, shippers millers
Chromium	Cancer of bronchus	Chronic dermatitis, chrome-perforated skin lesions and nasal mucosa	Chromate ore
Nickel	Cancer of nasal cavity, sinus, bronchus	Nasal polyps, chronic bronchitis, dermatitis	Nickel miners, shippers, refiners
Arsenic	Cancer of skin, bronchus, bladder, leukemias	Keratoses on palms and soles	Pesticide manufacturers lumber industry
Vinyl chloride	Hemangiosarcoma of liver		Chemical workers
Physical agents			
Ionising radiation	Cancer of skin, thyroid, tongue, tonsil, sinus, osteogenic sarcoma, leukemia	Radiation dermatitis	Therapeutic or accidental exposure
Ultraviolet radiation	Cancer of skin	Chronic active dermatitis, hyperkeratosis	Farmers, outdoor workers

These substances may also play a role in metastatic spread. In addition, many tumor cells appear to differentiate to terminal or mature cells that no longer grow. It is hypothesised that some tumor cells may accumulate so much genetic damage that they die, in a sense, of self-inflicted wounds.

All of the above abnormalities cause various functional derangements. Tumors may arise in organs that normally produce physiologically active substances, such as hormones. If the normal feedback mechanisms are interrupted by a tumor obstruction or by substances released by the tumor, then characteristic clinical illnesses will result. Pituitary tumors are an example; hormonal imbalances relative to pituitary output lead the clinician to the gland itself and eventually to a diagnosis. More commonly, neoplasms produce substances that induce inappropriate secretion of normal hormones. Tumor cells generally differentiate along lines similar to those of the cell populations from which they arose. The abnormality of their genetic material makes this impossible, and so normal processes, especially in self-renewing systems, are deranged, usually in the direction of a hyper-reaction. Table 1.2 and Boxes 1.3 to 1.9 list

Box 1.1   A short list of known and suspected carcinogens[17]

2-Napthylamine
4-Aminobiphenyl
Agent orange
Artificial sweeteners
Asbestos
Aspartame
Azathioprine
Benzene
Benzidine
Bis (chloromethyl ether)
Chlorambucil
Chromium
Conjugated equine estrogen
Contaminated drinking water (pesticides)
Contaminated fats
Cytoxan
Diethylstilbestrol (DES)
Electromagnetic fields
Formaldehyde
Melphalan
Methoxsalen
Mustard gas
Nitrates
Nitrites
Nitrosamines
Nuclear power plant emissions
Phenacetin
Radon
Saccharin
Some semi-permanent and permanent semi-dark
   and dark hair dyes
Thorium dioxide
Tobacco smoke
Ultraviolet radiation
Various food additives
Various herbicides
Vinyl chloride ·

Box 1.2   Common sites of metastases

Metastatic site	Primary site
Lung	Breast, colon, kidney, testis, stomach, melanoma, thyroid
Liver	Colon, breast, bronchus, stomach, pancreas
Ovary	Colon, stomach
Bones	Breast, lung, kidney, prostate, thyroid
Central nervous system	Lung, breast, colon, kidney
Serous cavities	Lung, breast, ovary, lymphoma

physiological abnormalities that may be present in the presence of a neoplasm.

DIAGNOSIS

The summary of a cancer diagnosis will include an anatomical or clinical diagnosis and a histologic/cytological diagnosis. These areas are combined in arriving at a diagnosis and prognosis, which then leads the physician or team to develop a treatment plan. Methods of definitive diagnosis include:

- surgical biopsy with tissue examination to give a clear picture of the extent of the tumor
- examination of tumor cells under a microscope to define the extent of the abnormality
- examination of tissue and cells obtained by fine needle aspiration or biopsy.

Fine needle aspiration (FNA) is used extensively in the diagnosis of many tumors including benign tumors. It involves the insertion of a hypodermic needle into the core of the tumor and aspirating tissue and cells for later analysis under a microscope. It provides a rapid diagnosis since results can usually be obtained the same day. False-negative results can occur when a small mass has few cancer cells, which are not picked up during the procedure.

Open biopsy is a common procedure for diagnosis. In smaller tumors this procedure may become the treatment as well; this is especially true in small carcinomas of the breast, cervix, lung (rare), and prostate. It is important in this technique that the margins around the excised tissue be completely free of cancerous tissue. If the margins are not clear or are very close to the lesion (<8 mm), this can become a problem in terms of spread and a lack of clarity regarding the remaining tissue. Often these excisional biopsies are done on an outpatient basis under local anesthesia

Table 1.2 Water and electrolyte disturbances

Manifestations	Mechanism	Neoplasm
Hyponatremia (volume expansion)	Ectopic vasopressin secretion	Lung, lymphoma, others
Hyponatremia (volume depletion)	Hypercalciuria, hypokalemia	Many tumor types, myeloma, lymphoma
Hypokalemia	Ectopic adrenocorticotropic hormone (ACTH) secretion	Lung, myeloma, leukemia
Hyperkalemia	Massive tumor breakdown, lactic acidosis	Leukemia, lymphoma
Metabolic acidosis	Renal tubular defects, lactic acidosis	Hematopoietic tumors
Metabolic alkalosis	Ectopic ACTH secretion	Lung, other types
Nephrotic syndrome	Amyloidosis, antigen–antibody complexes	Lung, kidney, ovary, lymphoma

---

Box 1.3   Connective tissue disorders

Neoplasm	Manifestations
Acute leukemia	Arthropathy
Bronchogenic cancer, intrathoracic tumors	Hypertrophic pulmonary osteoarthropathy with digital clubbing
Myeloma	Amyloidosis, rheumatic complaints, inflammatory signs, para-articular deposits, chronic tenosynovitis
Hematopoietic tumors, myeloma	Gout

Box 1.4   Neuromuscular disorders (non-metastatic)

Neoplasm	Manifestations
Several cancers, lung, ovary, breast	Encephalomyeloneuropathy
Lymphoma, leukemia	Leukoencephalopathy, demyelinating lesions
Several cancers especially lung	Carcinomatous myopathy, weakness and wasting
Several cancers, especially SCLC	Myasthenic syndrome, proximal limb weakness
Thymoma	Myasthenia gravis

Box 1.5   Gastrointestinal disturbances

Manifestations	Neoplasm
Peptic ulcer	Pancreas, carcinoids
Diarrhea, abdominal cramps, asthma	Carcinoid tumors
Watery diarrhea syndrome	Pancreas, lung, rarely others

Box 1.6   Metabolic disturbances

Manifestations	Neoplasm
Hypercalcemia	Lung, breast, kidney, colon, lymphoma
Hypocalcemia	Several tumor types, lymphoma, Burkitt's lymphoma
Osteomalacia	Mesenchymal tumors
Hyperuricemia, gout	Myeloproliferative disorders, lymphomas

---

depending on the location of the tumor. Many breast cancers are diagnosed in this way; liver biopsies, on the other hand, are always done on an inpatient basis.

Sometimes in non-palpable lesions where microcalcifications are present (as is often true in

---

Box 1.7   Endocrine syndromes due to ectopic hormone secretion

Manifestations	Neoplasm
Hyperadrenal corticism	SCLC, thymoma, carcinoid tumors, breast, ovary, prostate
Hyperthyroidism	Choriocarcinoma, placental tumors, testis
Hyperglycemia	Many tumor types
Hypoglycemia	Many tumor types
Feminisation – sexual precocity	Teratomas, lung, breast, melanoma
Virilisation – sexual precocity	Hepatoblastomia, melanoma, lung, breast
Hypertension	Lung, thymic, neurogenic tumors, renal

Box 1.8   Hematopoietic system

Manifestations	Neoplasm
Erythrocytosis	Renal, hepatoma, cerebellar hemangioma
Anemia:	
Normochromic	Stomach, prostate, breast, lung, pancreas, colon, thymoma, CLL
Hypochromic	GI and GU tract cancers, head and neck
Leukomoid reactions	Many tumor types
Leukopenia	Leukemia, lymphoma, others
Abnormal granulocyte function	Acute leukemia
Thrombocytosis	Myeloproliferative disorders, lymphoma, lung, others
Thrombocytopenia	Hematopoietic tumors
Prolonged bleeding	Many tumor types, prostate, plasma cell dyscrasias
Intravascular coagulation (DIC)	Many tumor types

Box 1.9   Infections and host resistance

Manifestations	Neoplasm
Localised infections	Several tumor types
Systemic infections	Leukemia, lymphoma, myeloma, others
Bacterial infections	Myeloma, chronic lymphocytic leukemia (CLL)
Salmonella bacteremia	Lymphoma, GI neoplasms
Tuberculosis, fungal, viral disseminated infections	Hodgkin's disease, others

---

breast cancers, for example) another FNA technique, called stereotaxic needle localisation, is used. A hooked wire is inserted into or adjacent to the lesion. Methylene blue dye is injected as a visual cue to the surgeon, as a precaution against the needle becoming dislodged. The excisional biopsy is then performed with the wire in place as a marker for deep and non-palpable microcalcifications found earlier, e.g. in mammography.

Routine studies are also done, often including a chest X-ray to rule out metastatic disease in the lung or mediastinum. X-ray or ultrasound may also be used to examine other parts of the body, including the abdomen and skeletal structures. A bone scan may be carried out, particularly if presentation is late and there is musculoskeletal pain. Blood testing will be done to look at liver and kidney function, hematopoietic abnormalities, and in some cases, hormone levels. Tumor markers may also be evaluated at this time.

Tumor size

There is often a direct correlation between tumor size and the risk of recurrence. Although this varies depending on the type and location of the primary tumor, generally, the larger the tumor, the greater the risk of recurrence.

Nuclear/histologic grade

The nuclear or histologic grade refers to the degree of cell differentiation within a tumor and is based on the pathologist's assessment of each cell's nuclear size and shape in the biopsy sample. It also refers to the number of mitoses (cell divisions), and the degree of tubule formation. Tumors of low malignancy are graded 1 and are associated with the best prognosis. Grade 3 tumors are associated with the worst prognosis. Cells that are well differentiated imply less mutation; those that are not differentiated, each looking different from the cell next to it, have probably been abnormal for a longer period of time.

S-phase fraction and DNA ploidy

Flow cytometry measures both DNA ploidy (DNA content) and the S-phase fraction (the fraction of cells actively cycling or synthesising DNA). Aneuploid tumors (the cells in the tumor contain an abnormal number of chromosomes) with a high percentage of cells in S-phase are more likely to recur than are tumors with a low S-phase fraction. These measurements assess the aggressiveness of a tumor, and this means the degree to which it is proliferating, based on the genetic action of the tumor cells.

Staging

Clinical staging includes physical examination, with careful inspection and palpation of the skin, the affected area, the local and regional lymph nodes. It also includes a pathologic examination of the tissue and any imaging done to establish the diagnosis. Operative findings are elements of clinical staging, including the size of the primary tumor and the level of invasion of that tumor, and the presence or absence of regional or distal metastasis.

Pathologic staging includes all data used for clinical staging and surgical resection as well as pathologic examination of the primary carcinoma, including total excision of the primary carcinoma with no tumor in any margin of resection. If there is tumor in the margin of the resection, it is coded TX, i.e. the extent of the primary tumor cannot be assessed.

A universal system has been put in place for the staging of cancers. There are also individualised systems in place for certain specific tumors that will be addressed in later chapters discussing those particular cancers. The current anatomic staging system, the TNM system, describes the anatomic extent of disease based on the assessment of three components:

T: the extent of the primary tumor
N: the absence or presence and extent of regional lymph node metastasis
M: the absence or presence of distant metastasis.

The addition of numbers to these three components indicates the extent of malignant disease: T0, T1, T2, T3, T4, N0, N1, N2, N3, M0, M1.

This is, in effect, a shorthand system for describing the extent of a particular malignant tumor.

Staging consists of all of the above procedures and assessments. It provides an anatomical, biochemical, and genetic map of the malignant disease in a given patient. It is important because it not only provides information concerning prognostic factors including potentials for recurrence, but also information concerning the therapies to be used in treatment for eradication of the cancer.

PRINCIPLES OF TREATMENT

Surgery

Surgery is the primary defense against any solid tumor. The purpose of surgery is to remove local and regional disease. When there is no metastasis surgery may be curative.

Radiation therapy

This is being used more and more for particular types of tumors. It is used in various delivery mechanisms for many situations in which residual tumor cells are a concern, or where the staging is too late for surgical resection and chemotherapy as a standalone therapy is not adequate. External beam radiation therapy is used in many solid tumor cancers and in some blood and lymph cancers. High-energy irradiation delivered by a linear accelerator is preferable to older cobalt-60 irradiation when using external beam irradiation.

The therapy is usually given five times per week for 33 sessions, with the last five to six sessions in the form of a boost treatment with higher-dose radiation targeted to just the scar and the tumor bed. A treatment simulator is now considered extremely desirable, and computerised planning is essential. Cautions in radiation therapy are pre-existing autoimmune disease, because the inflammatory components of these diseases are exacerbated by radiation, and pre-existing pulmonary or cardiac disease. Collagen vascular disease and uncontrolled diabetes are also probable contraindications for radiation therapy.

Concomitant radiation therapy and chemotherapy increase local tissue reaction and can cause greater damage. Therefore, radiation is often delayed until the end of chemotherapy in some cases, provided that the delay is not longer than 6 months. Delaying radiotherapy may result in local failure of treatment. However, there are some cases in which radiation therapy may be done first or concurrently with chemotherapy.

In advanced solid tumor cancer where surgery is no longer an option, radiation therapy can be used to consolidate or shrink a tumor in order to make it resectable. The aim may also be to control local disease in a non-resectable tumor. Here full-dose radiation is used and is sometimes supplemented by interstitial implantation of radioactive isotopes or seeds. In late disease, radiation is used to treat distant metastases, especially to the bone and brain. See Box 1.10 for some of the biologic effects of ionising radiation.

Chemotherapy and hormonal therapies

Chemotherapy and hormonal therapies have been used as adjuvant therapy for many cancers. The term adjuvant refers to treatment used in addition to and following primary treatment in order to cure, reduce, control, or palliate the cancer. The purpose of adjuvant therapy is to treat micrometastatic disease before it is clinically detectable, in the hope that the small tumor burden will be easier to eliminate. Patients at high risk for developing metastatic disease are treated

---

Box 1.10 Biological effects of ionising radiation

Tissue exposed	Clinical manifestations
Skin and mucosa	Early: erythema, desquamation, re-epithelialisation, fibrosis
	Later: atrophy, late necrosis, devascularisation (months)
	Still later: neoplasia
Hair	Epilation
Hematopoietic	Transient fall in reticulocytes, white blood cells, platelets, in several days
	Later may result in marrow aplasia, fibrosis
Eye	Conjunctivitis, ulceration, late cataract formation
Lung	Acute radiation pneumonitis, perhaps related infection
	Later: fibrosis
Heart	Acute and chronic pericarditis
Kidney	Delayed radiation nephritis due to vascular damage
Gonads	Sterility and mutational changes
Bone	Stops growth of ununited epiphyses, skeletal distortion
	Later: bone necrosis due to devascularisation
CNS	Delayed effects like radiation myelitis

after the primary tumor has been treated. The term neoadjuvant refers to therapy given before the primary treatment in order to shrink or otherwise affect the tumor prior to potentially curative treatment like surgery.

Chemotherapies are classified based on the cytotoxic action of the drug. They are generally grouped as vesicants or irritants. Vesicants are agents that cause blistering; irritants produce a local inflammatory reaction. These main groups are then broken down further into several subcategories:

- alkylating agents, e.g. platinum compounds, including cisplatin
- antibiotic agents, e.g. doxorubicin (Adriamycin)
- DNA intercalators, e.g. trastuzumab
- vinca alkaloids, e.g. vincristine
- epipodophyllotoxins, e.g. etoposide
- hormonal agents, e.g. tamoxifen
- enzymatic agents, e.g. asparaginase/ crisantaspase
- antimetabolites, e.g. cytarabine.

Many cytotoxic chemotherapeutic drugs were initially made from plant materials. Podophyllotoxins are made from the rhizome of *Podophyllum peltatum* and are used as a caustic. Box 1.11 lists some common antitumor drugs.

Non-cross-resistant therapies are combinations of multiple non-cross-resistant drugs. Their administration is based on the rationale that the presence of subsets of cells resistant to certain drugs requires a multi-pronged approach. The treatment principle is not unlike that for HIV infection. These combinations are given acronyms; many oncology texts have a list of acronyms in their addenda. The acronyms can become confusing as some include combined references to generic and brand names of drugs.

Hormonal or endocrine therapies are used to treat tumors that are associated with tissue that is, under normal circumstances, responsive to specific hormonal substances. Testosterone, progestins, antiadrenal drugs, and prednisone are hormonal substances commonly used to interact with or interfere with the proliferation of cells in specific types of tissue. Examples are the use of estrogen therapy in prostate cancer (leuprolide – Lupron), and the use of antiestrogenic therapy (tamoxifen) in estrogen-receptive breast tumors. Sometimes endocrine agents are used for up to 5 years after initial diagnosis, whereas chemotherapies are most commonly used for 4–6 months and up to 2 years.

Biologic therapies

Biologic therapies include different biological agents like BCG (bacillus Calmette Guerin), levamisole, polyA-polyU, *Corynebacterium parvum*, Azimexon, Basidiomycetes *Pleurotos pulmonarius,* interferon, interleukins, and colony-stimulating factors like Procrit.

Interferons
The interferons (IFN) comprise a family of naturally occurring proteins that were first recognised for their ability to confer resistance to viral infection on cells. The interferons are designated α-interferon, β-interferon, and γ-interferon. The genes encoding these proteins have been sequenced and cloned. The α- and β-interferons

---

Box 1.11 Commonly used antitumor drugs

Classification	Drug
Alkylating agent	Mechlorethamine, cyclophosmamide, melphalan, chlorambucil, busulfan, carmustine, lomustine, semustine, procarbazine, mitomycin, cisplatin
Antimetabolites	Methotrexate, 6-mercaptopurine, 6-thioguanine, 5-fluorouracil, ftorafur, cytosine arabinoside, hydroxyurea
DNA intercalators	Adriamycin, daunorubicin, bleomycin, actinomycin-d, mithramycin
Mitotic inhibitors	Vinblastine, vincristine, colchicine
Miscellaneous	Mitotane, L-asparaginase, epipodophylo toxins like VP-16, VM-26, anti-angiogenics

are class I drugs. Two recombinant human α-interferons are licensed for clinical use in the US. The broad classes of action for interferons are characterised as

- antiviral
- antiproliferative
- regulatory of differentiation
- modulatory of lipid metabolism
- inhibitory of angiogenesis
- antitumoral
- immunoregulatory.

All biologic activities of the interferons require binding to specific cell-surface receptors. All interferons usually act in a paracrine fashion and are present in high concentrations in the circulation. Antibodies to recombinant α-interferon are detected in two-thirds of patients receiving α-interferon. Administration of nonrecombinant α-interferon may restore responsiveness in patients whose disease (including cancer) has relapsed. It is also used in chronic myeloid leukemia (CML) and multiple myeloma. It has been used in cases of Kaposi's sarcoma, Hodgkin's disease and low-grade non-Hodgkin's lymphomas. It can be used with combination chemotherapies.

Interleukin-2

Interleukin-2 (IL-2) is one of a family of polypeptides that mediate interactions between leukocytes. It was initially called T-cell growth factor. It stimulates proliferation and enhances function of other T-cells, natural killer (NK) cells and B-cells. IL-2-activated B-cells generate secretory rather than membrane-associated IgM, and macrophages gain maturity and elaborate transforming growth factor-β (TGF-β) when stimulated with IL-2. These immunomodulatory effects are the rationale for studying IL-2 as an anticancer agent. Its toxicity has hindered widespread implementation. Anemia, thrombocytopenia, endothelial cell damage, and renal damage are all factors that need to be overcome. IL-2 has been used in treatment for renal cell carcinoma and metastatic melanoma.

Hematopoietic growth factors

Hematopoietic growth factors are a family of glycoproteins with important regulatory functions in the processes of proliferation, differentiation, and functional activation of hematopoietic progenitors and mature blood cells. They include erythropoietic factors, colony-stimulating factors, various interleukins, stem cell factor, thrombopoietin, and growth factors, including granulocyte CSF (G-CSF, filgastrim [Neupogen]), granulocyte-macrophage CSF (GM-CSF, sargramostim [Leukine]), multipotential CSF (multi-CSF, also known as IL-3), and monocyte macrophage CSF (M-CSF, also known as CSF-1), pegfilgastrim (Neulasta), and darbapoeitin alfa (Aranesp).

These growth factors interact at various levels of the hematopoietic differentiation cascade. They are present and produce growth factors at multiple sites in the body. They are used for the amelioration of myelosuppression after chemotherapy, and allow for dose escalation of toxic chemotherapeutic drugs by rescuing the patient from severe neutropenia. They are used in autologous bone marrow transplantation in the same way. They are also used in myelodysplastic syndromes that are iatrogenic – treatment-related; neoplastic clonal stem cell disorders caused by toxic treatment IL-3,4,5 plus GM-CSF and G-CSF have been studied. Some results are positive and some are not. G-CSF is commonly used as rescue therapy during and after chemotherapy in many cancers.

Retinoids

Retinoids are substances structurally or functionally related to vitamin A, or retinol. They reportedly induce differentiation and/or suppression of proliferation of many cell lines, including embryonal carcinoma, leukemia, melanoma, neuroblastoma, and breast carcinoma. Synergy has been seen when retinoids are combined with vitamin D and its analogs (like vitamin D_3), as well as in combination with other cytokines. These have been used most commonly to reverse or suppress carcinogenic progression to invasive cancer. Studies have also shown that in acute promyelocytic leukemia (APL), all-trans-retinoic acid (ATRA) has been used to achieve complete remission. Retinoids are highly teratogenic and must be used with extreme caution in women of child-bearing age. Retinoic acid syndrome (RAS) is seen in up to 20% of patients with APL treated with ATRA. It manifests as fever, respiratory distress, hyperleukocytosis, edema, pericardial effusions, hypotension, and renal failure.

Monoclonal antibodies

Monoclonal antibodies (MoAbs) are antibodies that are capable of binding with high affinity to specific determinants. They have the advantage of directly neutralising a target, indirectly mediating immune damage by means of complement activation, and activating cellular cytotoxicity by other immunocompetent cells. Many MoAbs have been conjugated with other agents that are cytotoxic, including chemotherapy. They may have the potential to improve targeted cell therapy. They are also used to target growth-factor receptors.

INTEGRATION OF CARE

Understanding the mechanisms and goals of these treatments is part of the integration of Chinese herbal medicine with conventional care. Therefore, these modalities have been investigated in some detail. It is important to be able to converse with conventional providers in the language they use and, when possible, to utilise this language when describing the interventions we use in an integrative approach. Each chapter in this book attempts to explain issues and treatment for an individual cancer according to the conventional and the Chinese approach. When possible the integration is shared in the text with the basic explanation. The cases serve as a means to more closely demonstrate the actual criteria used in the rationale for formula and/or herb choices based on the Chinese medicine analysis and the conventional medicine data and issues.

There are many issues that arise when treating patients with combined care. Most of the controversy arises on the part of conventional medicine and the concern that there will be an adverse reaction between herbs and drugs, including an undermining of the effectiveness of the conventional treatment by herbal medicine or supplementation. The main issues include the concept that antioxidant-like therapies may interfere with the free-radical effect of cytotoxic therapies and the concept that some herbs may be 'phytoestrogenic' and proliferative in effect. The concept of phytoestrogens is taken up in the breast cancer chapter. And although the idea that antioxidants scavenge free radicals is intuitive and logical, the vast majority of studies into whether or not antioxidants interfere with the free radical and,

therefore, cytotoxic effects of chemotherapy and radiation, report in favor of antioxidant use during conventional treatment for cancer. Over 98% of all studies show that, counter-intuitively, antioxidants enhance the free-radical effects of almost all chemotherapeutic regimens and radiation therapy. The best meta-analysis of the studies to date is by Lamson and Brignall.[18]

CHINESE MEDICINE APPROACH

From the Ling Shu, Chapter 81:

The Yellow Emperor asks Qi Bo . . . I do not understand the swellings and suppurations and that which follows their birth, the time of their success or defeat, the period of their death or birth. Qi Bo answers – Man's channels of blood [vessels] nourish and protect; they circulate and flow without stop. They resonate below the numerous rivers [ie the meridians which are more superficial]. When cold evil [due to external pathogens or injuries] is harbored in the middle of the major channels, it causes blood to settle [coagulate]. The blood settles, thus there is an obstruction [a clot or twisted area of microcirculation]. An obstruction causes the protective qi [immunity] to reverse, so it cannot re-circulate to oppose the evil [the infection or the injury or lesion or mutation], therefore, ulcers and swellings. When the cold qi is transformed [due to constraint] and made hot, the heat overcomes which causes putrefaction of the flesh [a mass or abscess]. The corrupted flesh thus makes pus. The pus not drained causes a rotting of the muscles. The muscles [flesh and viscera] rotting causes injury to the bones. The bones injured causes the marrow to melt so that it does not occupy the hollows of the bones and it cannot drain. The blood shrivels to emptiness and hollowness [all types of anemia]. This causes the tendons, bones, muscles, and flesh to be unsuitably malnourished. The major channels are defeated and leak [the meridians leak qi and the vessels leak blood]. Smoke is in the five viscera [the tissue is no longer clear and healthy due to metastatic disease]. The viscera injured causes death.

This description from the Ling Shu was written nearly 2000 years ago and is an almost complete and accurate description of the natural history of untreated cancer. As Chinese medicine has evolved into the 21st century the field of oncology has become one primarily of the integration between modern Western science and conventional medicine and classical and modern Chinese herbal medicine. Understanding the conventional approach to pathogenesis and treatment is important in this integration because Chinese medicine is primarily used as adjunctive care. In China and Korea, herbal medicine is used as adjunctive treatment to a very large extent. In the US, law prohibits the use of complementary forms of medicine for the direct and primary treatment of cancer. Patients may choose it but practitioners cannot provide it. The politics of these legal parameters are questionable and relate back to the early 20th century conflict between the regular doctors (chemical medicine) and the homeopaths, chiropractors, and naturopaths.

These early struggles for access to patients persist and have become embedded in the politics of medicine today. This is especially true in oncology. Adult patients are free to opt out of conventional care but it is a gray area, legally speaking, for practitioners to provide primary treatment to these patients. There are instances where Child Protective Services (CPS) have intervened and removed children with cancer from the care of their parents when the parents have looked to alternative treatments.

In many cases, the cytotoxic treatment utilised by conventional medicine may be necessary initially to save a life. There is controversy on this point and the main thrust of study and research in Chinese medicine has been in adjunctive or supportive care. Therefore, we are limited to adjunctive treatment by law and also by current available knowledge.

This is not to say that this is right, nor that there are not practitioners out there treating 'outside of the box'. These alternatives cover a broad spectrum, from John of God in Brazil to antineoplaston therapy to the Kelley–Gonzales enzymatic treatment to Gaston's 714X to miracles and so on.

Within the current milieu, the main thrust of research and knowledge in oncology in Chinese medicine is integrated care combining Chinese medicine and the standard of care of conventional medicine.

An understanding of the mechanism of cytotoxicity of conventional treatments is essential in order to know how to integrate herbal medicines. Herbal medicines are used to interface with the cytotoxic mechanism and to potentiate its effect. Formulas are also used to ameliorate the side effects of conventional treatment in order to enable the patient to remain as healthy as possible and to be able to maintain the treatment schedule for the cytotoxic intervention. Therefore, knowing the mechanism of action and the side effects of any given conventional treatment is necessary.

Herbal medicines are often chosen not for their classical usage but for their pharmacological actions. A great deal of research has been and is currently being done on individual herbs, herbal formulas, and their relationships to immunological function, organ protection, gastrointestinal function, hematopoietic function, and their ability to interact with various chemotherapies, radiation, hormonal therapies, and other biological therapies to potentiate or increase their effect.

Modern laboratory procedures are used to monitor the effects of Chinese medicine and conventional treatment. Therefore, the integration happens both between conventional and Chinese medicine and within Chinese medicine, where a mixed classical and Western scientific approach is combined. This makes Chinese medicine, in the specialty area of integrated oncology, a new hybrid medicine.

In classical Chinese medicine, many texts throughout history have addressed the subject of benign and malignant tumors. The Zhou Li[19] is a Chinese classical text that refers to the specialty of treating swellings and ulcers. These swellings are called zhong yang, and those with ulcerations and necrosis are called kui yang. Tumors are categorised according to their visual and palpable typing. They have traditionally not been separated according to malignant or benign characteristics. The general categorisations are shown in Box 1.12.[20,21]

There are many mechanisms by which these types of benign and malignant tumors evolve.

Box 1.12   Categories of tumors in Chinese medicine

Category	Definition
zhong yang	a swelling with ulceration
chuang yang	a lesion with ulceration
yin tumor	a glandular enlargement
liu	tumor
yan	a rock tumor that feels like a stone
jun	a fig- or pear-shaped tumor
zheng	a substantial mass
jia	an insubstantial mass (a boundariless mass as in a blood or lymph cancer)
ji	localised fixed mass attached to local tissue
ju	mobile mass that moves beneath the fingers
yi ge	hiccup, which is considered to be a local obstruction
fan wei	gastric regurgitation due to obstruction
chang tan	firm and immovable mass
pi kuai	distention and fullness due to mass
xuan pi	a cord-like swelling
kui	an ulcerous lesion
xi rou	a polyp
you zhi	warts and moles
zhui	a growth
rou liu	a myoma

PATHOGENESIS

In Chinese medicine, the pathogenesis of cancer is commonly, but not always, attributed to combinations of injuries. These injuries are multifactorial and have usually accumulated over time. Knowing the diagnosis for the end-stage of these injuries is important but, unlike conventional medicine, Chinese medicine will attribute more than one diagnosis to a single disease, based on the concept that these injuries are cumulative, usually developing over a long period of time within a certain constitutional environment. This multi-level approach views the entire history of the individual and those combinations of injury that led to the final disease of cancer. In other words, cancer is usually seen as a long-term evolutionary process rather than a single end-event. This process takes into account more than one functional organ system. The evolution of the cancer diagnosis is part of a complex of interaction, and is not only an anatomical, genetic and biochemical event. The pattern differentiations for any one type of cancer have usually at least two, if not more, distinct diagnoses present. One is the pattern differentiation within the individual that over time made for an environment in which the cancer was able to evolve and manifest. This pattern is usually called the constitutional diagnosis.

The second diagnosis relates to the diagnosis for the cancer itself and takes into account the current presentation of the patient. It may change from week to week or day to day depending on the staging of the cancer, the side effects of treatment, and other factors regarding performance status. The development of the more immediate diagnosis involves an evaluation of the symptom picture and the current signs. These signs are: the tongue, the pulses, the hara, the smell, the coloring, the sound of the voice, the spirit emanating from the face and eyes; all of the diagnostic parameters used in Chinese medicine. These parameters are considered to be objective signs. The inclusion of laboratory results including blood work, scans, cancer markers, staging and prognosis, and the analysis of conventional treatment mechanisms and side effects are also included. The symptoms are the subjective report of the patient, including pain, appetite, digestive symptoms, stools and their quality, thirst, sleep, temperature or sensation of temperature, energy level, abnormal sweating, spirit (mood).

In more cutting-edge conventional treatment of cancers (that is, Western treatment that takes into account prevention and causation as well as treatment) the current understanding of the pathogenesis of cancer is that there are carcinogenic events or exposures that occur as the primary causative factors. These events or exposures include all of those things that we now understand to be carcinogenic, including environmental exposures and hereditary predispositions. Beyond these primary causative factors are promoting factors. Promoting factors include lifestyle, alcoholism, poor diet, poor sleeping habits, poor exercise habits, chronic stress and unhappiness, and all of those diseases and conditions that result from these factors. In other words, they include the accumulation of good and bad as well as our inheritance. Diabetes, chronic heart disease, and hyperinsulinemia are examples of the effect of poor lifestyle on the body. Carcinogenic exposures can have a greater impact in those people who provide a promoting environment for proliferation of cancer cells and mutagenesis. We could say that, in terms of Chinese medicine, the carcinogenic hits are external factors that cause a mutation of the DNA, and the promoting factors are internal factors that create an internal environment in which a cancer is more likely to evolve given a carcinogenic hit.

Two factors form the cornerstone of a good prognosis in Chinese medicine. Good sleep and regular stools are essential to good health and play an important role in promoting factors for cancer. If a patient is not sleeping well it may mean that their ability to recuperate and regenerate is limited. Sleep allows the wei qi to circulate inwardly for 12 cycles during the night. This inward circulation, from a modern science perspective, allows for growth hormone to be released in order to foster tissue repair. Perhaps we could compare the circulation of wei qi to the passing when asleep in and out of delta sleep, which is the time that growth hormone is secreted. Growth hormone is primary in the rehabilitation of all body structure and function. Low growth hormone release due to poor sleep means that the body does not rebuild and recuperate optimally on a daily basis. This is a set-up for chronic diseases. The wei qi circulation also allows the liver (conventional) to detoxify itself both physiologically, from chemicals including chemotherapeutic agents, and emotionally (Chinese medicine – the Hun aspect). A peaceful spirit becomes part of healthy immunological function.

A well-formed and regular stool implies that stomach and spleen function is strong and that assimilation and absorption are optimal. Good nutrition is immensely important in everyday life and even more so during cancer treatment, when fast-growing cells including blood cells and the entire gastrointestinal mucosa are being killed off due to the cytotoxic effect of many anti-cancer agents. Rebuilding these tissues takes a tremendous amount of energy. The cancer itself also utilises qi and blood. Therefore, the need for qi and blood are increased in cancer. Good nutrition is essential for a better prognosis and for prevention of recurrence. Many patients who make profound lifestyle changes during treatment for cancer often report that they feel better after treatment than they ever have in their lives, even before the cancer diagnosis. This supports the theory that promoting factors are not carcinogenic in themselves but do contribute to the cancer environment. It also shows that good supportive care during treatment for cancer improve life both quantitatively and qualitatively. Regular and well-formed stool and good sleep are emblematic of the positive results of lifestyle changes and adjustments in regards to promoting factors in cancer pathogenesis and survival.

A malignancy spreads via blood and lymph circulation as in the conventional analysis of metastasis. However, the additional factor of qi circulation is also considered a mechanism of spread in Chinese medicine. The areas to which metastatic spread is often seen, depending on the type of cancer, are somewhat predictable. This predictability is part of monitoring in conventional care. In addition, it is possible to understand that the flow of qi in the body can be predictive for the area of spread beyond the region of the primary tumor. Monitoring and protection of distant predicted metastatic sites is part of treatment in Chinese medicine.

Main etiological factors in pathogenesis

Disharmony of qi and blood and emotions
If the qi and blood are imbalanced then stasis results. Qi is magnetised by the blood and vice versa. When the qi is not moving well and is not vitalising the functional processes of the body then the blood becomes sluggish. When the blood is sluggish for a long period of time it congeals or clots.[22] Conventional medicine describes an increase in fibrinogen levels and other clotting factors and a greater viscosity of the blood. Blood

clotting and platelet aggregation slows the circulation of qi and a vicious cycle begins. This disharmony is often part of a continuum that involves other pathogenic factors as well. These other factors can include unresolved emotional factors that drive the decisions made regarding diet, activity, and mental and emotional health, all of which are important to health and can lead to qi and blood disharmonies.

The mind/body connection remains intact in Chinese medicine via Five Phase theory. For example, the yin organ of the Metal phase is the lung. Lung function is damaged by continuous grief and the sorrow that comes from unresolved loss. On another level it can be damaged by other underlying organ injuries that lead a person to pathological perfectionism. When the lung is injured in these ways, the manifestations often have to do with repression that disallows deep breathing, and this leads to an inability to oxygenate the blood at a normal level. Breathing involves the action of the diaphragm and this action and the energetic function of the lungs moves qi and normal fluids up and down in the chest. The diaphragm is considered to be a dynamic heat exchanger in relation to the upper jiao.[23] When it is functioning in a lesser capacity the movement of qi is less, the fluid dynamism in the chest is less, and the exchange or ventilation of heat across the upper and middle jiaos is diminished. The lungs are the canopy of the human body and act, metaphorically, like the world's tropical rain forests. They cleanse the air, regulate temperature, hold and clean water, and form qi and oxygen. Injury at this level due to emotional constraint creates an environment that could be considered to be promotional for cancer if a mutagen is present.

The lungs are also responsible for a certain level of immunity – the wei qi, which circulates via the blood and the zheng qi. Therefore, in two ways, the immunity is affected by lowered lung capacity; lowered oxygenation of tissues and lowered wei qi levels. At the same time, if breathing is shallow and the hydraulic pumping mechanism of the diaphragm is diminished, normal fluids and blood tend to accumulate in the chest. This accumulation leads to stasis and loss of normal function. The lungs' ability to irrigate the upper jiao is intimately connected with breathing and with the heat-exchange mechanism. When there is injury at this level then internal heat and also static phlegm begins to accumulate. Blood stasis, pathogenic heat, and static phlegm are the foundations for most cancer pathogeneses.[24]

To paraphrase, whenever there is stasis of qi and/or blood, heat accumulates. Heat, as an element of stasis, will dry the blood, causing it to become sticky. It will also dry and burn normal body fluids, the jin ye and yin, and cause local stasis and eventually systemic heat. The main issues that can lead to this type of stasis are zang fu deficiencies and unresolved emotions.

Another manifestation of emotional injury is in the liver, which is said to be injured by the kind of frustration that leads to anger.[25] Emotional stresses of this kind when unresolved or not discharged also lead to stasis. The liver has an intimate relationship with the blood. Liver qi stasis can end in blood stasis.[26] In the case of breast cancers, the stasis of qi affecting the liver can, via the Five Phase cycle, affect the heart, stomach/spleen axis, and the lungs. All of these viscera are important to cancer pathogenesis because of their relationships with blood, with fluids, or with immunity. The liver channel runs through the axilla and the chest. The stomach channel runs directly through the middle of the breast. These kinds of stasis in the chest, along with other factors, can be part of a breast cancer diagnosis. Many western scientific studies have shown that stress and unresolved emotions lower immunity. Lowered immunity does not cause cancer, but can contribute to an environment in which cancers occur more readily. The mechanism for this is well explained in classical Chinese medical theory. Therefore, it becomes important to treat these underlying promotional mechanisms as part of treating the cancer. By changing the environment the course of the disease can be changed.

Other zang fu are also injured by emotional factors. Constant worry or obsessive-compulsive disorders, whether they are diagnosed or not, injure the spleen function, and can be indicative of stomach/spleen injury.[27] By considering the theory regarding spleen functions, we could say that the spleen is relative, biomedically speaking, to the stomach (enzymatic breakdown of foods), the gallbladder (fat metabolism), the pancreas (glucose metabolism), the jejunum portion of the small intestine (water metabolism), and the gastrointestinal lining (ying and absorption). When spleen function is injured it leads to:

- blood deficiencies that then affect the other zang fu
- damp accumulations due to impaired metabolic function relative to water, and then
- stasis arising out of deficiency and accumulation, another vicious cycle.

The spleen is yellow; it is the center of the body. Spleen injury occurs in many ways, some of which include childhood neglect, poor parenting, abuse, and lack of unconditional love wherein an individual does not learn how to care for her/himself. These kinds of injuries can lead to improper eating habits like anorexia and bulimia, over-eating, and craving sweets and high-fat diets that are inappropriate ways to rebalance the spleen function. This is another example of how a psychospiritual injury can lead to physical illness.

Dampness and phlegm accumulations
Normal body fluids, the jin ye, can accumulate under certain pathological conditions. When they do, like qi and blood, they tend to become sluggish, to stagnate, to generate heat, and to become sticky. There are many reasons why normal body fluids accumulate and become static. The swelling from local injury is one example. But internally, the pathological process relates to zang fu deficiencies due to other illnesses or improper living habits, qi and blood disharmonies, and failure of normal fluids to be transformed and evacuated properly as part of normal body qi transformation processes, as in spleen and kidney deficiencies.[28] Diet and especially irregular meals, wrong foods, high-fat foods, sweets, or eating in all the wrong circumstances, i.e. while working, while driving, under stress, all lead to stomach/spleen deficiencies which, in turn, lead to the loss of transformative and transportive functions in relation to water, fat, and sugar metabolism. This causes damp accumulations and then stasis, which thickens those damp accumulations into phlegm and heat and then into phlegm heat or phlegm cold and, under the right circumstances, to tumors.[29] In fact, dietary irregularity is considered a very

important promoting factor of cancerous tumors. Category I, II, and IV tumours commonly interweave and work hand-in-hand with one another to form a foundation for a future cancer.

Toxic heat pathogens, latent pathogenic factors, and fire poisons
Although modern physicians of Chinese medicine utilise the analysis of biomedicine, e.g. exfoliative cytology, obviously these techniques were not available in the 12th century. And yet cancers were diagnosed and treated and certain kinds of tumors were associated with various toxins and external pathogens based on discharges, suppurative fluids, bloody discharges and haemorrhages, and other bodily discharges. The cancers most commonly linked to toxins and infectious agents in the past were cervical, esophageal, colorectal, and breast. This is probably because of their presentation in the later stages of disease and because the presentation was visible to the naked eye, whereas more internal and visceral tumors were not. Today we know that these types (and many others) are linked to viral agents, in the case of cervical cancer with HPV and HSV and in the case of esophageal cancer with EBV. Breast cancer does not have a viral link but in later stages, when left untreated, it is often accompanied by local infection of the externally ulcerated mass. These kinds of presentations had observable symptomatic infectious qualities.

Fire poisons are exposures and unresolved infections (for example, latent viral infections and other infections, e.g. chronic malarial infection, which underlies Burkitt's lymphoma) that ultimately injure the yin and fluids and lead to stasis at the qi, fluid and blood level.[24] When stasis is present for a long period of time it also leads to a fire poison, sometimes called an inverted fire poison. Fire poisons effect the DNA and cause mutation. This can happen as part of a long-term process or it can happen immediately; perhaps this is part of what happens in childhood cancers like leukemia. Fire poisons also drain the zang fu and confound the wei and ying at various levels.

It seems safe to assume that within this category of causation are included chemical exposures such as certain ingredients in dark permanent and semi-permanent hair dyes, asbestos, nicotine derivatives, DDT and its break-down products, radiation, heavy metals such as lead, aspartame, nitrites, and fat-soluble organochlorines used in agriculture. Very few studies have been conducted on how combinations of chemicals and pathogens affect the human body. Most of the carcinogens fall into this category.

Zang fu deficiencies

The viscera and the gastrointestinal tube and their functions are undermined by any and all of the above mechanisms of injury. This continual assault and the onset of chronic disease as the result of aging all take their toll. For example, improper dietary habits can lead to adult-onset diabetes. Diabetes has recently been found to be a risk factor for certain types of cancers. There is a relationship between fluctuating insulin surges caused by unstable blood sugar levels and the proliferation of tumor cells. In Chinese medicine this is described as spleen-deficient dampness and is considered a promoting factor.[30] Cancer tends to develop in those aged over 40 years and in those suffering from various permutations of qi and blood deficiency. Cancers occur more frequently in those who eat a high-fat diet, and particularly a diet high in animal fat. This kind of diet leads to deficiencies of various kinds, especially spleen and kidney deficiency.[31] Fat molecules are receptacles for xenobiotics such as pseudoestrogens. These carcinogenic chemicals enter the body through the food chain via fat molecules. They take years to break down, and the accumulation of the carcinogenicity reaches a point where mutation occurs.

Chronic deficiencies are evolutionary disease processes that can affect all the organ functions of the body. When linked with toxin exposures their effect can be overwhelming. Strong and healthy qi within each organ and its functional orb of activity is what causes the movement and transformation that we call health.

Exhaustion due to overwork is a chronic condition especially in the West. Overwork leads to kidney and liver yin deficiency. Liver yin is the root of liver yang. Unrooted yang in the liver secondary to liver yin deficiency causes many pathologies including liver qi stasis. Liver qi stasis can overact on the spleen function via the Five Phase cycle and cause spleen and middle jiao defi-

ciencies. Liver qi stasis can transfer stasis, again via the Five Phases, to the heart and cause chronic heart qi stasis. The heart is the master of blood, and heart qi stasis can cause nodules to form on the physical level. On another level, the spirit, housed and anchored by the heart, can be harmed, leading to depression, insomnia and another vicious cycle. Chronic spleen deficiency drains the kidney qi for the same reasons.

In Chinese medicine no injury happens in a vacuum. Many vicious cycles turning on themselves and incorporating greater and deeper circles of pathology can cause serious, chronic, and life-threatening illness. When several factors come together with chronic exhaustion, the body's ability to transform qi properly, as in the many transformations that happen daily in the cells, can become injured. The zang fu deficiency category fits into the realm of promoting factors.

External pathogens

There is an overlap between the external pathogens and toxic heat pathogens. However, the reference here is to the six external pathogens (exterior pernicious influences; EPIs): wind, cold, heat, summer heat, dampness, and dryness. When the resistance to these pathogenic factors is low or when these factors are somehow abnormally strong then they may invade, usually via the channels and collaterals, but sometimes more directly.[24] When a pathogenic cold or wind (for example, via food contamination), enters the intestines, the wei and ying are impeded and made deficient at the same time. This can result in the beginning of the type of accumulation that in Chinese medicine is called damp stasis – a colon polyp. When the internal environment is already stressed and there is also organ deficiency with concomitant dampness or phlegm due to deficiency, then this EPI assault can become lodged at a deep level. It seems safe to say that this category, as well as the toxin and latent pathogenic factor (LPF) category, includes bacterial, viral, and parasitic invasions, and chemical carcinogens. Understanding the pathogenic factor, and therefore the treatment, is complex. These EPIs are present under normal circumstances. Reading the symptom picture of the early presentation, if at all possible, may give us clues as to how to diagnose and treat. It requires an in-depth case history.

Many childhood cancers appear to be of acute onset. Children's immune systems, depending on their age, are often not yet consolidated. Their lack of height results in greater exposure to carcinogens, e.g. from car exhaust fumes, that may be quantitatively greater than an adult's and qualitatively more problematic.[32]

Generally speaking, it is when combinations of the above factors are present in one individual that the internal environment for cancer is in place. However, only one factor may be present and cause underlying disease. This is true, for example, in cervical cancer, where certain types of HPV infection are commonly the underlying cause. When several of the above factors are present the resultant internal environment can also act as a catalyst for a transformation from a chronic benign condition to one that is malignant. In conventional medicine the transformation is said to occur at the level of the DNA. In Chinese medicine the transformation occurs because already-present external exposures or recent external exposures lead to a level of toxicity in a premalignant condition that results in a final transformation to malignancy where the last exposure becomes the final oncogenic hit.

THERAPEUTIC PRINCIPLES

Introduction

Conventional medicine treats the end stage of a disease process. All conventional medical interventions in cancer therapy are aimed at cytotoxicity. Chinese medicine considers the underlying condition of the patient and the long history of gradual debilitation (if present) and the deficiencies that are current at presentation. There are several different prongs to this approach.

If no deficiency underlies the cancer, the disease itself causes qi deficiency; it directly uses up qi and blood to sustain itself. It is important to remember that those cells that have run amuck are trying to survive, just as all life tries to survive. When considered in this way, it is those factors that caused the initial injury to the cell that are the real enemy, rather than the cancer itself. When approached from this perspective, therapy requires a more strategic intervention that changes over time and must be continually re-evaluated. This approach also includes eliminating the exposure(s) that caused the original injury.

The use of Western diagnostic techniques in detecting cancers in very early stages, especially precancerous and early cancerous conditions, is essential. There is no reason not to utilise these analytical techniques to monitor and diagnose precancers. For example, Pap smears can help monitor precancerous cervical abnormalities. Although the Pap is not foolproof, it is a useful tool, and has dramatically lowered the incidence of cervical cancer in the United States. In the case of cervical dysplasia or cervical intraepithelial neoplasia (CIN; a precancerous condition), Chinese medicine can treat the causative HPV infection directly when a surgical technique is unsuccessful. At the time of writing (2004) a new vaccine is about to be released to prevent the evolution of cervical cancer in women who are exposed to the high-risk types of HPV.

Laboratory analysis such as blood chemistries and tumor marker monitoring, used in conventional treatment, is another way that cancer therapy in integrative oncology is different from general Chinese medical practice. Using this information is a further way of understanding the effectiveness of the treatment of an individual patient. It is also useful in terms of determining a treatment plan and modifying a treatment plan already in place. The insidiousness and often asymptomatic but systemic reality of cancer makes it difficult to detect. The author refers you back to the conversation of Huang di and Qi Bo where Huang di asks how the pulse can appear perfectly normal but a month later the patient has died. Any and all information is extremely valuable in formulating better-integrated care.

The pharmaceutical analysis of specific herbs is added to the information regarding the choice of herbs in a given formula. For example, some fire poison herbs are specific to fire-poison-type tumors and some are not; some tonic herbs have an antineoplastic effect but others do not – astragalus and ginseng (white Chinese) are antineoplastic in various ways, but deer antler is not and may even be contraindicated in some cancers. The pharmaceutical properties of individual herbs have been studied for decades and continue to be studied. This analysis is becoming increasingly complex and, therefore, detailed. For this reason, it is important to keep reading in several areas of medicine, Western and Eastern, in order to keep up with pertinent information.

Fu zheng qu xie

This refers to the promotion and enhancement of the patient's immune mechanisms and total body function to eliminate external and internal pathology that has led to disease; in other words to dispel pathogenic factors by strengthening the patient's resistance. The herbs and formulas that are in this category can be considered to be biological response modifiers (BRMs). Therefore, this approach has the capacity to allow for intensified chemotherapy by treating the side effects of chemotherapeutic regimens.

Deficiency is commonly a predisposing factor for cancer. Cancer also causes deficiencies; one example is the utilisation of the blood supply by a tumor in order to feed itself. This treatment principle seeks to prevent these deficiencies caused by the cancer itself and by conventional treatment. The herbs and formulas in this category help to protect the bone marrow, mucosal lining of the gastroinestinal tract, and normal organ function. The cytotoxic effect of chemotherapies and radiation are said to defeat the normal qi. Therefore, maintaining normal qi is a primary aspect of fu zheng therapy.[33] Rarely, defeating the zheng qi is part of the conventional mechanism. For example, in bone marrow transplantation for leukemia treatment, destroying the bone marrow is a crucial part of the therapy. Utilising fu zheng formulas during this time would be contraindicated.

Maintaining the spirit of the patient falls into the realm of fu zheng as well. Patients who may be losing normal function and who are facing a life-threatening disease can be further injured by the loss of hope. Depression and anxiety are treated as part of maintaining the normal qi. Many cytotoxic therapies and support drugs in cancer treatment also affect mood in various negative ways. Insomnia is a common complaint in cancer patients undergoing treatment. Good sleep is an immensely important aspect of health maintenance, improving prognosis, and maintaining hope.

From a Western perspective, fu zheng herbs and formulas increase the rate of phagocytosis and lymphocyte transformation.[34,35] Some of these herbs promote the formation of antibodies, others prolong the time the antibody survives and show marked preventive action against leukopenia. Others improve phagocytosis of the reticuloendothelial system (RES). Many of the herbs in this category contain high levels of polysaccharides with strong immunopotentiating activity. Examples are *Eleutherococcus senticosus*,[36] *Astragalus mongolicus*,[37] and several mushrooms.[38]

Cancerous changes closely correlate with a decline in cyclic adenosine monophosphate (cAMP) content in cells. Many Chinese herbs are capable of elevating cAMP. Glycyrrhetic acid (from *Glycyrrhiza glabra* or *G. uralensis*) is an example of one of these, and can be used to treat both stomach ulcers and gastric cancer.

Many polysaccharides have strong antitumor activity against transplanted tumors in mice. *Ganoderma lucidum* has high polysaccharide content and strongly inhibits sarcoma-180 in mice.[39] It also increases the white blood cell (WBC) count, increases phagocytosis, reduces platelet aggregation thus slowing metastatic spread, and is a mild analgesic. Those herbs with very high polysaccharide content include aloe,[40] astragalus, codonopsis,[41] taraxacum, ginsengs,[42,43] hoelen (*Poria*),[44] laminaria,[45] lentinus,[46] and polyporus. These are just a few herbs and actions in the realm of fu zheng.

Huo xue qu yu

This term refers to the activation of blood circulation. Stasis is often a precursor condition for cancer and is always part of the end result. Masses and solid tumors are forms of congealed blood and often phlegm combined with toxin. Blood stasis syndrome is indicated when there are signs of poor microcirculation, which is characterised by abnormal capillary beds.[47] The tongue tip and nail beds can be viewed under a high-intensity light and with fairly low magnification for signs of poor microcirculation.[48] What is seen in normal circulation is a long line of blood cells moving through the circulation in an orderly and smooth manner. The capillaries are like rivers meandering through the tissue. In blood stasis syndrome the capillaries are twisted and knotted, preventing the blood cells from moving through and causing them to back up until they pile up on one another. High levels of platelet aggregation, high blood viscosity, high fibrinogen content and disseminated intravascular coagulopathy (DIC) are characteristics of sticky blood and blood stasis syndrome. Some common outcomes of this condition are deep vein thrombosis, coronary artery disease, and stroke. Scarring and adhesions are other forms of blood stasis. Blood stasis is part of the environment of cancer pathogenesis.

Signs of blood stasis, besides the above, are dark or purple coloration of the tongue. When the veins under the tongue are swollen and dark it indicates oxygen-deprived blood cells. A pulse presentation that is choppy or unsmooth in volume suggests congested circulation in certain organs or systemically. Palpable gross masses indicate blood and frequently phlegm stasis. All signs of blood stasis indicate a hypercoaguability of the blood. Regular exercise helps prevent this condition and this is one reason why exercise is important in cancer prevention.

Spontaneous bleeding can occur due to blood stasis syndrome. When the blood is prevented from moving according to its normal course then bleeding may occur. The vessels of patients with blood stasis syndrome are more fragile than those of an individual without blood stasis syndrome. Herbs that move blood are used to treat blood stasis and are generally divided into three categories:

- those that nourish the blood and move blood by increasing the volume
- those that invigorate the blood by helping it to course through the vessels more freely by mildly changing its viscosity
- those that act like dynamite and crack the blood when it is congealed by strongly changing its viscosity and by breaking down viscous membranes that surround tumors.

The herbs and formulas that regulate and activate the blood change the viscosity of blood, help maintain normal blood circulation, affect erythrocyte aggregation, affect platelet aggregation, help restore normal microcirculation, strengthen vasculature, and regulate blood flow.

Pan Mingji, a present-day Chinese researcher in cancer, states that 90% of cancer patients have abnormal circulation patterns. He has found that most cancer patients also have high fibrinogen levels in the blood and higher than normal coagubility of blood. Tumors are often surrounded by a fibrin coating that prevents immune cells from entering them. Blood-moving herbs help to break down this fibrin coating. Tumors cells often have a poorly developed circulation, and the cells that survive do so on low oxygen levels. These cells are less susceptible to radiation than those with an adequate oxygen supply. Therefore, there are many studies being done on the effects of blood-activating herbs on the oxygenation of tumor cells in order to make them more susceptible to radiation therapy. These herbs are used as radiosensitisers. The same process helps potentiate the effect of chemotherapy by allowing better access into the center of tumors.[49]

Metastatic cancer cells require the blood to have a specific viscosity in order to travel and then 'stick' in distant tissue. Some tumors secrete hormone-like substances that affect the blood and vasculature in certain ways that make metastasis easier. Studies are also being done on changing the viscosity of the blood with herbal medicine in order to prevent or slow metastasis. Some blood-activating herbs have direct cancer-inhibiting actions, and others promote immune surveillance.[50]

Qing re jie du

This category of treatment refers to the removal of heat toxins with clear heat herbs. Heat toxins are anything that transforms a simple abnormality into a very difficult-to-control disease process. Clear heat and toxin removing herbs may actually slow or prevent the mutation of the DNA by heat toxins. These toxins can be chemicals, viruses, pathogens, or the result of pathological internal imbalances. The herbs and formulas used to treat in this category often fall in the antibiotic spectrum of pharmaceutical drugs.[51] In fact, many chemotherapeutic agents are antibiotic in effect. Adriamycin, an early chemotherapeutic agent still in use today, is an antibiotic. The earliest conventional medical strategies for treating cancers, in the 1940s, were developed from the same concepts of medicine as antibiotic therapy.

Clear heat and toxin herbs do just that – clear heat, inflammation, accumulations, and toxins of various kinds, including those that result in fevers, inflammations, suppurations, and abscesses. They often also treat pain since inflammation often accompanies pain. These herbs are rarely used alone to treat cancers, but when added to complex herbal formulas appear to contribute significantly to the antineoplastic effect of the overall formula and also the cytotoxic conventional therapy.[52] Toxin and heat clearing herbs in this category include *Sophora flavescens* and *S. subprostrata*,[53] *Oldenlandia*,[54-55] *Scutellaria barbata*,[55] *Taraxacum mongolicum*, *Prunella vulgaris*,[55] and *Lonicera japonica*. In various ways they slow tumor cell growth.

Ruan jian san jie

This phrase refers to softening and dissolving hard masses. Many tumors that are hard in character, that is they feel like stone, are considered to be combinations of blood and phlegm stasis that are especially tightly intertwined. Herbs that transform phlegm are used along with herbs that are also very salty in taste. The saltiness of the herbs increases the dynamic flow of fluids into a tumor. This may help explain how they soften hardness. Many of these herbs also improve immunity and many are antineoplastic. The herbs used to treat lymphadenopathy, goiter, and abdominal masses are in this category. Many are sea vegetables such as *Laminaria* and other seaweeds.[56]

Yi du gong du

This refers to using a poison to combat a poison, the cancer. Generally, cytotoxic therapies are in this realm of treatment. The National Institutes of Health (NIH) have been in the process of testing many Chinese herbs for use as active agents against cancers, many of which fall into this category. These herbs are toxic from the point of view of Chinese medicine as well as conventional medicine. Rarely can we use them in a Western context. They are used in a formula context based upon pharmacological studies for activity against specific cancers.[57]

All of the above treatment principles are combined in various ways to address a cancer within the context of an integration of Chinese medicine and conventional treatment. The formula is like a chemotherapeutic regimen that is formulated to attack the cancerous environment from many different angles. The difference is that it also includes herbs whose action it is to protect and rehabilitate normal function and also potentiate the action of the conventional treatment. The choices made regarding the combinations of herbs are based on many factors including the tumor type, the conventional treatment's mechanism and side effects, the levels of blood and phlegm stasis, the Chinese medical diagnosis for the cancer, the staging of the cancer, the aggressiveness of the cancer based on the markers associated with it, the constitution of the patient, and the performance status of the patient (age, underlying or pre-existing conditions, overall vitality and strength).[58]

TREATMENT

The main principles in treating cancers include the following:[59]

- regulate the qi and harmonise the blood
- maintain the unobstructed flow in the channels and collaterals
- transform phlegm and drain dampness
- soften the hard and dissolve nodules
- dissolve toxins and stop pain
- tonify the qi and nourish the blood
- benefit the spleen and pacify the stomach
- replenish and tonify the liver and kidneys.

These principles and the therapeutic methods that follow are gleaned from various teachers from Beijing, Chengdu, and Shanghai, all of whom practice integrated oncology in hospital settings. The therapeutic methods garnered from the above principles draw from many categories of Chinese herbs.

- Regulate and activate blood:
    - qi-regulating herbs:
      chen pi (Citri reticulatae Pericarpium; *Citrus reticulata* pericarp)
      qing pi (Citri reticulatae viride Pericarpium; *Citrus reticulata* green pericarp)
      xiao hui xiang (Foeniculi Fructus; *Foeniculum vulgare* seed)
      mu dan pi (Moutan Cortex; *Paeonia suflruticosa* root cortex)
      xiang fu (Cyperi Rhizoma; *Cyperus rotundus* rhizome)

- blood-activating herbs:
  dang gui wei (Angelicae sinensis radicis Cauda; *Angelica sinensis* lateral roots; tangkuei tail)

  chuan xiong (Chuanxiong Rhizoma; *Ligusticum wallichii* root)

  dan shen (Salviae miltiorrhizae Radix; *Salvia miltiorhiza* root)

  chi shao (Paeoniae Radix rubra; *Paeonia lactiflora* root)

  tao ren (Persicae Semen; *Prunus* spp. seed)

  hong hua (Carthami Flos; *Carthamnus tinctorius* flowers)

  wu ling zhi (Trogopterori Faeces; *Trogopterus xanthipes* excrement)
- Maintain the unobstructed flow of the channels and collaterals:
  - gui zhi (Cinnamomi Ramulus; *Cinnamomum cassia* branches)
  - du huo (Angelicae pubescentis Radix; *Angelica* spp. root)
  - gao ben (Ligustici Rhizoma; *Ligusticum* root)
- Transform phlegm and drain dampness:
  - chen pi (Citri reticulatae Pericarpium; *Citrus reticulata* pericarp)
  - zhi ban xia (Pinelliae Rhizoma preparatum; *Pinellia ternata* rhizome)
  - sheng jiang (Zingiberis Rhizoma recens; *Zingiber officinale* fresh rhizome)
  - fu ling (Poria; *Poria cocos*)
  - chuan bei mu (Fritillariae cirrhosae Bulbus; *Fritillaria cirrhosa*)
  - zhe bei mu (Fritillariae thunbergii Bulbus; *Fritillaria thunbergii*)
  - jie geng (Platycodi Radix; *Platycodon grandiflorus* root)
  - huang bai (Phellodendri Cortex; *Phellodendron* cortex)
- Soften hardness and dispel nodules:
  - hai zao (Sargassum; *Sargassum*)
  - kun bu (Eckloniae Thallus; *Ecklonia kurome* thallus)
  - mu li (Ostreae Concha; *Ostrea* shell)
  - chuan bei mu (Fritillariae cirrhosae Bulbus; *Fritillaria cirrhosa*)
  - bai mao gen (Imperatae Rhizoma; *Imperata cylindrica* rhizome)
  - tian hua fen (Trichosanthis Radix; *Trichosanthes* root)
  - gua lou shi (Trichosanthis Fructus; *Trichosanthes* fruit)

- Dissolve toxins and stop pain:
  - tonify qi and move blood type:
    dang shen (Codonopsis Radix; *Codonopsis pilosula* root)

    tai zi shen (Pseudostellariae Radix; *Pseudostellaria heterophylla*)

    huang qi (Astragali Radix; *Astragalus membranaceus*)

    dan shen (Salviae miltiorrhizae Radix; *Salvia miltiorhiza* root)

    dang gui (Angelicae sinensis Radix; *Angelica sinensis*)

    ji xue teng (Spatholobi Caulis; *Spatholobus suberectus*)
  - harmonise the stomach/spleen type:
    bai zhu (Atractylodis macrocephalae Rhizoma; *Atractylodes macrocephala*)

    fu ling (Poria; *Poria cocos*)

    shan yao (Dioscoreae Rhizoma; *Dioscorea opposita*)

    gan cao (Glycyrrhizae Radix; *Glycyrrhiza*; licorice root)
  - warm and tonify kidney yang:
    fu zi (Aconiti Radix preparata; *Aconitum carmichaelii*)

    rou gui (Cinnamomi Cortex; *Cinnamomum cassia* cortex)

    lu rong (Cervi Cornu pantotrichum; *Cervus nippon*; deer velvet)

    yin yang huo (Epimedii Herba; *Epimedium grandiflorum*)

    rou cong rong (Cistanches Herba; *Cistanche*)

    tu si zi (Cuscutae Semen; *Cuscuta* seeds)
  - tonify liver and kidney yin:
    gou qi zi (Lycii Fructus; *Lycium chinensis* fruit)

    nu zhen zi (Ligustri lucidi Fructus; *Ligustrum lucidum* fruit)

    shan zhu yu (Corni Fructus; *Cornus officinalis* fruit)

    han lian cao (Ecliptae Herba; *Eclipta prostrata*)
  - clear toxin and heat toxin: many examples that are chosen primarily from pharmaceutical studies relating to specific cancers.
- Activate blood and remove stasis:
  - tao ren (Persicae Semen; *Prunus* spp. seed)
  - hong hua (Carthami Flos; *Carthamnus tinctorius* flowers)
  - chi shao (Paeoniae Radix rubra; *Paeonia lactiflora* root)
  - san qi (Notoginseng Radix; *Panax notoginseng*)

- dan shen (Salviae miltiorrhizae Radix; *Salvia miltiorhiza* root)
- chuan xiong (Chuanxiong Rhizoma; *Ligusticum wallichii* root)
- ru xiang (Olibanum; *Boswellia sacra;* frankincense; gum olibanum)
- mo yao (Myrrha; *Commiphora myrrha;* myrrh)
- wang bu liu xing (Vaccariae Semen; *Vaccaria segetalis* seeds)
  - Stop pain:
    - qi moving stop pain:
      chen pi (Citri reticulatae Pericarpium; *Citrus reticulata* pericarp)
      xiao hui xiang (Foeniculi Fructus; *Foeniculum vulgare* seed)
      mu dan pi (Moutan Cortex; *Paeonia suffruticosa* root cortex)
      xiang fu (Cyperi Rhizoma; *Cyperus rotundus* rhizome)
    - blood harmonising stop pain:
      chi shao (Paeoniae Radix rubra; *Paeonia lactiflora* root)
      bai shao (Paeoniae Radix alba; *Paeonia lactiflora* root)
      chuan xiong (Chuanxiong Rhizoma; *Ligusticum wallichii* root)
      yu jin (Curcumae Radix; *Curcuma longa* rhizome)
      yan hu suo (Corydalis Rhizoma; *Corydalis yanhusuo*)
      ru xiang (Olibanum; *Boswellia sacra;* frankincense; gum olibanum)
      mo yao (Myrrha; *Commiphora myrrha;* myrrh)
- Invigorate the spleen and pacify the stomach:
  - dang shen (Codonopsis Radix; *Codonosis pilosula* root)
  - bai zhu (Atractylodis macrocephalae Rhizoma; *Atractylodes*)
  - Si jun zi tang
  - Xiang sha liu jun zi tang
  - Xiao yao san
  - Ping wei san
  - Bao he wan
- Tonify the liver and kidneys:
  - nu zhen zi (Ligustri lucidi Fructus; *Ligustrum lucidum* fruit)
  - gou qi zi (Lycii Fructus; *Lycium chinensis* fruit)
  - tu si zi (Cuscutae Semen; *Cuscuta* seeds)
  - shan zhu yu (Corni Fructus; *Cornus officinalis* fruit)

- du zhong (Eucommiae Cortex; *Eucommia ulmoides* cortex)
- gui ban* (Testudinis Plastrum; *Chinemys reevesii* plastron)

These are only some of the examples of herbs used in these categories.

General treatment principles in integrated care require an analysis and differentiation of the cancer according to conventional and Chinese medicine. This will include staging, the degree of aggressiveness of the cancer, the differentiation and type of the cancer, the predicted side effects of the conventional treatment combined with the constitutional diagnosis of the patient, the Chinese medical diagnosis of the pattern for the specific cancer, and the presenting symptoms. An analysis of the balance of the excesses and deficiencies must take place in order to understand the thrust of treatment. This involves determining the root and the branches in any presentation. It may change through time. An example is an early-stage cancer that has aggressive markers where the conventional treatment will be quite strong. In this case, the classical treatment of the cancer may also be quite strong (unless the patient cannot tolerate it) with many clear heat and dissolve toxin herbs. In a later stage cancer in an elderly patient with complicating underlying chronic cardiovascular disease, the approach will be milder and include more fu zheng herbs. This is where the art of the medicine and the skill of the practitioner come in. This way of treating was imparted by Sun Gui Zhi of Guang An Men Hospital in Beijing.

All of the above general principles come together to provide information as to how to support the zheng qi, the source qi, the middle jiao function, and normal organ function in the presence of not only the constitution of the patient and the disease presentation but also the side effects of the conventional therapies being given. How much the technique of tonification is used versus the technique of clearing toxins depends on an analysis of all of the above. It will change depending on the patient's condition and the practitioner's ability to read the patient's capacity to utilise these strong herbs. All herbs require that a certain amount of qi be used by the body to metabolise them and also to activate the function for which they are intended. Qi is used in any restorative or clearing action, and this must be taken into account when deciding on which herbs to use.

At the same time, many conventional interventions are carcinogenic themselves. Therefore, it is sometimes difficult to know whether you are treating the cancer and its disease process or the side effects of the therapies used to treat the cancer. In this context, treating the side effects of conventional treatment with herbal medicine is as much antineoplastic as is treating the cancer directly with conventional cytotoxic treatment, because treating side effects allows for the conventional cytotoxic treatment schedule to be maintained and also helps to maintain normal health as much as possible. Thus patients are able to utilise their own internal mechanisms to change the environment in which the cancer originally evolved. These two contributions of herbal medicine treatment alongside conventional care cannot be stressed enough.

Writing a prescription

In the clinical management of a cancer, the treatment principles utilised and the resulting formulas are based on the observed injuries and the predicted injuries that will result from conventional care. Several factors are taken into account regarding the predicted injuries. These include the inherited constitutional diagnosis of the patient, the acquired constitutional diagnosis (what they did with their inheritance) that laid the foundation, if any, for the cancer to occur in the first place, and the current symptomatic presentation relative to the disease itself. In addition, the symptomatic presentation relative to the side effects from other therapies is taken into account. And then prophylaxis against metastatic spread is added to this complex list. All of these factors are weighed and addressed according to current necessity. For example, during certain kinds of chemotherapy the main issues in writing a script may relate to digestive dysfunction and myelosuppression. At this time, a formula may be used primarily to treat for anemia and nausea. At another time, a formula may be used to prevent recurrence.

Formulas should work alongside the cytotoxic treatment to support, rehabilitate and protect normal function, and also be anticancerous. Presurgery, the formula is used to build blood levels, speed tissue regeneration, decrease blood loss during surgery, and decrease swelling from trauma, while preventing the spread of the cancer during the procedure. After surgery the formula is changed to decrease wound healing time, decrease the amount of scar tissue and adhesion formation, facilitate normal bowel function, reduce pain, and prevent infection. During radiation treatment the purpose of the formula is to protect normal tissue while enhancing without interfering with the effect of the radiation. Radiosensitising formulas work by improving blood circulation to the tumor cells. Many studies have been done on dan shen, or *Salvia miltiorhiza* (Salviae miltiorrhizae Radix), in combined treatment with both chemotherapy and radiation. As a blood-activating herb, dan shen helps to make blood move, even into the dense areas at the center of a tumor mass. This action gives the chemotherapeutic agent better access to the target tissue. By providing better-oxygenated blood to the tumor it potentiates the radiation treatment while helping to reduce the amount of scar tissue (blood stasis) formation caused by radiation.[60]

Those formulas used during chemotherapy vary depending on several factors. The task is to understand the mechanism by which the agent or regimen is cytotoxic, the side effects of those agents, and then predict those areas of injury within the theory of Oriental or classical Chinese medicine. The formula should potentiate the mechanism of the chemotherapeutic regimen while treating the side effects. Formulas that protect bone marrow, the mucosal lining of the gastrointestinal tract and zang fu function are specifically designed for the regimen being used. When the normal function of healthy tissue is maintained as much as possible, this allows for two things: firstly the schedule for the chemotherapy can be maintained which, in turn, maintains a persistent level of cytotoxicity to kill every tumor cell, and secondly, the healthier and stronger the overall body function is, the greater the ability of the body itself to fight the cancer from the inside.

Within some health-delivery systems, there is greater flexibility regarding cancer care. For example, in Europe some treatment centers utilise higher doses of chemotherapy than in the United States. The combination of Chinese herbal medicine with higher dose chemotherapy allows for these higher dose cytotoxic treatments. In SCLC (small-cell lung cancer), there is an initial high sensitivity to chemotherapy but a poor prognosis, and early drug resistance makes the first courses of chemotherapy very important. The use of herbal formulas to allow for higher dose chemotherapy can give a better prognosis. These same formulas can also enhance or potentiate the effect of the chemotherapy.[61,62]

There are many complex factors, as stated above, that go into formulating the choice of individual herbs. No two people are the same, even with the exact same conventional medical diagnosis. The presentation of a given patient will change over time. The formula, therefore, is customised to meet an individual's needs. A portion of the formula will treat the constitution and the primary diagnosis for the cancer. Another portion will be combined with this main formula to address the primary symptoms. And another portion may be combined to address the primary predicted or observable side effects. And, finally, the formula attempts to be antineoplastic in the sense that it uses herbs whose pharmacology has been studied and found to have a specific anticancer effect. Therefore, a formula is tailored based on the following criteria, ubiquitous across systems of natural medicine. Not all of these will be used in any given formula.

1. Tumor load reduction or producing an anti-neoplastic effect by attacking, dissolving, moving, detoxifying, clearing pathogenic factors, warming, and cooling.
2. Prevention of the formation and development of a further cancer or cancerous spread by harmonising, strengthening ying and wei qi, clearing pathogenic factors.
3. Enhancement of immune function, including cellular and humoral immunity, by tonifying qi and nourishing blood, tonifying yang and generating yin, harmonising and promoting fluids.
4. Maintenance of the regulating function of the endocrine system by regulating qi and blood.
5. Enhancement and protection of the structure and function of the viscera by tonifying the yin and yang of the zang.
6. Strengthening of digestion and absorption by benefiting and tonifying the spleen.
7. Protection of the bone marrow and hematopoietic function by nourishing essence.
8. Increasing the efficacy of conventional treatments by harmonising the flow of qi and blood.
9. Prevention, amelioration, and control of adverse side effects and diseases caused by conventional therapy.

Chemotherapeutic regimens are given in a dosing schedule that usually allows for the regeneration of hematopoietic cells produced by the bone marrow. Since these cells turn over more quickly than many other cells in the body, they are affected by the cytotoxicity of conventional therapy. Chemotherapy kills not only tumor cells but also other fast-growing cells including those of the gastrointestinal mucosa, which naturally slough off approximately every 24 hours, and hair and blood cells. The loss of WBCs or red blood cells (RBCs) during treatment can lead to infection in the case of WBCs and extreme fatigue and loss of normal oxygenation of healthy tissue in the case of RBCs. Therefore, many chemotherapeutic regimens are scheduled in a way that will allow for maximum cytotoxicity but also time for the blood cells to reconstitute themselves. This is often every 21 days because this is the timing that allows the marrow to reproduce those blood cells impacted by chemotherapy. Not all chemotherapies act in this way. And not all regimens are dosed via this schedule. However, the dosing schedule, when higher amounts of chemotherapy are used over a longer interval between doses, can be used as a means for predicting an ebb and flow of physiologic activity in a given patient. This is another way in which formulas can be written.

For example, in a 21-day regimen containing Adriamycin, the first 6 days are the phase in which the main cytotoxic activity occurs. Fast-growing cells are eroded during this time, including those of the epithelial membranes, causing dry mouth, mouth sores, vomiting, nausea, loss of appetite, diarrhea, constipation, abdominal pain and distention, possibly cystitis, skin rashes, and possibly palpitations. Normal blood cells are also eroded during this phase. Therefore, the herbal approach at this stage is to increase blood circulation to promote distribution of the chemotherapy into the tumor site and into tumor cells, to promote clearing of toxins including cell debris, to nourish the yin especially to protect the mucosal lining of the gastrointestinal tract, to control nausea and vomiting, and to promote the appetite.

From days 7 to 12 in this same cycle, most of the cytotoxicity is accomplished, which means that the bone marrow damage is at its peak. The symptoms are generally fatigue, malaise, insomnia, possibly fever (from neutropenia), arthralgias, tachycardia, anemia and signs of anemia of various kinds, and possible cardiotoxicity (from Adriamycin). The role of the herbal formula changes to that of tonifying qi and yang, nourishing blood, yin and essence, protecting and restoring the zang fu and the bone marrow, promoting circulation and urination, restoring digestive function, and harmonising the ying and wei to prevent infection.

Days 12–21 become a time of regeneration and recovering. All signs and symptoms should be decreasing. Fatigue may persist and increase over time through treatment. Depression and anxiety may develop, persisting and increasing through time. This is primarily due to the fact that adjusting to the reality of having to go through this cycle again can be very depressing. Knowing that one will be physically debilitated in this cyclic fashion can be a hard pill to swallow. Treating the spirit of a patient is immensely important in helping to maintain overall health. The role of herbal medicine is the same here as in days 7–12 with the inclusion of calm the spirit herbs. This is another approach to designing formulas.

New treatment schedules include dose-dense and dose-intense drug delivery. In various ways the chemotherapy is delivered more frequently, either every week or every two weeks, at a lower dose per infusion. This way of dosing has a better outcome in some cases by maintaining a more consistent level of cytotoxicity. This is applicable to some patients where the type of cancer and the staging and the status of the patient allows for a more intensive schedule. This way of scheduling requires a different approach in herbal intervention than stated above. The approach is determined by the schedule and the side effects and remains more constant. This means that rather than writing two or three formulas for a 21-day infusion schedule, one formula is used that has a more generalised action, based on the fact that the chemotherapeutic action is more constant.

In some cases, patients are hospitalised for 3–5 days and undergo a more intensive high-dose chemotherapy with iv drip and maintenance drugs with fluids to help protect normal organ function. This approach can be 3–5 days on chemotherapy and then 3 weeks off to recover. Ordinarily it is very difficult logistically to apply herbal medicine in these conditions unless the patient brings the herbal preparation to the hospital and is insistent that they will take it regardless of any opposition. But once the patient has left the hospital then it is possible to resume a normal schedule of herbal medicine at home based on all of the precepts covered earlier. Access to patients is often determined by the relationship of the practitioner with the medical oncologist. Writing an introductory letter to a physician explaining your treatment to that provider is a good start to developing an interaction that then allows the complementary practitioner greater access to their patients when hospitalised. Many hospitals have criteria by which they allow non-credentialed providers access to their premises to see patients they have in common. The oncologist of a shared patient can be very supportive of the complementary provider if there is a strong and respectful relationship already in existence. Making these relationships can help provide better patient care.

Chemotherapy may also be delivered continuously, via an infusion pump that is strapped to the body. Drugs are delivered 24 hours per day at very low dose. Generally, the same rules apply here as in the dose-intense means of delivery.

Rules of treatment[63-65]

1. Alleviate acute symptoms first. This can include everything from referral to the primary oncologist or the emergency room for hemorrhagic bleeding to stopping acute nausea. This is the primary rule for all of medicine. Therefore, using one's best judgment is necessary.
2. In very weak patients, treat the symptom picture and the root (constitutional diagnosis) simultaneously. The strength of each prong is determined by the strength of the normal qi in the patient.

3. If the pathogenic factor (the cancer) and the body's normal qi are both weak, tonify the normal qi to push out the pathogen (if possible). This is especially important in later-stage disease.

4. If the body's normal qi is weak and the pathogen is strong (i.e. later-stage cancer or a very aggressive cancer), the pathogen must be eliminated without harming the normal qi.

5. As the qi, blood and yin become more engaged by the disease, a balance must be struck between eliminating and tonifying. In order to eliminate pathogens from the body adequate normal qi is required. In the case of chemotherapy, treatment is eliminative only and without rehabilitative function. In this case, herbal medicine becomes the balancing mechanism in the overall treatment by being almost entirely supportive.

6. Do not do anything to undermine the treatments chosen by patients for themselves. It is not our task as practitioners to make choices for patients in cancer treatment. We must honor and respect their own choices and evolve a treatment plan that will accommodate the continued efficacy of treatments from other systems of medicine. We can teach and provide as much information as we can to help patients make choices. To doctor is to teach.

7. Know the mechanism of the conventional treatment being used. The side effects can be treated without undermining the mechanism. Maintaining normal body functions as much as possible is one way of actually enhancing the effectiveness of the cytotoxic therapy.

Other concerns

Qi tonic herbs help resolve phlegm and this helps move qi. This is true in cancer treatment and in pain management.

Eliminating or detoxifying herbs are bitter, cold and pungent and can injure gastrointestinal function. They act in some ways just like chemotherapy or radiation.

Tonifying herbs are sweet and often sticky and can cause dampness. Dampness can be an underlying mechanism for the proliferation of cancers. Therefore, care must be used in choosing herbs, accurately diagnosing the constitution, and under-standing the overall environment in which one is hoping to work therapeutically.

Integrate Chinese with Western diagnostics and analysis. You must know more than classical Chinese medicine in order to treat cancer. This is especially true if you are working adjunctively alongside conventional medicine.

During chemotherapy the dose of anticancer herbs may be lowered. This depends on your expertise. If you feel unsure as to how to interface the antineoplastic herbs with a specific cytotoxic therapy, then treat only symptomatically for the 3 days prior to and 2 days after chemotherapy. Do not use antineoplastic herbs during the infusion period. Resume antineoplastic herbs after this time period. If you are confident in your understanding of the conventional cytotoxic mechanism, then go ahead and use antineoplastics.

Because of the extreme immune suppression during high-dose chemotherapy there is concern on the part of conventional providers about infection caused by herbal medicine that may have bacteria, molds, and other forms of contamination. This is especially true in the treatment of leukemias where high-dose chemotherapy and transplantation are possible treatments. This may automatically preclude treatment with any form of alternative medicine. If you are trusted by your patient and their providers, you may be able to treat with herbal medicine. Granulated herbs that have been packaged in single doses and then irradiated may be a means by which you can provide a safe herbal product to your patient. Patients undergoing transplantation still eat and herbs are designated as food. Therefore, work to ensure a pure herbal product and build strong relationships with conventional medical providers in order to continue providing care to your patients.

When using crude herbs that are prepared by the patient it is extremely important that the patient calls you during or after the first time of preparing the herbal soup. Have them describe to you what exactly they have done in the cooking process. Improper cooking can change the dose and allow for contamination of cooked soups. Any possible molds that develop as part of storage are to be avoided. If there is any question regarding contamination, the herbal soup must be discarded. Monitor your patients carefully in this respect.

When in doubt about your patient's ability to prepare soups use high-quality granulated herbs instead.

Do not allow patients to begin their herbal medicine during the first days of chemotherapy when nausea is high, as they may acquire a habituated negative response to the herbs. This can occur even with the patient on antiemetic drugs. Wait until the nausea has subsided to begin herbal treatment.

All of the formulas in this book are prescribed according to a gram dosage. This dosing method can be applied to either crude herbs or granulated herbs according to the usual means by which each are prescribed. The overall daily dose in oncology is usually at least twice that of the regular dose. For example, the typical dose per day for a non-cancer patient is 9 g. The typical dose for a cancer patient is at least 18 g, twice the normal dose. It is not uncommon for the dose per day to be increased to four times the normal dose. You will notice that the amounts for some of the herbs in many formulas are extremely high. The goal of all formulas in this context is to provide a very high circulating blood level of phytochemical materials over a constant period of time. This may mean that dosing three times per day may not be enough and dosing can be increased to five or six times per day. The schedule will rely upon the needs of the patient and their ability to absorb the herbs.

Use herbs supplied by a reputable pharmacist who can guarantee through batch assays that all of the herbs used for your patients are free of any form of contamination, including heavy metals, pesticides, bacteria, viruses, other biological contaminants, and chemical contaminants. It is impossible to guarantee that herbs are free of fungi or mold. Cooking will kill most spores and, therefore, crude herbs are free of spores at the end of cooking. But if more than one dose is cooked at a time, then storing cooked herbs must be done carefully in order to prevent contamination. Granulated herbs are less susceptible to contamination but are still at risk. In the case of a patient whose immunity is low and for whom the issue of biological contamination is of great concern, it may be best to supply the herbs in individual packs that have been irradiated. Herbs in cooked form can be purchased from various suppliers. However, these cooked herbal decoctions are packaged in a hot liquid form in plastic bags, which may release xenoestrogenic and other chemical contaminants. It is best, in my opinion, to avoid these prepared crude herb decoctions until the issue of plastic contamination can be resolved.

PREVENTION

No cancer is considered cured until there is a 5-year disease-free interval. In many cases, recurrence will occur during the first 2 years after the end of conventional treatment. Therefore, it is immensely important that patients continue treatment with complementary medicine for at least 2 years after finishing conventional care. During this time of monitoring by conventional providers no interventions occur that help to rehabilitate function lost as a result of the cancer itself or as a result of cytotoxic treatment. Very little information is given about things the patient can do to prevent a recurrence of their cancer.

Complementary providers frequently become the primary providers of support and information in this phase of cancer surveillance. It is important to convince patients that their cancer treatment is not finished. Diet, sleep, exercise, happiness, and peace are all necessary components of health that need to become a part of their life in the long term. Continuing with Chinese medicine and possibly supplementation will contribute to their ability to remain disease-free. Each chapter of this book has information and formulas used to prevent recurrence on each cancer type. The work to change the environment in which the cancer occurred continues after cytotoxic treatment. It cannot be stated strongly enough how important this ongoing treatment is in terms of overall survival. One chapter of this book has been dedicated to general prevention.

References

1. Silverburg E. Cancer statistics, 1995. American Cancer Society 1995; 40:9–26.
2. Dean M. Principles of molecular cell biology. In: DeVita VT, ed. Cancer: principles and practice of oncology. 3rd edn. Philadelphia: JB Lippincott; 1989.
3. Phillips RA. The genetic basis of cancer. In: Tannock IF, ed. The basic science of oncology. New York: Pergamon Press; 1987.
4. Minden MD. Oncogenes. In: Tannock IF, ed. The basic science of oncology. New York: Pergamon Press; 1987.
5. Roberts AB. Principles of molecular cell biology of cancer: growth factors related to transformation. In: DeVita VT, ed. Cancer: principles and practice of oncology. 3rd edn. Philadelphia: JB Lippincott; 1989:67–80.
6. Sager R. Tumor suppressor genes: the puzzle and the promise. Science 1990; 246:1406–1412.
7. Henshaw EC. The biology of cancer. In: Rubin P, ed. Clinical oncology. 7th edn. Philadelphia: WB Saunders; 1993:26.
8. Carson R. Silent spring. Boston: Houghton-Mifflin; 1962.
9. Epstein S. The carcinogenicity of heptachlor and chlordane. Sci Total Environ 1976; 6:103–154.
10. Infante PF. Blood dyscrasias and childhood tumors and exposures to chlorinated hydrocarbon pesticides. Proceedings from the 14–19 June 1976 Conference on Women in the Workplace. Washington, DC: Society for Occupational and Environmental Health.
11. National Academy of the Sciences, National Research Council, Advisory Center on Toxicology, Pesticide Information Review and Evaluation Committee. An evaluation of the carcinogenicity of chlordane and heptachlor. Washington, DC October, 1977.
12. Hoy C. The truth about breast cancer. Boston: Stoddart; 1995.
13. Raloff J. Menstrual cycles may affect cancer risk. Science News, 7 January 1995.
14. Raloff J. Breast cancer: environmental factors. Lancet 1992; 339:904.
15. Zurhasen H. Viruses in human cancer. Science 1991; 254:1167–1172.
16. Miller EC. Mechanics of chemical carcinogenesis. Cancer 1981; 47:1055–1064.
17. Altman R. The cancer dictionary. Facts On File 1992:319–320.
18. Lamson DW, Brignall MS. Antioxidants in cancer therapy; their actions and interactions with oncologic therapies. Altern Med Rev 1999; 4:304–329.
19. Zhou Li (The Zhou Rituals). Compiled in the Qin Dynasty. 221–207 BCE.52.
20. In: Shuo Wen Jie Zi (Discussing characters and explaining words).
21. In: Zheng Zi Tong (A comprehensive discussion of the correct use of characters).
22. Wang Qing Ren. Yi Lin Gai Gao (Corrections of errors among physicians). 1830 ACE. People's Health Publishing; 1985.
23. Kuwahara, Koei. Notes from Toyo Hari training, 1996.
24. Li Yan. Zhong Liu Lin Chuang Bei Yao (Essentials of clinical pattern identification of tumors). 2nd edn. Beijing: People's Medical Publishing House; 1998.
25. Larre C. The liver. Paris: Institut Ricci; 1989.
26. Jarrett L. Nourishing destiny. Spirit Path 1998:241–244.
27. Jarrett L. Nourishing destiny. Spirit Path 1998:279–290.
28. Sun Si Miao. Qian Jin Yao Fang (Presciptions worth a thousand gold pieces for emergencies). 652 ACE. People's Health Publishing; 1982.
29. Cleavey S. Fluid physiology and pathology in traditional Chinese medicine. London: Churchill Livingstone; 1995:167–168, 232–236.
30. Zhang Jing Yue. Jing Yue Yuan Shu (The complete works of Jing Yue). 1624 ACE. Shanghai Science and Technology Press; 1959.
31. Chao Yuan Fang. Zhu Bing Yuan Hou Lun (Generalised treatise on the etiology and symptomatology of disease). 610 ACE.
32. Huo Jinglun, ed. Treatment of pediatric diseases in traditional Chinese medicine. Academy Press (Xue Yuan); 1995:6–11.
33. Yu Rencun. Immune mechanism of Chinese materia medica in inhibiting cancer. Zhong Guo Zhong Liu (Chinese Journal of Oncology) 1993; 2:20–21.
34. Sun Yan. Results of double-blind clinical tests on Ligustrin in promoting the immune effect. Zhong Guo Lin Chuang Xao Li Za Zhi (Chinese Journal of Clinical Pharmacology) 1990; 2:1–3.
35. Wang Jin Yuan. Shen bai pian zhi liao bai xi bao jian shao zheng de lin chuang yi ji shi yan yan jiu (Clinical and laboratory study of Sheng bai pain (Restore the White Pills) in the treatment of leukopenia). Zhong Yi Zha Zhi (Journal of Traditional Chinese Medicine) 1988; 1:32–53.
36. Shan BE. Chinese medicinal herb, Acanthopanax gracilistylus, extract induces cell cycle arrest of human tumor cells in vitro. Jpn J Cancer Res 2000; 91:383–389.

37. Chu DT. Immunotherapy with Chinese medicinal herbs. I. Immune restoration of local xenogeneic graft-versus-host reaction in cancer patients by fractionated Astragalus membranaceus in vitro. J Clin Lab Immunol 1988; 25:19–23.

38. Zhang J. Antitumor active protein-containing glycans from the Chinese mushroom Songshan ling zhi, Ganoderma tsugae mycelium. Biosci Biotechnol Biochem 1994; 58:1202–1205.

39. Wang G. Antitumor active polysaccharides from the Chinese mushroom Songshan lingzhi, the fruiting body of Ganoderma tsugae. Biosci Biotechnol Biochem 1993; 57:894–900.

40. Pecere T. Aloe-emodin is a new type of anti-cancer agent with selective activity against neuroectodermal tumors. Cancer Res 2000; 60:2800–2804.

41. Hever D. The role of nutrition in cancer prevention and control. Oncology 1992; 6:9–14.

42. Duda RB. American ginseng and breast cancer therapeutic agents synergistically inhibit MCF-7 breast cancer cell growth. J Surg Oncol 1999; 72:230–239.

43. Kim SE. Ginsenoside-Rs4, a new type of ginseng saponin concurrently induces apoptosis and selectively elevates protein levels of p53 and p21WAF1 in human hepatoma SK-HEP-1 cells. Eur J Cancer 1999; 35:507–511.

44. Kaminaga T. Inhibitory effects of lanastane-type triterpine acids, the components of Poria cocos, on tumor promotion by 12-0-tetra-decanoylphorbol-13-acetate in two-stage carcinogenesis in mouse skin. Oncology 1996; 53:382–385.

45. Zheng S. Initial study on naturally occurring products from traditional Chinese herbs and vegetables for chemoprevention. J Cell Biochem Supplement 1997; 27:106–112.

46. Suzuki M. Antitumor and immunological activity of Lentinan in comparison with LPS. International J Immunopharm 1994; 16:463–468.

47. Sun Qingjing. Dan Shen Dui Gan Ai Zheng Sheng Wu Zhi Liao Xue (Current Biological Treatment of Cancer). Beijing: People's Military Press; 1995:2.

48. Huang Lizhong. Yuan fa xing gan ai zhong yi zhi fa de lin chuang yan jiu (Clinical study of primary liver cancer with Traditional Chinese Medicine methods). Hu Nan Zhong Yi Xue Yuan Xue Bao (J of Hunan TCM College) 1996; 16:14–17.

49. Pan Mingji. Cancer Treatment with Fu Zheng Pei Ben Principle. Fujian Science and Technology Publishing House; 1992:18–19.

50. Gao Jin. Xioa shu wei ai pi xia yi zhi hou zhong liu fa gou zheng zhong xue ye liu bian xue de guan cha (Study of blood rheology during tumor development after hypodermic implantation of stomach cancer in mice). Zhong Hua Zhong Liu Za Zhi (Chinese J Oncol, 1989; 6:429.

51. Bi Liqi. Zhong yao tian hua fen dan bai dui hei se su xi bao ji xi bao zhou qi de ying xiang (Effect of the proteins in tian hua fen, R. trichosanthes, on melanocytes and the cell cycle. Zhong Guo Zhong Yi Xi Jie He Za Zhi (J Integ TCM and Western Med) 1998; 18:35–37.

52. Zhang Liping. Ku shen jian dui K562 xi bao zhu huo xing he xi bao zhouqi de ying xiang (Effect of matrine on the activity of the K562 cell strains and the cell cycle). Zhong Hua Zhong Liu Za Zhi (Chin Oncolo J), 1998; 20:328–329.

53. Kojima R, Fukushima S, Ueno A, et al. Antitumor activity of Leguminosae plant constituents. I. Antitumor activity of constituents of Sophora subprostrata. Chem Pharm Bull 1970; 18:2555–2563.

54. Takagi S. Yakagaku Zasshi 1981; 101:657–659.

55. Huang KC. The pharmacology of Chinese herbs. 2nd edn. Boca Raton: CRC Press; 1999:478.

56. op. cit. 481.

57. op. cit. 480.

58. Huang Fuzhong. Ming Yi Zhi Zhang (A guide to famous physicians). 16th Century. People's Health Publishing; 1982.

59. Wani MC. Taxus. J Am Chem Soc 1971; 93:2325–2326.

60. Zhang Yize. Zhong yao zai e xing zhong liu fang liao zhong de jian du zeng xiao zuo yong (The role of Chinese materia medica in increasing the effectiveness and reducing the toxicity of chemotherapy in the treatment of malignant tumors). Shandong Zhong Yi Za Zhi (Shandong J of TCM) 1998; 17:488–490.

61. Cao Guangwen. Xian Dai Ai Zheng Sheng Wu Zhi Liao Xue (Current Biological Treatment of Cancer). Beijing: People's Military Press; 1995.

62. Liao Yuping. Tong qiao huo xue tang jia jian pei he fang liao zhi liao bi yan ai (Modified decoction for freeing the orifices and invigorating the blood combined with radiotherapy in the treatment of nasopharyngeal cancer. Zhong Xi Yi Jie He Za Zhi (J of Integrated TCM and Western Med) 1987; 7:214–216.

63. Zhang Daizhao. Zhang Dai Zhao Zhi Ai Jing Yan Ji Yao (A collection of Zhang Daizhao's experiences in the treatment of cancer). Beijing: China Medicine and Pharmaceutical Publishing House; 2001.

64. Zhang Daizhao. E Xing Zhong Liu Fang Hua Zhong Xi Zhi Liao (Chinese materia medica in the treatment of malignant tumors with chemotherapy and radiotherapy). Beijing: People's Medical Publishing House; 2000.

65. Bensky D. Formulas and strategies. Seattle: Eastland Press; 1990:7–8.

Chapter 2

Lung Cancer

CHAPTER CONTENTS

Risk factors and epidemiology   35

Small-cell lung cancer   36
   Biology   37
   Pathology   37
   Clinical presentation   37
   Current screening tools   38
   Natural history   39
   Staging   39
   Clinical evaluation   39
   Prognostic factors   40
   Treatment   40

Non–small-cell lung cancer   41
   Risk factors   41
   Subtypes of NSCLC   42
   Biology   42
   Clinical presentation   43
   Diagnosis   43
   Staging   44
   Treatment   44
   Stage III disease   45
   Stage IV disease   45

Chinese medicine   45
   Overview   45
   Etiology   46
   Diagnostic Patterns   47

> *Why should we cherish all sentient beings?*
> *Because sentient beings are the roots of the tree*
> *   of awakening.*
> *The Bodhisatvas and the Buddhas are the flowers*
> *   and fruits.*
> *Compassion is the water for the roots.*
>   From the *Avatamsaka Sutra*

RISK FACTORS AND EPIDEMIOLOGY

Lung cancer has been the leading cause of death from cancer until only recently. It accounts for 19% of all cancers in men and 11% of all cancers in women. The mortality from lung cancer in the United States has risen from 40 000 per year in 1965 to over 200 000 per year in 2000. The overall 5-year survival rate is still below 15%.[1,2] The incidence of lung cancer has begun to decline only recently, mainly because of a reduction in smoking. The main risk factor for lung cancer is smoking, and tobacco is considered a risk factor for many other cancers besides lung cancer, including esophageal, stomach, pancreatic, cervical, mouth, bladder, ureter, kidney, laryngeal and pharyngeal cancers and leukemia. Smoking-related diseases, including cardiovascular diseases, are reversible much more rapidly after quitting smoking.

The prevention and treatment of lung cancer have for too long been placed in a secondary role to other cancers. Even though lung cancer has consistently had the highest rate of death, it wasn't until recently that efforts were made to develop screening tools for earlier detection. Patients with lung cancer have been disregarded and sometimes maligned, not unlike early HIV/AIDS patients. For many people quitting smoking has been an ongoing, persistent, and failed effort over many years. At the same time, 20% of all lung cancers occur in patients who have never smoked or were exposed to those factors currently identified as high-risk.[3,4] The risk of lung cancer for a non-smoker living with a smoker is increased by 30%.

Smoking is the primary, but not the only, causative factor in lung cancer. It is certainly possible that air quality contributes to lung cancer, as there is a higher incidence of lung cancer in urban than in rural areas. The rates for asthma, especially in urban environments, are rising exponentially, and children are now at higher risk of asthma, which keeps them either at home or in the emergency room. Arsenic and asbestos exposure, a history of tuberculosis, pitchblende mining, certain chemicals and metals, radon, and radiation exposure are other risk factors for lung cancer.[5]

Lung-cancer patients deserve and require the same compassion given to other cancer patients; this remains true even if a patient has been diagnosed with lung cancer and still cannot quit smoking.

SMALL–CELL LUNG CANCER

There are two types of lung cancer; small-cell lung cancer (SCLC) and non-small-cell lung cancer (NSCLC). SCLC accounts for 20–25% of all new cases of lung cancer in the United States. Of the various histologic types of lung cancer it is the most sensitive to chemotherapy and radiation therapy, yet the overall outcome for this type is poor, with only 5–10% of patients surviving 5 years after diagnosis.

Cigarette smoking remains the major cause of SCLC. In men, 90% of cases are attributed to tobacco use.[6] In women, it is the most rapidly increasing type of lung cancer. People who smoke over a period of 40 years are 60–70 times more likely to develop SCLC. The chance of developing SCLC decreases with smoking cessation but, espe-

cially in the heavy smoker (20 pack years—20 years of smoking one pack of cigarettes per day), the risk may never return to the non-smoking level.[7] In fact, it is not until a former smoker has ceased smoking for more than 15 years that the risk will return to the same level as the non-smoking population.[7] Patients who are diagnosed with SCLC who continue smoking after the primary diagnosis are at a 32-fold increased risk of a second malignancy.

We now know that it is not just the particulate matter in cigarettes that is carcinogenic, but also the nicotine itself. In one study,[8] 100 healthy volunteer subjects were studied for early effects of smoking one or more of three substances—tobacco, marijuana, and/or cocaine. Most in the cohort were between the ages of 20 and 30 years. Bronchial mucosal biopsy specimens and brushings were analysed for histopathologic changes: for Ki-67 marker expression (cell proliferation), the p53 tumor suppressor gene, which is frequently knocked out in lung cancer and other cancers, and several other parameters. The conclusions were that smokers of any one substance or two or more of these substances exhibited more molecular abnormalities than non-smokers.

These findings suggested to researchers that smoking tobacco, cocaine, or marijuana exerts field cancerisation effects early on and after only 5 years of smoking any of these substances. These effects were on the bronchial epithelium and place smokers of these substances at significantly higher risk for development of lung cancer. This changes many people's perception about marijuana; perhaps the desired effects of smoking marijuana as a recreational drug are more complex than we have imagined, given that we now know that inhaling it in the form of smoke causes cancerous alterations in the epithelium of the lungs. Patients using medical marijuana for pain control and appetite enhancement should eat their medicine rather than smoke it.

In all types of lung cancer, exposure to industrial or environmental toxins, such as asbestos and radon, in combination with tobacco use, synergistically increases the risk of developing any type of lung cancer. As stated earlier, 20% of lung cancers occur in people who have never smoked. The majority of SCLC cases occur between the ages of 35 and 75 years, with a peak at 55–65 years.

BIOLOGY

Tumor suppressor gene products are negative growth regulators in the cell cycle. Refer to Chapter 1 for an in-depth discussion of cell growth regulators. Unlike oncogenes, tumor suppressor genes are oncogenic through loss of function rather than activation. The *Rb* gene on chromosome 13 is related to tumorogenesis, particularly solid tumors, through the frequent loss of heterozygosity in chromosome regions known to be loci for tumor suppressor genes. The loss of tumor suppressor gene activity is especially common in SCLC.

The *Rb* gene product is a phosphoprotein involved in cell cycle regulation. Frequent cytogenetic alterations occur at 13q14, the locus for this gene, in SCLC. Study data of SCLC mRNA and DNA support the concept of inactivation of the *Rb* gene as a key event in the pathogenesis of SCLC. Also mutations in the p53 tumor suppressor gene on chromosome 17p is the most commonly identified genetic alteration in human cancers and has been documented in 60–100% of SCLC cell lines and in 77% of tumors. The normal product of the p53 locus acts to suppress and control cell division, and its loss favors unregulated growth.

Drug resistance is one of the more difficult problems in the biology of SCLC.[9] Several events at the cellular level have been described in cell lines which have become resistant to repeated exposure to cytotoxic agents like chemotherapy. Drug resistance in recurrent SCLC is a major problem in treatment and is partially responsible for the high mortality rate of SCLC. There are probably multiple mechanisms at work. The early high sensitivity to chemotherapy followed by drug resistance means that early treatment of SCLC is the main window of opportunity for increasing survival. This is one important area where Chinese medicine contributes to patient outcomes in integrated care because of its ability to potentiate various chemotherapeutic regimens.

PATHOLOGY

There are many types of SCLC, including fusiform, polygonal, oat cell, intermediate small-cell, combined small-cell, and small-cell/large-cell. These types have made it difficult to come up with a meaningful staging system. The most commonly used system is that defined by the International Association for the Study of Lung Cancer (IASLC). This staging system was developed in 1984 and divides and classifies according to small-cell, variant (SC/LC), and combined.

Small-cell lung cancer expresses several markers of neuroendocrine differentiation, such as chromoganin and gastrin-releasing peptide. A new nomenclature is being defined relative to carcinoids, atypical carcinoids, large-cell neuroendocrine carcinoma, and SCLC. These form a spectrum of lung cancers, from the more indolent type of bronchial carcinoid tumor to the very aggressive small-cell anaplastic carcinoma. Knowing the type and aggressiveness of the carcinoma can help us define our strategies in combined care. For example, SCLC requires an aggressive approach with formulas that potentiate the chemotherapy regimen and also vigorously treat the side effects of that regimen. This approach allows for the overall environment of the patient to aid in defeating the cancer by maintaining normal blood levels and immune function. It also allows the patient to rehabilitate and return to normal function more quickly, and this aspect of combined care also contributes to a more successful outcome by lengthening the time between recurrences. More time between recurrences allows for a better response to the next regimen.

CLINICAL PRESENTATION

Patients report a relatively short duration of symptoms with this cancer, usually less than 3 months. The insidiousness of lung cancer and many other cancers makes the need for an early detection system mandatory. This is discussed with regard to NSCLC. Lesions are often centrally located and, therefore, can induce cough, wheezing, stridor, deep chest pain, hemoptysis, and dyspnea caused by airway obstruction. This obstruction can cause an inflammatory condition called pneumonitis.

Centrally located lesions occur in the mediastinum. The mediastinum comprises the tissues and organs separating the sternum in front and the vertebral column behind; the heart, the large vessels of the heart, the trachea, the esophagus, thymus and lymph nodes are enclosed. It is divided into anterior, middle, posterior, and superior regions. Mediastinal involvement is the hallmark of SCLC and can result in a variety of complications. Nerve entrapment can lead to recurrent laryngeal nerve paralysis and hoarseness. Phrenic nerve entrapment can cause paralysis and elevation of the diaphragm causing dyspnea. Tumor compression on the esophagus can lead to dysphagia. A right-sided hilar mass in the right mediastinal nodes compresses the superior vena cava causing superior vena cava syndrome. This obstruction of the venous drainage leads to dilation of collateral veins in the upper part of the chest and neck, edema of the face and neck and upper body, edema of the conjunctiva, orthopnea, and CNS symptoms such as headache and visual distortion. This is considered an urgent but not emergency condition. In Chinese medicine it is described as water edema due to the obstruction of the water pathways. Although it can be relieved with the use of diuretic herbs, the only curative approach is to resolve or lessen the mass with a cytotoxic intervention.

A variety of paraneoplastic syndromes can be produced by SCLC. Paraneoplastic syndrome refers to symptoms appearing elsewhere in the body caused by the tumor that would not ordinarily be associated with that cancer. For example, in lung cancer, hormones or hormone-like metabolites are produced by some cancer cells; one is argine vasopressin which acts on the kidneys causing a drastic reduction in sodium levels leading to hyponatremia. Excessive production of the precursor peptides of ACTH can lead to Cushing's syndrome. Cushing's causes a fat buildup in the face, back, and chest while the arms and legs remain very thin. This presentation is often seen in children being treated for leukemia. It may include high blood sugar levels, weak bones and muscles, and high blood pressure. Cushing's syndrome has more than one pattern associated with it in Chinese medicine. However, in this context it would probably be seen as a kidney qi and yin or essence deficiency.

Weight loss and anorexia occur in nearly one-third of patients with SCLC. No known causative mechanism has been found. However, the disharmony of stomach and spleen and spleen and kidney yang deficiency that may result from advanced and chronic illness would contribute to cachexia and anorexia in the theory of Chinese medicine.

CURRENT SCREENING TOOLS

Four randomised controlled trials including 40 000 participants have been conducted on lung cancer screening. All were male, smokers, and over the age of 45. Of all these men, the lung cancers detected in this population were stage I and II disease. The conclusions of these studies were that periodic chest X-ray (CXR) with sputum culture results in a dramatic reduction in lung cancer mortality. The recommendation was for the above screens to be applied to current and former smokers. Remember that after 5 years of abstinence, the lung cancer risk for those quitting smoking is still similar to that of current smokers. After 10 years of abstinence, the lung cancer risk among former smokers is 30–50% that of current smokers. It is not until a former smoker has ceased smoking for 15 years that the risk for lung cancer is the same as the general non-smoking population.[10] This means that, as providers, our obligation to our patients who have smoked is to encourage and even insist that they be screened for lung cancer. It also means that our obligation to our patients who are smoking is to help them quit no matter how long it takes. This can be a very complicated task, especially when some patients do not want to quit.

There are newer screening tools, including fluoroscopic endoscopy. A photosensitising drug is given which attaches to lipoprotein molecules. Cells undergoing rapid proliferation require more lipoproteins and this drug is delivered more quickly and in higher concentrations to these cells. This includes tumor cells. The endoscope is inserted and the 'photofrin' or photodynamic therapy can detect these cells and, thus, tumors that are still small and asymptomatic. When these cells are exposed to the white light at the tip of the endoscope the sensitising agent is activated and the cells are killed. The screening tool also becomes the treatment.

Early screening in any cancer is mandatory. In 1989, the American Cancer Society declared that 'it does not recommend any test for early detection of cancer of the lung . . .'. In the context of this policy, more than 90% of patients are symptomatic at diagnosis for lung cancer. Many past smokers think that if they quit smoking, they have reduced their risk for lung cancer. It is extremely important that they understand that this reduction takes a long time and is incremental. Therefore, they must continue to seek screening for lung cancer with chest computerised tomography (CT) or magnetic resonance imaging (MRI). Their best outcomes will come with earlier detection. Lung cancer is insidious in that it, like many other cancers, becomes symptomatic much too late for curative treatment.

NATURAL HISTORY

Small-cell lung cancer is characterised by a relentlessly progressive course and by the early development of metastatic disease. The median survival of patients with clinically apparent metastatic disease at presentation is usually 5–7 weeks while in patients with only regional thoracic involvement it is 12 weeks. Metastatic disease is assumed even in patients with no apparent metastatic disease. The Veterans Administration Lung Cancer Study Group (VALCSG) reported the use of adjuvant chemotherapy in this way and with these results has shown that SCLC is fundamentally a systemic disease at presentation.

STAGING

The VALCSG has come up with the best staging system, which is more clearly prognostic. This classification divides SCLC into limited disease (LD) and extensive disease (ED). This system is a division based on the clear survival rates between patients with regional disease and those with distant metastatic spread. Because mediastinal spread is a given in most circumstances, the definition of LD refers to tumors whose extent is within ipsilateral, mediastinal, and ipsilateral supraclavicular nodal parameters. This excludes contralateral supraclavicular nodes, and any pleural effusion (see below). This definition identifies patients who are likely to have disease amenable to combined treatment with chemotherapy and radiation. Extensive disease denotes tumors beyond these limits, and usually accounts for 60–70% of patients with SCLC. Survival of more than 3 years is almost exclusively confined to those patients with LD. Long-term survival in ED patients is uncommon. However, it is good to remember that these statistics are relative only to conventional care without a combined approach.

A pleural effusion is the buildup of fluid in the pleura of the lung due to inflammation and to cancer. This fluid buildup can put pressure on the lung parenchyma and close off the space between the lung lobe involved and the pleura. This contributes to atelectasis, or the local collapse of the lung. Both of these circumstances can cause pain and make it difficult to inhale and exhale because the pleural vacuum is compromised. This condition is usually treated with diuretic drugs or with a puncture through the chest wall and between the ribs with a hollow needle, thoracentesis, to aspirate the fluid. Sometimes drain tubes are placed although risk of infection is heightened with this procedure. The subject of treating pleural effusions is covered in Chapter 11.

CLINICAL EVALUATION

The most critical role in staging is identifying LD patients who will benefit from an aggressive combined approach of chemotherapy and radiotherapy (XRT) and Chinese medicine. The most important risk factor for treatment-related death is the initial performance status, and therefore it is very important to ascertain the physiologic condition of the patient. Sometimes and if at all possible, it may raise the efficacy of conventional treatment to prepare the patient with Chinese medicine prior to combined cytotoxic treatment. A complete history is taken including a physical exam, chest X-ray, blood studies, and the clinical work-up for staging. CT and MRI scans are frequently done in all SCLC patients to determine the extent of disease, especially in the chest.

Involvement of intra-abdominal organs is present in 30% of patients. Liver, adrenal gland, pancreas, and mesenteric and retroperitoneal lymph nodes are most frequently the sites of metastasis. Normal liver function tests of serum glutamic oxaloacetic transaminase (SGOT), lactate dehydrogenase (LDH) and alkaline phosphatase (AKP) do not exclude liver metastasis. CT is used to rule out liver metastases. Bone scans are important since 30% of SCLC patients present with bony metastasis. Bone marrow involvement is present in 20–25% of patients even with normal blood findings. Bone marrow aspiration may be warranted in SCLC. And brain metastasis may require the use of either CT or MRI. Serum markers for SCLC have little value at this time. Carcinoembryonic antigen (CEA) may correlate with tumor bulk and response to chemotherapy. With better monitoring and earlier detection, hopefully this clinical picture will change.

PROGNOSTIC FACTORS

- Female sex correlates with better response rates and survival; it is not known why.[10]
- Advanced age, supraclavicular nodal involvement in LD patients, and a large number of metastatic sites are predictive of a poorer outcome; the qi and blood have been depleted and there is overall yin and yang deficiency.
- Low hemoglobin, platelets, uric acid, and bicarbonate levels are poor prognostic factors; these could be indicators of underlying kidney qi and essence deficiency, which would be considered a deeper level of disease.
- High leukocytes, high LDH and CEA, indicating a larger tumor burden, have a poorer prognosis.
- Weight loss and slow response to therapy carry a poorer prognosis; the spleen and kidneys are injured and the overall wei qi is too low.[11]

TREATMENT

Almost two-thirds of patients with SCLC who have tumor dissemination beyond the thorax are presumed to have occult (asymptomatic) metastatic disease. SCLC is assumed to be a systemic disease at the time of presentation and, therefore, chemotherapy is the foundation of treatment.

The activity of single agents appears to be very dependent on prior therapy. For example, etoposide used as the primary single agent was only 9–15% effective in terms of response rate in patients who had already received chemotherapy for SCLC; yet in untreated patients the response rate was 40–60%. This illustrates again the value of treating with combined care during the early phase of treatment to enhance the effect of the chemotherapy, no matter what agent is used.

Generally in standard care single-agent chemotherapy is used as salvage therapy.

Combination chemotherapy has achieved complete response rates in previously untreated patients. Even so the search is still on for life-saving combinations. Cyclophosphamide, doxorubicin, and vincristine (CAV), and cisplatin and etoposide (PE) are two combination therapies used in SCLC. Another possible combination includes cisplatin, carboplatin, and etoposide. Cyclophosphamide, doxorubicin, and etoposide are also used. Paclitaxel is sometimes used as a single agent. The response rates for these combinations are quite similar and give a 40–60% complete response in LD SCLC, and 10–25% in ED SCLC. With these combinations the LD survival is 12–18 months. In ED the survival is 7–10 months. Iressa is a newer drug that has antiangiogenic mechanisms and is now approved in the US for the treatment of lung cancer. Currently there are no studies on this agent alongside blood-regulating herbs to potentiate its effect. None of the above statistics relate to the addition of Chinese herbal medicine.

Induction therapy is also commonly used in this cancer. Induction therapy is the first phase of therapy with chemotherapeutic drugs at high doses; it is an aggressive therapy to destroy the highest number of abnormal cells as quickly as possible. It can last from 4 to 6 weeks. The second phase of this type of therapy is called consolidation therapy. Consolidation therapy is used after a patient has been in remission for several weeks. It is a second course of chemotherapy to destroy any remaining cancer cells. Patients may receive repeated cycles of the same or varied drug combinations. The dose is not as high as the first, induction, dose, and the drugs are given over a shorter period of time. Maintenance therapy is treatment after remission after the consolidation therapy.

In SCLC CAV has been common treatment for induction. CEV, with etoposide substituted for doxorubicin, has become the standard with fewer side effects and high efficacy. PE lacks significant mucosal toxicity and is effective at dosages that are only minimally myelosuppressive, and it can be administered with thoracic radiation therapy.

However, despite high response rates, most patients with SCLC relapse with drug-resistant disease within months. Alternation of two equally effective non-cross-resistant therapies has demonstrated a small survival benefit in a small number of patients. When ifosfamide was added to cisplatin and etoposide (VIP) patients with ED showed superior survival; 13% vs 5% at 2 years.

Salvage therapy with PE, CAV, or carboplatin and taxol in patients in whom the cancer has recurred has better response rates when there is a drug-free interim period; the longer the period the better the response. Etoposide given orally over a protracted course produced response rates of 23–45%. These response rates were not relevant in patients who did not have a 3-month drug-free period. Because these two types are not specifically differentiated diagnostically in Chinese medicine, treatment options will be covered for both types together at the end of this section.

Thoracic irradiation

After chemotherapy-induced remission, the chest remains a significant site of failure in patients with LD. Chest radiation can reduce these recurrences by 10–20%, and the long-term survival rate can be increased up to 15%. The timing of thoracic radiation in combined-modality treatment of LD in SCLC is crucial. Early administration is superior when compared to late XRT. A benefit from radiation has been difficult to demonstrate when it is given following chemotherapy and as the last intervention in treatment. Therefore, XRT is given early on in treatment and in an alternating or sometimes concurrent schedule. A 2-year survival rate of 40% represents a significant improvement with the combination of these two therapies.

Surgery is elected in only a small subgroup. Those with no nodal involvement and no metastatic spread of any kind are candidates for surgery prior to chemotherapy and XRT. Even in these small tumors for which surgery is possible, the 5-year survival is 48%.

NON-SMALL-CELL LUNG CANCER

Non-small-cell lung cancer (NSCLC) accounts for 80% of new cases of lung cancer. As in SCLC over 70% of patients present with advanced disease at diagnosis.

RISK FACTORS

Cigarette smoking

Cigarette smoking is the most important risk factor for NSCLC. The N-nitrosamines and polycyclic aromatic hydrocarbons are the two main classes of tobacco-related inhaled carcinogens. N-nitrosamines are formed during tobacco processing and originate from nicotine and the alkaloid arecoline. The nitrosamines are activated through hydroxylation by the P450 enzyme system and then become active through the formation of DNA. This activity is directly related to the amount of cigarette consumption. These DNA products can remain in the system for as long as 5 years without significant change, and in heavy smokers may be responsible for as many as 100 mutations per cell genome. The polycyclic aromatic hydrocarbons benzo-α-pyrene and dimethylbenz-α-anthracene also lead to the DNA adducts.

The risk for developing lung cancer of any kind from passive smoke is difficult to assess but risk analysis has estimated that as many as 40% of lung-cancer deaths are caused by passive smoking.[12] In 1993 the Environmental Protection Agency (EPA) declared passive smoking to be a carcinogen, much to the chagrin of the tobacco industry. Later, after many political maneuverings, the EPA withdrew their declaration, much to the relief of the tobacco industry. Nevertheless, smoking in public buildings is now banned in the United States.

Asbestos

Asbestos exists in many natural forms and contains the silicate fiber, which has been implicated in carcinogenesis. It can remain in an individual's lungs for a lifetime. It has been confirmed that asbestos exposure is associated with certain lung diseases, including pulmonary fibrosis, mesothelioma, and lung cancer.[13] Shipyard workers, plumbers, and asbestos clean-up workers are at risk. People who live in buildings where asbestos has not yet been removed must take extreme care because the disturbance of asbestos-containing materials will release invisible particles, which are very fine and very easy to breathe in.

Asbestos works as a tumor promoter. Smoking prolongs the presence of asbestos in the pulmonary epithelium. When these two are combined, the risk for lung cancer is increased by 28.8 times, compared with 2.6 in non-smokers exposed to asbestos.

Diet

Diet may also be a risk factor for lung cancer. In retrospective studies of diet,[13] 14 out of 15 found an association between increased beta-carotene intake and decreased risk for lung cancer. However, two well-designed studies found an increased risk of lung cancer and death from lung cancer associated with beta-carotene supplementation.[13] A decreased risk was associated with increased vitamin C intake. A recent review of data suggests that if the general public increased its fruit and vegetable consumption to levels characteristic of the top 30% of individuals in the study, the risk for lung cancer would decrease by 31%. However, in one study of 30 000 male smokers aged 50–69 years, it was found that those who received beta-carotene had a higher incidence of lung cancer and heart disease and 8% higher mortality from lung cancer than those who did not receive beta-carotene[14,15]

Even though cigarette smoking is responsible for 90% of lung cancers in the United States, only a small fraction of smokers develop bronchial malignancy and only a portion of people exposed to common carcinogens responsible for lung cancer will develop lung cancer. Because of this the concept of a genetic predisposition has been posited. The genetic risk factors are poorly defined at this time but increasing data suggests the existence of a genetic component for lung cancer. Perhaps we should also be studying those people who are at high risk for lung cancer but never develop it.

SUBTYPES OF NSCLC

The distinction between SCLC and NSCLC is of major clinical significance. NSCLC subtypes include adenocarcinoma, squamous-cell carcinoma, and large-cell carcinoma. Adenocarcinoma constitutes 50% of all NSCLC. This type is associated with smoking but, at the same time, is especially predominant in women and non-smokers.

This type of NSCLC is usually peripheral in location and arises from the surface epithelium or bronchial mucosal glands and as peripheral scar carcinomas. On histologic examination, adenocarcinoma demonstrates gland formation, papillary structures, or mucin production. Adenocarcinomas stain positive for CEA.

Patients with this type of lung cancer will present with metastatic disease prior to the development of symptoms secondary to the local disease. Adenocarcinoma of the lung is associated with hypertrophic osteoarthropathy, Trousseau's syndrome, and cerebellar ataxia. Troussea's sign is carpopedal spasm caused by reduction of the blood supply to the hand and foot, in other words, a form of tetany. Cerebellar ataxia refers to a reeling ambulation and a wide-based gait in order to maintain balance. Both of these conditions are due to restriction of the blood flow caused by obstruction by tumors.

Squamous-cell carcinoma

Squamous-cell carcinoma accounts for 30% of NSCLC. This tumor arises most frequently in the proximal bronchi, and because of its central position and its tendency to exfoliate tumor cells it can be detected on cytologic examination at an early stage. These tumors tend to cause bronchial obstruction and atelectasis (collapse of a portion of the lung) or pneumonia. They tend to remain localised and form cavities. This type of tumor has the strongest association with smoking. Increased secretion of a parathyroid-like hormone can lead to hypercalcemia.

Large-cell carcinoma

Large-cell carcinoma is the least common subtype of NSCLC, accounting for 20% of cases. Previously, the histologic typing of other lung-cancer types was less accurate, and those that could not be differentiated were put into this category. It is still sometimes the case that those cancers in which the exact histologic type cannot be differentiated are put into this category.

BIOLOGY

The molecular biology of NSCLC is very similar to that of SCLC. The p53 gene is either deleted or mutated. Increased amounts of *p53* induce G1 arrest, thereby allowing time for DNA repair. Once repair has occurred, the cell is released and proceeds to S-phase and cell division. If the DNA cannot be repaired, the cell is diverted toward programmed cell death, apoptosis. When a mutation or deletion has occurred in the *p53* gene, G1 arrest cannot be achieved and the abnormal cell is allowed to proceed to S-phase, where it divides and propagates genetic damage which may lead to cancer. The *Rb* gene mutation is also connected to NSCLC. Mutations of codon 12 and the K-*ras* gene are commonly found in NSCLC.

CLINICAL PRESENTATION

The presenting symptoms in NSCLC can be very similar to those in SCLC. SCLC tends to be more centrally located than NSCLC, which tends to be peripheral (particularly adenocarcinomas, the most common type). Therefore, differences in presentation for NSCLC may include a lesion involving the intrathoracic nerves, which can become compressed resulting in Pancoast's syndrome. This is characterised by shoulder pain radiating to the arm in an ulnar distribution. This is caused by tumor invasion of the eighth cervical and first thoracic nerves. Horner's syndrome consists of enophthalmos, ptosis, meiosis, and ipsilateral dyshydrosis, and is caused by tumor extension into the paravertebral sympathetic nerves. Enophthalmos is a backward displacement of the eyeball into the orbit. Ptosis here refers to a drooping of the upper eyelid. Meiosis is a type of cell division that, in this situation, would be considered abnormal. Dyshydrosis refers to a dysfunction of the eccrine sweat glands on the same side of the body. Mediastinal involvement will lead to symptoms similar to those in SCLC.

Metastatic sites include the hilar and mediastinal lymph nodes, the pleura, the opposite lung, the liver, adrenal glands, bone, CNS, and abdominal viscera and structures, and the esophagus. Paraneoplastic syndromes common to NSCLC include hypercalcemia secondary to parathyroid hormone-related peptide or bone metastasis. Hypertrophic pulmonary osteoarthropathy may also be present. It presents as a symmetrical osteitis of the four limbs, especially the long bones of the forearm and leg.

DIAGNOSIS

A pathological diagnosis is essential because NSCLC is managed differently to SCLC. The studies common to SCLC are done but, in addition, sputum cytology is a first diagnostic step. If an easily biopsied lesion is not found and sputum cytology is negative, then a bronchoscopy is done. When lesions can be viewed in this way diagnoses are made 97% of the time. The biopsy of a viewed lesion is done via bronchial washings and brushings. These washings and brushings are very similar to a Pap smear procedure and the intent is to collect epithelial cells for analysis. It is a slightly invasive but non-surgical biopsy technique. When the lesion cannot be visualised 55% of cases can still be diagnosed through bronchial washings and brushings.

This histologic diagnosis is important. In its absence, a thorough bronchoscopy percutaneous transthoracic fine needle aspiration of pulmonary nodules located through X-ray or CT or MRI is performed. This same technique may be done to confirm supraclavicular adenopathy, pleural effusions, liver metastasis, bone or adrenal glands metastasis. When the above technique does not establish a diagnosis then a mediastinography with biopsy is done.

A solitary pulmonary nodule or mass is commonly found on routine chest X-ray. Having a baseline chest X-ray is often helpful at these times. In the absence of old films and in a patient with low risk factors, the film may help to evaluate the lesion. Very distinct margins and/or certain calcification patterns may rule out malignancy. For example, a diffuse or central core bullseye pattern usually suggests a granuloma from a previous illness; 'popcorn ball' lesions suggests hamartomas; concentric layers or very dense tissue on CT suggest a benign lesion of some other type, the most common of which is a granuloma which is usually an artifact from some previous illness.

In addition to the histologic diagnosis, the extent of the disease must be determined. A complete history and physical examination can confirm extrathoracic spread. Complete blood count (CBC) and routine electrolyte and blood chemistry tests with liver enzyme studies should be performed. A CT of the chest and upper abdomen including the adrenals is done. If abnormal blood chemistry results show elevations in serum calcium and alkaline phosphatase, and the patient reports pain, then bone scans should be done. Clinical staging will frequently underestimate the extent of disease.

STAGING

Staging for NSCLC is done within the context of the TNM system (see Box 2.1).

TREATMENT

Patients with stage I or II NSCLC should undergo surgical resection if possible. Please see the pre- and post-surgical formulas to apply here. Often resection via thoracotomy will show more extensive disease than thought. The 5-year survival rate for those patients who have pathologically proven stage I disease (T1–2N0) is 65%. For those with a completely resected T1N0M0 disease, the 5-year survival rate is 75%. In stage II with T1N1 the 5-year survival rate is 39%. This suggests that there may be microdisease elsewhere in the lungs and treating with Chinese herbs post-surgically, even in patients with no apparent disease, is very important.

Surgery is the standard treatment for stage I and II disease. Mortality in these patients is relative to metastatic disease and second primary tumors. Adjuvant chemotherapy has been explored in early-stage NSCLC and the results have been mixed. No differences in time to recurrence or overall survival were found. At present, adjuvant chemotherapy or XRT in patients with stage I or II NSCLC is administered but most frequently in the form of a trial. Currently what is known regarding locally advanced NSCLC is that only 15–17% of patients achieve histologic local control whether they receive XRT alone or sequential chemotherapy and radiation.

Local therapy will have no influence on survival if cells resistant to chemotherapy have escaped from the primary site. But at the same time, local control is a prerequisite for cure. Therefore, successful treatment regimens need to address both issues. This has been proven in SCLC management and applies also to the management of NSCLC. So even though the rate of distant metastases is higher in SCLC than in NSCLC, the

Box 2.1

- TX: positive sputum or washings with no tumor.
- Tis: carcinoma in situ.
- T1: tumor <3 cm.
- T2: tumor >3 cm; or involving main stem bronchus, or visceral pleura; or subtotal atelectasis, obstructive pneumonitis.
- T3: tumor invading the chest wall, diaphragm, mediastinal pleura; atelectasis or obstructive pneumonitis of entire lung.
- T4: tumor invading mediastinum, heart, great vessels, esophagus, vertebral body; ipsilateral malignant pleural effusion.
- N0: no regional lymph node metastases.
- N1: ipsilateral peribronchial or hilar nodes.
- N2: ipsilateral mediastinal or subcarinal nodes.
- N3: contralateral mediastinal or hilar nodes; any scalene or supraclavicular nodes.
- M0: no distant metastases.
- M1: distant metastases.

NSCLC staging

- Occult: TX N0 M0
- Stage 0: Tis N0 M0
- Stage I: T1–2 N0 M0
- Stage II: T1–2 N1 M0
- Stage IIIA: T3 N0–1 M0

T1–3 N2 M0

- Stage IIIB: T4 N0–2 M0

T1–4 N3 M0

- Stage IV: any T any N M1

addition of local therapy (thoracic XRT) to chemotherapy has resulted in improved survival.

As chemotherapy in lung cancer becomes more effective, the issue of local control becomes increasingly important. This means that innovative strategies are needed to more effectively eliminate local disease and potentially improve survival. Therefore, several new approaches include combined chemoradiotherapy, altered radiation fractionation schemes, and radiation dose escalation. One new chemotherapy approach is the use of induction therapy with chemotherapy and XRT. The regimen includes carboplatin and cisplatin; a very aggressive regimen. Another combined approach is the regimen combination of daily low dose carboplatin with VP-16 and XRT. This last combination improved the 4-year survival rates for NSCLC from 9% to 23%. Paclitaxel, ifosfamide, or gemcitabine, and Iressa and avastin are all single agents used as solitary treatments for NSCLC.

STAGE III DISEASE

Stage III disease has been delineated into stage IIIa (potentially resectable) and IIIb (not resectable). Stage IIIa patients have a 5-year survival rate of 15%, whereas those in stage IIIb have a 5-year survival rate of less than 5%. XRT has been considered a routine measure for patients with inoperable locally advanced disease. Currently, combined care with concurrent, rather than sequential, chemotherapy and XRT, shows better results. The 3-year survival in patients receiving concurrent mitomycin, vindesine and cisplatin (MVP) with XRT was 27% vs 12% in the sequential therapy.

As treatment regimens become more aggressive, the risk for normal tissue toxicity increases. These toxicities can result in breaks from treatment or dose reductions that may limit the success of the therapy. Esophagitis caused by both the chemotherapy and XRT is often a serious complication. A serious symptom is moderately extreme fatigue from combined therapy. Reduction in esophageal, lung, and upper gastrointestinal toxicities is a primary underlying management issue in this kind of aggressive treatment. Although overall survival may have increased, the benefit has come at a high price. One conventional rationale is to employ a radioprotector, amifostine, to reduce toxicity. Amifostine is an organic thiophosphate developed by the US Army. Free thiol acts as a potent scavenger of free radicals. Amifostine protects the bone marrow, skin, oral mucosa, esophagus, kidneys, and testes, and it protects against cisplatin-induced nephrotoxicity. It can cause hypotension. In the Chinese medical section of this chapter and in the Chapter 11 on concurrent issues, there are various formulas and other approaches that can be employed to reduce the impacts of toxicity from combined XRT and chemotherapeutic regimens for advanced local disease in NSCLC.

When treating NSCLC patients who are undergoing chemoradiotherapy concurrently, it is necessary for the Chinese medicine practitioner to combine formulas for XRT sensitising and protection with formulas designed specifically for certain chemotherapeutic regimens.

STAGE IV DISEASE

The presence of metastatic spread is ominous in NSCLC, as it is in almost every cancer. The most common sites of metastases are: hilar and mediastinal lymph nodes, pleura, opposite lung, liver, adrenal glands, bone, and CNS. In comparison to SCLC NSCLC is not sensitive to chemotherapy. One study showed that chemotherapy improved quality of life when compared to best supportive care. Oral etoposide, paclitaxel and vinorelbine are newer additions being studied in stage IV NSCLC. Many of these chemotherapeutic agents have fairly severe side effects and it may be that the use of Chinese herbal medicine can improve quality of life in late stage NSCLC without side effects.

CHINESE MEDICINE

OVERVIEW

Since cigarette smoking remains the primary cause of lung cancer, the injuries, from the point of view of Chinese medicine, lie in three areas. These include injury to the qi mechanism of the lung, the yin of the deepest level (and thus a resulting phlegm heat accumulation), and the heat exchange mechanism of the diaphragm. Phlegm heat, in this case, is due to yin deficiency combined with toxic heat. Lung tissue removed upon autopsy after death from lung cancer has a burnt leather consistency. The leathery quality is due to yin deficiency, and the dark color is due to phlegm heat and toxin.

The presentation of patients varies. The history, constitution, and underlying diseases or conditions that are present in an individual patient all combine to influence the presentation. Although the conventional medical approach is to narrow the focus of inquiry to the cancer, it is important to broaden the focus to include conditions that have been caused by smoking and other lifestyle factors. These conditions often include cardiovascular disease and diabetes. Cardiovascular diseases are common in older lung cancer patients; smoking and the resulting injuries to the lung parenchyma often preclude older and more symptomatic patients from exercising. A sedentary lifestyle leads to weight gain and often diabetes and diabetic conditions like hyperinsulinemia. Poor diet and a sedentary lifestyle are all risk factors for many cancers and for many conditions that contribute to a poorer outcome in cancer treatment. Lack of exercise and damp phlegm stasis also lead to blood stasis. Many cancer patients have been found to have hypercoagulability syndrome. This can lead to the cancer itself and also to coronary artery disease, a type of cardiovascular disease for which smoking is a risk factor. Therefore, the early management of these conditions is necessary in treating the lung cancer itself. This becomes more and more true the earlier the stage of the lung cancer.

ETIOLOGY

We can identify the pathways of injury by looking at the primary causative factor in lung cancer; smoking of tobacco/marijuana/cocaine. The toxic heat of smoking these substances causes constant irritation to the lung tissue.

The heat from the smoke and the resulting inflammation from toxicity burns yin fluids. Yin deficiency can be a precursor for phlegm heat accumulations and vice versa. The mucosal epithelium of the lungs responds to this heat and yin deficiency by misting or moistening the dry and hot tissue. This, in combination with the toxicity of exposure, leads to a drying of the mist, which leads to phlegm. The constant production of mucus (yin) to alleviate dryness leads to yin deficiency and qi deficiency (energy is used to produce more misting action), and a vicious cycle is begun.

The phlegm heat accumulation prevents the normal function of the lung in many ways. The constant production of mucus, which leads to phlegm, lowers the functional capacity of the alveolae, the parenchymal (qi-producing) tissue of the lungs. The phlegm heat accumulation also leads to the symptoms of cough and dyspnea, whereby qi is lost with every wheeze or cough. These also lead to qi deficiency. All of these processes lead to pathogenic internal heat from stasis. Because the patient does not breathe as deeply or exercise as well, the heat-exchange mechanism of the diaphragm is disrupted. Deep breathing through action of the diaphragm helps the lungs to mist and irrigate the upper and middle jiaos. This misting action also helps to clear heat from the chest where it tends to accumulate as a result of the physical law in which heat tends to rise. Diaphragmatic breathing is a natural process to prevent heat from accumulating in the chest. When this mechanism is disrupted then heat accumulates in the chest and a cascade of conditions can escalate, including cardiovascular diseases from phlegm stasis and blood stasis, yin deficiency, and phlegm heat in the lungs.

The local stasis of qi and blood, damp and phlegm, can result in stasis and pathogenic heat at deeper and deeper levels. Over time, these deeper levels of pathogenic heat can become systemic. One example is the quality and color of the skin of patients who are long-term smokers; it appears that what is happening invisibly to the lung tissue is happening simultaneously and visibly to the extension of the lung orb, the skin. The pathogenic heat can also bind with toxins and cause a malignancy. This appears to occur early. The malignancy spreads via the blood and lymph, via the water metabolism process of the lungs misting the chest and upper abdomen, and possibly via the circulation of qi, which is a function central to the lungs and liver.

The wei qi is significant to lung function and is circulated partially via the lung circulatory mechanism and via the heat-exchange mechanism of the diaphragm. When the lungs are injured on this level, the wei qi is not circulated well nor in normal quantities. This may help explain, at least partially, why smoking is a risk factor for other cancers. The lung is intimately involved in the immune response. Several vicious cycles become apparent when evaluating in this way the impact of smoking; the lung/kidney axis, the taiyang channels and organs, the lung/stomach axis in terms of yin fluids, and the lung/liver axis.

DIAGNOSTIC PATTERNS[16]

Lung heat with yin deficiency heat

This diagnosis is often seen in the central type of lung cancer with laryngeal nerve obstruction and infection.

Symptoms

- Dry and irritating cough.
- Sticky sputum that is hard to expectorate.
- Bloody sputum.
- Low-grade fevers.
- Night sweats.
- Chest distress and pain.
- Dry and hoarse throat.
- Irritability.
- Insomnia.
- Thirst.

Signs

- Tongue: red or purple with a thin, yellow coating.
- Pulse: rapid and weak.

Treatment principle

- Nourish the yin of the lung, clear pathogenic and toxic heat, add anticancer herbs.

Formula

Qing zao jiu fei tang jia jian[17]

bei sha shen (Glehniae Radix; *Glehnia*)	15 g
mai dong (Ophiopogonis Radix; *Ophiopogon*)	15 g
tian dong (Asparagi Radix; *Asparagus*)	15 g
gou qi zi (Lycii Fructus; *Lycium chinensis* fruit)	12 g
bai he (Lilii Bulbus; *Lilium* bulb)	12 g
huang qin (Scutellariae Radix; *Scutellaria baicalensis*)	10 g
shi hu (Dendrobii Herba; *Dendrobium*)	12 g
gua lou ren (Trichosanthis Semen; *Trichosanthes* seed)	25 g
chuan bei mu (Fritillariae cirrhosae Bulbus; *Fritillaria cirrhosa*)	9 g
bai hua she she cao (Hedyotis diffusae Herba; *Oldenlandia*)	25 g
ban zhi lian (Scutellariae barbatae Herba; *Scutellaria barbata*)	25 g
yu xing cao (Houttuyniae Herba; *Houttuynia*)	25 g
jiao gu lan (Herba Gynostemmatis; *Gynostemma*)	15 g

Bei sha shen clears lung heat, tonifies yin and stops cough. It acts as an expectorant and also helps to lower fevers. Mai dong, tian dong, bai he, and shi hu are all yin-nourishing herbs that generate fluids. Bai he also lowers fevers and helps to stop bleeding in the lungs. It has the added benefit of calming the spirit by clearing heat from the heart. Shi hu is the empiric herb of choice for treating dry mouth and throat. Gou qi zi is a blood-nourishing herb that also nourishes the yin and moistens the lungs. It can also help in treating wasting, which is a common condition in some cancers. Bai he alleviates the cough and dyspnea caused by lung heat. It is a broad-spectrum antibiotic which helps prevent infection caused by immune deficiency and by infection secondary to lung cancer. It also is a bronchodilator and improves many symptoms of middle- to advanced lung cancer.[18-20]

Gua lou ren is a primary herb in treating phlegm stasis tumors of any kind. It clears and transforms hot phlegm; it circulates knotted qi in the chest and dissolves phlegm damp accumulations. It promotes healing of sores and ulcerations, a condition not uncommon in this kind of cancer. At the same time, gua lou ren moistens the lungs. In higher doses, this herb is anticancer. Chuan bei mu also clears heat and transforms phlegm; it stops cough and nourishes the lung yin. It is an antitussive that also stops bleeding in the lungs. It has been found to be antineoplastic against some cancers, especially cervical cancer. It is not clear whether this effect can be extended to lung cancers but its other benefits make it a valuable herb in treating the symptoms of lung cancer.

Bai hua she she cao clears heat, resolves toxins and abscesses. It can be used to treat bronchitis, and it is antineoplastic in many cancers; when used with other antineoplastic herbs it has a synergistic effect, which has also been extended to some chemotherapeutic regimens. Ban zhi lian clears heat and toxins, clears blood heat, moves blood and stops bleeding. Yu xing cao clears heat and toxins and reduces swellings and abscesses in the lungs. It is antineoplastic especially in lung cancers. It is also antitussive and antibiotic. It is a hemostatic that also helps to prevent infections from surgery.

Phlegm/damp stasis in the lung

Symptoms

- Productive cough with thin, white sputum.
- Anorexia.
- General weakness.
- Loose stools.
- Edema of the upper body (superior vena cava syndrome).

Signs

- Tongue: white and sticky or thick coating.
- Pulse: rapid, slippery or soggy.

Treatment principle

- Tonify the general qi and support the spleen, transform phlegm and drain damp, antineoplastic.

Formula

Liu jun zi tang jia jian[21]

dang shen (Codonopsis Radix; *Codonopsis pilosula*)	15 g
bai zhu (Atractylodis macrocephalae Rhizoma; *Atractylodes macrocephala*)	12 g
fu ling (Poria; *Poria cocos*)	15 g
gan cao (Glycyrrhizae Radix; *Glycyrrhiza*; licorice root)	6 g
che qian zi (Plantaginis Semen; *Plantago*)	12 g
shan yao (Dioscoreae Rhizoma; *Dioscorea opposita*)	15 g
zhi ban xia (Pinelliae Rhizoma preparatum; *Pinellia ternata*)	10 g
chen pi (Citri reticulatae Pericarpium; *Citrus reticulata* pericarp)	10 g
qian hu (Peucedani Radix; *Peucedanum*)	10 g
zhu ling (Polyporus; *Polyporus – Grifola*)	20 g
ku xing ren (Armeniacae Semen amarum; *Prunus armeniaca*)	10 g
chuan bei mu (Fritillariae cirrhosae Bulbus; *Fritillaria cirrhosa*)	10 g
ze xie (Alismatis Rhizoma; *Alisma*)	8 g
yi ren (Coicis Semen; *Coix lacryma-jobi*)	20 g
zi wan (Asteris Radix; *Aster tataricus*)	10 g
qian shi (Euryales Semen; *Euryale*)	15 g

Dang shen, bai zhu, fu ling, and gan cao make up the formula Si jun zi tang, Four Gentlemen Decoction, which is the primary middle jiao tonic formula. The transformation of phlegm and dampness almost always clinically entails improving spleen function since its functional activities include transportation and transformation of fluids. Che qian zi is a drain damp herb that has the added function of transforming phlegm and controlling cough; in this sense it is an expectorant and antitussive herb. Shan yao is an especially good spleen qi tonic herb that also benefits the lungs by tonifying them and nourishing the kidney essence (the lung/kidney axis). Ban xia dries dampness and transforms phlegm and is mildly antineoplastic. Chen pi regulates the qi, tonifies the spleen in order to help it transform phlegm and dry dampness. Chen pi also regulates the qi of the lung in order to stop cough and it helps to improve appetite. Qian hu resolves phlegm heat and stops cough; the crushed fresh root has been found to reduce tumorous swellings. Zhu ling is a drain damp herb that also is an antitumor herb that protects the bone marrow and acts synergistically with chemotherapy of various types.[22] It improves T-cell transformation, increases phagocytosis, and decreases platelet aggregation which inhibits metastatic spread. Ku xing ren moistens the lungs to protect against the drying effect of the transform phlegm and drain damp herbs. It has been widely used and studied in lung and bronchial cancer treatment, and is especially valuable as a primary herb for stopping cough. Chuan bei mu helps resolve phlegm heat and stops cough. At the same time it moistens and nourishes.

Ze xie promotes urination to filter out dampness. Yi ren has multiple functions: it promotes urination and filters dampness, strengthens the spleen, transforms fluids, clears heat and toxins, and is anticancer against several different kinds of cancer. Zi wan resolves phlegm to stop cough and is also anticancer and antibiotic. It acts as an expectorant and an antitussive in chronic and acute bronchitis. Qian shi is an astringent herb that tonifies the spleen, dispels dampness, and strengthens the kidneys to retain essence. The overall effect of this formula is to resolve damp phlegm in the lung while protecting the yin of the lungs, to strengthen the ability of the spleen to resolve these fluid issues that are swamping the lungs, and to act as an antineoplastic agent against lung cancer.

Blood stasis with deficiency heat and pathogenic heat

This pattern reflects an advanced stage of lung cancer where infection (pneumonia or abscess) is present, there is pleural invasion with pleural effusion and atelectasis, and regional and probably distant metastatic spread.

Symptoms

- Hard cough.
- Yellow or green and bloody sputum.
- Chest distress and pain.
- Labored breathing.
- Whole body pain depending on metastatic sites.
- Intermittent fevers.
- Constipation.
- Dry mouth and throat.

Signs

- Tongue: very dark red with red points and yellow coating.
- Pulse: wiry and thready or choppy, rapid.

Treatment principle

- Regulate and invigorate the blood, clear heat from the blood level, nourish the yin, antineoplasm.

Formula
Special formula[23]

jin yin hua (Lonicerae Flos; *Lonicera* flowers)	10 g
cao he che (Bistortae Rhizoma; *Polygonum bistorta*)	15 g
chi shao (Paeoniae Radix rubra; *Paeonia lactiflora* root)	12 g
fu ling (Poria; *Poria cocos*)	15 g
mai dong (Ophiopogonis Radix; *Ophiopogon*)	15 g
bai mao gen (Imperatae Rhizoma; *Imperata cylindrica* rhizome)	15 g
xian he cao (Agrimoniae Herba; *Agrimonia pilosa* var. *japonica*)	30 g
shi hu (Dendrobii Herba; *Dendrobium*)	12 g
zhi mu (Anemarrhenae Rhizoma; *Anemarrhena*)	12 g
shi gao (Gypsum fibrosum; gypsum; calcium sulfate)	30 g
tai zi shen (Pseudostellariae Radix; *Pseudostellaria heterophylla*)	15 g
ba yue zha (Akebiae Fructus; *Akebia*)	15 g
bai mao teng (Solani lyrati Herba; *Solanum lyratum*)	15 g
bai hua she she cao (Hedyotis diffusae Herba; *Oldenlandia*)	20 g
yu xing cao (Houttuyniae Herba; *Houttuynia*)	20 g
da huang (Rhei Radix et Rhizoma; *Rheum*)	10 g
gua lou ren (Trichosanthis Semen; *Trichosanthes* seed)	20 g

Jin yin hua is a clear heat herb that clears heat from the lungs and is antineoplastic. Cao he che clears heat and resolves toxic heat. It resolves phlegm and decreases swellings and masses and is antineoplastic. Chi shao is a blood-regulating herb that also clears heat and cools the blood. It has some capacity to reduce masses. Fu ling is used in two ways: to drain damp by benefiting the spleen, and as an antineoplastic fungus that has many immunomodulating properties that can increase the effect of many antitumor agents.

Mai dong and shi hu both nourish the yin especially of the stomach and lung. They help alleviate the symptom of dry mouth and throat caused by yin deficiency. Bai mao gen and xian he cao work together to stop bleeding caused by heat in the blood level. Xian he cao also inhibits the growth of some tumors. Zhi mu clears heat and generates fluids; it enters the lung and kidney and nourishes yin and clears heat from the lungs. It is antibiotic against a broad spectrum of bacteria, an important contribution in lung cancer where complications due to pneumonia are common. Shi gao also clears heat from the qi level and the lung and with zhi mu is commonly used to treat pneumonia. Tai zi shen tonifies the qi while also generating fluids. It is neutral in temperature, which makes it a good choice for tonification when heat is present. Ba yue zha is a substitution for chuan shan jia (an animal product). It regulates the blood, moves the liver qi and blood and is antineoplastic. It does not contain the controversial aristolochic acid of mu tong, which is from the stems of the *Akebia* vine. Bai mao teng (or bai ying) clears heat and removes toxins and is antineoplastic. Bai hua she she cao is also antineoplastic and clears heat and reduces abscesses, especially of the lung. Yu xing cao clears heat and toxins and drains dampness (the pleural effusion) along with fu ling. It is especially good for lung infections and also is antineoplastic. Gua lou ren transforms phlegm and resolves infection. It is antineoplastic along with the last four herbs which all work together to resolve the toxins causing the cancer. Da huang helps to move stool and stop bleeding. It is considered antineoplastic for blood stasis tumors.

Spleen and kidney yang deficiency

This is a common presentation for any cancer at end stage. There is general debility; the patient will need to be ventilated; congestive heart and lung syndromes may appear; there may be metastatic bone pain with weakness and even fractures.

Symptoms

- Chest distress and dyspnea.
- Cough.
- Shortness of breath.
- Inability to exert oneself.
- Inability to expectorate.
- Rales.
- Orthopnea.
- White or gray complexion.
- Spontaneous sweats with fevers.
- Anorexia.
- Wasting/cachexia.

Signs

- Tongue: no color, no coat.
- Pulse: thready or minute.

Treatment principle

- Nourish the lung and kidneys, strengthen the spleen, mild antineoplastic effect.

Formula

Bu zhong yi qi tang[24] he Bai he gu jin tang jia jian[25]

tai zi shen (Pseudostellariae Radix; *Pseudostellaria heterophylla*)	15 g
fu ling (Poria; *Poria cocos*)	15 g
gou qi zi (Lycii Fructus; *Lycium chinensis*)	12 g
huang qi (Astragali Radix; *Astragalus membranaceus*)	15 g
bai zhu (Atractylodis macrocephalae Rhizoma; *Atractylodes macrocephala*)	12 g
wu wei zi (Schisandrae Fructus; *Schisandra*)	8 g
shan zhu yu (Corni Fructus; *Cornus officinalis* fruit)	9 g
bai ren shen (Ginseng Radix; *Panax ginseng*; white ginseng)	9 g
xi yang shen (Panacis quinquefolii Radix; *Panax quinquefolium*)	9 g
yu zhu (Polygonati odorati Rhizoma; *Polygonatum odoratum*)	12 g
ku xing ren (Armeniacae Semen amarum; *Prunus armeniaca*)	10 g
gan cao (Glycyrrhizae Radix; *Glycyrrhiza*; licorice root)	3 g
chen pi (Citri reticulatae Pericarpium; *Citrus reticulata* pericarp)	9 g
chuan bei mu (Fritillariae cirrhosae Bulbus; *Fritillaria cirrhosa*)	10 g
bai hua she she cao (Hedyotis diffusae Herba; *Oldenlandia*)	20 g
dong chong xia cao (Cordyceps; *Cordyceps*)	6 g

Tai zi shen is a qi tonic herb that also generates fluids. It especially tonifies the qi of the lung and spleen. Fu ling, bai zhu, and gan cao together form Si jun zi tang, or Four Gentlemen Decoction, which is the main qi tonic formula. This formula is often seen within many larger formulas for cancer treatment. Fu ling is antineoplastic as mentioned earlier. Gou qi zi nourishes the blood, and huang qi tonifies the qi of the lung and spleen. Huang qi, wu wei zi, shan zhu yu, bai ren shen, xi yang shen, and yu zhu are all herbs that could be used in a modified form in the formula Bu fei tang, or Benefit the Lung Decoction. Wu wei zi and shan zhu yu are astringents that astringe the qi of the lungs. Bai ren shen is a strong qi tonic herb that benefits the lungs and the kidneys and is immunomodulating. Xi yang shen is American ginseng and nourishes the yin, an important aspect in this formula, which has so many warming herbs to tonify the qi, while also tonifying the qi of the lungs and kidneys. Yu zhu is a lung yin-nourishing herb.

Ku xing ren is a primary herb for regulating the qi of the lungs; it helps to treat cough, shortness of breath, and orthopnea, all of which are symptoms of lung qi flushing upwards. Chen pi works in a similar way and also helps to tonify the spleen qi and aid in low appetite. Chuan bei mu is a phlegm-transforming herb that can used for a longer term than its relative zhe bei mu (*Fritillaria thunbergii*). It acts here like a lung tonic herb by helping to reduce those symptoms of lung qi flushing upwards. Bai hua she she cao is antineoplastic. Dong chong xia cao is a strong tonic herb that also acts as an antineoplastic herb.

The overall function of this formula strongly tonifies the qi of the middle jiao and the lungs. It works to improve appetite and to improve the function of the lungs. It is immunomodulating and mildly antineoplastic. It, therefore, acts as palliative therapy in order to ease a terminal stage of illness.

Preoperative formula

Weakened resistance, infection and complications from the cancer, can all contribute to risk for serious complications from surgery. When time permits, measures that strengthen resistance and also begin resolving pathogenic heat and toxin while simultaneously balancing yin and yang and supporting the zheng qi are of great benefit. The following formula tonifies the qi, especially of the lung, nourishes the yin, clears heat, transforms phlegm, relieves cough, reduces swelling and the formation of adhesions, and improves and hastens wound healing. This formula should be given 3 weeks prior to surgery and be continued until the day before surgery.

Formula

mai dong (Ophiopogonis Radix; *Ophiopogon*)	10 g
bei sha shen (Glehniae Radix; *Glehnia*)	10 g
jin yin hua (Lonicerae Flos; *Lonicera*)	10 g
fu ling (Poria; *Poria cocos*)	12 g
tai zi shen (Pseudostellariae Radix; *Pseudostellaria heterophylla*)	15 g
yu xing cao (Houttuyniae Herba; *Houttuynia*)	20 g
pi pa ye (Eriobotryae Folium; *Eriobotrya japonica* leaves)	10 g
jie geng (Platycodi Radix; *Platycodon gradiflorus* root)	10 g
chuan bei mu (Fritillariae cirrhosae Bulbus; *Fritillaria cirrhosa*)	12 g
zhu ru (Bambusae Caulis in taeniam; *Phyllostachys nigra*)	10 g
yu zhu (Polygonati odorati Rhizoma; *Polygonatum odoratum*)	15 g
shan zhu yu (Corni Fructus; *Cornus officinalis*)	6 g
bai hua she she cao (Hedyotis diffusae Herba; *Oldenlandia*)	25 g
huang qi (Astragali Radix; *Astragalus membranaceus*)	20 g

Mai dong, sha shen, yu zhu, and tai zi shen all nourish yin and generate fluids. Jin yin hua is an excellent clear heat herb, especially for the upper jiao, and it helps to reduce swelling resulting from inflammation. Tai zi shen, huang qi and all of the qi tonic herbs tonify the qi of the spleen and the lung. Huang qi also helps to protect against infection since its pharmacological functions include increased WBC counts and phagocytosis. Huang qi is also an excellent wound healer. It helps heal wounds and prevent the formation of adhesions.

Yu xing cao clears heat, reduces swellings and helps to clear abscesses in the lungs. It is also antineoplastic and helps prevent surgical infections. It is also mildly analgesic. Pi pa ye descends the lung to stop cough. It transforms phlegm and clears heat and is antibacterial. It contains amygdalin, which is an antineoplastic substance and mildly analgesic. Jie geng warms and transforms cold or hot phlegm. This makes it an excellent herb for regulating the qi of the lung and relieving cough.

Cough is a main symptom of many stages of lung cancer. Surgery can result in shortness of breath, coughing, and orthopnea, all of which are symptoms of lung qi flushing upward. Jie geng also directs the qi of the other herbs in a formula to the upper jiao. It is also antibacterial.

Chuan bei mu clears heat and transforms phlegm. It moistens and nourishes the lungs, stops cough, and is antineoplastic against phlegm fire tumors. Along with other herbs in this formula it is a component of Qing zai jiu fei tang (pi pa ye, yu zhu), a major formula to treat the symptoms of tuberculosis and various infectious diseases of the lung. Zhu ru also clears and dissolves hot phlegm. It helps to cool the blood and reduce bleeding. Yu zhu, shan zhu yu, and huang qi are possible components of a modified Bu fei tang formula. They astringe the qi of the lungs, tonify the lung and spleen qi, hasten wound healing, nourish yin. Bai hua she she cao is the only antineoplastic in the formula and helps to protect against local spread during surgery by containing the cancer through clearing heat and toxin.

Postoperative formula

Surgery causes injury in several ways. It weakens immune function through injury to the lungs from anesthesia. It injures soft tissue, causing yin and possibly blood deficiency (depending on the extent and site of surgery and the surgical technique); yin deficiency can lead pathogenic heat into deeper levels, especially the blood level. The anesthesia and trauma may also cause a damp/phlegm accumulation in the lung, even without infection. Trauma can cause blood stasis in the form of scarring and the formation of adhesions. It is important to treat as soon as possible after surgery in order to re-establish normal function and to begin the antineoplastic effect.

Formula
Special formula[26]

xi yang shen (Panacis quinquefolii Radix; *Panax quinquefolium*)	8 g
tai zi shen (Pseudostellariae Radix; *Pseudostellaria heterophylla*)	15 g
mai dong (Ophiopogonis Radix; *Ophiopogon*)	12 g
bei sha shen (Glehniae Radix; *Glehnia*)	10 g
shi hu (Dendrobii Herba; *Dendrobium*)	10 g
gou qi zi (Lycii Fructus; *Lycium chinensis*)	10 g
zhu ling (Polyporus; *Polyporus – Grifola*)	15 g
fu ling (Poria; *Poria cocos*)	15 g
chuan bei mu (Fritillariae cirrhosae Bulbus; *Fritillaria cirrhosa*)	10 g
pi pa ye (Eriobotryae Folium; *Eriobotrya japonica* leaves)	10 g
bai he (Lilii Bulbus; *Lilium* bulb)	10 g
jiao gu lan (Herba Gynostemmatis; *Gynostemma*)	15 g
bai hua she she cao (Hedyotis diffusae Herba; *Oldenlandia*)	25 g
huang qi (Astragali Radix; *Astragalus membranaceus*)	20 g

Xi yang shen, tai zi shen, mai dong, sha shen, shi hu, and bai he all nourish the yin. Gou qi zi nourishes and tonifies the liver and kidney yin. It nourishes the blood to replenish the yin. It moistens the lungs. Zhu ling and fu ling are drain damp herbs that, as mushrooms, act as immunomodulating herbs by increasing WBC counts, phagocytosis, and are mildly analgesic. They help prevent infection and also reduce fluid build-up as a result of the procedure. Chuan bei mu and pi pa ye regulate the qi of the lungs to prevent shortness of breath, coughing, wheezing, and orthopnea caused by the surgery. Huang qi also helps to prevent infection and tonifies the qi of the lung and the spleen. It is the premier wound healer. Qi ye dan and bai hua she she cao are two antineoplastics that continue to address the issue of toxin. They also clear heat.

Radiation formula

The side effects of radiation include initial local congestion and edema, inflammation of the bronchial mucosa, atrophy of lymph nodes, acute alveolitis, non-productive cough, dyspnea, low-grade fever, hemoptysis, rales. Many of these symptoms will begin after XRT and continue for some time (even years) after treatment. The side effects of XRT may require ongoing clinical attention and should be continued during other treatment modalities and during prevention of recurrence.

Radiation for lung cancer is used less and less because the damage done outweighs the cytotoxic effect and because new chemotherapies are becoming more comparable in effect without the long-term side effects of radiation.

Formula
Zha mei yi wei tang jia jian

zhu ling (Polyporus; *Polyporus – Grifola*)	15 g
mai dong (Ophiopogonis Radix; *Ophiopogon*)	10 g
bei sha shen (Glehniae Radix; *Glehnia*)	10 g
yu zhu (Polygonati odorati Rhizoma; *Polygonatum odoratum*)	12 g
gou qi zi (Lycii Fructus; *Lycium chinensis*)	12 g
jin yin hua (Lonicerae Flos; *Lonicera*)	10 g
yi ren (Coicis Semen; *Coix lacryma-jobi*)	20 g
pi pa ye (Eriobotryae Folium; *Eriobotrya japonica* leaves)	10 g
fu ling (Poria; *Poria cocos*)	15 g
tai zi shen (Pseudostellariae Radix; *Pseudostellaria heterophylla*)	20 g
dan shen (Salviae miltiorrhizae Radix; *Salvia miltiorhiza*)	15 g
chuan bei mu (Fritillariae cirrhosae Bulbus; *Fritillaria cirrhosa*)	10 g
gan cao (Glycyrrhizae Radix; *Glycyrrhiza*; licorice root)	4 g

Mai dong, sha shen, yu zhu, and gou qi zi all nourish the yin. Zhu ling potentiates the effect of radiation and can be used in even higher dose than given here. Jin yin hua clears heat. Yi ren clears heat and toxins and is also antineoplastic. It is a bronchodilator and mildly analgesic. Fu ling has a similar effect. It also potentiates radiation but not as strongly as zhu ling and both have an important contribution during radiation. Dan shen is a blood-regulating herb that also potentiates the radiation effect by increasing blood circu-

lation in general and to the local area. Tumor cells tend to be able to live in an environment that is less well oxygenated. Radiation is more cytotoxic in highly oxygenated cells. By increasing circulation and, therefore, oxygenation, the effect of the radiation is enhanced by this herb. Chuan bei mu dissolves phlegm and helps to regulate the qi of the lung, which is injured by the radiation treatment. Gan cao is a harmonising herb that benefits the spleen to enable it to metabolise the yin-nourishing herbs of this formula. It also regulates the lung qi and moistens the lung and throat.

Prevention

Guang An Men hospital in Beijing has researched and developed the following formula as an injectable intravenous formula during treatment for lung cancer. In a syrup form this same formula is used post-treatment as maintenance therapy and/or to prevent recurrence.

Formula
Fei liu ping (gao)[27]

huang qi (Astragali Radix; *Astragalus membranaceus*)	20 g
dan shen (Salviae miltiorrhizae Radix; *Salvia miltiorhiza*)	15 g
bei sha shen (Glehniae Radix; *Glehnia*)	12 g
mai dong (Ophiopogonis Radix; *Ophiopogon*)	12 g
xing ren (Armeniacae Semen; *Prunus armeniaca* seed)	12 g
jie geng (Platycodi Radix; *Platycodon grandiflorus* root)	12 g
chuan bei mu (Fritillariae cirrhosae Bulbus; *Fritillaria cirrhosa*)	12 g
bai hua she she cao (Hedyotis diffusae Herba; *Oldenlandia*)	25 g
shan ci gu* (Cremastrae/Pleiones Pseudobulbus; *Cremastra/Pleione* pseudobulbs)	20 g

Huang qi is a qi tonic herb that is especially tonifying for the lungs. It increases WBC counts and phagocytosis and is antineoplastic. Dan shen moves blood and helps to prevent spread of toxin. Sha shen and mai dong are both yin-nourishing lung herbs that nourish normal interstitial fluids in the lungs and help to heal the dryness that is the foundation for cancerisation of the lung tissue. Xing ren is a transform phlegm herb that is a main herb to prevent cough by regulating the qi of the lungs. The loss of qi through chronic cough is an important symptom to treat. Xing ren is also the seed from the *Prunus armeniaca* species from which laetrile has been made. It has some anti-neoplastic properties. Jie geng is a messenger herb that directs the 'qi of the formula' to the chest. Chuan bei mu is a phlegm-transforming herb that can be used over the long term. It regulates the qi of the lung and is mildly antineoplastic. Bai hua she she cao and shan ci gu* are both antineoplastic herbs used here in medium high dose to prevent a recurrence of lung cancer.

Case study 2.1

This is a 58-year-old female who presented with a dry intermittent cough and back and hip pain for 6 months. She had a history of smoking but had quit 14 years earlier. She was suffering from fatigue, depression, and anxiety. She also had a history of alcoholism and had been in recovery since the time she had quit smoking. Her signs and symptoms were quite typical for stage III to IV lung cancer.

Signs and symptoms

- Cough: intermittent and dry.
- Fatigue: 'ever since I found out [about the cancer]'.
- Energy: 5 out of 10; usually a 10+.
- Appetite: moderate to low.
- Weight: normal range.
- Digestion above the navel: normal.
- Digestion below the navel: mild gas and bloating for last several years.
- Stools: regular and formed.
- Throat: mucusy and difficult to expectorate.
- Sleep: was normal and 8 hours per night without interruption; now up a lot due to bone pain, thirst at night.
- Thirst: yes; dry mouth and general body thirst; drinking a lot of fluids without relief.
- Sweating: night sweats which began 5 months ago; mostly on lower extremities (spleen deficiency sign).
- Memory: normal.
- Dyspnea (shortness of breath): mild and only with mild to moderate exertion.
- Menopausal status: 9 years since last menses; taking hormone replacement therapy (HRT) for moderate flushing.

- Temperature: normal except at night when runs very hot.
- Fevers: low-grade lately on occasion; no infection found.
- Headaches: none.
- Menstrual cycle: first menses at age 11; three pregnancies with one abortion; two living children; no history of chronic reproductive infections or sexually transmitted diseases (STDs).
- Family: raised in alcoholic family; now stable and loving marriage; recovering alcoholic – clean and sober 15 years.
- Smoking: quit 14 years ago.
- Pattern of worrier – worry for family and 'whether I'm good enough'.
- Heritage: Irish.
- Bruxism: at night, chronic.
- Depression: long term, on sertraline (Zoloft) for several years.
- Pertinent history: alcoholism, smoking, thyroid nodule (benign).
- Tongue: long and thin, red body, wet, no coat, no distention.
- Pulse: liver sho, rapid and thin, slightly slippery, upper jiao pulses hard and stiff (almost leathery).
- Hara: very warm and dry; lung areas both tender; liver reflex tender on right from superficial to deep.

Specific diagnoses regarding the lung cancer

- Right pleural effusion: already drained twice; moderate size; each draining produced 1.5 L of fluid.
- Right upper lobe mass: 5 x 8 cm.
- Hemothorax: several round masses up to 8 mm.

Case study continues

- Right middle lobe: scarring with atelectasis.
- Bone metastases: T12, L1, L2, L3; upper cervical vertebrae; C3, 5, 7; sacrum, right acetabulum, right greater trochanter, right ischium.
- **Stage IV metastatic adenocarcinoma (NSCLC)**

Chinese medicine diagnosis

Lung and kidney qi and yin deficiency with latent pathogenic factor, underlying liver and kidney yin deficiency. The pleural effusion is also due to internal heat from yin deficiency.

The plan for this patient was chemotherapy in the form of carboplatin and paclitaxel (Taxol) every 3 weeks. This treatment could be considered only palliative. In this case, palliative meant preventing further spread, managing the effects of the cancer already present, and buying more time to live and prepare for the end of life. The chemotherapy regimen alone could manage all of these goals. Some pain relief was added in the form of acetaminophen (Vicodin). When the herbal medicine was added, the need for pain control was eliminated. There was also an immediate need to continue to manage the pleural effusion. When chemotherapy began, combined with the herbal formula this need also was eliminated.

The patient remained on the following formula for some time. Her constitutional diagnoses included lung and kidney qi and yin deficiency caused by the history of smoking and alcohol abuse, latent pathogenic factor in the form of toxin caused by smoking, and liver and kidney yin deficiency. The dose was 8 g granulated formula 3 times daily.

bai ren shen (Ginseng Radix; *Panax ginseng*; white ginseng)	15 g
bei sha shen (Glehniae Radix; *Glehnia*)	15 g
mai dong (Ophiopogonis Radix; *Ophiopogon*)	15 g
gou qi zi (Lycii Fructus; *Lycium chinensis*)	12 g
bai he (Lilii Bulbus; *Lilium* bulb)	12 g
huang qin (Scutellariae Radix; *Scutellaria baicalensis*)	10 g
gua lou shi (Trichosanthis Fructus; *Trichosanthes* fruit)	25 g
chuan bei mu (Fritillariae cirrhosae Bulbus; *Fritillaria cirrhosa*)	10 g
ban zhi lian (Scutellariae barbatae Herba; *Scutellaria barbata*)	25 g
bai hua she she cao (Hedyotis diffusae Herba; *Oldenlandia*)	25 g
yu xing cao (Houttuyniae Herba; *Houttuynia*)	25 g
zhu ling (Polyporus; *Polyporus – Grifola*)	20 g
ting li zi (Lepidii Semen; *Lepidium* seed)	15 g
jiao mu (Zanthoxyli Semen; *Zanthoxylum* seed)	10 g
yu zhu (Polygonati odorati Rhizoma; *Polygonatum odoratum*)	15 g
mai ya (Hordei Fructus germinatus; *Hordeum vulgare*; barley sprouts; malt)	15 g
huang qi (Astragali Radix; *Astragalus membranaceus*)	25 g
ji xue teng (Spatholobi Caulis; *Spatholobus suberectus*)	20 g
bu gu zhi (Psoraleae Fructus; *Psoralea*)	15 g
gu sui bu (Drynariae Rhizoma; *Drynaria*)	15 g
hong da zao (Jujubae Fructus; *Ziziphus jujuba*; red jujube)	10 g

The purpose of this formula is to treat the underlying constitution of the patient. This includes tonifying lung and kidney qi and yin deficiency, latent pathogenic factor, and liver and kidney yin deficiency. It is also meant to interface with the carboplatin and paclitaxel to stave off side effects and enhance the cytotoxic effect. The formula is meant to improve the overall parenchymal function of the lungs; resolve the pleural effusion and reduce fluid accumulation; improve cellular immunity, act antineoplastically, act as an antiemetic in the face of carboplatin, protect against neuropathies caused by paclitaxel, protect against cardiac toxicity from carboplatin, and help maintain normal blood levels in the face of myelosuppression.

White ren shen is a moderately strong qi tonic for the source qi, spleen and lungs. It concurrently tonifies the qi of the lungs and benefits the lung yin. It is a cardiotonic herb that helps protect the heart from the toxicity of carboplatin. It inhibits the growth of tumors, increases WBCs and helps to prevent lung infection, a serious threat in this

Case study continues

case. It also calms the spirit. Sha shen expels phlegm and clears lung heat while nourishing the lung yin. It is also cardiotonic. Mai dong nourishes the yin and clears heat, it moistens the lungs and nourishes the heart and calms the spirit. Gou qi zi nourishes the blood and nourishes the yin of the liver and kidneys, the main diagnosis in this patient. It also moistens the lungs, an important aspect of treating yin deficiency in the lungs while draining pathogenic fluids. Bai he moistens the lungs, clears heat and promotes urination to aide in draining fluids out from the pleural effusion. It also calms the spirit.

Huang qin clears heat and toxin, especially in the upper jiao and lungs; it dries dampness and cools the blood to stop hemorrhage, a common occurrence in lungs affected by lung cancer. Huang qin is also a broad-spectrum antibiotic and helps protect the lungs against infection. Gua lou shi transforms phlegm heat and circulates bound qi in the chest. It dissipates nodules and accumulations and is antineoplastic. It is mildly analgesic, useful especially for chest pain following thoracentesis to drain the effusion. Chuan bei mu has similar functions and also moistens and nourishes the lungs. It is also antineoplastic for phlegm fire tumors. Ban zhi lian is a clear heat and toxin herb that is antineoplastic. The same is true for bai hua she she cao. Even though this is a stage IV cancer, the patient is still moderately young and strong; there is an effort here to manage this cancer (versus cure) and gain some time.

Yu xing cao is a clear heat and toxin herb that is especially useful in treating lung abscesses. It is antineoplastic and also helps in draining dampness to aid the herbs used to treat the pleural effusion. Zhu ling is a mushroom that has many immunomodulatory properties. It drains dampness and helps the other draining herbs to reduce and resolve the pleural effusion. It is antineoplastic, increases phagocytosis, helps in T-cell transformation, is antibiotic, helping to prevent infection. Ting li zi redirects the lung qi downward and transforms phlegm; it is a cathartic to transform water and will strongly drain the water accumulation from the effusion. It enters the lung and the urinary bladder and provides a perfect route for water build-up to leave the lung. It is also a cardiotonic. Jiao mu, or the seed of the Sichuan pepper (chuan jiao; Zanthoxyli

Pericarpium; *Zanthozulum bungeanum*), works with the other drain damp herbs to guide out the retained fluids by warming the interior and spleen and stomach to help in transformation and transportation of fluids. It is also mildly analgesic.

Yu zhu nourishes the lung yin to protect the yin while draining abnormal fluids. Mai ya supports the spleen in the face of the cool or cold and bitter clear heat and toxin herbs and the chemotherapy. It increases the appetite and helps to ameliorate nausea and other digestive complaints caused by carboplatin. Huang qi also supports the spleen and digestion. It tonifies the lungs to increase parenchymal function of the lungs. It increases WBC counts, phagocytosis, NK cells, promotes urination, speeds healing from the surgical procedure, and is a cardiotonic. Ji xue teng mildly moves the blood by nourishing the blood; it is especially good for treating anemias caused by spleen deficiency. With bu gu zhi and gu sui bu, it helps to prevent peripheral neuropathies caused by paclitaxel. Hong (red) da zao tonifies the general qi, supports the spleen, harmonises the formula, generates fluids, and helps the medicine go down. It moistens the lungs and calms the spirit, increases endurance and also helps prevent allergic reaction to the chemotherapy.

Outcome

The patient did well on this formula and the combination of the herbs and chemotherapy resolved the pleural effusion, which was quite large at diagnosis. This took about 6 months but the effusion did not require another thoracentesis.

The first courses of the carboplatin and paclitaxel stopped the movement and further growth of the cancer for approximately 1 year. When the pleural effusion resolved, those herbs that were added to manage this initial primary issue were eliminated from the formula. Herbs were then added to manage the bone metastases. It was unclear at that moment and for some time if the patient would survive and if the chemotherapy would stop the progression of the cancer. Issues were prioritised based upon all of the issues present at diagnosis. When it was clear that the chemotherapy was working and the pleural effusion had resolved then Zuo gui yin plus

Case study continues

bai hua she (Agkistrodon; *Agkistrodon acutus*) was added to the formula in the place of those herbs used to resolve the effusion. The patient did well for almost 2 years post-diagnosis. The metastatic disease in the brain resolved with external beam irradiation at the time of diagnosis. There did not appear to be any side effects from the procedure (daily doses for 20 days) except for fatigue. However, at the end of year two metastatic disease was found in the liver. The chemotherapy

regimen, which had continued at lower doses as maintenance therapy, was changed to gefitinib (Iressa) because it became clear that the original regimen no longer held the cancer in check. However, the gefitinib did not work at all. The patient finally succumbed to liver and renal failure two and a half years after initial diagnosis with stage IV NSCLC. Her death came fast and was peaceful for her and her family.

Case study 2.2

This case involves a male aged 71, who presented with extreme fatigue during and after a downhill skiing vacation. He was a very active individual who had enjoyed all kinds of sports activities. He had taken good care of himself throughout his life, except for smoking. He had quit smoking 15 years prior to his diagnosis. He presented with mid- and lower-back pain and fatigue.

He was diagnosed with left lung adenocarcinoma NSCLC. All three lobes of the left lung were involved; he had a large pleural effusion, which was being managed with two indwelling drainage tubes; there was extensive pleural lesion and local metastatic spread. He had a non-metastatic calculus in his left kidney, which was asymptomatic. There were also multiple cysts in both kidneys that were not malignant. He was also diagnosed with benign prostatic hypertrophy (BPH) during his scans for lung cancer. His prostate was very enlarged and it was felt that he might also have prostate cancer because his prostate specific antigen (PSA) level was high. However, because of his diagnosis and the decisions he had made based on his prognosis, which was very poor, he decided not to seek treatment for the lung cancer nor to seek further analysis of the possible prostate cancer. Instead, he opted for palliative care and hospice.

Signs and symptoms

- Left lower lobe atelectasis.
- Left pleural effusion equaling one-third hemithorax.
- WBC: 17.8, indicating infection.
- Hematocrit (Hct): 32; RBC: 3.2; hemoglobin: 10; platelets: 427 (high).
- No bone metastases.
- PSA: 17.2 (high; see Chapter 5 on prostate cancer).
- Blood pressure: 154/75.
- Heart rate: 95 bpm.
- Temperature: 97°C.
- Appetite: very poor.
- Glucose: 152 (high); patient's family denies any history of diabetes, therefore, carcinoid syndrome?
- Digestion: mild nausea, metallic taste due to drugs (?).
- Stools: very dry stools, constipation (side effect of pain medications).
- Sleep: poor and restless, unable to breathe lying down.
- Thirst: severe, prefers slightly cold drinks.
- Energy: cannot walk down the hall but is restless and irritable.
- Urination: frequent and dribbling with start-and-stop stream.

Case study continues

- Sweating: moderate upper body sweats, only at night.
- Skin color: dark and slightly yellow.
- Breathing: labored, early stages of stridor.
- Cough: frequent.
- Sputum: green to clear but thick and difficult to expectorate.
- Lower extremity: pitting edema up to mid-lower leg.
- Tongue: scarlet, mirror coat, unrooted thick greasy brown coat only in center over stomach area (thrush).
- Pulse: leathery but soggy (on iv fluids), kidneys frail, overall slightly choppy, no doyo.

Medications

- Warfarin (Coumadin): low dose to maintain iv line.
- Megestrol (Megace): to improve appetite.
- Nystatin: oral candidiasis.
- Ceftriaxone: antibiotic (pneumonia).
- Oxycodone: pain.
- Mirtazapine (Remeron): antidepressant (sleep aid).

Plan

Palliative care and hospice.

Diagnosis

Lung phlegm heat with toxin, lung qi and yin deficiency, wind heat in the lung, kidney yang deficiency.

The laboratory work-up for this patient was not completed because the findings regarding the lung cancer were overwhelming. The large pleural effusion compressed the entire left lung and all three lobes were involved. Metastatic disease was probably greater than described as evidenced by thrombocytosis (the high platelet count). Abnormally high platelet counts are found in extensive metastatic disease, especially of the lung. The PSA implied prostate cancer, as well, and the start-and-stop stream was probably due to obstruction by cancerous tissue rather than BPH. The blood pressure was moderately low, given the other conditions the patient was dealing with, but

his lifestyle, which included hard exercise, probably stood him in good stead regarding this issue. However, the high heart rate demonstrated that the extent of the cancer in the lung and the obstruction by the pleural effusion, which was very large, were stressing the heart.

There are some drugs and conditions that predispose to hypothermia or low body temperature. These include sedatives and hypnotics and tranquilisers, congestive heart failure, hypothyroidism, starvation, pulmonary infection, sepsis, and any immobilising illness. One might expect a high temperature in the face of a bacterial pneumonia. But the combination of antidepressant, iv fluids, being bedridden, anorexia, possible congestive heart failure may have all contributed to the low body temperature of 97°C. The tongue does not match the temperature, but should not confuse the diagnosis.

High glucose levels can indicate diabetes but, in this case, the more obvious cause was carcinoid syndrome, which occurs in some cases when there is extensive metastatic disease The upper body sweats at night indicate upper jiao heat and probably yin deficiency. The green thick sputum is emblematic for a bacterial pneumonia (hence the wind heat diagnosis). There are several indicators for kidney yang deficiency: the frail pulse, cold sensation in the lower body, lower extremity edema (both kidney yang and water metabolism issues), irritability (here it is the kidney/heart axis and possible mixed upper jiao heat), frequent urination (kidney/bladder qi transformation), possibly the prostate cancer, and orthopnea (kidney/lung axis). The temperature cannot be accurately discerned within the parameters of Chinese medicine because the patient had been on iv fluids for over a week and the iv fluids probably lowered the temperature (see the above discussion). The wind heat diagnosis was made primarily on the sputum color and culture, the upper body heat and sweating, and extreme thirst.

It is not unusual for a terminal patient to present with mixed yin and yang deficiency. The relationship between yin and yang often unravels at the endstage of disease. Yang-deficient symptoms can be mistaken for yin deficiency as the yang floats to the surface in a yang-deficient

Case study continues

environment. The tongue of this patient indicates extreme heat and yin deficiency. These may be due to toxin. The toxin is relative to the upper jiao injuries. Even though there is also probable prostate cancer present, the prostate cancer is due less to toxin and more to internal spleen and kidney deficiencies that led to phlegm damp. These issues all require a judgment call. Generally at late stage, there is frequently little time to understand the whole picture. This is especially true when a terminal patient presents.

The lack of a middle pulse, or doyo, is a sign that death is imminent. The doyo is akin to the spleen pulse and demonstrates the middle jiao's ability to support and nourish all bodily function. It is the central pulse running through the larger tube of the radial vessel. When it is not present it means that the middle jiao and spleen function is no longer functional and cannot support the zheng qi. It is a death pulse. This patient's family had flown in from various parts of the country. They were deeply committed to being there in any way for their family member, but it was difficult for them to accept their loved one's decision to let go and 'not fight'. However, this patient was somehow conscious of the fact that his demise was imminent. He felt that he had to 'check out' of all of the discussions about what to do for him. He knew what needed to happen, and his incredibly loving family could not hear him voice his desires. Eventually they did, and it remains a mystery as to whether or not he hung onto life in order to wait for them to come to peace with this.

The following formula was used for only 1 week before the patient slipped into a coma and died the next day. He was taken off all other medications at his request, including iv fluids. He was very comfortable, without pain, there was no death rattle, he remained conscious until he slipped into the coma and then quietly away.

Formula

Fei liu ping jia jian
The herbs added to the base formula are:

fu ling (Poria; *Poria cocos*)	20 g
zhu ling (Polyporus; *Polyporus – Grifola*)	20 g
shi hu (Dendrobii Herba; *Dendrobium*)	15 g
bai zi ren (Biotae Semen; *Biota*)	15 g
ting li zi (Lepidii Semen; *Lepidium* seed)	15 g
yan hu suo (Corydalis Rhizoma; *Corydalis yanhusuo*)	20 g
xie bai (Allii macrostemi Bulbus; *Allium macrostemon*)	20 g

Fu ling and zhu ling are mushrooms that drain damp to relieve mildly the pleural effusion. They also increase WBC counts and phagocytosis to help fight the infection. They are mildly analgesic. Shi hu is the empiric herb for thirst and dry mouth, which was a major complaint in this case. Shi hu is a yin-nourishing herb that also helped moisten the stool along with bai zi ren. Bai zi ren also nourishes the heart and helps to calm the spirit. Ting li zi helps to drain downward fluids accumulated in the lungs and chest. Yan hu suo regulates the blood in order to treat pain. Xie bai directs the qi downwards and opens the chest; it reduces pain, especially in the chest.

References

1. Boring CC. Cancer statistics, 1999. Cancer 1999; 41:19–51.
2. Cancer facts and figures, 1998. American Cancer Society; 1998.
3. Wald NJ. Does breathing other people's tobacco smoke cause lung cancer? Br Med J 1986; 293:1217–1222.
4. NCI: Respiratory health effects of passive smoking: lung cancer and other disorders. The Report of the U.S. Environmental Protection Agency. Smoking and Tobacco Control Monograph No. 4. NIH Publication Number 93-3605, Bethesda, Maryland; 1993.
5. Salazar O. Lung cancer. Clin Oncol 1993; 31:646.
6. Richardson GE. Smoking cessation significantly reduces the risk of second primary cancer in long term cancer-free survivors of SCLC (abstract). Proc Am Soc Clin Oncol 1993; 12:326.
7. Surgeon General's Report. The health benefits of smoking cessation. 1990.

8. Barsky SH, Roth MD, Kleerup EC, et al. Histopathologic and molecular alterations in bronchial epithelium in habitual smokers of marijuana, cocaine, and/or tobacco. J Natl Cancer Inst 1998; 90:1198–1205.

9. Savaraj N. Multidrug resistance associated protein gene expression in SCLC and NSCLC (abstract). Proc Am Assoc Cancer Res 1994; 35:242.

10. Skarin AT. Analysis of long term survivors with SCLC. Chest 1993; 103:440–449.

11. Leblanc M. The Consensus Group for Prognostic Factors in SCLC. Verification of a multicenter prognostic model for SCLC. Proc Am Soc Clin Oncol 1993; 12:362.

12. Takahashi T. The p53 gene is very frequently mutated in SCLC with a distant nucleotide substitution pattern. Oncogene 1991; 6:1775–1778.

13. Kjuss H. A case-referent study of lung cancer, occupational exposures and smoking. Role of asbestos exposure. Scand J Work Environ Health 1986; 12:203–209.

14. Ziegler RG. Does beta-carotene explain why reduced cancer risk is associated with vegetable and fruit intake? Cancer Res 1992; 52 (suppl 7):2060–2066.

15. The Alpha-tocopherol, Beta-carotene Cancer Prevention Study Group. The effect of vitamin E and beta-carotene on the incidence of lung cancer and other cancers in male smokers. N Engl J Med 1994; 330:1029–1035.

16. Sun Gui Zhi. Kang Ai Zhong Cao Fang Xuan (Treatment of cancer with Chinese herbal medicine). Beijing Institute of Traditional Chinese Medicine 1992; 145–155.

17. Chang Y. Yi Men Fa Lu (Precepts for physicians). Qing Dynasty.

18. Kitamura K. Baicalin, an inhibitor of HIV-1 production in vitro. Antiviral Res 1998; 37:131–140.

19. van Loon IM. The golden root: clinical applications of *Scutellaria baicalensis* George flavonoids as modulators of the inflammatory response. Alt Med Review 1997; 2:472–480.

20. Takasuna K, Kasai Y, Kitano Y, et al. Protective effects of kampo medicines and baicalin against intestinal toxicity of a new anticancer camptothecin derivative, irinotecan hydrochloride (CPT-11), in rats. Japanese J Cancer Res 1995; 86:978–984.

21. Jiao Zhu Fu Ren Liang Fang (Revised fine formulas for women).

22. Aida Y. Chemical Pharmacology Bulletin, 1995; 43:859.

23. Sun Gui Zhi. Kang Ai Zhong Cao Fang Yuan (Treatment of cancer with Chinese herbal medicine). Beijing Institute of Traditional Chinese Medicine; 1992:150.

24. Li Dong Yuan. Pi Wei Lun (Discussion of the spleen and stomach). 1249 A.C.E.

25. Wang Ang. Yi Fang Ji Jie (Analytic collection of formulas). 1682 A.C.E.

26. Zhang Dai Zhao. Personal notes from training. Sino-Japanese Friendship hospital, Beijing; 1996.

27. Cheng JH. Treatment of 20 patients with terminal primary bronchogenic carcinoma using feiliuping. Jiangxi J TCM 1991; 22:344–347.

Chapter 3

Colorectal Cancer

CHAPTER CONTENTS

Epidemiology 61

Pathogenesis 62
Conventional medicine 62
Chinese medicine 63

Risk factors 65

Pathology 65

Clinical presentation 66

Diagnosis and screening 67

Diagnosis according to Chinese medicine 67
1. Damp heat 67
2. Toxin accumulation 68
3. Spleen and kidney yang deficiency 69
4. Kidney and liver yin deficiency 69
5. Qi and blood deficiency 70

Post-surgical formulae 71
Li qi kuan chang tang (rectify qi and loosen the intestine decoction) 71
Bu zhong yi qi tang 72

Radiation treatment 72
Retention enema 74
Suppositories 74

Chemotherapy 74

Later-stage colorectal cancer 76
Treatment principles 76

Prevention formula 77

> *For the inner flame to burn, one must feed it; one must watch over the fire, throw into it the fuel of all the errors one wants to get rid of, all that delays the progress, all that darkens the path. If one does not feed the fire, it smolders under the ashes of one's unconsciousness and inertia, and then, not years but lives, centuries will pass before one reaches the goal.*
>
> From Search for the Soul
> by The Mother (Mirra Alfassa)

EPIDEMIOLOGY

Thirteen percent of all cancers in the United States involve either the colon or the rectum. In 2003, 180 000 colorectal cancers were diagnosed. As a cause of cancer death, colorectal cancers rank second only to lung cancer. Approximately 60 000 deaths per year are attributed to colorectal cancer.[1]

The incidence of colorectal cancer is equal among men and women. Japan and Finland, countries with a high incidence of esophageal and gastric cancers, have very low rates of colorectal cancer. The highest rates of incidence are in the US, UK, Saskatchewan (Canada), New Zealand, Australia, Denmark, and Sweden. The lowest rates of incidence are in Colombia, Japan, India, South Africa, Israel, Finland, Poland, and Puerto Rico.

The 5-year survival rate of colorectal cancer is approximately 50%. Local disease generally has a higher survival rate, usually higher than 80%. Disseminated disease has a 5-year survival rate of less than 35%.

The natural history of colorectal cancer has changed over the last three decades. Colon carcinomas now constitute 70% of all cancers in the large intestine, and the right side of the proximal colon (the ascending colon) is the most common site.[2] This may be because of the more frequent use of sigmoidoscopy and polypectomy, which may have lessened the incidence of cancers in the rectum and the sigmoid (descending) colon. The incidence of colon carcinomas in Black Americans has increased by 30% since 1973 and is now higher than in Whites.[3] It is thought that dietary and environmental factors are responsible.

Five-year survival rates for patients with Duke's A, B, C colon carcinoma (TNM stages I, II, and III respectively) have improved. This may be due to the wider resections now performed, better examination of resected specimens, and better staging and abdominal exploration, which reveals clinically occult disease. Both adenomatous polyps and colon carcinomas should be detected early, when cure can be achieved by resection. Each death from this type of cancer must be viewed as a preventable tragedy.

PATHOGENESIS

CONVENTIONAL MEDICINE

Enterocytes are produced from stem cells in the colonic crypt. These cells mature and migrate towards the top of the crypt and then shed into the lumen of the colon at the end of their lifespan. Carcinogenesis in these cells results from a progressive loss of normal controls and balances in terms of proliferation, maturation, and apoptosis. This is a multistage process that may precede malignancy by 10 or more years. Mutational activation of the K-*ras* oncogene leads to enhanced cell growth, the inactivation of tumor suppressor genes (the APC gene), and generalised disorganisation of DNA methylation.[4-6]

Environmental, nutritional, genetic and familial factors have been found to be associated with colorectal cancers. Diets high in saturated fat, especially animal fat, and low in fiber and low in calcium, along with lack of exercise all contribute to colon cancer. The significant lower incidence and risk in Mormons and Seventh Day Adventists in the US points to the benefits of a diet low in meat intake and made up of mainly vegetables, fruits, and wholegrains.[7]

Dietary fat increases the endogenous production, bacterial degradation, and excretion of bile acids and neutral steroids, which are carcinogens, thereby promoting large bowel carcinogenesis. Excess lipids in the colon lead to an increase in the concentration of secondary bile acids, which stimulate protein kinase C (PKC), a major cellular communication pathway, resulting in the promotion of cancer. In colorectal cancer PKC may inhibit growth, while in normal mucosa it may stimulate growth through the action of bile acids. A diet high in fats can lead to the predominance of anaerobic bacteria in the intestinal microflora, and the enzymes in these bacteria activate carcinogens.[8]

Several world trials have found that a diet high in fiber from fruits and vegetables was more beneficial than fiber from cereals. Fiber decreases fecal transit time through the bowel, resulting in decreased exposure to fecal carcinogens, reduced carcinogenic microflora in the bowel, decreased fecal pH with a consequent decrease in bacterial enzymatic activity, and diluted carcinogens via an increase in stool bulk. It is also important to remember that sucrose increases the fecal concentration of both total and secondary bile acids. Along these same lines, insulin resistance and the associated changes in insulin and insulin growth factor (IGF) may promote colon tumor growth. Therefore, a high-fat, high-sugar, low-fiber diet results in the promotion of colorectal cancer.[9]

A protective role has been ascribed to calcium salts and calcium-rich foods because of their capacity to decrease colon cell turnover rates and reduce the colon-cancer-promoting effects of bile and fatty acids. Calcium inhibits proliferation of human colonic cells, and low calcium results in proliferation and diminished differentiation.[10] Selenium, vitamins C, D, and E, indoles, and beta-carotenoids also decrease cancer of the colon.[11] Reduced glutathione also plays a role in colorectal cancer. Glutathione protects DNA and the *p53* tumor suppressor gene. In colorectal cancer 50–75% of patients have lost the function of both alleles of the *p53* gene.[12] More than 80% of patients with advanced colorectal cancer harbor *p53* mutations.

In one study, selenium reduced the formation of new adenomatous polyps in 44% of patients, and there was a 61% reduction in the incidence of colorectal cancer in those who took selenium versus those who didn't. Omega-3 fatty acids lowered the incidence of colorectal cancer and decreased the formation of polyps.[13]

Vitamin D also inhibits the proliferation of human colorectal cancer. This effect of vitamin D is reduced by calcium channel blockers used to treat hypertension. Vitamin D and calcium in combination seem to work together synergistically.[14] Vitamin E enhances the cytotoxic effect of fluorouracil (5-FU) by inducing p53 in colorectal cancer. At the same time, vitamin E succinate arrests tumor cells in the G1 phase and leads, therefore, to apoptosis. When vitamin E was combined with omega-3 fatty acids the survival time in terminal cancer patients of any kind was significantly increased.[15] Non-steroidal anti-inflammatory drugs (NSAIDs) may inhibit the formation of adenomas (polyps) by Cox inhibition and by decreasing prostaglandin synthesis.

Low levels of the above vitamins and minerals may be risk factors for colorectal cancer when combined with a high-fat, high-sugar, low-fiber diet.

CHINESE MEDICINE

The colon and rectum are at the distal end of the gastrointestinal tube and are part of the fu aspect of the zang fu. This hollow tube is outside the body and acts as a conduit for the transfer of exogenous nutrition. Therefore, the mucosal lining of the tube is constantly exposed to whatever is passing through, not unlike the lungs, which are exposed to air. The lower intestine is also an aspect of the spleen function in that it continues to refine and separate pure from impure gu qi. In this regard, it mainly separates impure matter from water, and a certain amount of water absorption takes place in the colon across the bowel wall. The ying aspect carries through all of the gastrointestinal mucosa, including the bowel mucosa, and offers a level of immunity driven by the spleen and san jiao relationship.

For the above reasons, the colon is easily exposed to pathogenic factors, some endogenous and many exogenous. Damp heat and wind are the two main exposures. Damp heat can be synonymous with a diet high in unsaturated fats, sugars and refined foods, leading to damp heat in the middle and lower jiao, especially the large intestine. Wind refers to contaminated foods that carry exogenous pathogens into the large intestine via the fu organs. Nitrates and other carcinogens are probably in this classical category of pathogen. The colon is injured endogenously by upper gastrointestinal dysfunction and especially by spleen disorders. When spleen function is thought of in terms of anatomical features then fat metabolism and secretion of bile must be included. The overproduction of bile acids due to a high-fat diet falls into the realm of spleen function and spleen injury, because fats are a form of dampness. If we include the whole mucosal lining of the gastrointestinal tube within the function of the spleen, then it becomes more clear how middle jiao disorders involving the spleen can contribute to lower intestinal disorders like colorectal cancer.

Generally, the underlying environment that evolves into colorectal cancer is considered to be either organ toxin (zang du) or intestinal wind (chang feng). 'Du' refers to all of the expressions of toxic heat, pathogenic damp heat, inverted fire poisons, and latent pathogenic factors. The toxins that enter the digestion from contaminated food and water are all a form of external toxin exposure. These toxins can also form endogenously as a result of improper diet, especially as relates to a diet high in animal fat (excess bile acids, the generation of anaerobic bacteria) and low in fiber, which increases the exposure of the bowel wall to these toxins.

Chang feng refers to the accumulation of wind heat in the intestines where it forms toxins. Wind heat is usually considered an external pathogen, and it is interesting to consider that wind heat is usually a lung or wei level pathogen.[16] The lungs and the large intestine are coupled organs and it may be that they share this relationship because they are both sensitive organs that must incorporate the outside, air and food, into the body. As a result they share special tissue types that can act as an exchange mechanism between outside and inside and act as an integral part of immunity.

Wind heat enters from external pathogens entering the body via food and water. Wind heat may also evolve from endogenous exposures that generate anaerobic bacteria that accumulate because of internal environmental imbalances. Therefore, zang du and chang feng are inter-related.

Blood in the stools is traditionally divided into two categories: intestinal wind and toxin in the yin organs.[17] Bright red bleeding, which precedes defecation or is present in the stool, indicates intestinal wind. Dark purple blood with clots indicates toxin in the yin organs. This type of obstruction injures the yin collaterals in the lower body, which causes blood to seep into the intestines. It seems logical to say that intestinal wind is the early manifestation of colorectal cancer while toxin in the yin organs is a later manifestation for colorectal cancer through metastatic spread. As the lung and large intestine are coupled organs they share an energetic relationship and structural similarities. They are the only organs in the body that are continually exposed to the outside. The manner in which they each respond to exogenous factors is somewhat similar in that they tend to form phlegm and various accumulations of phlegm obstruction. In fact, it is the essential nature of these tissues, secretory and epithelial, to form natural mucus that is continually shed and replenished. This turnover makes the lung and large intestine more susceptible to damp phlegm accumulations.

Obstruction in the flow of qi and blood by wind, wind heat or damp heat in the intestines will manifest as a red tongue and a wiry, rapid, or soggy rapid pulse. Therefore, formulas that treat these kinds of conditions will typically clear heat in the intestines, cool the blood, and disperse wind in order to resolve the disease. When wind, heat, dampness, and toxin are resolved, the disease should resolve.

Endogenous injury to spleen function is exemplified by symptoms that arise below the navel. Symptoms that arise above the navel are attributed to the stomach. This kind of injury is often caused by unresolved emotional material haunting the patient and leading to a transverse rebellion or to spleen deficiency disorders. These can, over time, end in spleen and kidney yang deficiency and/or in heat accumulation in the intestines due to stasis from dampness and phlegm or to stasis from qi and blood deficiency, which

results in qi and blood stasis. These emotional injuries often begin in early childhood. The spleen (digestive fire) is the last system to consolidate in the young human body. Children are often fed improperly and with foods that they cannot yet assimilate.[18] This can lead to a lifetime of improper eating habits that are equated with comfort and nurturance on the emotional level. Early spleen deficiency caused by familial eating habits and familial emotional coping mechanisms through food choices can be handed down from generation to generation. Type II diabetes is a preventable condition that often begins with the early pattern of spleen deficiency that deepens through a lifetime of poor eating.

The spleen is the middle and the mother of the body.[19] It is most easily injured by neglect and poor parenting and by the lack of unconditional love in many families. The spleen's intimate relationship with the liver also feeds into this scenario. If the spleen function is weak, even when the liver is not reactive, it can invade transversely. This leaves the spleen weaker, which leads to blood deficiency and then to liver blood deficiency. If the liver blood is not sufficient then the liver will function less smoothly and possibly with more heat. It can then invade the spleen more forcefully and thus begins a vicious cycle. All of these stresses can lead to yin deficiency in the spleen, which also contributes to liver yin deficiency and thereby to the same pattern. Food and emotional nourishment are intimately connected. Changing dietary habits is a complex and life-changing path.

When these spleen patterns manifest, they generally do so with symptoms below the navel. Spleen dysfunction will manifest below the navel with sinking qi symptoms. Damp accumulations are a form of sinking spleen qi manifestation. Polyps are a form of damp accumulation that are partly the result of sinking spleen qi.

In transverse rebellion the symptoms of the spleen injury will manifest as combinations of excess and deficiency.[19] Inadequate food consumption, as in anorexia or bulimia, or in going too long between meals, sporadic eating, and then bingeing due to fluctuating blood sugar levels, is exceptionally hard on the middle burner and the spleen. The spleen and the middle jiao are four-square organs; they require routine, constancy, and regular nurturing.

The extremes cause serious injury to assimilative processes that may lead to food allergies, chronic constipation and/or loose stools, low digestive fire, qi and blood deficiency, kidney yang deficiency and issues with water metabolism. Water metabolism transportive and transformative deficiencies can lead to damp accumulations[20] that cause stasis and, therefore, heat. This heat stasis leads then to damp phlegm and then to substantial or substantive phlegm. Adenomatous polyps are a form of phlegm stasis. When they are smaller and newer formations they are purely phlegm accumulations. But when they are left untreated, they can transform into malignancy, especially in the presence of wind heat or toxin. Therefore, the internal and external contributions to colorectal cancer are intertwined and complex.

Spleen deficiency can also lead to sinking qi and dampness pouring down.[21] This inhibits the immunity of the mucosa of the large intestine. It also allows for pathogenic accumulations (polyps, anaerobic bacteria, increased bile acids), particularly intermittent diarrhea and constipation, both of which disrupt the bowel's ability to separate the pure from the impure, mucus in the stool, hemorrhoids, and blood stasis in the intestine. All of these problems either expose the intestinal wall to constant pathogens or scrape away the mucosal lining of the intestinal wall (as in diarrhea) lowering immunity. Accumulations of dampness and toxin injure the qi and enter the blood level and cause stasis, which leads to the development of polyps and toxins and malignancy.

RISK FACTORS

- Advancing age, over the age of 40: this may indicate an advancing spleen/kidney yang deficiency that leads to damp/phlegm stasis with associated toxin.
- Family history of colorectal cancer, especially first-degree relatives (Lynch syndrome type I); risk = 2–3 × higher
- Cancer family syndrome (Lynch syndrome type II); includes adenocarcinomas of the ovary, endometrium, breast, and pancreas: this may indicate an inherited disposition for a damp/phlegm constitution as all of these tumor tissue types are essentially damp/phlegm and secretory in nature.
- A personal or family history of multiple adenomatous polyps after age 10 (familial polyposis): this may indicate a constitutional characteristic of common dietary habits.
- Previous history of polyps of the colon or rectum: the underlying acquired environment has not yet been addressed.
- Inflammatory bowel syndrome (IBS), that is ulcerative colitis and ileitis (Crohn's disease); the risk in ulcerative colitis for colorectal cancer is 20 times the average; increased risk for ulcerative colitis occurs in gynecological cancer, prostate cancer, or any pelvic cancer where radiation therapy is utilised: IBS frequently indicates a liver/spleen disharmony, which needs long-term intervention as a preventive to colorectal cancer.
- Diet high in saturated fat and sugar and low in fiber and various nutrients, including calcium: see above.
- High consumption of charcoal-broiled foods: charbroiled foods change normal oils into carcinogenic substances through exposure to high heat and these then become wind heat toxins that transform normal bowel tissue.
- Chronic inactivity of the bowel and constipation: these can lead to a longer transit time and increased exposure of the bowel wall to toxins of various kinds depending on the diet.
- Asbestos exposure: asbestos is a known carcinogen and enters via the lungs and skin that are related to the large intestine in Five-Phase theory. Perhaps we could call asbestos a wind heat pathogen.

PATHOLOGY

Polyps gradually increase in size and disorganisation until they are able to invade the bowel wall and spread. There are two major groups:

- Non-neoplastic, which are further divided into:
  - hyperplastic
  - inflammatory
  - lymphoid.
- Neoplastic.

Neoplastic adenomas or polyps all have the potential to become malignant. Those with the highest probability of developing into a malignancy are those of greater size, those with a higher percentage of villous component, and those with a presence of dysplasia. The majority of colorectal cancers arise in pre-existing neoplastic polyps.[22]

Tubular adenomas are a type of neoplastic adenoma that account for 75% of all neoplastic polyps. They are generally found at or after the age of 60 and twice as often in men than in women. This type accounts for 75% of all distal colon cancers and for 50% of rectosigmoid colorectal cancers. There is a 40% chance of finding more of this type of colorectal cancer within 5 years of original diagnosis. Therefore, treatment for prevention is important. However, the overall incidence of this type of carcinoma is 3–5%, since these types of polyps, with proper monitoring, are usually found when small.

Villous adenomas are the least common type, the largest, and the most ominous. They are found equally in both sexes and usually around the age of 60–65 years. Of these, 75% are found in the rectum and rectosigmoid colon. This type can be found in precancerous lesions that harbor invasive cancers in 30% of cases. Villous adenomas are more frequently symptomatic. Rectal bleeding is common, and protein-rich mucus secretions indicate hypoproteinemia, hypoalbuminemia, or hypokalemia. It is also possible to find a combined type of polyp that contains tubulovillous components.

Familial polyposis syndrome refers to an inherited autosomal dominant type of polyposis. It is frequently identified between the ages of 20 and 30. There is a literal carpeting of the entire colon with polyps (500–2500). The majority are tubular and the rate of transformation to malignancy is very high; there is a 100% risk of cancer if they are not removed.[23]

Colorectal tumors usually appear either ulcerating (left-sided; 75% of all tumors) or stenosing or fungating (right-sided; 25% of all tumors). Adenocarcinomas make up 90% of colorectal tumors. These tumors consist of cuboidal or columnar epithelium with multiple degrees of differentiation. Mucinous adenocarcinoma is a histologic variant containing large quantities of extracellular mucus in the tumor.[24]

Colorectal cancer has a tendency for local invasion by circumferential growth and for lymphatic, hematogenous, transperitoneal, and perineural spread.[25] The most common site for non-lymphatic spread is the liver. It commonly metastasises to the lungs, bone, kidneys, adrenals, and brain.[26]

In the US, lesions are more common in the rectum and sigmoid, with a gradual increase in those in the right colon. This is probably due to the removal of suspicious-looking polyps via sigmoidoscopy. Left-sided colorectal cancer accounts for 62% of colorectal cancers. It begins as an in situ lesion, becomes annular, and then an encircling lesion. It produces 'napkin-ring' constrictions, which are an early sign of obstruction. It may take 1 to 2 years to totally encircle the lumen of the bowel. These lesions infiltrate the bowel wall, flatten, and then cause ulcerations of the mucosa.

Right-sided colorectal cancer accounts for 38% of colorectal cancers. This location tends to produce a lesion that is fungating with bulky cauliflower tumors that protrude into the lumen. They will eventually circumvent the bowel wall, extend into the mesentery, and spread to the regional nodes and distant sites. Because the cecum is large and capacious, right-sided colorectal cancer does not usually cause obstruction and remains clinically silent for long periods of time.

CLINICAL PRESENTATION

Symptoms will vary depending on the anatomic region involved. Early stages may be asymptomatic or there may be vague complaints of abdominal distention, pain and bloating with flatulence. The presentation may look like a peptic ulcer or gallbladder disease or spleen deficiency of various types. Minor changes in the bowel movement, with or without rectal bleeding, may be seen but are often ignored. Colorectal cancer occurring on the left side of the colon can cause constipation alternating with diarrhea, abdominal pain, and thin stools (pencil stools). There may be nausea and vomiting. Qi circulation throughout the gastrointestinal tube is generally downward. If the lower end of the tube is obstructed, this causes the qi at the other end to flush upward and this causes nausea. Right-sided lesions produce vague abdominal aching and may also be palpable. Anemia resulting from bleeding may accompany right-sided colorectal cancer. As a result, there may be weakness and weight loss. Pelvic pain usually indicates that the lesion has infiltrated nerve tissue. This is a sign of later stage disease.

DIAGNOSIS AND SCREENING

Fecal occult blood tests (FOBTs) are of great use in detecting bleeding from lesions. Those using guaiac, which detects the peroxidase-like capacity of hemoglobin, are inexpensive and easy to perform. However, a false-negative rate of up to 30% is possible because intermittent bleeding is typical and this type of FOBT requires blood to be present at the time of the testing. Newer FOBTs, including Hemoccult SENSA and HemoQuant appear to have better sensitivity.[27] Using these types of tests has decreased the mortality rate from colorectal cancer in Europe by 33%. Digital rectal examination (DRE), can detect lesions up to 7 cm from the anal verge. The American Cancer Society (ACS) has recommended that this procedure be done once a year after the age of 40 and in populations at high risk.[28]

Proctosigmoidoscopy uses a flexible 60 cm sigmoidscope. Almost 50% of all colorectal cancer is within reach of this scope.

Colonoscopy provides information about the mucosal lining of the entire colon, except perhaps the cecum. It can be used to collect biopsy specimens and allows for excision of adenomatous polyps. There are some blind corners and mucosal folds that limit the effectiveness of colonoscopy and sometimes the cecum cannot be reached. But colonoscopy remains the definitive tool for diagnosis after positive screening tests.

Barium enemas can have a false-negative rate of 2–18% owing to misreading, poor preparation, and difficulties in detecting smaller lesions.[26]

Beta-2 microglobulin and CA 19-9 may be a sensitive indicator of tumor bulk and may indicate metastasis. Carcinoembryonic antigen (CEA) levels are directly related to the size of the primary tumor and the extent of spread. Higher CEA levels have been found in 19–40% of colorectal cancers that are detected earlier. Of large metastatic neoplasms, 100% have elevated CEA. The CEA can also be elevated in lung, breast, ovary, bladder and prostate cancers. It is also elevated in other disease like alcoholic cirrhosis, pancreatitis, and ulcerative colitis. Its greatest use is in assessing possible recurrence after resection. If total removal has been accomplished the CEA level will disappear. Its return is a highly probable indicator of recurrence. It can also be a rough indicator of the effectiveness of chemotherapy.[29]

DIAGNOSES ACCORDING TO CHINESE MEDICINE

In patients who appear to be at higher risk for colorectal cancer it is advisable to refer them for screening to their primary care provider. Those who would be considered at risk are patients with signs and symptoms of spleen deficiency that have persisted for more than 6 months (a careful history is very important), in combination with having eaten a poor diet for a long period of time, who have a family history of colorectal cancer, are pre-diabetic or diabetic, whose stools have changed over the past 6 months, and who have many of the risk factors stated earlier for colorectal cancer. Final diagnosis relies on conventional screening tools but, as complementary providers see their patients more frequently, it is our responsibility to advise patients when conventional screening is in their best interest.

Although intestinal wind and organ toxin are underlying evolutionary elements in colorectal cancer, once a patient has been diagnosed there are five different discernable patterns associated with the diagnosis.

1. DAMP HEAT

Signs and symptoms

- Paroxysms of abdominal pain.
- Dysentery.
- Tenesmus.
- Possible fever and aversion to cold.
- Mun.

- Thirst.
- Tongue: a yellow greasy coat and probable red body.
- Pulse: slippery and rapid.

Treatment principles

- Clear heat, drain dampness.

Formula

Huai hua di yu tang jia jian[30,31]

huai hua (Sophorae Flos; *Sophora* flowers)	10 g
di yu (Sanguisorbae Radix; *Sanguisorba*)	10 g
mu tou hui (Patriniae Herba; *Patrinia*)	30 g
ma chi xian (Portulacae Herba; *Portulaca*)	30 g
huang bai (Phellodendri Cortex; *Phellodendron* cortex)	10 g
yi ren (Coicis Semen; *Coix lacryma-jobi*)	30 g

Huai hua cools the blood and stops bleeding. It is especially good for clearing damp heat in the large intestine. It has the added advantage of lowering the blood pressure and lowering cholesterol. Di yu also cools the blood and stops bleeding and can help to stop diarrhea. Mu tou hui (bai jiang cao; Thlaspi/Patriniae Herba) clears heat and toxic heat and pus. It also moves and regulates blood that has been congealed by heat. Ma chi xian cools the blood, clears heat and toxins, and controls diarrhea. Huang bai clears heat, dries dampness, especially in the lower jiao, eliminates toxins and has the added advantage of reducing ascending kidney fire (HTN). While it dries dampness, as in damp heat, it is also an astringent and helps to protect normal fluids, an important action in a yin-deficient patient. Yi ren promotes urination and filters out dampness while benefiting the spleen. It clears damp heat and is antineoplastic, especially in gastrointestinal cancers.

2. TOXIN ACCUMULATION[32]

Signs and symptoms

- Irritable heat.
- Thirst.

- Diarrhea with purulent bloody feces.
- Tenesmus.
- Low abdominal pain and cramping.
- Tongue: purple body with yellow coat and ecchymotic spots, may be red points.
- Pulse: thready and rapid.

Treatment principles

Regulate stasis and clear toxins.

Formula

Tao hong si wu tang jia jian (from the Golden Mirror of the Medical Tradition)

dang gui wei (Angelicae sinensis radicis Cauda; *Angelica sinensis* lateral roots; tangkuei tail)	10 g
bai shao (Paeoniae Radix alba; *Paeonia* lactiflora root)	20 g
tao ren (Persicae Semen; *Prunus* ssp. seed)	10 g
hong hua (Carthami Flos; *Carthamnus tinctorius* flowers)	10 g
jin yin hua (Lonicerae Flos; *Lonicera* flowers)	20 g
mu tou hui (Patriniae Herba; *Patrinia*)	35 g

Dang gui wei is a blood-nourishing herb that is also blood-regulating when the tails of the root bulb are used. It helps to relieve spasm and pain. It cannot be used in this diagnosis in high quantity because it also moistens the stool. If diarrhea persists the formula must be modified. Bai shao nourishes the blood and consolidates the yin, which is an important adjustment to be made when treating toxin. Bai shao also adjusts the ying and wei levels helping to protect against infection in a serious condition. It calms the liver and helps to relieve irritability and pain. Tao ren regulates the blood and is antineoplastic in abdominal tumors. Because it is an oily seed it also must be used with caution when diarrhea is present. It is analgesic and its blood-regulating and blood 'cracking' capacity helps open the tumor to allow chemotherapeutic agents better access.

Hong hua regulates the blood and relieves pain, is mildly antineoplastic, and will help to prevent the formation of adhesions. Jin yin hua clears heat and toxins, clears damp heat in the lower jiao, and dispels wind heat, which is one of the underlying pathogenic components in colorectal cancer. It can lower fevers and is antiviral, antifungal, and antibacterial. It is also antineoplastic in some cancers. Mu tou hui (bai jiang cao; Thlaspi/Patriniae Herba) clears heat and toxin, vitalises the blood congealed by heat, dissipates pus, and is antineoplastic.

3. SPLEEN AND KIDNEY YANG DEFICIENCY

Signs and symptoms

- Cold limbs.
- Loose stools.
- Shortness of breath.
- Abdominal pain better with heat and pressure.
- Cock-crow diarrhea.
- Tongue: pale body with thin white coat or no coat.
- Pulse: deep thready, weak.

Treatment principles

- Warm and tonify the spleen and kidneys.

Formula

Shen ling bai zhu san[33] plus Si shen wan[34] jia jian

dang shen (Codonopsis Radix; *Codonopsis pilosula* root)	30 g
bai zhu (Atractylodis macrocephalae Rhizoma; *Atractylodes macrocephala*)	15 g
fu ling (Poria; *Poria cocos*)	20 g
yi ren (Coicis Semen; *Coix lacryma-jobi*)	30 g
rou dou kou (Myristicae Semen; *Myristica fragrans*; nutmeg seed)	10 g
bu gu zhi (Psoraleae Fructus; *Psoralea*)	15 g
wu zhu yu (Evodiae Fructus; *Evodia*)	10 g
he zi (Chebulae Fructus; *Terminalia chebula* fruit)	10 g

Dang shen, bai zhu, and fu ling form the basis of the formula, Si jun zi tang. The doses are slightly different but this formula is the main middle jiao or spleen tonic formula. Yi yi ren supports the spleen to drain dampness; it is also antineoplastic, hence the large dose. Fu ling is also antineoplastic and will increase natural killer (NK) cells, white blood cells (WBCs), and phagocytosis.

Fu ling, yi ren, he zi, and bu gu zhi are the main antineoplastic herbs in the formula. Spleen and kidney yang deficient patterns generally imply that one is seeing a later-stage presentation. Therefore, the antineoplastics in this formula for late stage disease are milder and less about clearing toxin. They are more about draining and astringing in order to provide a palliative treatment that helps the patient live longer and more comfortably.

Rou dou kou astringes the intestines and controls diarrhea. It warms the spleen and circulates qi in the middle jiao and helps to reduce pain. Along with bu gu zhi, it is especially good at treating diarrhea caused by spleen and kidney yang deficiency. Bu gu zhi is also one of the herbs highest in genistein, an anticancer substance. Bu gu zhi is a kidney yang tonic herb. Wu zhu yu dispels cold and relieves pain. It warms the spleen to stop diarrhea caused by cold stasis and dampness in the middle jiao. Wu zhu yu can also be used to treat oral candidiasis and ulcers when present as a result of chemotherapy. He zi is an astringent herb that helps to treat diarrhea. It protects the mucosal lining of the digestive tract and is antineoplastic in colorectal cancer.

4. KIDNEY AND LIVER YIN DEFICIENCY

Signs and symptoms

- Five centers heat.
- Dizziness and blurred vision.
- Bitter taste.
- Dry throat.
- Low back pain.
- Constipation.
- Tongue: red and dry.
- Pulse: wiry and thready, possibly rapid.

Treatment principles

- Nourish the yin of the liver and kidneys, clear heat and toxin.

Formula

Special formula

zhi mu (Anemarrhenae Rhizoma; *Anemarrhena*)	15 g

huang bai (Phellodendri Cortex;   15 g
    Phellodendron cortex)

shu di (Rehmanniae Radix preparata;   15 g
    Rehmannia)

gou qi zi (Lycii Fructus; *Lycium*   20 g
    chinensis fruit)

nu zhen zi (Ligustri lucidi   20 g
    Fructus; *Ligustrum lucidum*
    fruit)

fu ling (Poria; *Poria cocos*)   20 g

ze xie (Alismatis Rhizoma;   15 g
    Alisma)

This formula resembles Zhi bai di huang wan,[35] the main formula for treating yin deficiency heat. This formula nourishes yin and also clears heat. Zhi mu clears heat and fire from the qi level. It also generates fluids, an important contribution in this diagnostic pattern. When coupled with huang bai, it clears deficiency heat. Huang bai reduces ascending kidney deficient fire, eliminates toxins and clears heat and dries dampness in the lower jiao. Shu di nourishes the blood and the liver and kidney yin. It also has some antineoplastic actions. Gou qi zi nourishes the blood and the yin of the liver and kidney. Nu zhen zi also nourishes the yin of the liver and kidneys. It can increase the WBCs during chemotherapy and radiation therapy. It is also antineoplastic and is a cardiotonic that may be an advantage with some chemotherapeutic agents that are cardiotoxic.

Fu ling is a mushroom that drains dampness. It benefits the spleen and harmonises the middle jiao, and calms the spirit. It is antineoplastic, increases WBC counts, phagocytosis, and is mildly analgesic. Ze xie promotes urination and filters dampness. It also drains deficiency fire, its main use in this presentation.

5. QI AND BLOOD DEFICIENCY

Signs and symptoms

- Shortness of breath.
- General fatigue.
- Frequent loose stools or watery diarrhea.
- Pallor.
- Prolapse of various kinds.
- Hemorrhoids (sinking spleen qi).
- Tongue: very pale or even white.
- Pulse: thready or even minute.

Treatment principles

- Tonify qi and nourish the blood.

Formula

Ba zhen tang[36] plus Dang gui bu xue tang[37] jia jian

dang gui (Angelicae sinensis Radix;   15 g
    Angelica sinensis)

bai shao (Paeoniae Radix alba;   15 g
    Paeonia lactiflora root)

shu di (Rehmanniae Radix   10 g
    preparata; *Rehmannia*)

tai zi shen (Pseudostellariae Radix;   30 g
    Pseudostellaria heterophylla)

bai zhu (Atractylodis macrocephalae   12 g
    Rhizoma; *Atractylodes macrocephala*)

fu ling (Poria; *Poria cocos*)   15 g

huang qi (Astragali Radix; *Astragalus*   30 g
    membranaceus)

dan shen (Salviae miltiorrhizae   30 g
    Radix; *Salvia miltiorhiza* root)

Dang gui, bai shao, and shu di are all blood-nourishing herbs. When combined with tai zi shen, bai zhu, and fu ling they form a variation of Ba zhen tang. Without the qi tonic herbs, the blood-nourishing herbs in this presentation might be too cloying. The high dose of tai zi shen, a qi tonic and neutral temperature, helps the middle jiao to assimilate the phytochemical components of the blood-nourishing herbs. Huang qi at high dose also tonifies the middle jiao, the source of qi and blood. *Astragalus* increases the WBC and RBC counts and, thereby, increases immune function. It is also an excellent wound-healing herb and this formula might be appropriate post-surgery in some cases. Dan shen is added here for two reasons; it makes sure that blood stasis does not occur in the deficient environment, and it increases access of the chemotherapeutic regimen to the tumor by increasing circulation. In this sense it is an antineoplastic herb in this formula.

These diagnostic patterns are the basis of the Chinese medical approach. It is important in adjunctive care to include portions of the correct pattern formula when treating in relation to all of the conventional medical interventions. The conventional treatment will work cytotoxically to eliminate the cancer itself; the Chinese medical treatment will interface with those treatments and also treat the overall environment in which the cancer evolved. Treating the overall environment is immensely important in treatment outcomes and in prevention of recurrence. It must begin as soon as possible and continue throughout treatment.

There are times when treating only to ameliorate side effects may be necessary in order to allow the patient to remain on schedule with conventional treatment. This is especially important, for example, during chemotherapy, when the whole thrust of the treatment is to kill off any micrometastatic disease. Timing is important in this task and skipping an infusion because blood levels are low, or for other reasons, is a difficult interference in staying on top of the cancer. However, in the long term, treating the environment in which the cancer came about is immensely important and must be reinstituted as soon as possible.

POST–SURGICAL FORMULAE

LI QI KUAN CHANG TANG (RECTIFY QI AND LOOSEN THE INTESTINE DECOCTION)

Abdominal surgery of any kind, and particularly of the intestinal tube, will shut down peristalsis. It is important, even when there has been a resection and anastomosis of the bowel, to re-establish normal bowel function. Rectifying the qi flows relative to digestion will aid in rehabilitation and healing. The following formula adjusts all of the qi flows, nourishes the blood and stops bleeding, improves appetite, and warms the lower jiao. Warming the lower jiao is important because the surgical procedure opens the abdomen and allows exposure to cooler air and fluids. This is part of what slows or disinhibits peristalsis.

dang gui (Angelicae sinensis Radix; *Angelica sinensis*)   15 g

xiang fu (Cyperi Rhizoma; *Cyperus rotundus* rhizome)   10 g

chuan xiong (Chuanxiong Rhizoma; *Ligusticum wallichii* root)   10 g

chen pi (Citri reticulatae Pericarpium; *Citrus reticulata* pericarp)   10 g

bai shao (Paeoniae Radix alba; *Paeonia lactiflora* root)   10 g

huang qi (Astragali Radix; *Astragalus membranaceus*)   15 g

wu yao (Linderae Radix; *Lindera*)   10 g

hou po (Magnoliae officinalis Cortex; *Magnolia officinalis* cortex)   10 g

zhi gan cao (Glycyrrhizae Radix; *Glycyrrhiza uralensis* pan fried)   8 g

Dang gui is a blood-nourishing herb, which also gently moves the blood by increasing its volume. It works with chuan xiong and bai shao to re-establish normal blood levels where blood has been lost due to surgical trauma. Dang gui, bai shao, and huang qi all work together to heal the anastomosis and the surgical wound. Xiang fu regulates the qi flows of the whole digestive tract and works with chen pi to regulate the qi in the middle jiao. Many channels are broken during the surgical procedure. The abdomen is laid open and colder air is allowed to penetrate the lower jiao. This stops peristalsis. Qi-regulating herbs help to re-establish the channels and the normal flow of spleen qi upward, stomach qi downward, and the liver/gallbladder qi in a circular direction. It cannot be overstressed how important it is to manage the qi at this time. Acupuncture is very beneficial.

Wu yao is a warming herb, especially to the lower jiao. Warming the intestines enables all of the other actions of this formula to engage. Wu yao also protects the lower jiao from cold and wind invasion. Hou po promotes qi circulation, descends the qi, warms and transforms phlegm in all three jiaos, and disperses food stagnation. It enables the patient to regain normal nutritional status and promotes bowel function. All of the herbs in the formula help to re-establish normal bowel function.

During the time prior to surgery it is appropriate to treat the main constitutional diagnosis for the cancer. The patient has not yet started chemotherapy unless there is an effort to use this form of cytotoxic therapy to reduce a tumor. Therefore, there is no need to interface with side effects of chemotherapy. This time should be utilised for treatment of the cancer itself and to help and address any symptomatic issues. This formula anticipates the injuries caused by surgical trauma. Blood-nourishing herbs are used to reduce blood loss without increasing bleeding. Qi tonics help to reduce swelling and aide in the healing of the wound for better recovery and reduced risk of infection.

After surgery it is important to prevent the formation of adhesions that are a form of blood stasis and also contribute to local blood stasis. Since blood stasis is part of the end process of cancer formation, one way to prevent recurrence is to prevent blood stasis by maintaining the normal flow of qi and blood.

BU ZHONG YI QI TANG[19]

Surgery for colorectal cancer is quite extensive and, therefore, a period of time anywhere from 2 weeks to 1 month is given prior to chemotherapy for the patient to recuperate. This time gives the body a period in which to heal from the surgical trauma and to re-establish normal qi and blood flow and rebuild qi and blood. A very common formula to aid in this process follows.

huang qi (Astragali Radix; *Astragalus membranaceus*)	20 g
chai hu (Bupleuri Radix; *Bupleurum*)	10 g
dang shen (Codonopsis Radix; *Codonopsis pilosula* root)	15 g
sheng ma (Cimicifugae Rhizoma; *Cimicifuga*)	10 g
bai zhu (Atractylodis macrocephalae Rhizoma; *Atractylodes macrocephala*)	12 g
chen pi (Citri reticulatae Pericarpium; *Citrus reticulata* pericarp)	5 g
dang gui (Angelicae sinensis Radix; *Angelica sinensis*)	10 g
zhi gan cao (Glycyrrhizae Radix; *Glycyrrhiza uralensis* pan fried)	5 g

The previous formula can be used with Xiao yao san:[38]

bai zhu (Atractylodis macrocephalae Rhizoma; *Atractylodes macrocephala*)	10 g
chai hu (Bupleuri Radix; *Bupleurum*)	10 g
fu ling (Poria; *Poria cocos*)	10 g

dang gui (Angelicae sinensis Radix; *Angelica sinensis*)	10 g
bai shao (Paeoniae Radix alba; *Paeonia lactiflora* root)	10 g
bo he (Menthae haplocalycis Herba; *Mentha haplocalyx*)	5 g

The modified combination of these two formulas together will lift, tonify, smooth, and regulate the qi. Also the blood-nourishing and qi tonics in the formulas will nourish the blood and move it in a way so as to prevent stasis without precipitating bleeding. The actual amounts of the herbs in the combined formula will depend on the needs of the patient for whom it is being written. Some patients may need a higher dose of qi tonics and others may enter surgery already anemic and will require more blood nourishing. If constipation persists, then more qi tonics and mild laxatives may be needed to further modify the formula. When the diaphragm is stopped during abdominal surgery, this interferes with the lung qi circulation. Some forms of constipation are the result of the lung and colon losing their relationship as coupled organs. Jie geng acts as a bridge in this case to get the colon peristalsis engaged again.

During this post-surgery time, and depending on the regimen that is planned for the given patient, it is still important to address the constitutional diagnosis for the cancer. A small part of the constitutional formula may be given as part of the above combined formula. For example, if the constitutional diagnosis for the cancer is damp heat, then lower jiao damp heat draining herbs can be added to modify the formula for post-surgery. Another example would be to add herbs that are specific to blood stasis or damp phlegm, depending on the constitutional diagnosis, and then combine specifically anticancer herbs for colorectal cancer. If damp phlegm is part of the constitutional diagnosis, then gua lou shi (Trichosanthis Fructus; *Trichosanthes* fruit) and tian nan xing (Arisaematis Rhizoma preparatum; *Arisaema erubescens* rhizome) would be good additions.

RADIATION TREATMENT

Radiation burns local tissue and, as a result, causes scarring. Scarring and adhesions are considered to be forms of blood stasis. The main injury in radiation is blood stasis in the long term and yin deficiency, qi deficiency, and wei qi deficiency in the shorter term. The immediate response will result in local pain and burning, erythematosus, and then scarring and adhesions. Often systemic reactions look like qi and yin deficiency. In radiation to the colon, acute to chronic diarrhea is a manifestation of these injuries and can even persist for years after the end of the intervention. Radiation is cumulative in effect. On the positive side, this means that protection against local recurrence can persist for some time. On the negative side, it means that the side effects can become more severe over time, usually up to 4–6 months, or longer in radiation therapy for colorectal cancer.

It is very important to monitor for signs and symptoms of radiation injury. It is also much easier to prevent these injuries than it is to treat them after the fact. Many side effects are not preventable and must be managed over the long term. Good management can change long-term quality of life. Some signs that there is radiation injury in colorectal cancer include lower abdominal aching, irregular stools, urinary dysfunction, chronic and frequent diarrhea. In women who have been treated with radiation there may be a disturbance of the normal menstrual cycle if they are not or have not been made menopausal by treatment.

A formula that is specifically yin-nourishing may be required to heal and resolve injuries from radiation. Local application can be applied in the case of rectal cancer where local irradiation is commonly used as primary treatment. Suppositories made from a base of cocoa butter and infused with vitamin E or with aloe vera are used. These can be used at night when the patient is in a prone position and danger of leakage due to gravity is lessened. Retention enema can also be used as long as the anastomosis is completely healed and there is no friability of the bowel wall that might allow the pressure of added fluid to break through the wall. This might require a conversation with the surgeon or medical oncologist to determine. This technique can be used if a patient is having bowel movements without pain or bleeding. Variations of the following herbs can be combined in groups of four to five herbs that can be powdered and

infused in a suppository, or decocted in crude herb form to use as a retention enema:

mai dong (Ophiopogonis Radix; Ophiopogon)	15 g
shu di (Rehmanniae Radix preparata; Rehmannia)	15 g
tian dong (Asparagi Radix; Asparagus)	15 g
zhi mu (Anemarrhenae Rhizoma; Anemarrhena)	10 g
bei sha shen (Glehniae Radix; Glehnia)	15 g
nu zhen zi (Ligustri lucidi Fructus; Ligustrum lucidum fruit)	20 g
he shou wu (Polygoni multiflori Radix preparata; Polygonum multiflorum root)	15 g
bai hua she she cao (Hedyotis diffusae Herba; Oldenlandia)	20 g
gou qi zi (Lycii Fructus; Lycium chinensis fruit)	10 g
ban zhi lian (Scutellariae barbatae Herba; Scutellaria barbata)	20 g

The herbs listed can be used as a formula for oral use to treat the yin deficiency caused by radiation to the abdomen. Of course, it must be modified to treat the presentation of the patient. If chronic diarrhea is present, as is common, then this formula will need to be modified to slow the stool. However, it is well to remember that the primary cause of the diarrhea in this case is yin deficiency. A nutritional approach to frequent acute diarrhea caused by radiation is the use of fresh aloe vera juice; 100 ml drunk four times daily will help to heal the burns from radiation therapy. Fresh aloe juice can be purchased at many natural food stores (it is kept in the refrigerator section).

Mai dong, tian dong, sha shen, and nu zhen zi are all yin-nourishing herbs. He shou wu, gou qi zi, and shu di are all blood-nourishing herbs. Yin- and blood-nourishing herbs potentiate each other. The blood-nourishing herbs can help to prevent the formation of adhesions through their mild blood-regulating effect. Zhi mu is a clear heat herb that also generates fluids. It might seem strange to use yin-nourishing herbs to treat chronic diarrhea, however, in this case, it is exactly what is required to heal the tissue injured by radiation burns. Until this tissue can heal there will be an inability of the bowel to function properly through peristalsis, absorption of fluids, and the normal formation of stool. Bai hua she she cao and ban zhi lian are both antineoplastic herbs that clear heat and help to prevent recurrence.

RETENTION ENEMA

The herbs listed can also be used in smaller portions and, as stated earlier, as a retention enema. To retain an enema the colon must first be cleared of all fecal matter at least to the level of the splenic juncture. This may require a few passes with clean and warm water until all that is being released is clear fluid from the enema water. Have the patient lie on the left side and apply the water until the descending colon is clean. Then rolling the patient onto the back, apply the water again in the same way to clear as much as possible from the transverse colon. To reiterate, in the case of post-surgical care, it is important not to stress the anastomosis or any other surgical injures. If there is concern that injury will occur, do not use this technique.

After the colon is cleared, apply the decocted formula as high as possible and in a quantity to comfortably fill the sigmoid colon. The decocted fluid should be warm or body temperature. Hotter fluid may stimulate a release or may burn the bowel wall. If possible, the fluid should be retained for several hours, even overnight. The amount of water used for the decoction and the enema should equal approximately two quarts. Do not overfill the bowel. Do not use this technique if it is too difficult for the patient. Some patients will do well and others will not.

The value of an herbal retained enema is that a higher dose of herbal material can be delivered systemically and locally. The phytochemicals will cross the bowel wall and be absorbed locally into the vessels. This will help to heal the radiation damage and also treat the cancer and prevent spread of the cancer.

SUPPOSITORIES

Suppositories are made with clean and non-rancid cocoa butter. The cocoa butter is melted at low heat on the stove. Then herbs or vitamin E or other substances of your choice are added to the melted cocoa butter. If herbs are added, they must be as finely powdered as possible. This allows for more exposure of the whole area to the powdered herb. Then the melted cocoa butter is poured into a mold and refrigerated to harden. Molds can be purchased or made as needed. The suppositories are wrapped in foil or another wrapper to keep them clean and airtight. They are refrigerated until use. Body temperature will melt the cocoa butter and spread the preparation internally. This is why it is best to deliver the preparation to the area while the patient is lying prone.

CHEMOTHERAPY

The main chemotherapeutic regimen for colorectal cancer is 5-FU plus levamisole[39,40] Levamisole (an anthelmintic) and/or Leucovorin are added as chemotherapy-enhancing drugs to potentiate 5-FU in the treatment of CRC. The side effects are:[41]

- myelosuppression: anemia, leukopenia, thrombocytopenia, with a general nadir at 14 days post-infusion
- nausea and vomiting
- stomatitis
- diarrhea
- gastrointestinal bleeding
- renal toxicity
- cardiac arrhythmias and possible myocardial infarction
- headache and visual disturbance
- hair loss and skin hyperpigmentation
- maculopapular rash.

The evidence of injury from the point of view of Chinese medicine is written in these side effects. The main injuries are to the spleen and kidney levels of blood production, to the stomach qi from the cold nature of the clear toxin drugs, to the kidney/heart axis, and to the liver and kidney yin. Therefore, a herbal formula to address these injuries is necessary in order to support the normal function systemically and to allow for normal nutrition, normal blood levels, renal and cardio-protection, and any symptoms that may be particular to the patient. A representative formula follows:

huang qi (Astragali Radix; *Astragalus membranaceus*) — 20 g

mai dong (Ophiopogonis Radix; *Ophiopogon*) — 15 g

tian dong (Asparagi Radix; *Asparagus*) — 15 g

gou qi zi (Lycii Fructus; *Lycium chinensis* fruit) — 15 g

shu di (Rehmanniae Radix preparata; *Rehmannia*) — 12 g

ji xue teng (Spatholobi Caulis; *Spatholobus suberectus*) — 20 g

tai zi shen (Pseudostellariae Radix; *Pseudostellaria heterophylla*) — 15 g

zhu ling (Polyporus; *Polyporus – Grifola*) — 15 g

gan jiang (Zingiberis Rhizoma; *Zingiber officinale*) — 8 g

wu wei zi (Schisandrae Fructus; *Schisandra*) — 10 g

rou dou kou (Myristicae Semen; *Myristica fragrans*; nutmeg seeds) — 10 g

ban zhi lian (Scutellariae barbatae Herba; *Scutellaria barbata*) — 25 g

bai hua she she cao (Hedyotis diffusae Herba; *Oldenlandia*) — 30 g

xian he cao (Agrimoniae Herba; *Agrimonia pilosa* var. *japonica*; agrimony) — 15 g

hong da zao (Jujubae Fructus; *Ziziphus jujuba*; red jujube) — 10 g

Huang qi is a qi tonic herb that increases WBC and RBC counts by tonifying the spleen. Mai dong and tian dong are yin-nourishing herbs that are potentiated by the blood-nourishing herbs gou qi zi, shu di, and ji xue teng. Tai zi shen is a neutral temperature qi tonic that tonifies the lung and spleen and also generates fluids. Zhu ling is a drain damp herb that is a mushroom and acts somewhat like fu ling (Poria; *Poria cocos*) in a tonic formula by benefiting the spleen to prevent the formation of dampness when using qi tonic herbs. It also has immunomodulating properties and is used to increase WBC counts, NK cells, and to act antineoplastically.

Gan jiang is a dried form of ginger that can help to ameliorate nausea. It works with rou dou kou to warm the middle jiao and prevent chemotherapy-induced nausea. It also works well with the qi tonic herbs that increase blood cells and tonify the middle jiao to protect the spleen from chemotherapy-induced injury. Wu wei zi is an astringent that helps protect the yin from the drying effect of the qi tonics, which are warm. Ban zhi lian and bai hua she she cao are both antineoplastics that potentiate the effect of 5-FU and levamisole. Xian he cao is a stop-bleeding herb that does so by cooling the blood. Here it is the third antineoplastic herb that is also a cardioprotective herb. Hong (red) da zao is used as a harmonising herb that also tonifies the spleen qi to enable it to improve the spleen's ability to absorb and assimilate the formula.

For severe nausea and vomiting add the following herbs to the above formula or use as a separate formula during the period when nausea is most severe, i.e. for the 5 days post-chemotherapy. Then start the patient again on the original formula.

xuan fu hua (Inulae Flos; *Inula* flowers [wrapped]) — 10 g

zhi ban xia (Pinelliae Rhizoma preparatum; *Pinellia ternata* rhizome) — 10 g

yu zhu (Polygonati odorati Rhizoma; *Polygonatum odoratum*) — 15 g

chen pi (Citri reticulatae Pericarpium; *Citrus reticulata* pericarp) — 10 g

mu xiang (Aucklandiae Radix; *Saussurea*) — 10 g

zhu ru (Bambusae Caulis in taeniam; *Phyllostachys nigra*) — 10 g

shen qu (Massa medicata fermentata; medicated leaven) — 30 g

Xuan fu hua is a warming herb that transforms cold phlegm, a result of spleen injury caused by cold and bitter clear toxin chemotherapy. It redirects the qi downward, stops vomiting, and has the added benefit of softening hardness. Ban xia dries dampness and transforms phlegm, conducts rebellious qi downward to stop vomiting, and is antineoplastic against phlegm tumors. Yu zhu nourishes the yin, especially of the lung and stomach, and increases body fluids. Although we are working to reduce phlegm and dampness as the main underlying causative factor in this nausea, it is important to protect the normal fluids of the stomach and upper digestive tract. Patients suffering from nausea often cannot eat or drink; even water can cause nausea. Nourishing yin is always an important aspect of treatment for nausea.

Chen pi is a primary herb in regulating qi. It also tonifies the spleen, injury to which is part of the mechanism of nausea. It reverses the upward flow of qi to stop vomiting. Mu xiang promotes the circulation of qi in the spleen and stomach, harmonises the stomach, and regulates stagnant qi in the intestines. When antiemetic drugs are used to treat nausea they often have the side effect of causing constipation. This stasis at the far end of the digestive tube contributes to back flow and disrupts the downward flow of qi, thus contributing to nausea, the very symptom they are meant to treat. Mu xiang treats this side effect of many antiemetics and helps them to work better.

Zhu ru clears and dissolves hot phlegm. It helps to stop vomiting caused by heated phlegm that can be the result of stasis caused by damp or cold phlegm in the middle burner. Often the symptom of nausea can worsen with each round of chemotherapy. When the original stasis caused by cold phlegm is perpetuated it can transform to hot phlegm. Hence a combination of different approaches is included in this formula. Zhu li (Bambusae Succus; *Bambusa* dried sap) is a possible substitute in the place of zhu ru when hot phlegm is present or when a heart-calming herb is called for in this context. Finally, shen qu relieves food stagnation. It harmonises the stomach and aids in digestion. This herb enters the stomach and spleen. It is often a disharmony between stomach and spleen that causes nausea. The spleen becomes deficient and the stomach becomes excess, causing the stomach qi to flush upward. Harmonising the stomach/spleen axis, transforming damp or phlegm, moving food stagnation, and tonifying the middle jiao are all part of treating nausea and vomiting.

LATER-STAGE COLORECTAL CANCER

For recurrent and/or metastatic colorectal cancer, where resection or radiation is no longer an option or where chemotherapy is refused by the patient (as sometimes happens in later stage patients who have already been through several rounds of chemotherapy), it becomes necessary to find other options. In these later stage cases treatment is considered palliative, and quality-of-life issues are foremost for the patient and their family. These cases will generally include supporting the spleen and kidney yang, boosting the kidneys, regulating qi and blood to reduce pain, and clearing pathogenic heat. The following formula is generally appropriate.

TREATMENT PRINCIPLES

- Tonify spleen and kidney yang, regulate qi and move blood strongly, clear pathogenic heat, reduce pain.

huang qi (Astragali Radix; *Astragalus membranaceus*)	20 g
dang gui (Angelicae sinensis Radix; *Angelica sinensis*)	12 g
dang shen (Codonopsis Radix; *Codonopsis pilosula* root)	15 g
bai shao (Paeoniae Radix alba; *Paeonia lactiflora* root)	10 g
bai zhu (Atractylodis macrocephalae Rhizoma; *Atractylodes macrocephala*)	10 g
hong teng (Sargentodoxae Caulis; *Sargentodoxa cuneata*)	15 g
bai bian dou (Lablab Semen album; *Dolichos lablab* seeds)	15 g
bai hua she she cao (Hedyotis diffusae Herba; *Oldenlandia*)	20 g
yi zhi ren (Alpiniae oxyphyllae Fructus; *Alpinia oxyphylla* fruit)	10 g
ban zhi lian (Scutellariae barbatae Herba; *Scutellaria barbata*)	20 g
dan shen (Salviae miltiorrhizae Radix; *Salvia miltiorhiza* root)	10 g
gua lou ren (Trichosanthis Semen; *Trichosanthes* seed)	15 g
yi ren (Coicis Semen; *Coix lacryma-jobi*)	15 g
mu xiang (Aucklandiae Radix; *Saussurea*)	10 g
hong da zao (Jujubae Fructus; *Ziziphus jujuba*; red jujube)	5 g

Huang qi is an antineoplastic herb that tonifies the central qi and increases WBC and RBC counts. It also heals wounds and helps to prevent infection, both risk factors in later stage colorectal cancer where ulceration of the bowel leading to infection is common. Dang gui combines with huang qi to form a formula within the formula (Dang gui bu xue tang) to tonify the qi and blood. Dang shen and bai zhu are one-half of Si jun zi tang, the main formula to support the spleen. Bai shao nourishes the blood and also combines with huang qi to heal wounds and calm spasm. Therefore, it helps to stop pain. Hong teng clears heat and cools the blood. It moves blood and is antibacterial, thus helping to prevent infection. It is also mildly antineoplastic. Bai bian dou clears summer heat and tonifies the spleen to filter dampness. It can also help to relieve diarrhea.

Bai hua she she cao is a clear heat herb that is also antineoplastic. It is cardioprotective and also reduces damage to the liver (certain chemotherapies used in colorectal cancer may cause damage to both these organs). Yi zhi ren tonifies the yang of the spleen and kidneys and helps to stop diarrhea. It is astringent and helps to prevent diarrhea and the resulting dehydration. Ban zhi lian is a clear-heat-and-toxin herb that is antineoplastic. It clears blood heat and blood stasis to stop bleeding. Dan shen is a blood-cracking herb that breaks down the fibrinogen outer layer of a tumor and changes the viscosity of the blood to allow chemotherapy to enter a tumor. Here it is used to allow the other herbs in the formula to access all tissues and to treat pain. Gua lou ren clears heat and transforms hot phlegm. It dissipates phlegm-type accumulations and promotes the healing of abscesses and sores. It is antineoplastic and antibacterial. Care must be taken not to use too much of this seed in the formula as it can cause diarrhea (already present).

Yi ren is a drain damp herb that has many antineoplastic properties. It also supports the spleen and helps to prevent spleen yang deficiency and sinking spleen qi symptoms like diarrhea. Mu xiang regulates the qi of the spleen and stomach, alleviates pain, controls diarrhea, and harmonises the middle jiao to prevent stasis from tonic herbs. It is important to regulate the central qi using a formula that tonifies the spleen and kidney yang. Hong (red) da zao harmonises the formula, tonifies the middle jiao, and generally helps the medicine to go down.

After conventional treatment and assuming a state of remission, the patient will be seen periodically (in the beginning, every 3 months) by their oncologist or surgeon for monitoring of various markers, especially CEA[42] and the CA19-9.[43] A physical exam will be given at each visit, all palpable nodes will be palpated, a DRE may be given, possibly an abdominal ultrasound will be performed, and, on a less frequent basis, a chest X-ray and possibly an abdominal and pelvic computerised tomography (CT) scan will be given. Liver and kidney function tests may be administered via common blood chemistries since metastatic spread in the abdomen is not uncommon. Kidney function abnormalities can show obstructive disease around the ureters or in the kidneys. Raised transaminase levels can indicate possible liver metastases. A repeat colonoscopy may be performed if tumor markers indicate recurrence. Most recurrence of many cancers occurs during the first 2 years after the end of treatment. A period of a disease-free remission of 5 years is necessary for most cancers to be considered cured. Even though this period is considered extremely important in terms of recurrence, conventional care does not include any treatment for prevention. The following formula is used for this purpose along with instituting all of those dietary, lifestyle, and supplemental factors mentioned in the beginning of this chapter under causative or risk factors for colorectal cancer. It cannot be emphasised enough how important these things are, because colorectal cancer is generally a very preventable cancer when heritable issues are not present.

PREVENTION FORMULA

huang qi (Astragali Radix; *Astragalus membranaceus*)	30 g
tai zi shen (Pseudostellariae Radix; *Pseudostellaria* heterophylla)	20 g
bu gu zhi (Psoraleae Fructus; *Psoralea*)	15 g
dang shen (Codonopsis Radix; *Codonopsis pilosula* root)	15 g
nu zhen zi (Ligustri lucidi Fructus; *Ligustrum lucidum* fruit)	15 g
fu ling (Poria; *Poria cocos*)	15 g

tu si zi (Cuscutae Semen; *Cuscuta* seeds)	15 g	gou qi zi (Lycii Fructus; *Lycium chinensis* fruit)	15 g
bai zhu (Atractylodis macrocephalae Rhizoma; *Atractylodes macrocephala*)	10 g	zhi gan cao (Glycyrrhizae Radix; *Glycyrrhiza uralensis* pan fried)	8 g

Case study 3.1

Male, 53 years

Presentation

Abdominal pain, frequent stool four to five times per day mixed with blood and pus, diarrhea, mucus at the end of the stool, the blood is bright red without clots.

History

Stomach ulcer 10 years ago resolved with pharmaceutical treatment; hypertension controlled with medication; normal childhood illnesses; polyps; acid eructation and heartburn for several years; chronic constipation with dry stool; dizziness and thirst; low back pain; poor diet— high fat and greasy foods, few vegetables, high in ice cream and dairy; high in animal fats; little exercise; 30 lb overweight; work is high stress and sedentary.

Work-up

- Stool sampling for parasites: negative.
- Barium imaging: positive for 3 cm mass in transverse colon.
- Abdominal and pelvic CT: localised mass without metastatic spread has invaded the muscle layer but not beyond.
- Chest CT: negative.
- Liver and kidney function tests: normal.
- CEA = 13; CA19-9 = 25.
- Complete blood count (CBC): slight anemia; RBC = 3.5; haematocrit = 34.
- Tongue: slight red, swollen, yellow greasy coat striped in posterior area, vein distention: +3.
- Pulse: wiry, forceful, slight slippery, spleen position weakest.
- Hara: cool over spleen reflex area, hot over kidney area, lung area sticky and clammy, blood stasis reflex at mid and deep position tight and tender.

Symptoms

- Abdominal pain, especially with stool.
- Diarrhea with red blood.
- Thirst for cool drinks.
- Dizziness.

Diagnosis

- Damp heat with liver and kidney yin deficiency.

This patient has a long history of upper and middle digestive complaints. His lifestyle has contributed to an internal environment of yin deficiency. We know that a yin-deficient environment has a tendency to attract latent pathogenic factors inward and that damp heat can develop more readily as a latent pathogenic factor in this environment. These issues have evolved from spleen deficiency due to an improper diet and from yin deficiency due to a high stress and inactive lifestyle. No mechanism for discharge of emotion was developed, and the patient may have used food as a means of coping. These two factors led to hypertension. The use of pharmaceutical drugs, rather than lifestyle changes, to manage these conditions (the gastric ulcer and hypertension) probably contributed to the environment in which colorectal cancer came about. The hypertension in this case was due to liver and kidney yin deficiency and to the accumulation of plaque caused by phlegm heat. All of these conditions, and therefore the colorectal cancer, were preventable, as there was no family history or heritable genetic component to the diagnosis.

Prevention of recurrence is dependent upon helping this patient understand his relationship to food, exercise, stress reduction, and self-care. The same diet that would prevent cardiovascular disease in the patient will also prevent a recurrence of colorectal cancer. Diet and exercise,

Case study continues

a healthy work situation, and healthy relationships at work and at home are all part of the path of colon health for this patient. The changes toward prevention of recurrence and survival all must begin during conventional treatment. It is essential that patients start making dietary changes, changes in exercise habits, and reducing stress at the beginning of their treatment. This begins the most important aspect of changing the internal environment to one in which colorectal cancer does not occur. These changes will help improve the outcome of treatment and also the decrease the risk of recurrence. Patients must begin to understand the important role their own actions have in their health.

Surgical plan

Presurgery

1. Prevent spread by treating the constitutional diagnosis, using antineoplastic herbs, increasing immune function.
2. Reduce blood loss by mildly nourishing the blood and utilising mild blood-regulating herbs that prevent bleeding.
3. Stop swelling and pain by utilising blood- and qi-regulating herbs, tonifying qi and using antineoplastic herbs.
4. Treat the cancer to begin direct treatment; this is part of the first point.

Formula: Li qi kuan chang tang jia jian

dang gui (Angelicae sinensis Radix; *Angelica sinensis*)	15 g
xiang fu (Cyperi Rhizoma; *Cyperus rotundus* rhizome)	10 g
chuan xiong (Chuanxiong Rhizoma; *Ligusticum wallichii* root)	10 g
chen pi (Citri reticulatae Pericarpium; *Citrus reticulata* pericarp)	10 g
ce bai ye (Platycladi Cacumen; *Biota orientalis*)	10 g
tian hua fen (Trichosanthis Radix; *Trichosanthes* root)	20 g
wu yao (Linderae Radix; *Lindera*)	10 g
hou po (Magnoliae officinalis Cortex; *Magnolia officinalis* cortex)	10 g
bai shao (Paeoniae Radix alba; *Paeonia lactiflora* root)	10 g

huang qi (Astragali Radix; *Astragalus membranaceus*)	20 g

This formula has been analysed earlier in the chapter. Two herbs have been added: ce bai ye and tian hua fen. Ce bai ye cools the blood and stops bleeding. It is used here to stop bleeding from surgical trauma. Tian hua fen clears heat and toxins, transforms hot phlegm, generates fluids and is antineoplastic. It helps to prevent surgical spread of the cancer, it addresses the diagnosis of damp heat/phlegm heat, it helps to prevent dehydration post-surgically.

Post-surgery

1. Prevent spread.
2. Stop swelling and pain.
3. Reduce healing time.
4. Re-establish normal bowel function.
5. Treat the cancer.

Formula: Bu zhong yi qi tang

add:

huo ma ren* (Cannabis Semen; *Cannabis sativa* [sterilised] seeds)	15 g
zhe bei mu (Fritillariae thunbergii Bulbus; *Fritillaria thunbergii*)	10 g
yan hu suo (Corydalis Rhizoma; *Corydalis yanhusuo*)	15 g
bai jiang cao (Thlaspi/Patriniae Herba; *Thlaspi/Patrinia*)	20 g

Huo ma ren is a mild laxative. Zhe bei mu transforms hot phlegm and clears heat and dissipates masses that are phlegm in nature. It is antineoplastic. Yan hu suo is a blood-moving herb that is the main herb to relieve pain caused by blood stasis. It is also antineoplastic especially for abdominal tumors. Bai jiang cao clears heat and toxins while moving blood congealed by heat. It is also antineoplastic and will help to prevent gastrointestinal abscess and infection.

Chemotherapy plan

Post-surgically the tumor markers went down. They were still not in the normal range but it is common, once tumor debulking has occurred, for

Case study continues

the tumor markers to decrease. Gemcitabine is a chemotherapeutic agent used often in gastrointestinal cancers. Its side effects are neutropenia, thrombocytopenia, nausea, stomatitis, liver and renal toxicity. Gemcitabine was combined in this case with 5-FU, which has been the standard of care for colorectal cancer for several years. The side effects of 5-FU are leukopenia, thrombocytopenia, nausea, stomatitis, severe diarrhea, liver and renal toxicity, cardiotoxicity, lethargy, weakness and photophobia. Assessing this combination, it becomes clear that the treatment principles guiding the formula are to:

1. Maintain normal blood levels, especially RBC, WBC, and platelet counts.
2. Protect heart, kidney and liver function.
3. Maintain normal digestive function, especially prevent nausea and diarrhea.
4. Treat antineoplastically by potentiating the gemcitabine and the 5-FU and using antineoplastic herbs for colorectal cancer.
5. Treat the constitutional diagnosis (liver and kidney yin deficiency) and the Chinese medical cancer diagnosis (damp heat). Treating for damp heat in a yin-deficient constitution is a complex thing.

Formula

huai hua (Sophorae Flos; *Sophora* flowers)	15 g
di yu (Sanguisorbae Radix; *Sanguisorba*)	10 g
mu tou hui (Patriniae Herba; *Patrinia*)	30 g
ma chi xian (Portulacae Herba; *Portulaca*)	30 g
huang bai (Phellodendri Cortex; *Phellodendron* cortex)	15 g
yi ren (Coicis Semen; *Coix lacryma-jobi*)	30 g
zhi mu (Anemarrhenae Rhizoma; *Anemarrhena*)	15 g
shu di (Rehmanniae Radix preparata; *Rehmannia*)	15 g
nu zhen zi (Ligustri lucidi Fructus; *Ligustrum lucidum* fruit)	15 g
fu ling (Poria; *Poria cocos*)	20 g
bai hua she she cao (Hedyotis diffusae Herba; *Oldenlandia*)	20 g
huang qi (Astragali Radix; *Astragalus membranaceus*)	20 g
xian he cao (Agrimoniae Herba; *Agrimonia pilosa* var. *japonica*)	15 g
bu gu zhi (Psoraleae Fructus; *Psoralea*)	15 g
ji nei jin (Gigeriae galli Endothelium corneum; *Gallus gallus domesticus*; chicken gizzard lining)	15 g
zhi ban xia (Pinelliae Rhizoma preparatum; *Pinellia ternata* rhizome)	15 g
shen qu (Massa medicata fermentata; medicated leaven)	15 g

Huai hua cools the blood and stops bleeding. It clears damp heat from the lower jiao and also cools liver heat, thus treating elements of both the underlying diagnosis and the cancer pattern and protecting liver function. Di yu also cools the blood and controls bleeding. It helps to slow diarrhea and works well with huai hua to treat the dysentery-like symptoms of this cancer. Mu tou hui (or bai jiang cao) vitalises blood congealed by heat. It clears heat and toxin and dissipates pus; it is antineoplastic. Ma chi xian is a clear heat and toxin herb that also cools the blood and controls diarrhea. It clears damp heat toxins from the skin (epithelial tissue similar to the mucosal lining of the bowel wall—polyps are damp stasis masses). Huang bai clears damp heat from the lower jiao. It also brings down ascending kidney deficient fire and, therefore, treats both parts of the diagnosis. It also protects renal function. Yi ren is a drain dampness herb that seeps damp through benefiting the spleen. Yi ren is added here in high dose because it is also antineoplastic, especially for damp phlegm masses. Mu tou hui, ma chi xian, yi ren, and bai hua she she cao are the main antineoplastics in this formula and help to potentiate the chemotherapeutic regimen by detoxifying damp phlegm toxin.

Zhi mu is a clear heat herb that generates fluids, which in a yin-deficient patient is important. It not only treats the yin-deficient heat, it also helps to protect yin while clearing damp heat. Nu zhen zi is a yin-nourishing herb for the

Case study continues

liver and kidney. At the same time, it increases the WBC count and has antitumor activity; therefore, it treats the cancer, the constitution and the side effects of the chemotherapy by protecting liver and kidney function. Blood- and yin-nourishing herbs are synergistic. Shu di and nu zhen zi in concert with zhi mu all work to increase fluid and blood volumes. Shu di is also an antitumor herb.

Fu ling helps the spleen to assimilate the complex combination of yin-nourishing and damp heat-clearing herbs. It protects the middle jiao from damp accumulation, an important contribution in a damp heat diagnosis. It is antineoplastic and hence it is used in high dose. Huang qi would ordinarily be contraindicated in a yin-deficient environment because it is a warming herb. It would also be contraindicated in a damp heat pattern, but here its benefits outweigh its negatives. Huang qi helps maintain normal blood levels, is antineoplastic and increases NK cells and WBC counts and phagocytosis. Its pharmacologically oriented actions are of great value in this chemotherapeutic regimen. Since it is surrounded by other herbs of complex cooling and blood- and yin-nourishing qualities its negatives are considered to be ameliorated.

Xian he cao cools the blood to stop bleeding, inhibits colorectal cancer cell growth, and clears heat from the liver, thus treating the yin-deficient heat and acting as a liver protectant. Bu gu zhi is traditionally not used in yin-deficient heat since it is a yang tonic. However, it astringes and nourishes the essence and warms the spleen yang both of which are attributes of value in this presentation. But its main contribution to this formula is the fact that it is higher in genistein than any other known herb. This anticancer action is of great value and demonstrates again how sometimes a pharmacological finding outweighs the classical usage of a herb.

Ji nei jin, ban xia, and shen qu all work to ameliorate the side effect of nausea. Nutrition is of great importance in any cancer. Here, the accumulation of dampness and phlegm has contributed to the phlegm heat component of hypertension and the colorectal cancer. Allowing dampness to accumulate now would add insult to injury. Nausea is most often a symptom of spleen deficiency leading to dampness obstructing the middle jiao and creating a stomach/spleen

disharmony. The stomach qi flushing up is only a symptom of further injury. Managing nausea is important for many reasons, including helping the patient be comfortable and well-nourished and, in this case, managing the cancer (and hypertension) by disallowing further accumulation of dampness and phlegm stasis. The dosage for this formula was 6 g three times per day.

Outcome

This patient went through four rounds of gemcitabine with 5-FU. He maintained normal blood levels and blood chemistries showed no abnormal organ function. He was never given colony-stimulating factors (CSFs) to maintain WBC or RBC counts. He was given antiemetics for two rounds and then he decided to discontinue the antiemetics because of the side effect of severe constipation. He was treated for the last two rounds with herbal medicine alone to manage the nausea and all other side effects. This worked well. He has been monitored now for 4 years post-treatment without signs of recurrence. His CEA and CA19-9 levels are normal. He has dramatically changed his diet and exercises daily for 1 hour. His weight is in the normal range for his height and frame. He sleeps well and reports that he is grateful for the cancer diagnosis because he now feels more alive than he ever has in his adult life. He continued on herbal medicine for prevention of recurrence for 2 years post-treatment with conventional medicine. The formula has changed in small ways based on his presentation. It has included variations on Liu wei di huang wan with damp phlegm stasis antineoplastic herbs. A supplement regimen was also instituted that included:

calcium di-glucarate	800 mg daily
selenium	100–400 µg daily
vitamin C	1000 mg daily
vitamin D	500 mg daily
vitamin E succunate	800 iu daily
glutathione	recommended daily dose
an omega-3 fatty acid, e.g. fish oil	1 tbsp. daily
CoQ10	800 mg daily

He is now seen by a Chinese medicine practitioner once every 6 months for monitoring of his lifestyle habits, pulse, and tongue.

Case study 3.2

Female, age 40

Presentation

Diagnosed when she was 38 years of age with an adenocarcinoma (tubular adenoma, which means there is a higher incidence of finding other polyps of this type within 5 years) in the sigmoid colon after screening for rectal bleeding. She was diagnosed with recurrent metastatic disease on her liver and possibly the left lower lobe of her lung 6 months after ending the initial treatment.

History

This patient had two idiopathic seizures when she was 16 years of age and has been on carbamazepine (Tegretol) since then for seizure control. She also uses oral contraception started at the age of 25 after two pregnancies (norethindrone and ethinyl estradiol; Ortho-Novum). Chemotherapy interrupted her menstrual cycle during the first courses of treatment and it has never been reconstituted. She is now considered post-menopausal as a result. She has a small right renal cyst, which is considered to be benign, and uterine fibroids, which have never been treated and have now shrunk in size due to her iatrogenically-induced menopausal status. She was considered borderline anemic for several years due to bleeding from the fibroids.

She was treated for 6 months – once per week for 6 weeks and then 2 weeks off – with 5-FU and leucovorin. Six months after treatment ended a recurrence was found as part of an abdominal and chest CT scan for monitoring. At this time the tumor markers were in the normal range. She began treatment with oxylaplatinum infused every 3 weeks and capecitabine (Xeloda) given orally twice daily for 2 weeks. The side effects of oxylaplatinum are fatigue, lowered RBC and WBC counts, nausea, and peripheral neuropathy. The antiemetic treatment for this agent contributed to fatigue, which was the main complaint when coming for treatment at this time in the history of disease for this patient.

Work-up

The original work-up for this patient was exactly the same as for Case study 3.1.

The second work-up at the time of the recurrence showed

- RBC = 3.1; WBC = 2.7; haematocrit = 34.2.
- Alk/Phos: low.
- Potassium: low.
- Calcium: low.
  These signs show spleen and kidney deficiency.
- Tongue: pale with a dry white coat and 3+ vein distention.
- Pulse: tight and thready, slight fast, a liver/kidney sho (Japanese).
- Hara: tight and clammy over lung reflexes, cold over spleen and kidney reflexes, blood stasis reflex tight and tender through all levels.

Symptoms

The patient presented during the chemotherapy regimen (round three of a four-course regimen).

- Appetite: low but eating.
- Digestion: no upper gastrointestinal symptoms; lower abdominal gas with slight bloating.
- Stools: regular but 3 x daily and looser than normal, had hemorrhoids.
- Sleep: waking 1–2 x nightly and then cannot get back to sleep.
- Temperature: cold hands and feet, runs cold.
- Thirst: never thirsty, has to force fluids.
- Pain: none.
- Sweating: normal but history of night sweats prior to first surgery, no history of flushing.
- Menstrual cycle: began at age 16, two pregnancies during early 20s, no premenstrual syndrome (PMS).
  - Last menstrual period: 18 November 2003; bleeding for 6 days, light bleeding, bright red blood, sometimes cramping but low back pain.
- Wore orthodenture braces for 2 years in early 20s.

Case study continues

- Exercise: walking on occasion; no organised exercise pattern.

Diagnosis

- Spleen and kidney yang deficiency.

This patient presented for treatment after having failed earlier treatment with conventional medicine. She continued with her conventional care but wanted to add a level of complementary care to improve her chances for survival. Even though her diagnosis placed her at Stage IV colorectal cancer she was a very young woman with a different prognosis to a 70-year-old person with the same diagnosis. Spleen and kidney yang deficiency is often a diagnostic pattern of later-stage disease but, in her case, this was her constitutional diagnosis of long standing and not related to her age or status with the cancer. She is very slight, weighing only 95 pounds on a good day, runs cold, has a chronically low appetite, and very pale white skin.

Treatment plan

Continue chemotherapy with oxalyplatin, prepare for surgery to remove one lobe of her liver, and then a second surgery to remove and biopsy the probable lung metastases. Because of the fairly immediate recurrence and the higher risk of recurrence with this type of colorectal cancer the plan should include prevention of recurrence and strong treatment with antineoplastics. Removing part of the liver is an unusual management strategy. Removing the metastases in the lung is also an unusual strategy, but this patient has a good chance of surviving this cancer, even with stage IV disease.

The initial course of chemotherapy is most commonly thought of as the time to save a patient's life. The first treatment, and especially surgery, is an extremely important time in the overall survival of the patient. In this patient's case, it is possible that the patient may survive cancer-free. Therefore, all efforts are being made to try and achieve this outcome. The object of treatment with Chinese medicine is to underline that effort by potentiating all interventions and by maintaining normal health and establishing a new robustness for the patient given her spleen/kidney

yang deficient foundations. This is an extremely important time.

Chemotherapy

The primary side effects of oxalyplatin are fatigue, myelosuppression, including low WBC and RBC counts, nausea, and peripheral neuropathy. Oxalyplatin is a platinum-based agent that binds to DNA and prevents protein synthesis. It is not specific to any part of the cell-cycle. The half-life is 5–10 days. There is no evidence with this newer drug that there is any interference between it and the herbal formula used. An assumption had to be made regarding efficacy of combining care; the decision was made with the patient's consent that using this herbal formula did more good than harm (if any). Blood levels remained normal, kidney function (conventional) remained normal and all other liver and kidney function tests were normal. The patient did not require CSFs or any other support treatment while undergoing this chemotheraputic regimen with Chinese herbs. The dose for this formula was 6 g three times per day.

Treatment principles

- Tonify spleen and kidney yang, improve appetite, maintain normal blood levels, prevent peripheral neuropathies from beginning, act antineoplastically.

Formula

dang shen (Codonopsis Radix; *Codonopsis pilosula* root)	20 g
bai zhu (Atractylodis macrocephalae Rhizoma; *Atractylodes macrocephala*)	10 g
fu ling (Poria; *Poria cocos*)	25 g
yi ren (Coicis Semen; *Coix lacryma-jobi*)	30 g
rou dou kou (Myristicae Semen; *Myristica fragrans*; nutmeg seeds)	20 g
bu gu zhi (Psoraleae Fructus; *Psoralea*)	30 g
he zi (Chebulae Fructus; *Terminalia chebula* fruit)	25 g
ji nei jin (Gigeriae galli Endothelium corneum; *Gallus gallus domesticus*; chicken gizzard lining)	30 g

Case study continues

hong ren shen (Ginseng Radix; *Panax ginseng*; red ginseng)	20 g
huai hua (Sophorae Flos; *Sophora* flowers)	25 g
gu sui bu (Drynariae Rhizoma; *Drynaria*)	20 g
dan shen (Salviae miltiorrhizae Radix; *Salvia miltiorhiza* root)	25 g
chuan xiong (Chuanxiong Rhizoma; *Ligusticum wallichii* root)	20 g
bai hua she she cao (Hedyotis diffusae Herba; *Oldenlandia*)	35 g
huang qi (Astragali Radix; *Astragalus membranaceus*)	35 g
ji xue teng (Spatholobi Caulis; *Spatholobus suberectus*)	30 g
ling zhi (Ganoderma; *Ganoderma*)	30 g
long kui (Solani nigri Herba; *Solanum nigrum*)	25 g

Dang shen, bai zhu and fu ling form the basis for Si jun zi tang the traditional formula to treat spleen deficiency. These herbs address part of the underlying diagnosis for the environment in which this cancer evolved. These herbs also protect middle jiao function and protect against nausea or other gastrointestinal injury predicted with this chemotherapy. Yi ren potentiates the Si jun zi tang portion and also protects against damp accumulation. Since damp phlegm stasis is part of the diagnosis for the cancer this herb helps to protect the spleen and that portion of the fu and, in this way, acts as an antineoplastic in the formula. This explains the high dose of the herb.

Rou dou kou astringes the intestines and helps to control diarrhea. It also warms the spleen and works to circulate qi and reduce pain in the middle jiao, including the middle and lower abdomen. Bu gu zhi tonifies the spleen and kidney yang and, therefore, treats the diagnosis. It is also antineoplastic and contains the highest levels of genistein, an anticancer substance, of any herb yet studied, including soy (*Glycine max*). He zi also astringes the intestines to control diarrhea. It is an astringent and helps to lift and hold the qi. It protects the intestines from ulcerations. Ji nei jin in a high dose is added to improve appetite.

Red Chinese ginseng acts as an immunomodulator to improve energy, calm the spirit, protect the heart, improve lung function and protect the lungs against further spread. Huai hua cools the blood to stop bleeding and clears damp heat in the large intestine. It also cools liver heat and is added here to prevent possible bleeding and to ameliorate the warming from the large number of warming herbs. Gu sui bu, chuan xiong and dan shen all work together to prevent the occurrence of peripheral neuropathy, which is very difficult to treat once it becomes established. These are preventive herbs used in this capacity. They also move blood and many studies show the ability of dan shen to improve circulation and thereby improve access of chemotherapeutic regimens to all tumor cells.

Bai hua she she cao is an antineoplastic that is especially active against colorectal cancer. Long kui is also an antineoplastic that is especially active against liver cancer. The cancer in the liver is not liver cancer per se, it is metastatic colon cancer. But utilising this herb in this circumstance is an appropriate use to prevent further spread. Ji xue teng helps to improve the WBC and RBC counts in maintenance of the normal blood levels. Ling zhi does the same and acts as an analgesic. It is antineoplastic by increasing NK cells and phagocytosis. The dose for this formula was 8 g three times per day.

The CEA and CA 19-9 levels were in the normal range after treatment with this regimen. CT scans showed no spread of the tumors and the liver metastases and lung metastases had shrunk. The blood levels remained in the normal range during treatment, even without CSFs. The patient was given 4 weeks off treatment, and then the surgery to remove a portion (one lobe) of her liver was performed. During the month between chemotherapy and surgery the patient was placed on the following formula.

Treatment principles

- Prevent spread of the cancer, improve digestive capacity by tonifying spleen, increase immune function, calm the spirit.

dang shen (Codonopsis Radix; *Codonopsis pilosula* root)	15 g

Case study continues

bai zhu (Atractylodis macrocephalae Rhizoma; *Atractylodes macrocephala*)	10 g
fu ling (Poria; *Poria cocos*)	15 g
yi ren (Coicis Semen; *Coix lacryma-jobi*)	20 g
rou dou kou (Myristicae Semen; *Myristica fragrans*; nutmeg seeds)	10 g
bu gu zhi (Psoraleae Fructus; *Psoralea*)	15 g
ji nei jin (Gigeriae galli Endothelium corneum; *Gallus gallus domesticus* chicken gizzard lining)	15 g
tai zi shen (Pseudostellariae Radix; *Pseudostellaria heterophylla*)	15 g
huai hua (Sophorae Flos; *Sophora* flowers)	15 g
dan shen (Salviae miltiorrhizae Radix; *Salvia miltiorhiza* root)	15 g
huang qi (Astragali Radix; *Astragalus membranaceus*)	20 g
bai hua she she cao (Hedyotis diffusae Herba; *Oldenlandia*)	20 g
gua lou ren (Trichosanthis Semen; *Trichosanthes* seed)	25 g
hong ren shen (Ginseng Radix; *Panax ginseng*; red ginseng)	20 g
he huan pi (Albiziae Cortex; *Albizia*)	15 g

Dang shen, bai zhu, and fu ling form the base for Si jun zi tang, the main spleen tonic formula. Yi ren is a drain damp herb that benefits the spleen and is one of three herbs in this formula that is directly antineoplastic. Rou dou kou warms the spleen and helps to circulate qi. Bu gu zhi is a kidney and spleen yang tonic herb that is also high in genistein, an antitumor constituent. Ji nei jin helps to improve digestion and appetite and is added to help this patient continue eating and, hopefully, gain weight. Tai zi shen is a middle jiao tonic herb with neutral temperature. It helps to improve digestion without adding yet another warming herb to the formula. It also generates fluids and ameliorates the drying nature of the formula. Huai hua cools the blood and treats dysentery-like intestinal disorders. Dan shen moves the blood and improves circulation of the chemotherapy into the tumor cells by changing the viscosity of the blood.

Huang qi is antineoplastic and most importantly here helps to maintain normal blood levels injured by the myelosuppressive actions of the chemotherapeutic regimen. Bai hua she she cao and gua lou ren are both antineoplastic in the case of colorectal cancer. The red ginseng is more warming than white and is called for in a young patient with yang deficiency. The ginseng is immunomodulating and tonifies the zheng qi and the lungs, helping to protect the lungs from further spread. It is also cardioprotective and is used in a relatively high dose because the patient can tolerate the dose and needs this level of support. He huan pi calms the spirit by nourishing the heart. Both it and ginseng calm the spirit and help this patient through a difficult time.

The patient did well on this regimen and was ready for surgery 4 weeks after finishing chemotherapy. She had gained 5 lb, not an easy task for her given her lifelong struggle to maintain her weight. Her blood levels were all normal, she was sleeping well, and scared but optimistic about the surgery. The surgery went very well with little blood loss (one concern in liver surgery) and she was hospitalised for only 5 days post-surgery. There was no weight loss post-surgery. She stayed at home for 1 month before returning to work part-time. Over the next 2 months she was able to gradually return to a full-time work schedule. The above formula was used during this time with no changes.

Four months after the liver surgery the liver had healed and was growing back the portion removed. The liver is the only visceral organ that can regrow itself. Liver function tests were all normal, blood levels were normal, the weight gain was stable, tumor markers remained in the normal range. The patient was ready for the next phase of treatment – removal of the probable lung mets. The second surgery was performed. This surgery was more complex. It required entering from the posterior thorax, spreading the ribs, and resecting the two lower lobes of the left lung to ensure that no metastatic disease was present. The surgery lasted many hours and the recuperation was long and slow. There were complications re-establishing the negative pleural space; a bubble developed that would not resolve, and fluid build-up (pleural effusion) complicated healing. A tube had to be placed to allow for drainage of the pleural space; the stoma where the tube had been placed

Case study continues

became infected before the patient left the hospital.

Treatment principles

- Resolving the pleural effusion, healing the surgical wound and the lung, tonifying the lungs, preventing the spread of the cancer post-surgery, preventing infection.

bai ren shen (Ginseng Radix; *Panax ginseng*; white ginseng)	15 g
huang qi (Astragali Radix; *Astragalus membranaceus*)	20 g
shu di (Rehmanniae Radix preparata; *Rehmannia*)	10 g
wu wei zi (Schisandrae Fructus; *Schisandra*)	10 g
zi wan (Asteris Radix; *Aster tataricus*)	10 g
sang bai pi (Mori Cortex; *Morus alba*)	10 g
sha ren (Amomi Fructus; *Amomum*)	5 g
fo shou (Citri sarcodactylis Fructus; *Citrus sarcodactylis*)	10 g
ji nei jin (Gigeriae galli Endothelium corneum; *Gallus gallus domesticus* chicken gizzard lining)	15 g
chong lou (Paridis Rhizoma; *Paris*)	20 g
zhu ling (Polyporus; *Polyporus – Grifola*)	20 g
yuan hua (Genkwa Flos; *Daphne genkwa*)	15 g
xie bai (Allii macrostemi Bulbus; *Allium macrostemon*)	15 g
dong chong xia cao (Cordyceps; *Cordyceps*)	5 g

The first six herbs in this formula make up the formula called Bu fei tang, or boost the lungs decoction. It adjusts the qi of the lungs and tonifies the overall function of the lungs. The high dose of huang qi helps the lung tissue and surgical wound heal from surgical trauma. Sha ren is a fragrant herb used to transform dampness. This capacity enlivens the spleen to awaken appetite, circulate qi in the middle jiao, and stop nausea. It was used in this case to prevent nausea and increase appetite in a post-surgical patient with little appetite in the first place. Fo shou moves the qi and reduces pain, harmonises the stomach and improves spleen function, and it regulates the qi of

the lungs and disperses phlegm. All of these actions are important post-surgically. Ji nei jin also prevents food stasis and improves appetite. Without the ability to nourish herself, this patient would not have been able to recuperate quickly.

Chong lou is an antineoplastic herb used to prevent metastatic or local/regional spread of the cancer due to the surgical procedure. Zhu ling is an antineoplastic fungus playing double duty as a drain damp herb. Along with the yuan hua and xie bai it works to drain the pleural effusion, treat the local infection, increase cellular and humoral immunity to prevent further infection, and stop the spread of the cancer. Dong chong xia cao nourishes the lungs and strengthen the kidneys treating the lung/kidney axis. It stops post-surgical bleeding, controls cough, helps resolve phlegm, and is antineoplastic.

Over the next 2 weeks the infection and the pleural effusion resolved. Antibiotics were also given. Appetite gradually returned although the patient lost 8 lb during the procedure and weight gain was slower than before. The tube was removed. A slight cough persisted for 2 weeks and then resolved with a new variation of the above formula and with herbal cough syrup (Chuan bei pi pa lu). Chuan bei mu (Fritillariae cirrhosae Bulbus; *Fritillaria cirrhosa*) and xing ren (Armeniacae Semen; *Prunus armeniaca* seed) were added to the formula and gradually the pleural effusion resolving herbs were decreased in dose. The patient stayed on this formula for a total of 1 month. The dose was 7 g three times per day.

It has now been 6 months since the surgery. There is no sign of tumor in the abdomen, liver, or lung. The lung masses were biopsied and found to be colorectal cancer metastases. The call had been correct and removal of these potential seeds for further metastatic disease was the right thing to do. The patient has regained 5 lb of the 8 lb lost. The tumor markers are normal and CT scans are done every 3 months. She is once again working full-time and feeling well. Her diet is good, she is now exercising more and engaging in daily yoga. In a year's time, the plan is to taper the dosage of the seizure medication. She has found a neurologist who agrees that staying on seizure control medications for life may not be necessary. This patient is currently on the following formula for prevention of recurrence.

Case study continues

You gui yin plus the following herbs:

bai ren shen (Ginseng Radix; *Panax ginseng*; white ginseng)	15 g
huang qi (Astragali Radix; *Astragalus membranaceus*)	30 g
bu gu zhi (Psoraleae Fructus; *Psoralea*)	15 g
shu di (Rehmanniae Radix preparata; *Rehmannia*)	15 g
dang shen (Codonopsis Radix; *Codonopsis pilosula* root)	20 g
bai zhu (Atractylodis macrocephalae Rhizoma; *Atractylodes macrocephala*)	15 g
fu ling (Poria; *Poria cocos*)	25 g
ji nei jin (Gigeriae galli Endothelium corneum; *Gallus gallus domesticus* chicken gizzard lining)	25 g
bai shao (Paeoniae Radix alba; *Paeonia lactiflora* root)	15 g
he huan pi (Albiziae Cortex; *Albizia*)	15 g
chong lou (Paridis Rhizoma; *Paris*)	30 g

You gui yin treats the underlying kidney yang deficiency, which is part of the constitutional diagnosis. A small portion of Bu fei tang remains in this formula with a high dose of huang qi to act antineoplastically and to increase NK cells and phagocytosis. It also aids in the final healing of the wounds from the abdominal and thoracic surgeries. Bu gu zhi acts as a spleen and kidney yang tonic and also as an antineoplastic. Si jun zi tang remains a main part of treatment in a young woman who shows such strong signs of middle jiao insufficiency. Ji nei jin continues to work to increase appetite. It helps to prevent food stasis and transforms phlegm in a colorectal cancer patient where dampness and phlegm are the pathogenic factors. Huang qi and bai shao work together to heal the surgical injuries, huang qi tonifying the qi, and bai shao nourishing the blood. He huan pi acts almost like an antidepressant to stabilise and lift the spirit of this patient who has gone through so much. And chong lou works as the main antineoplastic to prevent recurrence. The patient will remain on a variation of this formula for the next 2 years unless a recurrence occurs.

References

1. Wingo PA. Cancer statistics, 2000. Cancer 2000; 45:8–30.
2. Miller BA. Cancer statistics review 1979–2000. National Cancer Institute, National Institutes of Health Publication N 92 – 2789; 2000.
3. Boring CC. Cancer statistics for African Americans. CA Cancer J Clin 1992; 42:7–17.
4. Forrester K. Detection of high incidence of k-ras oncogenes during human tumorogenesis. Nature 1987; 327:298–303.
5. Su LK. Association of the APC tumor suppressor protein with catenins. Science 1993; 262:1734–1737.
6. De Cosse JJ. Colorectal cancer: detection, treatment and rehabilitation. CA Cancer J Clin 1994; 44:27–42.
7. Burkitt DP. Dietology and prevention of colorectal cancer. Hosp Pract 1984; 19:67.
8. Maclennan R. Dietary fibre, transit time, fecal bacteria, steroids, and colon cancer in two Scandinavia populations: reports from the International Agency for Research in Cancer Intestinal Microecology Group. Lancet 1977; 2:207–211.
9. Thun MJ. Risk factors for fatal colon cancer in a large prospective study. J Natl Cancer Inst 1992; 84:1491–1500.
10. Baron JA. Calcium supplements for the prevention of colorectal adenomas. Calcium Polyp Prevention Study Group. N Engl J Med 1999; 340:101–107.
11. White E. Relationship between vitamin and calcium supplement use and colon cancer. Cancer Epidemiol Biomarkers Prev 1997; 6:769–774.
12. Bounoc G. Whey protein concentrate and glutathione modulation in cancer treatment, Anticancer Res 2000; 20:4785–4792.
13. Combs GF. Chemopreventive agents: selenium. Pharmacol Ther 1998; 79:179–192.
14. Garland CF. Calcium and vitamin D. Their potential roles in colon and breast cancer prevention. Ann NY Acad Sci 1999; 889:107–119.
15. Shklar G. Experimental basis for cancer prevention with vitamin E. Cancer Invest 2000; 18:214–222.
16. Wu Ju Tong. Wen bing tiao bian (Systematic differentiation of warm diseases). 1798 ACE.
17. Gu XZ. Modern oncology. Beijing: PHOF PUMC Press; 1993:448–457.
18. Hou Jinglun. Treatment of pediatric diseases in traditional Chinese medicine. Beijing: Academy Press; 1992.

19. Li Dong Yuan. Pi Wei Lun (Discussion of the spleen and stomach). 1249 ACE.

20. Zhang Jing Yue. Jing yue Quan Shu (Complete works of Jing Yue). 1624 ACE. Shanghai Science and Technology Press; 1959:531.

21. Chao Yuan Fang. Zhu bing yuan hou lun (Generalised treatise on the etiology and symptomatology of disease), 610 ACE. Annotated Version, Nanjing TCM College; People's Health Publishing; 1983.

22. Sugarbaker JP. Colorectal cancer. In: DeVita VT, Hellman S, Rosenberg SA. Cancer: principles and practice of oncology. Philadelphia: JB Lippincott; 1985:800–803.

23. Fuchs CS. A prospective study of family history and the risk of colorectal cancer. N Engl J Med 1994; 331:1669–1674.

24. American Joint Committee on Cancer. Manual for staging of cancer. 4th edn. Philadelphia: JB Lippincott; 1993.

25. Socco GB. Primary mucinous adenocarcinomas and signet-ring cell carcinomas of the colon and rectum. Oncology 1994; 51:30–34.

26. Takahashi T. Tumors of the colon and rectum: clinical features of surgical management. In: Moossa AR, Schimpff SC, Robson MR, et al, eds. Comprehensive textbook of oncology. 2nd edn. Baltimore: Williams and Wilkins; 1991:904–933.

27. St John DJB. Screening tests for colorectal neoplasia. J Gastroenterol Hepatol 1991; 6:538–544.

28. Selby JV, Friedman GD, Quesenberry CP Jr, et al. A case-control study of screening sigmoidoscopy and mortality from colorectal cancer. N Engl J Med 1992; 326:653–657.

29. Winawer SJ. Colorectal cancer screening. J Natl Cancer Inst 1991; 83:243–253.

30. Xue Shen Bai. Shi re tiao bian (Systematic differentiation of dampness and heat). 1740 ACE.

31. Xu Shu Fei. Pu ji ben shi fang, or Lei zheng pu ji ben shi fang (Formulas of Universal Benefit from my practice). 1150 ACE.

32. Wu Qian. Yi zong jin jian (Golden mirror of the medical tradition). 1742 ACE. People's Health Publishing; 1992.

33. Wang ang. Yi fang ji jie (Analytic collection of formulas). 1682 ACE.

34. Wang Ken Tang. Zheng zhi zhun sheng (Standards of patterns and treatment). 1602 ACE.

35. Qin Zhi Shen. Zheng yin mai zhi (Symptoms, cause, pulse and treatment). 1706 ACE.

36. Zheng ti lei yao (Catalogued essentials for correcting the Body).

37. Li Dong Yuan. Nei wai shang bian huo lun (Clarifying doubts about injury from internal and external causes). 1231 ACE. Jiangsu Science and Technology Press; 1982.

38. Chen Si Wen, ed. Tai ping hui min he li ju fang (Imperial grace formulary from the Tai Ping era). Imperial Medical Department, 1107 ACE.

39. Moertel CG, Fleming TR, Macdonald JS, et al. Levamisole and fluorouracil for adjuvant therapy of resected colorectal cancer. N Engl J Med 1990; 322:352–358.

40. Moertel CG. Fluorouracil plus levamisole as effective adjuvant therapy after resection of stage III colon carcinoma: a final report. Ann Intern Med 1885; 122:321–326.

41. Physician's Desk Reference. 57th ed. Montvale, NJ: Medical Economics Company; 2003.

42. Hine KR. Serum CEA testing in post-operative surveillance of colorectal cancer. Br J Cancer 1984; 49:689–693.

43. Gupta MK. Measurement of a monoclonal-antibody-defined antigen (CA 19-9) in the sera of patients with malignant and non-malignant diseases. Cancer 1985; 56:227–283.

Chapter 4

Breast Cancer

CHAPTER CONTENTS

Epidemiology 90

Risk factors 90
  Family history 90
  Age 91
  Reproductive history 91
  The Pill 92
  Hormone replacement therapy 94
  Phytoestrogens 96
  Mammography 97
  Breast implants 98
  Chemoprevention/tamoxifen as
    prevention 98
  Common medications and risks 99
  Obesity 100
  Dietary fat 101
  Dietary contaminants 101
  Nuclear emissions 102
  Hyperinsulinemia 102
  Pseudoestrogens and endocrine
    disruptors 103
  Contamination of the food supply 104
  Food packaging 105
  Food dyes 105
  Meat and sex hormones 105

Anatomy 106

Breast cancer types 106
  Non-invasive 106
  Invasive 107

Etiology 107
  Chinese medicine 107

Prognostic factors 110
  Tumor size 110

Nuclear/histologic grade 110
Hormone-receptor status 111
HER-2/neu status 111
Other markers 111

Detection 111
  Diagnostic procedures 112
  Chinese medicine 113

Staging 115

Principles of treatment 115
  Surgery 115
  Radiation therapy 117
  Chemotherapy and hormonal therapies 120
  Hormonal therapy: post-chemotherapy
    and/or as prevention 128

Metastatic breast cancer 130

Formula bases for constitutional
    patterns 132
  Kidney yang deficiency pattern 132
  Kidney yin deficiency pattern 132
  Liver and kidney yin deficiency pattern 133
  Liver qi stasis pattern with constraint as
    main feature 133
  Liver qi stasis with spleen deficiency
    pattern 134
  Liver qi stasis with spleen deficiency leading
    to rebellious stomach qi pattern 135
  Liver qi stasis leading to latent liver heat
    pattern 136

Prevention 137
  Chinese medicine 138

> *We stand now where two roads diverge. But unlike the roads in Robert Frost's familiar poem, they are not equally fair. The road we have long been traveling is deceptively easy, a smooth superhighway on which we progress at great speed, but at its end lies disaster. The other fork of the road – the one 'less traveled by' – offers our last, our only chance to reach a destination that assures the preservation of our earth.*
>
> From *Silent Spring* by Rachel Carson, 1962

EPIDEMIOLOGY

The death of Rachel Carson from breast cancer two years after the publication of *Silent Spring* is emblematic of the predicament in which we currently find ourselves. In 1950 in the United States the rate of incidence of breast cancer was 1 in 20 women; there has been a 50% increase since 1965;[1] and today the rate is 1 in 8 women, and in California, the bread basket of America, the rate in 2001 was 1 in 7 women. The higher rate in California has prompted the California State Legislature to fund the first state-funded study in medicine to find out why the incidence of breast cancer has risen so dramatically in California.

As of 1999 breast cancer accounted for 32% of all cancers in women.[2] The mortality rate is 28 per 100 000 and remained unchanged for 50 years until only recently. Between 1990 and 1995 the mortality rates decreased by an average of 1.7% per year. Decreases were more pronounced among white women and younger women.

Breast cancer is the leading cause of death in women between 40 and 55 years of age. Not accounting for gender, 66% of women who are diagnosed with breast cancer have no risk factors.

RISK FACTORS

One percent of all breast cancers occur in men. The major risk is being female. An individual with no family history is no longer placed in a low-risk category. A history of previous breast cancer increases the risk fivefold.[3] It also increases the risk of endometrial, ovarian, and colon cancer. Menopause before the age of 45 reduces the risk by 50% compared to those who enter menopause after age 55. Nulliparity increases risk by perhaps 30%. Having a first full-term pregnancy after the age of 27 increases the risk by 40% when compared to a first pregnancy before age 20.[3] This information is rarely shared with women when making reproductive decisions. It is true that 85% of women diagnosed with breast cancer have no family history of breast cancer.

Most forms of cancer, including breast cancer, are multifactorial diseases, having many different risk factors or potential causes that may interact with one another in ways that are still not completely understood. For example, genetic, familial, environmental and lifestyle factors can all work together to create the conditions necessary for a cancer to develop. A woman with no familial or genetic risk factors may be hit by so many environmental carcinogens that she does develop breast cancer. A woman with genetic risk factors may never develop breast cancer depending on other factors. This implies that there are factors that one can avoid in order to reduce one's risk for breast cancer.

FAMILY HISTORY

The *BRCA1* and the *BRCA2* genes are tumor suppressors. Women with an abnormality in these genes run a very high risk for developing breast cancer – a fourfold increased risk. A woman carrying one of three alterations in the *BRCA1* or the *BRCA2* genes has a 56% increased risk for developing breast cancer by the age of 70.

Another gene affects breast cancer through its influence on estrogen production. This gene is called the *CYP1* gene and is carried by about 40% of women. It may be involved in some way in 30% of all cases of cancer. A variation of this gene causes women to enter puberty and start producing estrogen earlier (~5 months) than women without the variation. Women with breast cancer who carried the variation to *CYP1* were two and a half times more likely to have disease that had spread than were women without the variation to this gene.[4]

Women with denser breasts have a significantly higher risk for cancer than women with less dense breasts.

About 1–2% of American women carry a rare gene called ataxia-telangiectasis (A-T), which markedly increases their sensitivity to X-rays, including mammography, and thus their risk for breast cancer.

The National Breast Center of Australia published the following overview of genetic risks in 1995:[5]

1. At or slightly above average risk: women who have (a) no family history, or (b) a first- or second-degree relative diagnosed with breast cancer after the age of 50. Most women fall into this category. Their lifetime risk is between 1 in 13 and 1 in 8.
2. Moderately increased risk: women who have (a) one or more first- or second-degree relatives diagnosed with breast cancer before the age of 50, or (b) two first- or second-degree relatives on the same side of the family with breast cancer, especially those diagnosed before the age of 50. Less than 4% of women fall into this group. Their lifetime risk is between 1 in 8 and 1 in 4.
3. Potentially high risk: women who have three or more first- or second-degree relatives on the same side of the family diagnosed with breast or ovarian cancer. Less than 1% of women fall into this category. Their lifetime risk is between 1 in 4 and 1 in 2.

The vast majority of breast cancer cases are not genetically linked. At this time, even the 4% of women who do inherit a predisposition are not necessarily fated to develop breast cancer. Environmental influences have an impact on genes. DNA is not stable and is sensitive to environmental influences. DNA constantly alters its structure in response to changes in the cellular environment. In other words, it is more important where you live and how you nurture yourself than to whom you were born.[6]

Chinese medicine

The gene factors refer to kidney jing and yuan qi factors that cannot be changed, but for which compensation can be made.

AGE

The risk for breast cancer increases with age[7,8] More than 80% of breast cancer occurs in women over the age of 50.[5] The median age to date is 64 years, which means that half of all women who get breast cancer will get it after the age of 64 and half will get it before the age of 64. Younger age is, however, not a safety net against breast cancer. I am currently treating women aged 21, 19, and 14 years, all with breast cancer. The age factor relates to kidney yin and yang deficiencies that evolve as a result of the wear and tear of life. The idea of cause and effect in classical Chinese medical theory adds an additional element, that of time. Everything transforms in time. The changes that come as a result of time will eventually involve the deeper levels of the body, the kidney yin and, therefore, the yang.

Chinese Medicine

Kidney yang deficiency can affect the Chong and Ren channels, leading to inversion fire and then to fire poison. Kidney yin deficiency affecting the Chong and Ren channels can also lead to inversion fire and then to fire poison. When women lose the downward draining action of the menses, a mechanism of clearing heat and other contaminants from the body, then heat can rise to the upper jiao more easily. Also the circulation of blood in the whole, but especially the upper, jiao is changed. A natural evolution of heat and blood stasis in the upper jiao can occur, especially in women who are not active and do not exercise regularly. Diet also plays a role in this evolution of blood stasis and heat.

REPRODUCTIVE HISTORY

One major culprit often involved either directly or indirectly in breast cancer is estrogen. The longer one is exposed to estrogen, and the greater the amounts of estrogen in the blood circulation, the greater the risk for developing breast cancer. The risk is higher in a woman who menstruates for more than 40 years than for a woman who menstruates for 30 years or less. Because pregnancy influences the amount of estrogen that the body produces, it also has an impact on breast cancer. Women who have never become pregnant have a higher risk than do those who have a child before the age of 30,[7] because breast cells complete maturation only with a full-term pregnancy. After pregnancy, the breast cells stabilise and become less affected by menstrual cycle hormones, developing greater resistance to breast cancer until menopause. Partially-matured breast cells have unstable DNA that is more susceptible to the process of cancer.[3] However, women who get pregnant for the first time after the age of 30 have a greater risk for breast cancer than do those who never get pregnant.

During pregnancy, the hormone estriol (a weak, short-acting, protective estrogen) is secreted by the placenta at about 1000 times the level that exists in the body before pregnancy. Serum estriol concentration may be increased by 14–25% for many years following a first pregnancy. After a first pregnancy, there continues to be an elevated ratio of estriol to estradiol and estrone. Estriol is able to bind to estrogen receptors in breast cells and competitively prevent the stronger estrogens, estradiol and estrone, from binding where they would promote cell division and potentially tumor growth.[9–12]

One of the reasons that breast cancer rates are rising may be due to the extra exposure to estrogen that now occurs as a result of the use of the birth control pill and estrogen replacement therapy after menopause. There are medical, dietary, and environmental risk factors that promote breast cancer largely by influencing either the amount of estrogen to which women are exposed or the way that estrogen behaves in their bodies.

Chinese Medicine

There are sociological and philosophical questions that arise from the meaning of gender in societies. Males and females have different expectations placed upon them based upon gender; these expectations are philosophically based in sociological and historical perspectives. The Chinese believe that the constraints placed on women due to societal expectations make them more at risk for diseases caused by unresolved emotional material in their lives. Reproductive decisions are placed in this realm of societal constraints that lead to emotional constraints.

Liver qi constraint is a common outcome of this kind of constraint. Lung qi stasis also can arise from suppressed emotions. And when liver qi constraint leads to heart qi stasis via the Five Phase cycle then liver and heart qi stases arise. When liver and heart qi stases combine with lung qi stasis then a form of clumping arises in the chest that leads to blood and phlegm stasis, a precursor condition for cancer. The liver channel runs through the flank. The area of the axilla relates to the Jueyin. Liver constraint due to unresolved emotional issues is commonly part of the overall presentation for breast cancer. Liver qi stasis due to or leading to kidney yin deficiency also contributes to abnormal hormonal levels.

THE PILL

The safety of the oral contraceptive pill has yet to be established, especially prolonged use and use starting in one's teens. The origin of the contraceptive pill is the Mexican wild yam (*Dioscorea floribunda*), from which diosgenin provides the basis from which estrogen, progesterone and other hormones can be synthesised. The first oral contraceptive pills contained high doses of mestranol, which is a relatively weak estrogen. In the 1970s, a second-generation pill was developed, one that delivered low doses of ethinyl estradiol. Because the doses of estrogen and progestin are lower in the second-generation pill than in the first, the pharmaceutical industry claims that they are safer. There are several factors to take into account when evaluating the risks for developing breast cancer.

- The type of estrogen (mestranol) used in the first-generation pill is half as potent as the type used in the second-generation (ethinyl estradiol). Unlike ethinyl estradiol, mestranol does not bind to estrogen receptors in the breast.
- Most women who used the first-generation pill did so for a relatively short time and usually starting in their 20s, whereas women using the second-generation pill have tended to do so for much longer, sometimes starting in their teens and continuing until menopause, thus putting breast tissue under constant hormone stimulation.

Most of the studies done on the oral contraceptive pill have been done on the first-generation form. Most women for the past 25–30 years have been using the second-generation pill. A third-generation pill that uses progestin alone is becoming popular. Other forms of hormonal contraceptives, such as the implant Norplant, the injectable Depo-Provera, and morning-after pills, are used around the world. They each contain differing amounts of estrogens, progestins, or both, having different potencies, and each with its own set of side effects and level of breast-cancer risk.

Since the 1930s, studies have shown that estrogen induces breast and other cancers in a wide variety of rodent species. In the 1960s, researchers at the National Institutes of Health (NIH) reported to the Food and Drug Administration (FDA) that they had found precancerous changes in the breasts of monkeys given standard doses of oral contraceptives. In 1969, the chief of endocrine cancer at the National Cancer Institute (NCI) warned about the potential danger of birth control pills. The NCI Medical Letter, in a 1976 issue, emphasised that estrogen causes cancer of the breast, endometrium, cervix, pituitary gland, ovaries, testes, kidney, and bone in mice, rats, hamsters, squirrel monkeys, and dogs. Since that time, more than 20 well-controlled studies have demonstrated the clear risk of premenopausal breast cancer with the use of oral contraceptives. The estimates from these studies predict that a young woman who uses oral contraceptives has up to 10 times the risk for developing breast cancer than a non-user, especially:

- if she uses the pill during her teens and early 20s
- if she uses the pill for 2 years or more
- if she uses the pill before her first full-term pregnancy
- if she has a family history of breast cancer.

Furthermore, several studies from the late 1980s showed that the risk of breast cancer is long-lasting. This means that postmenopausal women are also at increased risk for developing breast cancer many years after first using oral contraceptives.[13–19]

The above information is partially taken from the 1995 book, The Pill: A Biography of the Drug that Changed the World, by B Asbell.

Evidence is growing that the third-generation pill, which contains only synthetic progestin, may be just as dangerous. A study from 1986 quoted in the New England Journal of Medicine reported a 30% increased risk of breast cancer with the third-generation pill. Norplant contains high levels of progestins released over time for up to 5 years. Depo-Provera is an injectable progestin that protects against pregnancy for 3 months and increases the risk for breast cancer in a relatively short period of time. Studies reported in the Journal of the National Cancer Institute and the Lancet all support this fact. The first study was reported in 1973. It was not until 1989 that the FDA acknowledged the breast-cancer risk of Depo-Provera.[20–23]

Morning-after pills like Desogen have never been studied at all. Therefore, the avoidance of hormonal contraceptives is, if at all possible, an important element of advice in terms of helping our patients reduce risks for breast cancer. Safe and effective alternatives to the pill must be taught so that patients can make informed decisions.

A recent study of the newer forms of oral contraceptive pills showed that women utilising the pill had a lower incidence of breast cancer. The reason given for this lowered rate of incidence is that women who use hormonal contraception are exposed to less estrogen as a result of the fact that they are regulating their cycles via a chemically hormonal means rather than the body's own regulating mechanism. The study results and conclusions make it difficult to understand the logic of hormonal therapy for contraception versus hormonal therapy for menopausal syndrome, one of which finds less incidence in breast cancer and the other which finds more incidence of breast cancer, utilising the same hormones.

Chinese medicine

The Jueyin has a direct relationship with hormonal levels. The Jueyin also has a relationship with the Chong and Ren embryonic channels. The liver and kidney axis is the primary interface relating to hormonal levels and interacts with the Chong and Ren. Supplementing this axis of relationship with exogenous substances interferes with normal balance and causes abnormal function, which can lead to yin deficiency and blood stasis. Yin deficiency and blood stasis contribute to latent pathogenic factors and inverted fire poisons.

HORMONE REPLACEMENT THERAPY

There are three principal natural estrogens in the human body: estradiol, estrone, and estriol with estradiol being the most potent and active form. Estrogen replacement therapy (ERT) consists of varying amounts of these estrogens, alone or in combination, and of either natural or synthetic formulas. Natural estrogens are produced in the laboratory from animal sources and they are almost identical to those found naturally in the human body. Synthetic estrogens are more potent and are used chiefly to make birth-control pills, because higher doses are needed to suppress ovulation. Hormone replacement therapy for menopausal women is usually made from natural estrogen sources and is currently opposed with progesterone.

Premarin is the most commonly prescribed brand of estrogen in the US and is made from the urine of pregnant mares. The offspring produced from this means of producing estrogen are usually slaughtered not long after birth. There are currently citizen actions taking place (primarily in Canada where most of the American Premarin supply is produced) to save the foals born as a result of estrogen production from the urine of pregnant mares. It is important to know all of the ramifications of one's pharmaceutical choices.

Estrace is manufactured by Bristol-Myers Squibb and is made from the more potent estrogen estradiol.

Opposed hormonal therapy (HRT) includes progesterone, which inhibits cell division in the uterus and counteracts the stimulation of cell growth caused by estrogen. Progestins can be either natural or synthetic. In synthetic form progesterone actually increases the risk of breast cancer.[24,25]

A newer trend is to add testosterone to the HRT mix in order to increase the libido and increase sex drive.[26] Lowered libido is a normal occurrence in menopause. Very few long-term studies have been done on testosterone. A woman's body fat converts testosterone to estrogen, and therefore the addition of testosterone almost always results in higher levels of estrogen and in estrogen stimulation, especially in overweight women. In 1996, a study in the *Journal of the NCI* showed that this increase in estrogen levels elevates the breast cancer risk.[27] More research is necessary to assess the long-term risks of testosterone.

Hormone replacement therapy is usually prescribed to mimic a woman's menstrual cycle. Estrogen alone is taken orally for 12 days and then opposed in combination with progestin for about 13 days. At day 25, both pills are discontinued and bleeding occurs. Osteoporosis and heart disease have been thought to be factors related to 'estrogen deficiency' and that treating preventively for both far outweighed the risks of using HRT. It is now clear that heart disease and osteoporosis are not impacted by HRT. Even if it is true that HRT could impact cardiovascular and bone health, there are many other ways to reduce risk for these two diseases, including diet, exercise, and better control of conditions that exacerbate heart disease, like diabetes and hypertension.[28,29]

Osteoporosis has now reached epidemic proportions, affecting 15–20 million women per year. Osteoporosis also affects men but is greatly underreported. About 50 000 elderly women die each year from complications from hip fractures. Many women undergoing chemotherapy for cancer treatment (not just breast cancer treatment) leave cytotoxic treatment osteopenic. It has been thought that estrogen helps protect bones from being robbed of calcium because it stimulates the production of the hormone calcitonin, which helps bones take up calcium. Estrogen also helps to produce and maintain collagen, which is a component of bone. However, there continues to be a debate as to whether HRT provides efficient and sufficient protection against osteoporosis. The studies are confusing: one showed that women who begin HRT in their 60s showed slowed bone loss, but actually increased bone mass within 3 years. Another study showed that estrogen alone was ineffective and that estrogen/progestin combinations were better. It also stated that women with the greatest bone density had more than double the risk of breast cancer than women with the least bone density. Taking HRT for 30 years or more to prevent osteoporosis may not be the best choice for many women.[30]

On the positive side, studies from 1995 show that HRT may reduce the risk for colorectal cancer by as much as half. This reduction is maintained for about 10 years after a woman has stopped HRT. Also some studies have shown that women who take HRT had only a 7% incidence of Alzheimer's disease versus 18% incidence in those who did not.[31] It is believed that nerve growth factor and estrogen work together somehow to protect brain cells from degenerating. Estrogen also appears to protect brain cells from various toxins, including amyloid, the protein that accumulates in the brain of patients with Alzheimer's disease. Estrogen may also help to improve memory and mental function.

Urinary tract problems, including incontinence and infections, occur more often as estrogen is lost because estrogen plays a role in maintaining healthy body tissue. The outer membrane of the urethra and bladder becomes thin, weak, and more prone to infections and dysfunction. HRT appears to help these problems in older women.

Estrogen also helps to maintain the skin and mucous membrane of the vaginal wall. It reduces flushing, night sweats, sleep disturbances, and mood swings, all of which are commonly present in postmenopausal women whether their menopause is natural or iatrogenic, induced by treatment for breast or another cancer.[32]

The risks for hormone replacement need to be weighed in with the benefits. HRT may alleviate some medical problems; it may exacerbate others. Until the turn of the century, HRT was one of the most commonly prescribed drugs in the US. In addition to breast, endometrial, liver, and ovarian cancers, HRT also promotes the development of other conditions, including benign breast disease, uterine fibroids, blood clots, and gallstones. Other side effects include weight gain and premenstrual symptoms like cramping and mood changes. HRT is currently rarely used because of the risks for breast cancer. However, women who have been on HRT remain at risk for some time even when they have stopped HRT.

A 1991 study reported in the *American Journal of Epidemiology* showed that HRT was responsible for 8% of all postmenopausal breast cancers in the US.

A series of well-controlled studies over the last two decades shows that extended use of estrogen increases the risk of breast cancer by 30–70%. This means that a 70-year-old woman on HRT may have an increased risk of breast cancer from 1 in 14 to 1 in 5. This information is rarely shared with patients who are deciding whether or not to use hormonal therapy. The FDA-approved package insert for Premarin, for instance, states that the 'majority of studies . . . have not shown an association with breast cancer with the usual doses for estrogen replacement'. It is obvious that one cannot always trust the state of the evidence regarding these issues. One must educate oneself and make informed decisions for oneself.[33,34]

The addition of progestins, testosterone, or both, to the HRT mix makes matters more confusing. Since 1979, the World Health Organization (WHO) has known that synthetic progestins enhance the carcinogenic effect of estrogen and increase a woman's risk of breast cancer. A joint study between the United States and Sweden published in 1989 in the *New England Journal of Medicine* reported that taking progesterone as part of HRT increased the risk by more than 400%. Testosterone added to HRT increases the risk by about 60%.[35]

Alcohol consumption increases estrogen levels in women taking hormones. The circulating level of estrogen surges upwards by 300% in women on HRT who drink 4–6 oz (118–177 ml) of alcohol per day. These effects are almost immediate and last for up to 5 hours.

The rates for ovarian cancer increased by 40% after 6 years of HRT and by 70% after 11 years or more in one study.[36] The long-term risk for uterine cancer increased by more than fifteenfold with estrogen use. HRT more than doubles the risks of lung cancer in smokers. And the risk of liver cancer appears to be slightly elevated in women who take HRT.

Currently in the United States, HRT is rarely prescribed because of the risks associated with its use. This new attitude regarding HRT evolved out of many years of research in large cohorts of women. However, many women have taken HRT and continue to be at risk for the effects of this use. Therefore, it is as well to know the history, the studies, the risks, and the alternatives for these patients.

Chinese medicine

All of the issues in breast-cancer risks and causation that have the potential of raising hormonal levels relate to liver and kidney, Chong and Ren patterns. The overexposure that results from hormonal therapies and exposures from other means may also fall into the category of latent pathogenic factor. See Chapter 14 on cancer prevention. These patterns have physiological and psychoemotional components. Developing the ability to recognise all of the potential components in an individual patient gives the practitioner the capacity to work with and specifically advise that patient regarding these issues. The capacity of the patient to empower themselves through resolution and understanding of these issues contributes to their survival.

PHYTOESTROGENS

The term 'phytoestrogen' is misleading, in that it implies that plant materials contain estrogen. Phytoestrogens are substances with a chemical structure similar to estrogen. Isoflavones are so-called phytoestrogens found in soy (*Glycine max*) and some other legumes and in several herbs. Lignans are a second class of phytoestrogen found in flax seeds (*Linum*), berries, and some vegetables and grains. The chemical structure of these phytoestrogens is close enough to human estrogen that estrogen receptors in the human body are filled by these exogenous substances.

Genistein and daidzen are isoflavones that bind to breast cell estrogen receptors. This blocks the body's own endogenous estrogens, in the form of estradiole and estrone, from binding to these same receptors. This interruption of body estrogen acts as an antiestrogenic influence, helping to increase the levels of estrone and estriol, which have a weaker influence on breast cell turnover, while simultaneously preventing osteoporosis.[37–39]

Genistein has many positive properties. It is an antioxidant and influences enzymes that regulate cell growth and division. It helps to reverse the proliferative process of cancer and turns off certain breast cancer genes.[40] It inhibits platelet aggregation, which is often central in the cancerisation process. It also lowers estrogen production stimulated by the pituitary and the ovaries and reduces the bioavailability of sex hormones, once again lowering estrogen levels.[41] Differentiation is induced in cancer cells by genistein and this slows the mutational process. Tyrosine kinase is also inhibited, which slows the mutational process and mitosis. Protein tyrosine kinases activate breast cancer genes.[42]

When phytoestrogenic foods that contain genistein, daidzen, and lignans are eaten, the intestinal bacteria convert these phytoestrogens to other substances such as equol and enterolactone, which then bind to estrogen receptors and have weak estrogenic acitvity. These substances have a protective effect against breast cancer and possibly ovarian cancer. Women who have been diagnosed with breast cancer have lower levels of equol and enterolactone excreted in their urine. Women who eat a macrobiotic diet excrete much higher levels of dietary phytoestrogens than do women eating the standard American diet (SAD). Diets high in animal fat decrease equol production.

Genistein induces apoptosis, or programmed cell death, which is often one major point of dysfunction in cancers. It is also antiangiogenic.[43,44] It inhibits topoisomerase II, which stops or slows the proliferation of tumor cells.

There are several common sources of phytoestrogenic foods. Soy in its many forms is very helpful in breast cancer prevention for all of the reasons stated above. Soy foods, like tofu, miso, tempeh, are probably preferable to soy concentrated powders. Some people are allergic to soy and some have developed Hashimoto's thyroiditis after heavy use of soy concentrate supplementation. Freshly ground flax seeds, raw pumpkin seeds, clover sprouts, and mungbean sprouts are all good sources.

There is no evidence that consuming phytoestrogens during treatment for breast cancer contributes in any way to cancerogenesis. There is a great deal of evidence, as stated above, that there is a protective effect in consuming phytoestrogens during treatment for breast cancer. Currently there are several studies on this subject, particularly with soy products, to understand better the influence of phytoestrogens on breast cancer during treatment. Several European studies have already shown that using phytoestrogenic substances during treatment with various chemo-therapeutic regimens (AC) actually enhances the effect of these regimens. In vitro studies (unpublished) have shown that black cohosh (*Cimicifuga racemosa*) alongside tamoxifen significantly decreases the rate of proliferation of breast cancer cells. Studies on borage (*Borago*) oil and tamoxifen show similar decreases in proliferative rates of breast cancer cells. A study is now being conducted at UC San Francisco Medical Center on the use of soy (*Glycine max*) alongside tamoxifen for use in prevention of recurrence of breast cancer.

MAMMOGRAPHY

The discussion regarding mammography swings back and forth. One argument was that mammography screening did not change the death rates from breast cancer. The NCI reached the decision to favor mammography amidst vocal dissension amongst its own staff. One dissenter stated that, at most, 1.5% of women in their 40s who have annual mammograms receive any benefits.

Before menopause, the dense, highly glandular structure of the breast is maintained by relatively high levels of estrogen production. This density tends to mask small early tumors and shield them from X-rays. After menopause, the progressive reduction of glandular tissue makes the detection of early tumors much easier. Recent developments, including techniques based on digitised mammography and computer enhancement, provide better images, especially of the denser premenopausal breast. These techniques include PET scans and MRI and RODEO scans.

Displacement mammography is a screening method for women with silicone implants. The implant is displaced away from the chest wall, allowing the breast to be compressed more effectively and preventing tissue from being shadowed by the implant.

Mammography narrowly focuses X-rays (electromagnetic radiation capable of penetrating solid material) on the breasts. Rads equal the radiation-absorbed dose. In the past, mammography exposed women to up to 50 rads during a mammography session. We know that radiation is carcinogenic. In 1977 the average single dose was 8 rads, and in the 1980s the dose was around 3 rads. One week in Denver (the mile-high city) equals a whole-body exposure of 1 millirad. Mammographic exposure per shot is around 300 milli-rads, and the number of shots varies depending on the size and density of the breast. Usually at least two shots per breast are taken. So most women are receiving much more than 300 milli-rads per breast at each mammogram screening session. Today the average dose to each breast from mammography is 340 millirads.

A Swedish study showed that screening with a single view every 2–3 years achieved a 34% reduction in postmenopausal breast cancer mortality. This result is similar to that achieved with American procedures using two or more views per breast each year. There is no evidence that more views at more frequent intervals reduces mortality.[45,46]

Mammography is put forth as an early screening tool for prevention of breast cancer. But by the time a mammogram can detect a cancer, the cancer can be up to 8 or 9 years old, can reach 1 mm in diameter, and may have spread to distant sites, especially in premenopausal women. A 1 cm mass is usually detectable by the woman herself using self-examination. Although there is also controversy regarding breast self-examination (BSE), in my experience breast cancers are found by the woman herself rather than through mammography. The best palpators for breast cancer are breast surgeons and the woman herself.

Radiation may trigger the very cancer it is meant to detect.[47] The link between radiation and breast cancer is strong.[48] In Nagasaki and Hiroshima a 39% increase in breast cancer was found for every rad of exposure in those survivors who were 10 years old or younger at the time of the bomb. There was a two-decade time lag because usually breast cancer takes a long time to develop. John Gofman, MD, the leading international expert on medical radiation, claims that past medical radiation is probably the single most important cause of the modern breast cancer epidemic. This is in no way meant to advise a practitioner to discourage patients from seeking mammography. However, it is important that patients have as much information regarding their condition as is currently possible.[49–51] All decisions are their own to make. It is the role of the practitioner to teach, heal, and support.

Chinese medicine

Exposure to ionising radiation is an exposure to a fire toxin. This fire toxin is not an endogenous factor but is exogenous. It apparently goes straight to the ying and blood levels and there ferments into a deep level fire toxin. Ionising radiation may also be a latent pathogenic factor.

BREAST IMPLANTS

If rupture occurs in a saline implant, the fluid portion is naturally absorbed. However, the empty silicone envelope must then be surgically removed. If rupture of a silicone gel implant occurs, the viscous gel may ooze out so slowly that the woman may be unaware of a problem in her breast. Even intact gel implants leak microscopic amounts of gel into surrounding tissue. The blood levels of silica or silicon are five-times higher in women with perfectly performing implants. These particles can be carried to distant sites and are found in joint lining tissue, lung cells, skin, and in tissue surrounding the implants. Chronic inflammation in the breast or anywhere can cause autoimmune disease.

Hardening of the gel or saline implants causes capsular contraction and often the formation of adhesions around the local area. This can be extremely painful and require surgery to remove the adhesions. The implant material seems to cause the body to produce antibodies that are abnormal. These autoantibodies are attracted to normal cells, which can lead to rheumatiod arthritis (RA), systemic lupus erythematosus (SLE), and scleroderma. A 1993 study in the *Archives of Internal Medicine* reported that 35% of women with implants develop autoantibodies.

Silicone gels are carcinogenic in rats. The tumors caused by silicone gel were found to be highly invasive and rapidly lethal. The studies were performed by Dow Corning and immediately Dow and the FDA buried these facts in their confidential files. The information was released by the Freedom of Information Act in 1990. A 1994 study in the *Journal of the NCI* showed that injections of silicone gel into the abdominal cavities of mice induced a high incidence of plasma cell

tumors (related to multiple myeloma). Silicone degrades in the body to crystalline silica, a known potent carcinogen in both animals and humans. It also acts like estrogen in animals. The polyurethane foam used to cover some silicone gel implants is even more carcinogenic than the gel. These implants are still available to women today.[52–54]

Chinese medicine

Silica acts both like an exterior pernicious influence (EPI) and latent pathogenic factor (LPF). The EPI action most probably is similar to a wind heat pathogen. The reaction to the EPI is long term and often so low grade that it appears asymptomatic, which is why it may also be a latent pathogenic factor.

CHEMOPREVENTION/TAMOXIFEN AS PREVENTION

Tamoxifen (Nolvadex) is the first generation of a group of drugs known as selective estrogen receptomodulators (SERMs), which have both estrogenic and antiestrogenic effects. Tamoxifen is antiestrogenic to the breast and estrogenic to the uterus, and to a lesser extent, the heart, blood vessels and bone. Tamoxifen prevents estrogen from binding to receptor sites on breast cells. Women with breast cancer are usually treated with surgery, chemotherapy, radiation and then hormonal therapy in the form of tamoxifen. Tamoxifen therapy usually lasts for 5 years posttreatment with the other modalities of surgery and chemotherapy.

There is currently a belief that the antiestrogenic effects of tamoxifen in relation to breast cancer can be used to prevent breast cancer from developing in healthy women. In 1992 the NCI began a large trial in Canada and the US using this drug to treat women with a strong family history of breast cancer or who were at risk for breast cancer for other reasons. In other words, a supposed preventive drug is being tested to prevent breast cancers that may have been induced by chemical pollutants, medical technology (radiation), and carcinogenic/estrogenic drugs in the first place. Instead of attempting to reduce the carcinogenic chemical burden under which we struggle to maintain our health, the solution is proposed by adding more chemicals to the mix.[55]

This study makes no attempt to give guidance on alternative measures, such as increasing exercise, maintaining a healthy body weight, eating a protective diet, and avoiding exposures to environmental carcinogens. It also does not fully inform participants about the serious risks of tamoxifen. A 1992 study report in the *New England Journal of Medicine* emphasised that tamoxifen may reduce the incidence of contralateral cancer, but only in premenopausal women, and then in only three of eight trials. In another study from the same year, it was shown that tamoxifen not only failed to reduce contralateral cancers in premenopausal women; it actually increased their incidence.[56,57]

A 1995 audit of long-term trials by the NCI showed that tamoxifen provides no advantage for preventing contralateral breast cancer in women treated for more than 5 years. The NCI further admitted that tamoxifen might actually be detrimental. Several trials showed that tamoxifen has no effect on bone density and that tamoxifen does not appear to reduce total cholesterol levels and thus the idea that it protects cardiovascular health is no longer clear.[58]

Complications of tamoxifen therapy for breast cancer prevention include menopausal symptoms, eye damage, blood clots, hepatitis, liver, uterine and other cancers. Tamoxifen binds tightly and irreversibly to the DNA, causing a cancerous mutation to take place. The warning is that no amount of tamoxifen is safe when it comes to carcinogenic effects. When cancer develops in the other breast of patients treated with tamoxifen, the cancer tends to be highly aggressive and rapidly fatal. Patients treated with tamoxifen run a 50% increase in risk for developing other cancers, particularly of the digestive tract. Risks of aggressive uterine cancers are sharply increased by tamoxifen.[59]

Recently American studies have shown that the population gaining the greatest advantage from prophylactic therapy with tamoxifen comprises premenopausal women with node-positive breast cancer. Their risk of recurrence was reduced by 30%. There is a study ongoing at UC San Francisco on the combined effect of tamoxifen and soy (*Glycine max*) in reducing breast cancer recurrence.

Is it possible that utilising only natural means to reduce estrogen levels is good prevention of recurrence? Is it possible that xenoestrogenic influences stored in fat tissue contribute to the overall load and that treating to reduce this stored load of estrogenic influence should be part of prevention of breast cancer in the first place and as prevention of recurrence in women who have already been diagnosed?

There may also be a relationship between tamoxifen and ovarian cancer.

Chinese medicine

Tamoxifen is a heat toxin that injures the yin and causes yin deficiency heat. This injures the liver and kidney axis and impacts the Chong and Ren. These impacts can lead to menopausal symptoms. The loss of the menses either prematurely or as an iatrogenic event can exacerbate blood stasis syndrome in the chest and in the lower jiao, both of which are the result of Ren and Chong injuries. Blood stasis in the chest can lead to cardiovascular disease like deep vein thrombosis (DVT). Blood stasis in the lower jiao can lead to uterine cancer.

COMMON MEDICATIONS AND RISKS

Antihypertensive drugs may increase breast cancer risk. Reserpine, hydralazine, spironolactone and atenolol are all antihypertensives that have different mechanisms for treating high blood pressure. For various reasons they should all be taken only following careful consideration.[60–62]

Two types of antibiotics appear to increase breast cancer risk. They are metronidazole (Flagyl) and nitrofurazone (Furacin). Flagyl kills trichomonas and giardia. Animal studies show a significant excess of breast cancer in rodents with normalised levels of Flagyl. Furacin is used to treat wounds, burns, and skin infections. It is available in pills, creams, ointments, powders, solutions, sprays, suppositories, and surgical dressings. Furazolidone (similar to nitrofurazone; Furoxone) is used to treat gastric ulcers caused by *Helicobacter pylori*. These drugs have also been found to affect breast cancer risk in rodents. No follow-up studies have ever been done.[63,64]

Some tranquilisers, like diazepam and alprazolam (Xanax), appear to increase blood levels of estrogen and the development of invasive breast cancer. Amitriptyline (Elavil) and fluoxetine (Prozac) are used to treat depression, OCD (obsessive-compulsive disorder), and panic attacks. Both drugs promote the growth of breast cancer in rodents after the administration of a chemical carcinogen. Haloperidol (Haldol) is used to treat psychotic disorders such as schizophrenia. It triggers the release of the cancer-promoting hormone prolactin and induces significant increases of breast cancer in rodents.[65] Pravastatin (Pravachol) is a cholesterol-lowering drug which causes a reported 12 times higher rate of breast cancer in women taking this drug. Bristol-Myers Squibb, the manufacturer, calls this a 'statistical fluke'. An article in the *Journal of the American Medical Association* (JAMA) recently concluded that the fibrates and statins can cause breast cancer and other cancers in rodents and should be avoided.[61]

Cimetidine (Tagamet) is now available over the counter and appears to alter the body's metabolism of estrogen, decreasing the levels of good estrogen and increasing the levels of bad estrogen. These estrogenic impacts explain the higher rates of gynecomastia in men who take this drug.[66]

OBESITY

Obesity increases a woman's risk for developing postmenopausal breast cancer by 50–100%. This percentage increases the older a woman gets and the longer she remains obese. The inclusion of other possible risk factors for any given individual can raise the risk to 600%.[67,68]

Estrogen is produced not only by the ovaries and adrenal glands, but also by abdominal fat cells that convert other hormones (especially testosterone) into estrogen. The more weight a woman carries, particularly around the abdomen, the more estrogen circulates in her body and the higher the risk for breast cancer.[69] In premenopausal women, obesity appears to offer about a 10–20% decrease in breast cancer risk. Obesity in younger women is associated with lower overall estrogen levels, which results in irregular menstruation and ovulation and with higher levels of estrogen-binding proteins that reduce free estrogens. However, such decreases in risk must be counted against the negative effects

of obesity-related health problems, such as heart disease and diabetes.[70]

Obesity in postmenopausal women has the opposite effect. The fat in the buttocks, thighs and breasts contains an enzyme called aromatase that can convert testosterone and other steroid hormones into estrogen. After menopause the activity of aromatase increases, which means that heavy women secrete more estrogen into the blood stream and breast tissue. Postmenopausal obese women have a higher proportion of 'bad' estrogen and lower levels of estrogen-binding protein.[71]

Obesity keeps the estrogen window open longer than usual. Obesity lowers the age at which a young girl first menstruates and raises the age at which a woman enters menopause. Also the estrogen window opens sooner than usual after breastfeeding if a woman is obese. She misses fewer periods and starts ovulating sooner when breastfeeding than her counterparts. Also, obesity almost always coexists with inactivity, which is itself a risk factor for breast cancer.

When these factors are combined with the issues covered in the next sections on dietary fats and food contaminations the insults in terms of estrogen overload can be overwhelming. Xenoestrogens coming through the food chain from pesticides and synthetic fertilisers are all fat-soluble compounds. They accumulate in the environment and then in the internal environment of the human body, especially in fat cells. More fat cells means more storage of endogenous and exogenous estrogens. We don't know what the effect would be if the exogenous estrogens coming through the environment were to be eliminated.[72-75]

Chinese medicine

The stomach and spleen are coupled organs. The stomach channel runs directly through the breast. Spleen deficiency can be caused by improper eating habits that lead to damp accumulation, which in turn can lead to heat, which traverses the middle jiao invading the liver and causing a form of deficiency constraint. This is another way by which liver qi constraint can evolve. Also, spleen deficiency can lead to the blood failing to be nourished. This form of blood deficiency also can cause liver qi constraint and the Five Phase cycle of upper jiao constraints that can cause blood and phlegm stasis in the chest via liver/heart qi constraint and liver/lung qi constraint.

The stomach and spleen also have a relationship to the Ren and Chong channels or seas. For example, liver qi stasis affecting the spleen and stomach can lead to dampness pouring down and then to damp heat, which contributes to stagnant blood and then to stomach heat with fluid deficiency. The next injury in this vicious cycle is congealment of blood. Another example is that of liver qi stasis with spleen deficiency leading to qi and blood deficiency and then blood stasis and then blood dryness and then blood heat and finally to fire poison. There are many examples of liver and stomach/spleen injuries that end in fire poisons and inverted fire and in blood stasis. See primary constitutional patterns under Etiology.

DIETARY FAT

Recent studies have shown that there was no difference in the rates for breast cancer between those who consumed diets containing <25% of fat and those who consumed diets containing >40% fat. However, these studies failed to look at several linked issues. First, a high-fat diet often leads to obesity, which is linked to breast cancer. Second, consuming a low-fat, high-complex-carbohydrate diet reduces breast density, and dense breasts are a risk for breast cancer. Finally, none of the studies looked at the role that food contaminants, many of which are cumulative and concentrate in dietary and body fat, play in breast cancer pathogenesis. Dietary fats contain a wide range of contaminants, like pesticides, other industrial pollutants, sex hormones, and antibiotics. These contaminants tend to accumulate and concentrate in body and breast fat at levels thousands of times greater than in food, thus putting the breast and other hormonally sensitive tissues at special risk.

Chinese medicine

Some of the contaminants that effect body and breast fat can be categorised as external pathogens and others as latent pathogenic factors. No one knows if and how all of these contaminants work in combination to cause disease.

DIETARY CONTAMINANTS

Packaging and shipping depletes the nutritional value of many foods. Potent and potentially toxic chemicals are used to grow and market the enormous quantities of agricultural and other products we have available to us. These are then sold at what are enormous profits for the middlemen but not the growers. Sex and growth hormones, plastic wrapping and packaging, food coloring dyes, and radioactive pollutants from nuclear power plants all contaminate our food. These issues regarding our food supply are relevant not only to breast cancer but to many other cancers as well.

Dietary contaminants affect breast tissue in two different ways.[76] They may be carcinogenic and trigger cancer in healthy cells by deranging their DNA. Or they may be pseudoestrogenic, which means that they act like female sex hormones, although they are structurally different. Atrazine is an organochlorine pesticide made from petroleum products that is both carcinogenic and pseudoestrogenic. When the Israelis eliminated atrazine and two other organochlorine pesticides from their agricultural practices the breast cancer rate in Israeli women decreased by 30% over 10 years.[77,78] The studies done on the subject of breast cancer and dietary contaminants fall into three categories: those that show that some of these contaminants, especially pesticides, induce breast cancer in rodents; those that show that dietary contaminants selectively concentrate in breast tissue; and those that show higher concentrations of contaminants in the blood of breast-cancer patients.[75,79]

Pesticides pose special dangers to the food supply. They enter the body through contaminated food and water, through inhalation, and through absorption through the skin. Pesticides are sprayed, powdered or dropped as pellets in and around places where humans live. A 1985 study in the *Lancet* showed that pesticide residues are commonly found in the fatty tissue of almost everyone in the United States, and in human breast milk and cows' milk. In 1993 another study showed a strong association between high blood concentrations of DDE (a breakdown product of DDT) and breast cancer compared with women without breast cancer.[76,80] The risk for breast cancer was four times greater for women with the highest levels of DDE compared to those with the lowest levels. In 1994 another study published in the *Journal of the NCI* showed that concentrations of a wide range of carcinogenic and estrogenic pesticides and industrial pollutants were higher in the fat and blood of women with estrogen-receptor-positive breast cancers than in healthy women.[79]

In 1997, the same research group showed that there was a strong relationship between concentrations of estrogen receptors in the breast cancers of these women and DDE levels in their breast fat.[76] This suggests that exposure to DDT-type estrogenic pesticides explains, at least in part, the increase in estrogen receptor levels in breast tumors observed during the past two decades. One might say that breast tissue is like the canary in the coal mine, since it acts as a harbinger of a negative environment.

Chinese medicine

Pesticides and their breakdown products after metabolisation in the human body appear to be latent pathogenic factors and fire toxins. They seem to remain latent until a critical mass of cumulative effect is reached when they can cause transformation at the blood level. This causes a fire toxin trigger to breast cancer and probably other cancers. Xenoestrogenic pesticides, like atrazine and DDT and DDE, affect the Chong and Ren and disturb their natural function.

NUCLEAR EMISSIONS

Every day nuclear power plants release carcinogenic by-products into the atmosphere. These by-products then contaminate grasses and water on which dairy cows feed. They enter the food chain in the form of dairy products, the most concentrated form of any kind of ingested contamination. Some types of radiation are stored in the bone where they can damage the marrow that produces many blood cells including immune cells. They are also stored in breast tissue. There is a general denial that nuclear by-products invade the environment. But the *International Journal of Health Sciences* published an article that cited that the 'highest emissions of airborne and liquid fission products ever released from any nuclear power plant in the Unites States' were released in an area around the Millstone I reactor in Waterford, CT, in 1993. The levels were 15 times higher than those that existed at Three Mile Island after the nuclear accident. Even before this release, the milk produced in Waterford in 1976 contained levels of strontium-90 that were higher than levels recorded during the height of nuclear weapons testing. Other examples of high-risk nuclear by-products involve communities on Long Island. A 1993 study claims that the risk of dying from breast cancer there has risen sharply as strontium-90 levels have risen. Long Island has one of the highest rates for breast cancer in the United States.[81]

Chinese medicine

Nuclear exposures are clearly fire toxin exposures. They may also be considered as latent pathogenic factors because we are now aware that fetuses exposed during the Nagasaki and Hiroshima atomic explosions did not exhibit incidences of cancer until later in life and often only when hormonally mature, that is, when the Chong and Ren had consolidated. These and many other exposures in utero are considered endocrine disruptors and the study of endocrine disruptors is a new area of research. Fetal toxicology is an arm under which this research is being done. One might think of these exposures as insults to the yuan qi or the source qi. The fact that they do not surface until the yin and yang have consolidated may indicate that the Chong and Ren are damaged in some way never thought of in classical Chinese medicine. This is probably true of all of these exposures that act as latent pathogenic factors. They are not latent pathogenic factors in the sense that Zhang Zhong Jing thought of LPFs. But, in function, they act very much as LPFs. They entered the body from outside and could not be cleared. As a result, they moved to deeper levels where they smoldered for a period of time, and then, when the environment was correct for their emergence, they surfaced symptomatically. It was only when symptomatic that their presence was known.

HYPERINSULINEMIA

Hyperinsulinemia is a risk factor for breast cancer. Breast tumors were found to have 1.9–3.0 times as many insulin-like factors. Glucose is considered the preferred substrate for cancer cells. Sucrose and retinol carbohydrates are a risk factor for breast cancer. Mice injected with aggressive mammary tumors were placed on three diets. After 70 days 95% of the mice on the low-sugar diet were alive. Of the mice on the moderate-sugar diet 67% were alive. And only 33% on a high-sugar diet were alive. Also 'moderate' alcohol consumption is associated with elevation in the risk for breast cancer from 50 to 100%. Alcohol consumption is associated with a linear increase in breast cancer in women over the range of consumption reported by most women.[82]

Chinese medicine

Prediabetes and diabetes are conditions on a spectrum that relates to spleen deficiency and the cumulation of damp fluids in the middle jiao, which gradually cause deeper levels of injury to the middle, the upper, and the lower jiaos. Spleen deficiency leads to blood deficiency and blood stasis. Spleen deficiency also leads to damp/phlegm stasis. Blood stasis and phlegm stasis are foundational environments for cancers of any kind. Spleen deficiency can be considered to be a promoting factor for a cancerisation environment. Blood deficiency caused by underlying spleen deficiency can lead to liver and kidney yin deficiency. The liver and kidney axis is related to the Chong and Ren and to reproductive hormonal balance. All of these interfaces of activity have their roots in the spleen function and the middle jiao's foundation for whole-body health. Diet is key to maintaining normal spleen function and the circle of health in which it is central.

PSEUDOESTROGENS AND ENDOCRINE DISRUPTORS

Some species are becoming extinct not due to loss of habitat but due to pseudoestrogens contaminating the environment, and then feminising the sex organs of the males.[83] Wild gulls in the Great Lakes area are born with deformed beaks that prevent them from eating properly. Their eggshells are abnormally thin. What is harming other animals is also harming us. The estrogenic effects of industrial dietary contaminants act like natural estrogen once in the body, attaching to the same receptors on cell membranes intended for

natural estrogen and then inducing similar but weaker hormonal responses in the body. In the breast, estrogenic chemicals cause cells to grow and divide more quickly than normal, and also promote the growth of any abnormal or premalignant cells that might be present. Certain chlorinated pesticides, including DDT, and packaging materials, such as the plastic linings in canned foods have been documented to have estrogenic effects.[84–86]

DDT was banned in the early 1970s in the United States but is still used widely throughout the rest of the world usually as a result of exportation of American-made DDT, which is still produced here. Much of the food we import is contaminated with DDT making the banning of DDT in the United States a moot point.[87] And DDT persists in the environment. Some studies have shown that female dogs remained in heat even after their ovaries were removed, an effect caused by DDT exposure. DDT binds to human breast estrogen receptors. Pseudoestrogens influence a woman's risk of breast cancer in various interrelated ways:

- Although much weaker than natural estrogens, they may concentrate in a wide variety of foods, and in such high levels, that their cumulative effect is substantial.
- While the body eliminates natural estrogen within 24 hours, pseudoestrogens may persist in the body for decades because they are unable to bind to proteins that would then eliminate them from the body. They then concentrate in body and breast fat. Organochlorines are fat soluble.
- Pseudoestrogens trigger the body to metabolise more estrogen into the 'bad' form, and this increases the risk of breast cancer even further.

Chinese medicine

It is difficult to say exactly what category of pathogen would apply to pseudoestrogens. They act somewhat like an LPF but also have effects that are fairly immediate, making them look more like a fire toxin. Please see Chapter 14 on prevention. Whatever we call them, these pathogens affect the liver/kidney axis and the reproductive capacity of both the male and female.

CONTAMINATION OF THE FOOD SUPPLY

Pesticide regulations in the US are stringent but, at the same time, full of loopholes. Manufacturers continue to legally export banned pesticides, and then the food industry imports the food grown with these pesticides from countries where pesticide use is not banned, and sells them back to consumers. We eat squash from Mexico and the Netherlands that is contaminated with dieldrin, a carcinogenic and pseudoestrogenic pesticide. Benzene hexachloride-, DDT-, and lindane-contaminated nuts and grains are imported from India. Norwegian farm-raised salmon contain these same carcinogens. Fish farming worldwide remains unregulated, and the industry frequently uses fat supplements to hasten growth, as well as veterinary drugs and pesticides to combat illness and bacterial contamination due to overcrowding. Fish caught in industrialised portions of Europe's major rivers and the Baltic Sea are usually highly contaminated by pesticides and other pollutants known to cause breast cancer. Most of the pollutants are manufactured in the United States. At the same time, there are many pesticides that are legal in this country but banned in many European countries. The main markets for American chemical pesticides and fertilisers are developing countries and oftentimes these markets are coerced into utilising these products rather than their own traditional agricultural practices.[87]

Pork is a relatively lean meat and so contains much lower levels of pesticides than beef. But pork products, like ham and bacon, contain nitrite preservatives that combine with other chemicals in the meat or in the human body to form nitrosamines, which are highly potent cancer-causing chemicals. Sulfa drugs, known to be carcinogenic to the thyroid gland, are also likely to contaminate pork products. Pesticides are also found in chicken, but at lower levels than in beef because the fat content is lower in poultry. Antibiotics that can cause low-level allergic reactions and can breed super strains of bacteria, also taint chicken. Turkey is the least comtaminated type of commercially raised meat. Wild venison and wild boar also tend to be safe. Bison is gaining popularity on the exotics market but many bison growers are now managing their animals in the same way that they would beef. Animals fed grain to fatten them up have higher fat content and lower levels of omega-3 fatty acids. They also have higher levels of conjugated linoleic acid (CLA).

It is now thought that all fish in Europe and in the United States may be contaminated. The list is long of the carcinogens and the pseudoestrogens found in fish in our waters. They include benzene hexachloride, chlordane, dieldrin, endrin, heptachlor, lindane, toxaphene, mirex, atrazine, DDT, PCBs, PBBs, and mercury.

When the Environmental Working Group conducted a recent sampling of water in the Midwest, Maryland, and Louisiana, they found that tap water in 28 of 29 cities contained atrazine.[84,88–90] Atrazine not only is a probable cause of breast cancer but also of human ovarian cancer. Studies done by the Environmental Protection Agency (EPA) have shown associations between pesticide contamination of water and increased breast cancer rates.

Even baby food contains carcinogenic and pseudoestrogenic chemicals. A 1984 study in the journal *Cancer* noted that 'Numerous studies have found that there is a greater risk of developing cancer if exposure to carcinogens begins in infancy rather than later in life'.[91] As stated earlier, numbered amongst my current patients are young women aged 14–21 with breast cancer. A new field of study is evolving that looks at endocrine disruptors through time. This research is finding that, in many cases, exposures at certain moments in utero are more profound than longer term exposures in children and adults. Sandra Steingraber, fetal toxicologist, has written several papers on this subject and is one of the main researchers in this area of endocrine disruptors and how they work to injure the DNA in developing fetuses. As stated many times, no one knows how combinations of contaminants work together or if they do. This is a whole new field of inquiry. It is amazing to think that of the 85 000 new chemicals developed since the 1940s only 1500 have been studied in any way for individual health impacts. It is overwhelming to consider the various combinations of all 85 000 chemicals, plus the new ones constantly being developed, and how these chemical 'soups' might be causing harm in our world and in our bodies.

FOOD PACKAGING

Packaging materials such as styrene cups, trays for microwaving prepared foods, and the lining of cans for canned foods also contain pseudoestrogens and carcinogens. Alkylphenols, nolylphenol, and bisphenol are used in packaging materials and all migrate into foods, especially when stored for long periods of time or heated at high temperatures. All plastics are considered suspect unless proven otherwise.[86]

FOOD DYES

Red dye no. 3 is a carcinogen that can bind to estrogen receptors on breast cells and damage the cells' DNA. Currently about 80% of our food supply has been processed by the food industry, and the use of food additives in these products continues at a rate of 45% annually. Red dye no. 3 is widely used and hard to replicate. It is used to color maraschino cherries, bubble gum, a wide range of snack foods and baked products. Researchers estimate that the average woman receives a daily dose of red dye no. 3 about 1000–2000 times the amount that would derange cellular DNA. In 1990, the FDA discontinued the use of all 'lake' forms of red dye no. 3 used to make external drugs and cosmetics because of reports that the chemical caused thyroid cancer in rats. It is still allowed for use as a 'food' dye.[92]

MEAT AND SEX HORMONES

Sex hormones fed to livestock increase body weight by about 10% before slaughter. Hormones in beef, the most commonly eaten form of hormone-fed meat, have serious estrogenic and carcinogenic effects. The FDA has been aware of these effects for several decades.

Women prescribed diethylstilbestrol (DES) in the 1950s developed increased rates of breast cancer, their daughters developed increased rates of vaginal cancers, and their sons developed increased rates of reproductive and urinary tract abnormalities. The FDA approved the use of DES as a cattle growth promoter in 1947. In the 1950s ranchers began implanting DES in the ears or muscles of cattle as a way of forcing them to gain weight in feedlots. This resulted in high residues in meat. By 1971, ranchers used DES in 75% of cattle nationwide. DES was finally banned in 1979, 40 years after scientists knew of the carcinogenicity of DES. Even after the FDA was forced by Congress to ban DES, its illegal use continued until 1983, when inspectors found DES contamination in 1500 veal calves from five farms in upstate New York. The pharmaceutical and food industries exposed the meat-eating population of the US to DES from the 1940s to the 1980s.[93,94]

The US meat industry switched from DES to natural sex hormones like estradiol, progestins, and testosterone, or to their synthetic variants. Today, the FDA allows their unregulated use by implantation of pellets under the skin of the ear in all cattle raised in feedlots. The theoretical and nonenforceable requirement is that residue levels in meat should be less than 1% of the daily hormonal production in children. Residues of natural hormones can only be detected by highly specialised analytic methods that make routine monitoring an extremely difficult and expensive process. A large-scale national survey, published in the April 1997 issue of *Pediatrics*, revealed that 1% of Caucasian and 3% of African-American girls show signs of pubic hair and/or breast development by the age of 3 years. A random survey in 1986 showed that up to half of all cattle sampled in feedlots in Kansas, Colorado, Texas, Nebraska, and Oklahoma had hormone pellets illegally implanted in muscle tissue rather than under the skin of the ear. This practice leads to higher absorption of hormones from the implants and very much higher residues than even the FDA admitted could have adverse effects. Hormone treatment increases the profits by up to $80 per animal. Records obtained from the FDA through the Freedom of Information Act show that even with a single implant beneath the ear skin, levels of estradiol and other hormones in meat and organs are more than triple the levels found in non-implanted controls. When intramuscular implants are used these levels increase up to 300-fold.[94]

Recombinant bovine growth hormone (rBGH) is used in milk production to increase output by about 10%. The FDA approved for sale in 1993 milk from cows that had been treated in this way. The hazards include:

- increased fat concentrations in milk
- contamination with rBGH
- mastitis and other udder infections in cows treated with rBGH resulting in pus and bacteria in the milk supply
- antibiotics to treat the above forms of mastitis in the milk supply
- milk contaminated with high concentrations of a potent growth factor: insulin-like growth factor 1 (IGF-1).

These levels are further increased through pasteurisation. IGF-1 is a hormone that regulates cell division and growth. It resists digestion in the human gut and when it passes into the blood stream it can produce abnormal or premature growth-promoting effects.[95,96]

ANATOMY

The breast is composed of glandular tissue within a dense fibroareolar stroma. The glandular tissue consists of approximately 20 lobes, each of which terminates in a separate excretory duct in the nipple. The breast lymphatics drain by way of three major routes: axillary, transpectoral, and internal mammary. Intramammary lymph nodes are considered with the axillary lymph nodes for staging purposes. Metastasis to any other lymph nodes – including supraclavicular, cervical, and contralateral internal mammary nodes – are considered distant (M1).

The regional nodes are:[97]

1. Axillary (ipsilateral): interpectoral nodes and lymph nodes along the axillary vein and its tributaries:
   a) level I or the low axilla: lymph nodes lateral to the lateral border of the pectoralis minor muscle
   b) level II or the mid-axilla: lymph nodes between the medial and lateral borders of the pectoralis minor and the interpectoral lymph nodes
   c) level III or apical axilla: lymph nodes medial to the medial margin of the pectoralis minor including those designated as subclavicular, infraclavicular, or apical.

2. Internal mammary (ipsilateral): lymph nodes in the intercostal spaces along the edge of the sternum in the endothoracic fascia.

BREAST CANCER TYPES

NON-INVASIVE

DCIS

Ductal carcinoma in situ (DCIS) is found more now due to screening mammography. Fine microcalcifications are seen, and perhaps 15–20% found through mammography are of this type. Not all DCIS progresses to invasive cancer. Carcinomas in situ are considered to be premalignant conditions. Those that do progress to an invasive malignancy most commonly do so 7–10 years from their inception. A 2% rate of positive axillary nodes has been reported in DCIS; this occurs usually in patients with extensive areas of DCIS, as opposed to one area. The risk of carcinoma in the opposite breast is not high. DCIS can metastasise, and it can recur even up to 15 years after discovery. The distribution is usually segmental and unicentric. On mammography slide it has a characteristic appearance of a line of marching individuals.

Local excision alone has a 13–60% chance of recurrence, with 50% of recurrences being invasive carcinoma.[98,99] Mastectomy is curative in 98% of patients. There is a morphological marker for risk. For example, the comedo type refers to necrosis of cancer tissue within the DCIS and almost always a higher nuclear grade (see below). Approximately 80% of this type of DCIS tumor are aneuploid, estrogen receptor negative, and express *HER-2/neu* highly, all of which are markers that carry a poorer prognosis.[100] The risk for developing infiltrating ductal carcinoma is 8–10 times higher in the comedo type. There is also a higher rate of local recurrence with comedo DCIS. The non-comedo is the most common type of DCIS. The cribiform non-comedo type carries the best prognosis.

LCIS

Lobular carcinoma in situ (LCIS) follows a different course than DCIS. It tends to be multicentric and may be bilateral. It does not produce a mass and, therefore, has no clinical or mammographic presentation. The risk of invasive cancer in the opposite as well as the ipsilateral breast is increased. In fact, LCIS is considered a marker for increased risk of developing invasive breast cancer. The risk is equal in both breasts. And the risk increases by approximately 1% each year. Management of this kind of breast cancer has ranged from bilateral mastectomy to complete excision with careful observation. LCIS is undoubtedly a risk factor for invasive cancer but the course can be indolent, and, therefore, conservative surgery has been considered a reasonable approach.

INVASIVE

Infiltrating ductal carcinoma (DIC) accounts for 75% of all breast cancers. It more frequently metastasises to bone, lung and liver.

Infiltrating lobular carcinoma (LIC) accounts for 5–10% of all breast cancers. It more often metastasises to the meninges, serosal surfaces, ovaries and the retroperineum.

Medullary carcinoma accounts for 5–7% of all breast cancers. There is commonly a younger age at diagnosis. Typically this type is estrogen receptor (ER) and progesterone receptor (PR) negative and p53 positive.

Tubular carcinoma is also known as 'well-differentiated carcinoma' and accounts for 2% of all breast cancers. It carries a better prognosis than DIC. Axillary metastasis is rare and it is typically ER/PR positive.

Inflammatory carcinoma of the breast (IBC) accounts for 1% of all breast cancers and is an aggressive form of a locally advanced breast cancer. Clinical features include erythema and edema of the breast with or without an associated mass. It often has a characteristic appearance of 'orange-peel skin'. Dermal invasion of lymphatics is the histologic hallmark. Twenty-five percent of patients have breast or nipple pain. This is considered a stage IIIB breast cancer with a rapid onset. All IBC patients are considered to have nodal involvement, and the incidence of systemic disease at presentation is very high. Patients have a 25–50% probability of developing contralateral breast cancer. It is typically ER/PR negative. And it is more common in Northern Africa and Tunisia,

where it is associated with pregnancy and lactation. Initial treatment with radical mastectomy is contraindicated. The usual treatment has been high-dose chemotherapy. The prognosis is very poor.

Paget's disease presents as an eczematoid, crusted lesion of the nipple or areola. It is characterised by large cells with large nuclei in the epidermis. It is almost always associated with underlying non-invasive or invasive cancer. Treatment depends on the underlying pathology.

Pregnancy and lactation concurrent with breast cancer does not appear to have a poorer prognosis. Mastectomy can be safely performed during pregnancy. If it is late enough in the pregnancy, often induction of birth is performed so that chemotherapy, if an appropriate treatment, can begin. There are some forms of chemotherapy that can be safely used during pregnancy.

ETIOLOGY

See the section on risk factors above. Breast cancer is a multifactorial disease that is probably caused by a combination of several factors that, having reached critical mass in terms of the number of 'hits' an individual has suffered, creates an environment in which cancer then develops.

CHINESE MEDICINE

Once broken, breast nodes seldom result in survival. The breasts are where the yangming (the stomach channel) passes, the nipples are ascribed to the jueyin (liver or pericardium channel). Improper food and unresolved emotional issues will result in qi blockage and then the portals will be blocked. The blood of the yangming will become hot and transform into pus. Cumulative results of constant worry will end in a dormant node developing, hard like a turtle shell but with no pain or itching. This takes 10 years to develop into a sunken sore. It is incurable. If, at the end stage of its generation, one eliminates the root of the disease by keeping the heart tranquil and the spirit calm and administers certain treatment, recovery is possible.[101]

In relation to the various qi disorders, anger makes the qi ascend, fright makes the qi chaotic, apprehension makes it descend, taxation makes it dissipate, sorrow makes it disperse, joy makes it slack, and thought makes it bind.[102] The alteration of qi movement, for whatever reason, leads to blood stasis, which can lead to fire and to fire poisons and then to malignancies.

It is difficult to squeeze classical Chinese medicine into a comparative analysis of breast cancer causation with modern biomedicine. Zhu Dan Xi's ideas regarding diet, although unable to take into account pesticides, xenoestrogens and chemical toxins, seem straightforward. However, the mind/body connection has steadily been removed from Western science starting during the Age of Enlightenment. The removal of all inter-relationships is the basis upon which the double-blind placebo study is devised; all definitions and, therefore, treatments, of disease rely on this process. The process itself is the antithesis of the theory and clinical practice of Chinese medicine. Therefore, Zhu Dan Xi's inclusion of unresolved emotional factors becomes problematic for the Western practitioner but not for the practitioner of Chinese medicine. There is no comparable arena of disease causation in Western science except in the realm of psychoneuroimmunology. Please see the earlier parts of the chapter on liver qi stasis and spleen and stomach disharmonies. All of the research done in breast cancer is aimed largely towards finding new treatments and not towards identifying causative factors that can be utilised by patients to prevent an occurrence or a recurrence. Except in the area of exercise and diet, patients learn little about how to protect themselves.

The problem of ascribing emotional material to disease causation is complex for other reasons. Patients may begin to blame themselves for being sick. This is especially true of women; women are often programmed to take care of others and to never be sick themselves. It also may appear that others are blaming the individual for their own cancer; this may especially be true if the woman is unable to meet the demands of daily life that often involve caring for others. Blame cannot be healing. It is important to remember that, as a multifactorial disease, breast cancer has many contributing elements that come together. Unresolved emotional material and the physical injuries it can cause, if present at all, is only one factor. There-fore, it is better to present this idea more as a factor of healing and cure than one of causation. To approach and help make visible to a patient emotional issues that are not promoting health is of tremendous value in freeing up energy that could be utilised for healing. Cancer patients who make deep and true changes in their approach to life seem to do better than those who do not. It may or may not be true that unresolved emotional material contributes to breast cancer but it is certainly true that resolution of those same issues contributes to overall health.

Overwork leads to liver and kidney yin deficiency. The liver yin is the root of liver yang. Stasis in the liver is a secondary effect of liver yin deficiency, which roots the yang. Breast distention preperiod is often due to liver stasis secondary to liver blood or yin deficiency. Liver qi stasis due to deficiency rather than excess can be differentiated by a forceless wiry pulse rather than a forceful wiry pulse. In women, liver qi stasis is most commonly due to deficiency.

Overwork often results in inadequate sleep and is a major problem in the West. It is part of a whole complex of problems that are interrelated. Sleep and relaxation are related to detoxification on the physical and emotional levels. From the conventional biomedical viewpoint, liver function can bypass many daily functional activities at night during sleep. At this time it can perform the work of detoxification, particularly of its own parenchymal tissue – one of its major tasks. Also, during sleep growth hormone is released to help in the rehabilitation of all body tissue. The loss of these two functions due to inadequate sleep helps lay the foundation for chronic illness. Overwork often leads to poor sleep. The two are bed partners, so to speak. Many people do not know when to rest and when to be active. The wei qi circulates inwardly for 12 cycles each night and outwardly for 12 cycles each day. There may be a correlation between this circulation of wei qi in Chinese theory and the detoxification and rehabilitation cycle of biomedicine.

There have also been journal articles speculating on the issue of etiology from sociological perspectives. The modern woman has many more menstrual cycles than her 19th century counterpart. She begins menses earlier – at the age of 12 versus age 17. Her first child, if any, is born much later, even in her thirties or forties versus age 18 or 19 years. She often does not breastfeed, thus initiating her cycle not long after giving birth, and the breast cell maturation that occurs as a result of breastfeeding does not occur. She has one or two children rather than four or six. Her adult life is spent having as many as 200–300 hundred cycles versus 10–20. The modern woman lives longer and starts menopause at the age of between 45 and 55. Her counterpart was often menopausal by the age of 35 years. The combination of these changes in lifestyle not only increases estrogen exposures but adds stress and emotional factors to which biomedicine does not relate. The modern woman juggles parenting, having a career, a spouse, housework, and often care for aging parents all into one lifetime. It is a difficult life that is highly complex, fraught with decisions and choices with which women in simpler times were not confronted. It is here that the rubber meets the road regarding emotional factors and physical illness, and Chinese medicine has a great deal to offer in the clarification and healing of these factors.

Disharmony of the Chong and Ren appears in menopause and leads to disharmony of blood, especially in the chest. The uterus and heart/pericardium and breast are connected internally by the Chong channel. When the downward flow of blood through the menses stops at menopause there is a propensity, especially with other underlying injuries, for the blood to stagnate in the chest. It is thought that, over time, tamoxifen aggravates this condition, leading to a higher incidence of uterine cancer and clotting disorders. Therefore, we must treat to prevent heart qi constraint and blood stasis, especially when postmenopausal women are treated to prevent recurrence or prophylactically with tamoxifen. Blood stasis is a condition that generally the body cannot heal on its own. It requires outside intervention to change. However, exercise is a major tool in preventing and treating blood stasis, no matter what its origin.

The primary constitutional diagnoses for breast cancer are (I Cohen, pers. comm.):

1. Kidney yang deficiency can affect the Ren and Chong and lead to fire poison. Kidney yang deficiency is a factor of aging and menopausal status in most cases.

2. Kidney yin deficiency can affect the Ren and Chong and lead to fire poison. Kidney yin deficiency is also a factor of aging and menopausal status in most cases.
3. Liver qi stasis can affect the spleen and stomach function, leading to dampness pouring down, which transforms to damp heat and then to blood stasis (caused by heat) and then stomach heat (caused by a transverse rebellion and heat causing the qi to flush upwards) with fluid deficiency, blood dryness, and then congealed blood. This pattern is primarily due to a combination of emotional constraint and dietary issues that lead to liver blood deficiency and liver qi stasis or unresolved emotional material and stress. This is a promotion factor in cancer, in my opinion.
4. Liver qi stasis with underlying spleen deficiency can lead to qi and blood deficiency and then to blood stasis, which in turn can again lead to blood dryness and then to blood heat, which transforms finally to fire poison. This is similar to the above pattern but without the dampness aspect as more substantial. It is also a promotional factor in cancer.
5. Liver qi stasis with underlying spleen deficiency can lead to stomach and spleen disharmony and stomach qi rebellion then food stasis (common GERD-presentation), which leads to stomach heat and then to injury of fluids and then blood heat and finally fire poison. This is very much a promotional factor in cancer pathogenesis.
6. Liver qi stasis can lead to depressive fire and then blood stasis and blood heat in the diaphragm (the heat exchange mechanism is disrupted), which in turns causes kidney yin deficiency, which then injures the Chong and Ren and leads to uncontrolled inversion fire.

Some of these diagnostic patterns have to do with aging and chronic overwork that deplete the liver/kidney axis. Some have to do with chronic deficiencies that evolve out of poor eating habits and unresolved emotional material and probably chemical exposures of various kinds. In older women, they all can diverge into post-menopausal breast cancer. There is evidence now that stress contributes to aging. It is not clear if aging contributes to cancerogenesis, but it probably contributes to the role of promoting factors. None of the above patterns discusses the formation of fire poisons from outside exposures. It is my belief that both internal and external exposures to estrogens and xenoestrogens are necessary for a cancerisation process to be turned on. Xenoestrogenic exposures are not factored into most analyses in Chinese medicine from the classical point of view. These exposures are rampant in our modern world and need to be incorporated into modern Chinese medicine's etiological analysis of cancers. There is currently evidence that biological factors may be useful in decontamination of pesticide-laden soils. If this is true, might it also be true that herbal medicines could also help to clear these burdens from human fat tissue? At any rate, it is my opinion that carcinogenic exposures are necessary for breast cancers to evolve. All of the more typical etiologies for breast cancer do not take into account carcinogenic exposures.

PROGNOSTIC FACTORS

Breast carcinoma has a long natural history and a wide variation in its clinical course. There are many different kinds of breast carcinoma. And the underlying constitution and medical history of the patient, separate from cancer, also contributes to and affects the course of the disease. The spread of primary cancer occurs by direct infiltration into breast parenchyma, along mammary ducts, and through the breast lymphatics and blood vessels. Some practitioners in the East are of the opinion that qi movement or lack of it also affects the way in which a cancer spreads. Studies have been done on the question of whether or not acupuncture treatment to move the qi actually spreads the cancer. The outcomes of these studies, all done in Japan, showed that patients receiving acupuncture as part of treatment for cancer had no different incidence in metastatic spread than those who never received acupuncture. In fact, the studies showed, counterintuitively, that patients receiving acupuncture treatment had less spread. The most frequent site of regional involvement is the axillary lymph-node region. Patients who are node positive with axillary node involvement have a worse prognosis than those who are node nega-

tive. Prognosis progressively worsens as the number of disease-positive lymph nodes increases. The rate of disease-free survival for 5 years with one to three positive nodes is 62%, for four to nine positive nodes is 58%, and for 10 or more positive axillary nodes is 29%.[103] It is important to remember that all statistics quoted in this book, except when stated, do not take into account any changes in outcomes that may result from combined care. The most widely accepted prognostic factors for node-negative breast cancer are:

- tumor size
- nuclear/histologic grade
- estrogen- and progesterone-receptor expression
- CA 27.29 status
- BR CA 15-3
- *HER-2/neu* oncogene expression
- *Ki-67* expression
- *p53* tumor suppressor gene mutation.

TUMOR SIZE

There is a strong correlation between tumor size and the risk of recurrence. Overall the 5-year survival was 99% in patients with tumors less than 1 cm in diameter, 91% in patients with tumors 1–3 cm in diameter, and 85% in patients with tumors >3 cm in diameter. Node-negative patients with tumors of 1 cm or less had a recurrence rate of 14%, while patients with tumors of 1.1–2 cm had a 20-year recurrence rate of 31%.[104]

NUCLEAR/HISTOLOGIC GRADE

The nuclear or histologic grade describes the degree of tumor differentiation and is based on the pathologist's assessment of each cell's nuclear size and shape, the number of mitoses (cell divisions), and the degree of tubule formation. Tumors of low malignancy are graded 1 and are associated with the best prognosis. Grade 3 tumors are associated with the worse prognosis. Cells that are well differentiated imply less mutation; those that are not differentiated have been running amuck for a longer period of time or are more aggressively mutating. Under a microscope these cells all look different from one another, thus they are undifferentiated. This lack of organisation in the tissue growth is a poor sign.

HORMONE-RECEPTOR STATUS

Estrogen- and progesterone-receptor positivity correlate with prolonged disease-free and overall survival. Measurement of hormone-receptor levels is valuable in both node-negative and node-positive patients for identifying patients likely to benefit from adjuvant hormonal therapy. These receptors are cytoplasmic proteins that form complexes with the respective hormone. They are translocated to the cell nucleus to produce the final hormonal effect. Estrogen-receptors are found in 60% of breast cancers in women under the age of 50 and in 75% of those over the age of 50. See the discussion in this chapter on phytoestrogens.

HER-2/NEU STATUS

HER-2/neu (or *c-erbB-2*) is an oncogene that, when present, reflects an increase in the proliferative activity of a tumor. Overexpression has been demonstrated in 15–30% of patients with breast cancer and has been found to be associated with shorter survival. However, this overexpression was also associated with significantly longer disease-free and overall survival in those who received higher doses of anthracycline-containing adjuvant chemotherapy. Doxorubicin (Adriamycin) is an example of an anthracycline antibiotic used in breast-cancer treatment.[105]

Trastuzumab (Herceptin) is a recombinant, DNA-derived, humanised monoclonal antibody that binds to the c-erbB2 protein. It is among the first biological approaches to cancer cytotoxic therapy. The HER2 is a transmembrane growth factor receptor that has tyrosine kinase activity. HER2 is structurally similar to the epidermal growth factor receptor and both are members of the type-1 growth factor receptor gene family. Herceptin can be used as a single agent in patients who are *HER-2/neu* positive and who have already received one or more chemotherapeutic agents. It can also be used in combination with a taxoid agent, like paclitaxel (Taxol) or docetaxel (Taxatere), for first-line treatment in patients who

have relapsed after anthracycline-based adjuvant chemotherapy.

OTHER MARKERS

The CA 15-3 or CA 27.29 is a marker that has useful sensitivity for breast cancer, but lacks specificity. It is used more as an indicator to determine the efficacy of treatment that is being utilised. So it is not necessarily prognostic immediately post-diagnosis but rather prognostic in terms monitoring. The range for the CA 27.29 marker is 0–38. Numbers above 38 indicate that there is probably cancer activity in a patient who has already been diagnosed with breast cancer. Laboratories use both designations in their printouts but are referring to the same marker.

DETECTION

Self-breast examination (SBE) is an important means of detection. Several studies have shown no change in survival with the use of SBE. However, in my practice many women with breast cancer have detected their own tumors through palpation and in spite of annual mammography. Therefore, I teach self-breast examination as part of prevention and prevention of recurrence. It only makes sense that the better one knows one's own body the more opportunity there is to prevent disease of any kind.[106,107]

Screening mammography has the potential to detect lesions before they become palpable. Mammographic findings that indicate malignancy are clustered microcalcifications, an irregular mass, a solid nodule with ill-defined borders, an enlarging solid well-defined mass, a developing density (in comparison to previous screenings), and an asymmetric density. In 40 to 49-year-old patients, the number of cancers found in the first year after a negative mammogram was 40% of the number found in unscreened controls, and this increased to 70% in the second year. No matter what a woman's decision regarding X-ray exposure with mammography, it is probably good to have at least a baseline mammogram in one's forties. See the mammography section under risks and causation.

RODEO, or rotating delivery of excitation off-resonance, is a new nuclear magnetic resonance imaging (MRI) technique. It has demonstrated promise for improving the sensitivity of breast cancer detection for disease not visualised by mammography.

PET, or positron emission tomography, is an imaging technique that requires a 'hot' laboratory for producing short-lived positron emitting radioisotopes and special twin headed PET scanners. This imaging technique is used to monitor the efficacy of treatment regimens because it is more able to visualise smaller changes in tissue than a CT. The parameters it can image include oxygen consumption and extraction efficiency, regional blood flow and volume, glucose consumption, pH, amino acid uptake/protein synthesis, metabolic effects of antitumor therapy, and binding of agents to receptors, like estrogen receptors and estrogen binding. The PET scan is the monitoring device of choice for later stage breast cancers and for IBC. Because sugar is the preferred substrate for cancer cells sugar consumption pre-PET scan is sometimes advised in order to enhance uptake by cancer cells, which then show up more strongly during the scan. Some practitioners even advise their patients to increase sugar intake prechemotherapy in order to magnetise the chemotherapy to the cancer cells.

DIAGNOSTIC PROCEDURES

Fine needle aspiration or FNA is used extensively in the diagnosis of benign and malignant breast lesions. If a lumpectomy appears possible, then this procedure is appropriate. Usually the tumor is small, less than 3 cm. It provides a rapid diagnosis since results regarding malignancy versus benignity can usually be obtained in a day. False negatives are rare and occur when a small mass has few cancer cells and they have not been picked up during the procedure. The FNA should be considered the first step in a series of others.

Core needle biopsy provides more information than FNA and has a significantly higher diagnostic yield. It is a procedure often done with ultrasound guidance. For non-palpable lesions a stereotactic biopsy can be done of an abnormality. This is the least invasive technique. A wire is localised with ultrasound guidance for placement to determine the exact area for excision by the surgeon. The surgeon follows the wire for margins and depth of excision. A blue dye is also used in case the wire moves during the procedure.

Open breast biopsy is the most common procedure for diagnosis. If a lumpectomy is an option then the margins around the excised tissue must be free of cancerous cells. The diagnostic technique becomes the treatment as well. When the surgical margins are not free of cancerous cells or the margin ends up being very close to the lesion (usually <8 mm), this becomes a problem in terms of spread. There is a lack of clarity regarding the remaining tissue. This biopsy is done as an outpatient procedure under local anesthesia.

Sentinel node biopsy is a newer procedure where the first mammary node or several mammary nodes nearest to the tumor site are injected with an imaging dye. The flow of this dye is an indicator as to whether or not there is spread to the adjacent nodes in the axilla. Not all patients are good candidates for sentinel node biopsy. In those who are, this procedure can mean an axillary node sparing procedure. If the axillary nodes are not involved, there is no need to remove any or all of them. If they are involved, then this procedure indicates how many should be removed. Doing breast massage prior to the sentinel node biopsy procedure probably gives clearer results.

Routine studies include chest X-ray, complete blood count (CBC), and liver function tests (LFTs). A bone scan is included if LFTs are abnormal, the alkaline/phosphatase levels are elevated, or there are positive nodes. For example, if a patient is anemic before entering chemotherapy, which often suppresses bone marrow, we need to treat more strongly those zang fu that are found to be deficient regarding blood nourishment. Knowing this prior to therapy is important because it helps us understand the baseline and original injuries the patient has suffered before cytotoxic treatment, which causes more injury.

ER and PR analysis is performed on the specimen from either mastectomy or excisional biopsy. Flow cytometry looks at the s-phase, mitotic rate, and other DNA activity (like *HER-2/neu*, *p53*, *ki67* status) to determine a grade for the cancer tissue found. The ER/PR analysis helps to determine types of therapy to be used; for example, in an

ER-negative tumor hormonal therapy is not of use since there are no receptors to which to bind a therapeutic drug. If the tumor is ER positive then more specific choices are made regarding single herbs in a formula; some may increase estrogen levels slightly, others will reduce estrogen levels slightly. One example is Liu wei di huang wan which reduces estrogen levels in premenopausal women but increases estrogen levels (by about 1–2%) in post-menopausal women. In a HER-2/neu positive tumor Herceptin may become a choice for therapy. HER-2/neu positive tumors carry a worse prognosis and so our formulas for the patient carrying this expression should be stronger and more aggressive.

There are other studies that are often done within the context of alternative treatment for cancers. For example, specific immune parameters can be identified, like the T-cell and natural killer (NK) counts, which help the practitioner understand the specific injuries that may be present in any individual patient. Also, analysis of specific chemical exposures for heavy metals, pesticides, and other toxic chemicals are done to determine if there are alternative means for clearing these toxins as part of overall treatment and prevention of recurrence. Many cancer patients tend to be hypothyroid. A simple thyroid panel allows the practitioner to know if this is an issue that needs addressing as part of general health care. Patients who are hypoglycemic or prediabetic or even outright diabetic need special care in terms of resolving these conditions. Usually this arena of activity includes very specific dietary and lifestyle guidance and follow-up.

CHINESE MEDICINE

The Chinese tongue can be utilised to develop or analyse a diagnosis of cancer. In breast cancer, the chest areas are the same as the breast, that is, the sides and the middle tip. The color of the body is indicative; purple in any of these areas alone may indicate stasis of blood in the chest. This is considered to be a poor prognosis. If there are lumps in the breast without purple areas on the tongue relative to the breast, this is considered to be a good prognosis. If the veins under the tongue are dark and distended this can indicate stasis of blood in the chest and in women in the breast.

Looking at the veins is helpful because changes here are seen before the tongue body changes. The veins also show phlegm damp stasis. If the connective tissue on and around the veins is whitish, swollen and extensive this indicates phlegm damp. It is not uncommon to see this more frequently than blood stasis signs. Red points in any of the tongue body areas relative to the chest along with a sticky yellow tongue fur indicates fire poison in the breast. If the coat is stripped in any of these areas, the prognosis is poor. The right side of the tongue refers to the right breast, and so on. It is very important to remember that the tongue will change as a result of conventional treatment. If at all possible, viewing the tongue and analysing the tumor before intervention is highly preferable to later analysis.

For those with skill in abdominal diagnosis, the use of palpation can aid in determining the constitutional environment of the patient. Are the liver reflexes positive? Is only one liver reflex positive and does this correlate with the breast involved? If both are positive, should the other breast be considered in the overall evaluation. Is the blood stasis reflex positive? To what degree and level? These are very important signs in evaluating a cancer diagnosis. What channels are restricted? And at what level is there discomfort and signs of stasis or constraint. Yin wei and Ren mai patterns in the abdomen are also useful. Cupping Ren 8 may be helpful in determining the levels of systemic blood stasis.

The Chinese use a procedure whereby a high white light is shone, with minor magnification, on the tip of the tongue and the nailbeds. The microcapillary system is visible at these sites and can be observed under these conditions. If the red blood cells (RBCs) are moving well through the vessels this shows that blood stasis is not present. If the RBCs are not moving well and the vessels are twisted and torturous, then blood stasis is present and requires attention. There are descriptive analyses of types of tumors, benign and malignant. In the case of a patient who comes to you post-surgery it may not be possible to analyse a tumor via this method. Sometimes a patient will be able to describe to you exactly how the lump felt. Sometimes the patient's constitution will enable you to predict the type of tumor that was present. Liver and kidney yin deficient constitutions will often present with a blood stasis type of tumor. A woman with a more spleen deficient constitution that hasn't led to blood deficiency but has led to damp phlegm will more often present with phlegm or damp type tumors. There may be combinations of types, for example, it is common to see a knotted form of blood and phlegm stasis tumor. In fast-growing and aggressive tumors, one can assume fire poison as the type.

Types

1. Blood stasis: a hard, palpable, non-movable lump, which doesn't change and may or may not be painful.
2. Phlegm stasis: soft lumps, can be moved with palpation, possible watery discharge from the nipple, no pain.
3. Fire poison: fast-moving, erythema on breast surface over the area involved, possible 'orange-peel skin', probable local and regional node involvement, can be IBC. If later stage of any type the breast will be hard, swollen, hot and very painful; there may be open sores with a secondary infection.
4. Dampness: swellings with oozing, soft movable lumps, similar to phlegm but less nodular.

Knowing the type of tumor (versus the pattern) at presentation enables us to fine tune our formulas to treat the underlying constitution and the type of breast cancer from the classical Chinese point of view. Following are listings of herbs that are used in combination with the constitutional formula and with other specifically designed formulas for use during conventional treatment.[108–110]

Phlegm-resolving breast herbs

- zhe bei mu (Fritillariae thunbergii Bulbus; *Fritillaria thunbergii*)
- chuan bei mu (Fritillariae cirrhosae Bulbus; *Fritillaria cirrhosa*)
- gua lou shi *or* ren (Trichosanthis Fructus *or* Trichosanthis Semen; *Trichosanthes* fruit *or* seed)
- tian hua fen (Trichosanthis Radix; *Trichosanthes* root)
- huang yao zi (Dioscoreae bulbiferae Rhizoma; *Dioscorea bulbifera*)

- tian nan xing (Arisaematis Rhizoma preparatum; *Arisaema* erubescens rhizome)
- ai ye (Artemisiae argyi Folium; *Artemisia argyi* leaves)
- mao gen (Ranunculi japonici Radix; *Ranunculus japonicus* root – not bai mao gen, which is Imperatae Rhizoma; *Imperata cylindrica* rhizome)
- pi pa ye (Eriobotryae Folium; *Eriobotrya japonica* leaves)

Blood-regulating breast herbs

- ru xiang (Olibanum; *Boswellia sacra*; frankincenze; gum olibanum)
- mo yao (Myrrha; *Commiphora myrrha*; myrrh)
- san leng (Sparganii Rhizoma; *Sparganium* rhizome)
- e zhu (Curcumae Rhizoma; *Curcuma zedoaria*; zedoary)
- wang bu liu xing (Vaccariae Semen; *Vaccaria segetalis* seeds)
- yu jin (Curcumae Radix; *Curcuma longa* rhizome)
- xue jie (Daemonoropis Resina; *Daemonorops draco*; Resina Draconis; dragon's blood)
- si gua luo (Luffae Fructus Retinervus; *Luffa cylindrica*; loofah)
- wu ling zhi (Trogopterori Faeces; *Trogopterus xanthipes* excrement)
- ban mao (Mylabris; *Mylabris*)
- xian he cao (Agrimoniae Herba; *Agrimonia pilosa* var. *japonica*; agrimony)

Fire poison/toxin-clearing breast herbs:

- xia ku cao (Prunellae Spica; *Prunella vulgaris*)
- pu gong ying (Taraxaci Herba; *Taraxacum mongolicum*)
- ban bian lian (Lobeliae chinensis Herba; *Lobelia chinensis*)
- tian kui zi (Semiaquilegiae Radix; *Semiaquilegia adoxoides* root)
- ban zhi lian (Scutellariae barbatae Herba; *Scutellaria barbata*)
- ba jiao lian (Podophylli Rhizoma; *Podophyllum pleianthum* rhizome)
- zao jiao ci (Gleditsiae Spina; *Gleditsia* spines)
- lu feng fang (Vespae Nidus; *Vespa* wasp/hornet nest)

- she mei (Herba Duchesneae indicae; *Duchesnea indica*)

Soften hard mass breast herbs

- mu li (Ostreae Concha; *Ostrea* shell)
- hai zao (Sargassum; *Sargassum*)
- kun bu (Eckloniae Thallus; *Ecklonia kurome*; kelp thallus)
- shan ci gu* (Cremastrae/Pleiones Pseudobulbus; *Cremastra/Pleione* pseudobulbs)
- long kui (Solani nigri Herba; *Solanum nigrum*)

STAGING

Clinical staging includes physical examination with careful inspection and palpation of the skin, mammary gland, and the lymph nodes (axillary, supraclavicular, and cervical), pathologic examination of the breast and other tissues, and imaging to establish the diagnosis of breast cancer. The extent of the tissues examined pathologically for clinical staging is less than that required for pathologic staging. Operative findings are elements of clinical staging, including the size of the primary tumor and chest wall invasion and the presence or absence of regional or distant metastasis.

Pathologic staging includes all data used for clinical staging and surgical resection as well as pathologic examination of the primary carcinoma, including not less than excision of the primary carcinoma with no tumor in any margin of resection. If there is tumor in the margin of resection, it is coded TX, i.e. the extent of the primary tumor cannot be assessed.

The chest wall includes the ribs, intercostal muscles, and serratus anterior muscle, but not the pectoral muscle.

Dimpling of the skin, nipple retraction, or any other skin change ('orange-peel skin') except those described under T4b and T4d may occur in T1, T2, or T3 without changing the classification. The current anatomic staging system is reproduced in Box 4.1. The TNM system for describing the anatomical extent of disease is based on the assessment of three components:

This is, in effect, a shorthand system for describing the extent of a particular malignant tumor.[97]

Box 4.1   TNM system

T: the extent of the primary tumor
N: the absence or presence and extent of regional lymph node metastasis
M: the absence or presence of distant metastasis

The addition of numbers to these three components indicates the extent of malignant disease:

T0, T1, T2, T3, T4, N0, N1, N2, N3, M0, M1

The staging work-up consists of all of the above procedures and assessments. It provides an anatomical, biochemical and genetic map of the malignant disease in a given patient. It is important because it not only provides information concerning prognostic factors including potentials for recurrence, but also information concerning the therapies to be used. Knowing the staging helps us to know and therefore predict future treatment, the side effects of that treatment, the strength of treatment necessary on our part to overcome these side effects in that given patient, and the strength necessary to overcome the cancer itself. We can also understand the mechanism of the therapy chosen so that we do not undermine its effect.

PRINCIPLES OF TREATMENT

SURGERY

Surgery is considered to be the primary conventional defense against almost any solid tumor. The purpose of surgery is to remove local and regional disease. When there is no metastasis surgery may be curative. The belief has been that breast cancer underwent an orderly progression from primary site to regional lymph node involvement to distant metastasis. The Halsted radical mastectomy was designed with this in mind. It removed the entire breast and all of the tissue down to the ribs. It was a disabling procedure. However, patients with negative lymph node status died despite this radical procedure. It has been suggested that distant metastasis can occur independent of lymph node metastasis. Therefore, less radical procedures including modified radical mastectomy and lumpectomy have evolved. The staging of breast cancer has become much more sophisticated.

Partial mastectomy has been subcategorised into lumpectomy, wide excision, or segmental mastectomy (quandrantectomy). The local recurrence rate after lumpectomy alone has been reported at 39%. If post-surgical radiation is added the rate falls to 10% recurrence at 8 years. The standard now is lumpectomy with radiation post-surgery in tumors less than 4 cm.[111]

In a total mastectomy the whole breast including the axillary tail is removed. If the axillary node dissection is performed in continuity with the mastectomy, it is called a modified radical mastectomy. The pectoralis muscle is left intact. In a lumpectomy or quandrantectomy, the axillary lymph node dissection is done through a separate incision and suction drains are placed. The radiation therapy in the latter procedure is usually done 3 weeks following the surgery. In total mastectomies, separate foci of cancer have been found in 27% of patients. However, 57% of these foci were in the same quadrant as the primary tumor, suggesting multifocality. Lumpectomy with post-surgical radiation is usually considered to be equally curative as mastectomy alone.[111] The clinical examination of axillary nodes is not especially accurate. There is no evidence that removal of benign nodes leads to improved survival. But when clinically and pathologically positive nodes are removed the recurrence rate is reduced.

Every day women are exposed to more and more carcinogens. It may be that as time passes the nature of the breast cancers we see will become more complex. There is a great deal yet to be known about how this cancer happens. With so few resources being assigned to prevention, the main thrust has been on more and more specific and genetically-oriented treatment. The lack of research in prevention implies a lack of information regarding causation. We don't know if these cancers are becoming more aggressive and, if so, why. We do know that the rates of incidence have risen so astronomically that breast cancer is now considered an epidemic disease.

Chinese medicine

The side effects of surgery are:

- General anesthesia during mastectomy causes general qi stasis and lung qi stasis; herbal medicine and supplements are used to help hasten recovery and prevent digestive sluggishness including constipation.
- Local trauma and swelling leading to fluid stasis.
- Blood loss depending on the procedure; the initial incision through the skin utilises a scalpel but the rest of the surgery involves the use of a cautery stick to reduce bleeding. A mastectomy usually will result in more blood loss.
- A lumpectomy will result in a hole in the breast, which initially will fill with fluid which gets resorbed; this resorption can be resolved more quickly with herbal medicine and local applications.
- Axillary dissection will also result in fluid build-up; tubes are used when appropriate to drain this fluid; there is also local pain and often a loss of range of motion, which can be treated with acupuncture and herbal medicine.
- The scarring that results from any surgical technique is considered to be a form of blood stasis; acupuncture and herbal techniques are used to prevent the formation of adhesions and keloids (in patients with this propensity).

There is now enough evidence to indicate that surgery during the last part of the menstrual cycle is preferable to surgery during the follicular phase. The follicular or yang and qi moving half of the cycle has more hormonal activity relative to the breast tissue. Surgery during that time may enhance the possibility of spread of tumor cells during the surgical procedure itself. This activity is not present during the yin half of the cycle, and now women are recommended to have breast surgical procedures after days three to twelve after the end of their menses. The standard now is to avoid surgery from days three to twelve.

Pre- and post-surgical formulas

When time permits it is always appropriate to use anticancer formulas according to the patient's diagnosis. This will help to prevent the movement of tumor cells during surgery and it also prompts the patient towards cure. To this formula can be added qi and blood tonic herbs like *Astragalus membranaceus* (huang qi), *Angelica sinensis* (dang gui), and *Spatholobus* (ji xue teng), all of which improve blood levels and wound healing. If surgery is scheduled sooner than in one month then use the following guidelines:[112]

- in a premenopausal woman who has an ER/PR positive stasis use Liu wei di huang wan
- in a premenopausal patient with deficiency symptoms use Ba zhen tang or Shi chuan da bu tang
- in a weak and postmenopausal patient with blood deficiency, anxiety, and no inflammatory signs use Gui pi tang or Shi chuan da bu tang
- post-surgically use Shi chuan da bu wan (Ten herb tonify the great decoction)

Three weeks post-surgery the following formula can be given to address the tumor more directly:

xia ku cao (Prunellae Spica; *Prunella vulgaris*)	15 g
dang gui (Angelicae sinensis Radix; *Angelica sinensis*)	9 g
zhu ling (Polyporus; *Polyporus – Grifola*)	15 g
shan ci gu* (Cremastrae/Pleiones Pseudobulbus; *Cremastra/Pleione* pseudobulbs)	12 g
jin yin hua (Lonicerae Flos; *Lonicera* flowers)	12 g
san qi (Notoginseng Radix; *Panax notoginseng*)	1.5 g
huang qi (Astragali Radix; *Astragalus membranaceus*)	15 g
tai zi shen (Pseudostellariae Radix; *Pseudostellaria heterophylla*)	15 g
gua lou shi (Trichosanthis Fructus; *Trichosanthes* fruit)	20 g
fu ling (Poria; *Poria cocos*)	15 g
bai shao (Paeoniae Radix alba; *Paeonia lactiflora* root)	10 g
tian dong (Asparagi Radix; *Asparagus*)	15 g
bai hua she she cao (Hedyotis diffusae Herba; *Oldenlandia*)	20 g

The above formula takes into account the healing process necessary post-surgically and the urgency of beginning to treat the cancer directly after surgery. Xia ku cao and jin yin hua are both heat-clearing herbs that clear heat from the qi level and are specific to the chest (breast). Zhu ling and fu ling help drain fluids from the area; they are fungi that increase WBC counts, increase phagocytosis, and are mildly analgesic. San qi helps stop bleeding and has anticancer properties. Dang gui improves the quality of blood and acts mildly as a laxative. Tai zi shen is a neutral-temperature qi tonic herb that also generates fluids; it improves lung function and aids in improving general digestive function. Bai shao and tian dong work together to nourish fluids and nourish the blood; they also soothe the liver to calm the spirit. Huang qi is the master herb of wound healing; it also tonifies the general qi, increases WBC and phagocytosis to clear cellular debris post-surgically; it helps prevent infection along with jin yin hua and xia ku cao. Shan ci gu, bai hua she she cao, and gua lou shi are all anti-neoplastics. They work with the heat-clearing herbs to prevent spread of cancerous cells.

RADIATION THERAPY

Radiation therapy is used in treating smaller tumors following partial mastectomy. Radiation is used at this stage when breast preservation is appropriate. High-energy irradiation delivered by a linear accelerator is now the standard of care in lumpectomy, mastectomy, and axillary dissections where cancer is found. A treatment simulator is considered extremely desirable, and computerised tatooing and planning is essential. Cautions in radiation treatment are pre-existing serious pulmonary disease or serious cardiac disease. Collagen vascular diseases (usually autoimmune diseases such as SLE) and uncontrolled diabetes are also probable contraindications for radiation therapy.[113] Many centers use a boost to raise the dose in the immediate vicinity of the tumor. The boost includes the entire breast scar and the tumor bed below. Preoperative and postoperative mammograms are helpful to determine the site and depth of the tumor bed. Many surgeons will mark the tumor bed with clips at the time of the lumpectomy in order to guide the radiation oncologist in setting the field for delivery of radiation therapy.

If there is gross axillary node involvement or an inadequate dissection, then postoperative irradiation will improve control of the local disease.

This usually includes irradiation of the supraclavicular area. However, the morbidity for lymphedema from axillary irradiation is very high. Lymphedema caused by axillary dissection and irradiation can become a lifetime management issue, requiring careful avoidance of infection from mosquito bites and the nicks and bruises common in everyday life. Many people believe that acupuncture is contraindicated in patients with axillary dissection followed by irradiation because of the risk of infection not by the needle but via the hole left by the needle. This does not preclude acupuncture needling on the ipsilateral arm or other techniques within the scope of acupuncture like moxibustion without burning, tui na, cupping, and other manual therapies. The very high risk of lymphedema from axillary irradiation is reason for some women to decide against this procedure. The evidence for axillary irradiation is still not clear. The data show there is no change in survival after 10 years from those who do and don't have axillary irradiation. In general, if nodes have confined and encapsulated cancer present but with no spread outside the node, then many radiation oncologists now tend not to do axillary radiation.

Concomitant radiation therapy and chemotherapy increase local tissue reaction and may worsen both the cosmetic and the therapeutic result. Radiation therapy destroys tissue and the capillary system that carries chemotherapy; and it can cause scarring and the formation of adhesions, both of which reduce blood circulation. This reduced circulation limits the access of chemotherapeutic drugs to the local area. Therefore, radiation is often delayed until the end of chemotherapy, provided that the delay is not longer than 6 months. Sometimes three to four cycles of chemotherapy are given and then radiation and then a resumption of chemotherapy. The most common scenario is surgery followed by chemotherapy and then radiation.

In advanced breast cancer where surgery is not an option because the cancer is no longer localised then systemic therapy is usually the initial approach. Radiation is sometimes used as consolidation therapy. The aim is local control in a non-resectable tumor or reduction of a larger tumor to a resectable size. Full-dose radiation is used. Regional nodes are also treated vigorously but care must be taken not to risk injuring the lung tissue or the brachial plexus. In late disease radiation can also be used to treat distant metastases, especially those to the bone and brain. Treating bone to stop the disintegration of the bony structure by cancerous cells helps to stop the advance of the disease and also helps to treat pain associated with bony invasion. The same is true with metastatic disease in the brain; very low dose and specifically oriented radiation beams to specific sites in the brain that are involved can stop the cancer in that area. Amazingly, the side effects are usually mild or non-existent depending on the number of sites that are irradiated, the dose of radiation, and the amount of steroidal drugs that are used to manage swelling as a result of radiation. Currently, gamma knife irradiation is becoming the standard of care for the management of smaller brain metastases.

Radiation therapy usually begins after chemotherapy and lasts for approximately 35 daily treatments. The treatment session lasts for about 15–20 minutes including set-up time. Symptoms usually begin to show at about the middle of the treatment schedule at day 15–20. Then redness, possibly blistering, and second- or third-degree burning may occur. The skin will be tender and red and an unpredictable level of fatigue will set in.

Chinese medicine

Radiation therapy during breast cancer treatment causes:

- systemic qi deficiency that may persist for some time; radiation therapy (XRT) is cumulative and the effect lasts up to 6–9 months after treatment has ceased
- local yin deficiency that, depending on the field of XRT, may cause throat and mouth dryness due to either superficial or deeper level injury to fluids in the lung and stomach or esophagus
- local yin deficiency caused by burning of the tissue can lead to red and blistered skin and the underlying tissue
- blood stasis and scarring due to yin deficiency and the burning effect of XRT.

Formulas are designed and modified to treat the level of injuries caused by XRT. The dosage and field used in treatment with XRT for a lumpectomy is much less than that used in treating a mastectomy or a lumpectomy with axillary irradiation. XRT to the supraclavicular nodes will also require a modified formula that takes into account the inflammation of the esophagus and trachea.

The purpose of XRT is to kill local and regional cancer cells mainly by making cell-damaging free radicals. Antioxidants, and by extension Chinese herbs that clear heat, are thought to possibly inhibit radiation from having its full effect. The scientific data shows that, counterintuitively, antioxidants, and by extension Chinese herbal formulas that clear heat and nourish yin, actually improve the efficacy of both chemotherapy and XRT.[114,115] There is no current evidence that herbal medicines will decrease the effect of XRT. I refer you to a meta-analysis of many of the studies done on antioxidants relative to XRT and specific chemotherapeutic regimens by Davis Lamson, ND, from the October 1999 issue of *Alternative Medicine Review*. The vast evidence from research regarding herbal medicine and antioxidant therapies during radiation shows that especially blood-regulating herbs like dan shen enhance the effectiveness of radiation.

Formula for radiation treatment

pu gong ying (Taraxaci Herba; *Taraxacum mongolicum*)	15 g
jin yin hua (Lonicerae Flos; *Lonicera* flowers)	12 g
dan shen (Salviae miltiorrhizae Radix; *Salvia miltiorhiza* root)	15 g
tai zi shen (Pseudostellariae Radix; *Pseudostellaria heterophylla*)	15 g
fu ling (Poria; *Poria cocos*)	15 g
zhu ling (Polyporus; *Polyporus – Grifola*)	15 g
tian dong (Asparagi Radix; *Asparagus*)	15 g
mu dan pi (Moutan Cortex; *Paeonia suffruticosa* root cortex)	10 g
ling zhi (Ganoderma; *Ganoderma*)	15 g
bei sha shen (Glehniae Radix; *Glehnia*)	15 g
nu zhen zi (Ligustri lucidi Fructus; *Ligustrum lucidum* fruit)	15 g
shan yao (Dioscoreae Rhizoma; *Dioscorea opposita*)	12 g
zhi mu (Anemarrhenae Rhizoma; *Anemarrhena*)	12 g

This formula clears heat and moves toxins out via the skin and sweating and through the stool and urine. It also nourishes yin and helps generate normal interstitial fluids. It increases blood circulation and improves the oxygenation of the cells; radiation therapy works best in highly oxygenated cells, but tumor cells are usually very poorly oxygenated. Improving the supply of blood with oxygenated RBCs to the local area to be irradiated actually improves the effect of the XRT.

Pu gong ying and jin yin hua are both herbs that clear heat and remove toxin. They are also emperic detoxifying herbs for the breast. Dan shen is a blood-moving herb that has been highly studied for its ability to enhance the effect of XRT through improving the oxygen levels to cancer cells. Tai zi shen is a neutral qi tonic herb that improves energy, generates fluids and with fu ling potentiates the XRT effect. Zhu ling and fu ling and tai zi shen all work together to potentiate the radiation effect. Fu ling and zhu ling are both fungi that increase WBC counts and phagocytosis. Tian dong, nu zhen zi and bei sha shen all nourish yin and protect normal cells from the effects of XRT. Mu dan pi helps clear heat from the blood level. Zhi mu helps clear heat from the qi level and benefits fluids. Ling zhi is another fungus that potentiates the effect of radiation, increases WBC counts and macrophage activity. It is also mildly analgesic.

There are several different local applications that can be used to promote healing to the surface tissue during XRT. Ching wan hung, or Ten thousand brights, cream is especially helpful in preventing blistering and painful burning which usually begins to appear after day 15–20 of local XRT. Also the Spring wind herbs product Burn creme is especially beneficial in preventing blistering and reducing pain. It is being studied at Kaiser Permanente Hospitals in the San Francisco Bay Area and preliminary results are extremely positive.

CHEMOTHERAPY AND HORMONAL THERAPIES

Chemotherapy and hormonal therapies are considered systemic adjuvant treatments for breast cancer. The purpose of adjuvant therapy is to treat micrometastatic disease before it is clinically detectable in the hope that the smaller tumor burden will be easier to eliminate. Patients at high risk for developing metastatic disease may be treated before their primary tumor is treated. Neoadjuvant chemotherapy and hormonal therapies have been used as adjuvant therapy.

There are two main groupings of adjuvant combination chemotherapy for the treatment of breast cancer: those consisting of CMF (cyclophosphamide, methotrexate, and fluorouracil) and those containing doxorubicin (Adriamycin). Doxorubicin-containing regimens (which may also include Cytoxan, Taxol or Taxatere, Herceptin, or Navelbine) are generally used for high-risk patients with more than four positive nodes and negative ER status. There is evidence from the Early Breast Cancer Trial's Collaborative Group (a worldwide collaboration) that even in node-negative disease there was a 26% reduction in recurrence and a 17% reduction in mortality when adjuvant therapy was used (in this study it was tamoxifen).[104] However, in node-negative early stage breast cancer patients, the role of adjuvant chemotherapy is less clear. Most commonly, women with early stage breast cancer in the United States are treated with three to four courses of the AC regimen or with surgery and radiation alone.

In node-positive patients the benefit of adjuvant therapy is clearly established. However, the rates of reduction are equal to the rates using oophorectomy.[104] The advantage of tamoxifen over oophorectomy has always been stated as an advantage of sustained ovarian ablation over time. Tamoxifen is often given for up to 5 years after surgery, chemotherapy, and radiation. I refer you to the earlier discussion on tamoxifen relative to risk factors for breast cancer.

Doxorubicin plus Cytoxan, or AC, is a common regimen for women with earlier stage breast cancer (stages I and IIA with negative lymph nodes. This regimen is commonly given intravenously in a 21-day cycle of administration for four to six cycles. Symptoms may vary in individuals and with the progression of the therapy. If we analyse the activity and symptoms caused by Adriamycin and Cytoxan, we can understand better how to interface with this stage of therapy.

Chinese medicine

From day 1 of chemotherapy to day 6 the greatest cytotoxic effect takes place. As a result, cancerous and non-cancerous fast-growing cells are killed off. There is erosion of the epithelial mucous and serous membranes. This relates, therefore, primarily to the entire gastrointestinal lining from mouth to anus. Resulting symptoms include:[116]

- dry mouth
- ulcerations and sores in the mouth; mucositis, apthous ulcers
- in prone patients herpetic lesions in the mouth may proliferate
- vomiting and nausea
- anorexia
- diarrhea and/or constipation
- abdominal discomfort
- possibly cystitis or even hemorrhagic cystitis (rare)
- pericarditis in patients who are prone because Adriamycin is a cardiotoxic drug.

The functional impact of a formula at this time should be:

- to increase qi and blood circulation in order to promote the circulation of the chemotherapeutic agent
- to enable the elimination of metabolites from the chemotherapy and cell debris from kill off
- to nourish the yin and protect the gastrointestinal mucosa
- to control nausea and promote appetite so that the patient can continue to nourish herself
- to promote urination and normalise stool.

There is an old saying in Chinese medicine that states that normal stools and good sleep are the prerequisites for health. These things need to be treated before any others so that the body can rehabilitate itself while healing. The need for adequate nutrition and sleep while suffering from cancer and undergoing treatment for cancer becomes much greater, since cancer takes qi and blood to sustain itself and since cytotoxic treatment takes even more because of the general impact on hematopoiesis, digestion, and other organ functions. From days 7 to 12 the cytotoxic effect is mostly over and damage to the bone marrow and the organs peaks. This stage is marked by:[116]

- fatigue and malaise; 'chemo brain', as it is called by patients
- insomnia
- possible fevers caused by neutropenia, possible infection, cytotoxic reactions
- alternating hot and cold sensations
- possible dry cough
- possible tachycardia, palpitations, and other signs of anemia
- cardiac, liver, or renal signs due to toxicity.

The need here is to tonify qi and yang, and nourish blood, yin, and essence. Organ function needs protection and restoration depending on the presentation. The wei and ying need harmonising and nourishment in order to increase immune function on whatever levels blood work indicates (to prevent infections). The most common injuries are to the WBC counts.

From day 12 to 21 the body is regenerating and recovering. The signs and symptoms will gradually improve and some will leave off completely. Fatigue, malaise, insomnia and joint pain may persist. Usually starting at day 14 of the first course of the AC regimen the hair will begin to fall out. Many women have their heads shaved in order to avoid the emotional experience of gradually losing their hair. There may also be hyperpigmentation in some patients' nailbeds. And at this point, and especially later in the courses of treatment, anxiety and depression can set in as an individual looks ahead to yet another round of cytotoxic treatment.

The role of the formula at this stage is to tonify qi and yang, nourish yin and blood and promote the recovery and regeneration of all body structures. It is very important to support the spirit. Without spirit the patient loses hope and this has a profound impact on the prognosis. The complexity of writing a formula to interface with a specific chemotherapeutic regimen is obvious. When possible always address the constitutional environment of the patient in some part of the formula. Constitutional formulas are included for

each diagnostic pattern. The construction of the formula is based on the:

- presentation of the patient including the symptom picture, medical history, emotional status
- Western analysis including blood work; is any organ function test abnormal and how does that translate into Chinese medicine; is the patient already anemic prior to cytotoxic treatment; is there underlying chronic disease
- staging; is this early stage or advanced cancer with metastatic disease and where and to what effect
- ER/PR status and other markers that might change the selection of herbs based on the pharmaceutical analysis of their effect
- ability of the patient to assimilate and absorb oral medication; you must chose specifically based on the patient's gastrointestinal status
- predicted side effects and the mechanism of the chemotherapeutic regimen.

Single herbs may be added because of their antineoplastic effect as measured by pharmaceutical studies. Single herbs are also added according to the tumor type (phlegm stasis, blood stasis, etc.). Usually the constitutional formula as a whole acts as the chief of the whole formula and the symptomatic formula is the deputy, with the additional single herbs being assistants or messengers. However, sometimes the side effects of the conventional treatment are so severe that addressing them becomes primary. Then the constitutional aspects of the formula take second place. Once a patient has committed to undergoing conventional cytotoxic treatment the support of Chinese medicine can help them undergo that treatment more comfortably and with less damage. Maintaining normal function allows the patient to maintain the cytotoxic schedule for administration. It can also allow for a higher dose of cytotoxic treatment; the greater the cytotoxic effect without injury the greater the possibility of resolving the cancer.

It is important, if at all possible and no matter what the staging of the cancer, to address the constitutional environment even in a small way. By doing so there is a continual prompt towards healing the memory or spirit of the disease. This memory can be thought of as genetic, acquired, physiological and emotional, and even karmic. It is the memory, the roots, of the disease at the cellular level and within the emotional or subtle body of the patient. The continual prompting is essential, even in the terminally-ill patient. The etheric or subtle level of every disease is important to heal even in death. The patient will be more comfortable and move through death with greater ease if some kind of healing has happened within the subtle body.

Formula base for the AC regimen[117]

huang qi (Astragali Radix; *Astragalus membranaceus*)	20 g
dan shen (Salviae miltiorrhizae Radix; *Salvia miltiorhiza* root)	15 g
bai zhu (Atractylodis macrocephalae Rhizoma; *Atractylodes macrocephala*)	12 g
fu ling (Poria; *Poria cocos*)	12 g
ze xie (Alismatis Rhizoma; *Alisma*)	12 g
tian dong (Asparagi Radix; *Asparagus*)	12 g
gou qi zi (Lycii Fructus; *Lycium chinensis* fruit)	15 g
huang jing (Polygonati Rhizoma; *Polygonatum*)	15 g
mai dong (Ophiopogonis Radix; *Ophiopogon*)	12 g
san qi (Notoginseng Radix; *Panax notoginseng*)	10 g
ji xue teng (Spatholobi Caulis; *Spatholobus suberectus*)	15 g
he shou wu (Polygoni multiflori Radix preparata; *Polygonum multiflorum* root)	10 g
bei sha shen (Glehniae Radix; *Glehnia*)	10 g
zhi ban xia (Pinelliae Rhizoma preparatum; *Pinellia ternata* rhizome)	12 g
wu zhu yu (Evodiae Fructus; *Evodia*)	10 g
shi di (Kaki Calyx; *Diospyros kaki* calyx)	10 g
shen qu (Massa medicata fermentata; medicated leaven)	12 g
xi yang shen (Panacis quinquefolii Radix; *Panax quinquefolium*)	10 g
nu zhen zi (Ligustri lucidi Fructus; *Ligustrum lucidum* fruit)	15 g
da zao (Jujubae Fructus; *Ziziphus jujuba*; jujube)	6 g

Adriamycin is an antitumor antibiotic made from the culture broth of various species of *Streptomyces*. It is metabolised by the liver and causes myelosuppression with the nadir at days 10–14. Nausea and vomiting are moderate risks. Alopecia is universal. Hyperpigmentation of the nail beds occurs and is temporary. Adriamycin is associated with acute and chronic cardiotoxicity. Pretreatment cardiograms including a MUGA-scan to establish the baseline ejection fraction is important. This is repeated every three courses, or at least at the end of treatment with Adriamycin.

The AC regimen injures the spleen qi thus causing a damp stasis that can lead to nausea and vomiting. The spleen injury also leads to spleen failing to nourish the blood, which manifests as anemia in the form of neutropenia. This regimen also injures the essence and leads to general bone marrow suppression, which can manifest as a low hemoglobin count and RBC counts that are decreased. The spleen injury can cause disharmony between the stomach and spleen leading to stomach qi flushing upwards manifesting as nausea and vomiting and either stomach heat or cold, which can cause mouth sores, mucositis, inflammation/ulceration of the gastrointestinal mucosa, and headaches. This regimen also injures the kidneys, which can manifest as painful urinary dysfunction (PUD) and essence deficiency. The injury to the liver can cause injury to the heart via the Five Phase cycle.

Huang qi is a prime herb in maintaining spleen and lung function; it raises WBC counts and increases phagocytosis and NK cells. Dan shen works as a blood-cracking herb to improve the blood circulation generally in order to increase the overall effect of the AC regimen. Huang qi, bai zhu and fu ling are the primary elements of Si jun zi tang, the main formula to tonify the spleen qi. This formula can be found in many formulas designed to treat the side effects of chemotherapy. Ze xie clears heat and generates fluids. Gou qi zi, huang jing, tian dong, mai dong, ji xue teng, he shou wu, nu zhen zi and bei sha shen all work together to nourish the blood and generate fluids. Blood- and yin-nourishing herbs potentiate one another since the yin and blood are in some ways one and the same; the blood plasma is the yin component of blood, the WBCs and the RBCs are the qi component of blood – the active component of the fluid. The yin-nourishing herbs in this cluster also nourish the yin of the zang fu and help clear heat manifesting as inflammation along with ze xie. These herbs together help maintain normal organ and digestive function.

The digestive injuries caused by the AC regimen are also ameliorated by the herbs that warm the middle jiao. Ban xia is the empiric herb for nausea and vomiting. It redirects the stomach qi, along with wu zhu yu and shi di, both of which are warming herbs that treat nausea. Xi yang shen is a yin-nourishing herb that also tonifies the qi. This makes it a very valuable herb for treating the fatigue that is common with certain kinds of chemotherapeutic agents. Da zao is added as a harmonising herb that also generates fluids. Although chemotherapies are heat- and toxin-clearing drugs from the classical point of view and would, therefore, be cold in nature, they are so strong and have such an intense cumulative effect that it is only in the very early phase of treatment that we see injury by cold. That same injury transforms to heat soon in the first course of treatment depending on the constitution of the patient. Thus the need for yin-nourishing herbs not only to nourish blood but also to cool and detoxify.

Formula base for the CMF regimen[117]

huang qi (Astragali Radix; *Astragalus membranaceus*)	20 g
dang shen (Codonopsis Radix; *Codonopsis pilosula* root)	15 g
bai zhu (Atractylodis macrocephalae Rhizoma; *Atractylodes macrocephala*)	12 g
fu ling (Poria; *Poria cocos*)	15 g
ze xie (Alismatis Rhizoma; *Alisma*)	12 g
nu zhen zi (Ligustri lucidi Fructus; *Ligustrum lucidum* fruit)	15 g
ji xue teng (Spatholobi Caulis; *Spatholobus suberectus*)	15 g
he shou wu (Polygoni multiflori Radix preparata; *Polygonum multiflorum* root)	12 g

shu di (Rehmanniae Radix preparata; *Rehmannia*)	12 g
gou qi zi (Lycii Fructus; *Lycium chinensis* fruit)	15 g
huang jing (Polygonati Rhizoma; *Polygonatum*)	15 g
bei sha shen (Glehniae Radix; *Glehnia*)	12 g
du zhong (Eucommiae Cortex; *Eucommia ulmoides* cortex)	15 g
bu gu zhi (Psoraleae Fructus; *Psoralea*)	15 g
bai mao gen (Imperatae Rhizoma; *Imperata cylindrica* rhizome)	12 g
di yu (Sanguisorbae Radix; *Sanguisorba*)	10 g
san qi (Notoginseng Radix; *Panax notoginseng*)	6 g
yu jin (Curcumae Radix; *Curcuma longa* rhizome)	12 g
wu yao (Linderae Radix; *Lindera*)	12 g
mai dong (Ophiopogonis Radix; *Ophiopogon*)	12 g
zhi ban xia (Pinelliae Rhizoma preparatum; *Pinellia ternata* rhizome)	12 g
shi di (Kaki Calyx; *Diospyros kaki* calyx)	10 g
wu zhu yu (Evodiae Fructus; *Evodia*)	10 g
da zao (Jujubae Fructus; *Ziziphus jujuba*; jujube)	6 g

The side effects of the CMF regimen are slightly different than those for the AC regimen. These side effects include more severe renal toxicity, which can lead to hemorrhagic cystitis and even renal failure caused by all three chemotherapies. Mesna is an assisting drug to help prevent bladder damage. Therefore, herbs to protect and repair kidney and bladder function are included. Cardiotoxicity is present with cyclophosphamide and 5-FU. Platelet levels and hemoglobin can be impacted by methotrexate and so essence-restoring herbs are also included. And various kinds of rashes can evolve as a result of the use of methotrexate and 5-FU. 5-FU is excreted in the tears and increased lacrimation and photophobia can be side effects of 5-FU. Side effects from 5-FU used singly can change, depending on whether it is used as a continuous infusion or as a bolus. Continuous infusion usually results only in gastrointestinal mucositis and diarrhea. The bolus schedules are more likely to produce marrow suppression. Myelosuppression will occur in the form of leukopenia and thrombocytopenia with the nadir generally around day 15. Nausea and vomiting are common symptoms. All of these conditions require a slightly different approach in designing the formula. 5-FU also can produce hand/foot syndrome, which manifests as scaling and hyperpigmentation and paresthesias on the palms and soles. Vitamin B_6 at 50 mg three times daily helps the paresthesias, and bag balm® helps the hand/foot syndrome. Vitamin B_{12} injections are also beneficial.

Huang qi tonifies the lung and spleen function; it increases WBC counts and increases phagocytosis. Dang shen, bai zhu and fu ling are the main components of the formula, Si jun zi tang, which is a main spleen tonic formula. This formula helps protect and support digestive function, especially spleen function. Ze xie helps clear heat and as a diuretic provides a downward draining action that helps clear toxicity. Nu zhen zi, ji xue teng, he shou wu, shu di, gou qi zi, huang jing, mai dong and bei sha shen work as a potentiating unit to nourish yin and blood and help to maintain normal blood levels. Most of these herbs also nourish liver and kidney yin and, therefore, help to protect organ function.

The renal toxicity of the regimen requires amelioration. Du zhong and bu gu zhi work together to nourish the kidney qi and yang and protect renal and bladder function. Bu gu zhi contains the highest levels of genistein of any herb studied to date. Genistein has strong antitumor properties. Bai mao gen and di yu help clear heat from the urinary bladder and also stop urinary bleeding. San qi is a strong cardiotonic herb that also stops bleeding without causing blood stasis. It can improve platelet levels in patients who are otherwise not blood deficient. It also has antitumor properties. It works in four different ways in this formula.

Yu jin has several functions, including moving blood, clearing blood heat in the bladder, protecting the heart, especially from blood stasis due to blood deficiency, and acting as a diuretic. Yu jin is a highly valued herb in breast-cancer treatment

since it enters the liver channel and moves blood. Some practitioners use this herb in every formula to treat breast cancer. Some use it as a single in the form of Curcumin. Wu yao enters the kidney and urinary bladder channels. It helps protect the kidneys and urinary bladder from injury by cold and deficiency. Ban xia is the empiric herb for treating nausea and vomiting. Shi di enters the stomach and helps stop nausea. Wu zhu yu is a warm-the-interior herb that helps prevent nausea and vomiting, diarrhea due to cold, and mouth sores.

Formula base for Taxol or Taxol-based regimens[118]

huang qi (Astragali Radix; *Astragalus membranaceus*)	20 g
dang shen (Codonopsis Radix; *Codonopsis pilosula* root)	15 g
bu gu zhi (Psoraleae Fructus; *Psoralea*)	12 g
gu sui bu (Drynariae Rhizoma; *Drynaria*)	12 g
chuan xiong (Chuanxiong Rhizoma; *Ligusticum wallichii* root)	12 g
dan shen (Salviae miltiorrhizae Radix; *Salvia miltiorhiza* root)	15 g
ling zhi (Ganoderma; *Ganoderma*)	20 g
long kui (Solani nigri Herba; *Solanum nigrum*)	15 g
nu zhen zi (Ligustri lucidi Fructus; *Ligustrum lucidum* fruit)	15 g
ji xue teng (Spatholobi Caulis; *Spatholobus suberectus*)	20 g
he shou wu (Polygoni multiflori Radix preparata; *Polygonum multiflorum* root)	10 g
gou qi zi (Lycii Fructus; *Lycium chinensis* fruit)	15 g
huang jing (Polygonati Rhizoma; *Polygonatum*)	15 g
tai zi shen (Pseudostellariae Radix; *Pseudostellaria heterophylla*)	15 g
fu ling (Poria; *Poria cocos*)	15 g
ze xie (Alismatis Rhizoma; *Alisma*)	10 g
bei sha shen (Glehniae Radix; *Glehnia*)	10 g

shu di (Rehmanniae Radix   12 g
    preparata; *Rehmannia*)

bai zhu (Atractylodis macrocephalae   10 g
    Rhizoma; *Atractylodes*
    macrocephala)

gan cao (Glycyrrhizae Radix;   6 g
    Glycyrrhiza; licorice root)

Taxol induces fairly severe granulocytopenia, cardiac rhythm anomalies, sometimes anaphylactic reactions in persons who are allergic, peripheral neuropathies, especially of the hands and feet, sometimes nausea, peripheral joint pain and neuritis, shifts in blood pressure, and insomnia and mood changes. There may be fairly severe muscle and joint pain especially in the lower extremity. Depression and insomnia seems to be more severe in women undergoing treatment with Taxol. The myelosuppression is often treated prophylactically with colony stimulating factors (CSF) like Procrit and Neupogen.

Huang qi increases the WBC count. Dang shen increases the RBC count and supports the spleen function. Bu gu zhi is anticancer and also works with gu sui bu, chuan xiong, dan shen and nu zhen zi to increase the WBC and simultaneously help prevent peripheral neuropathy (a main side effect of Taxol). Ling zhi and long kui are both anticancer and work together with chuan xiong to increase granulocytes. Nu zhen zi, ji xue teng, he shou wu, gou qi zi, bei sha shen, shu di and huang jing are all important in protecting yin, yin and blood, and the yin organs. Tai zi shen is a qi tonic herb with a neutral temperature that also generates fluids; it is a very valuable herb in treating cancer where deficient heat and cold exist alongside each other. Fu ling and ze xie act as diuretics to help flush cell debris and toxins. Bai zhu and gan cao are part of Si jun zi tang to help protect and improves digestive function and absorption.

Specific herbs can be added to the above formulas that potentiate specific chemotherapeutic regimens and also treat their side effects. These herbs can added as needed depending on the reactions of the individual patient. Many of them are already included in the previous formulas.

During the CMF regimen the following herbs potentiate the mechanism of the agents while addressing side effects (I Cohen, pers. comm.):

- dang shen (Codonopsis Radix; *Codonopsis pilosula* root)
- gou qi zi (Lycii Fructus; *Lycium chinensis* fruit)
- nu zhen zi (Ligustri lucidi Fructus; *Ligustrum lucidum* fruit)
- tu si zi (Cuscutae Semen; *Cuscuta* seed)
- bai zhu (Atractylodis macrocephalae Rhizoma; *Atractylodes macrocephala*)
- bu gu zhi (Psoraleae Fructus; *Psoralea*)

During methotrexate:

- shi hu (Dendrobii Herba; *Dendrobium*)
- mai dong (Ophiopogonis Radix; *Ophiopogon*)
- rou cong rong (Cistanches Herba; *Cistanche*)

During 5-FU:

- ba ji tian (Morindae officinalis Radix; *Morinda officinalis* root)

During Adriamycin:

- dan shen (Salviae miltiorrhizae Radix; *Salvia miltiorhiza* root)
- ji xue teng (Spatholobi Caulis; *Spatholobus suberectus*)
- san qi (Notoginseng Radix; *Panax notoginseng*)

During cyclophosphamide:

- ya dan zi (Bruceae Fructus; *Brucea*).

Generally:

- to raise the RBC counts tonify the qi and blood
- to raise the platelet counts tonify the yin and essence
- to raise the WBC counts invigorate the yang.

Writing formulas according to staging

There is another way that formulas are written, and that is according to staging. The staging, constitutional pattern differentiation, and symptom picture should be included. In classical literature regarding cancer treatment, there are two different approaches to treating early and late stage cancers. One approach states that the treatment of early stage cancer should be primarily a fu zheng approach. This means that, since the pathogen is less in the early stage, then the herbs of choice should be those that enhance immunity. In late stage cancer, since the pathogen is larger (a larger tumor burden), then the herbs of choice should be detoxifying and antineoplastic. The other approach is the opposite and states that during early stage cancer the patient is still strong and one should treat with the strongest antineoplastic approach at this time. In late stage, the patient is weak and cannot utilise as well the heat-clearing and detoxifying herbs that are usually very cold in nature. Therefore, one should use primarily a fu zheng approach. It is up to you to determine the ability of your patient to utilise your approach.

There are laboratory analyses that can be used to measure the status of the immune system within the context of biomedical parameters. When tests are done to measure T-cell counts and so on, most patients are not found to have severely damaged immune systems. Whether this has meaning in the context of Chinese medicine is difficult to say. But my personal approach is to treat as strongly as possible at all times. This means different things in different patients based on their staging, age, performance status and underlying conditions, digestive ability to metabolise the herbs, conventional treatment, and the aggressiveness of the cancer itself. The treatment must be individualised.

Early stage base formula[118]

chai hu (Bupleuri Radix; *Bupleurum*)	10 g
dang gui (Angelicae sinensis Radix; *Angelica sinensis*)	15 g
bai shao (Paeoniae Radix alba; *Paeonia lactiflora* root)	15 g
yu jin (Curcumae Radix; *Curcuma longa* rhizome)	12 g
fu ling (Poria; *Poria cocos*)	12 g
gua lou shi (Trichosanthis Fructus; *Trichosanthes* fruit)	20 g
chen pi (Citri reticulatae Pericarpium; *Citrus reticulata* pericarp)	10 g
xia ku cao (Prunellae Spica; *Prunella vulgaris*)	20 g
chuan bei mu (Fritillariae cirrhosae Bulbus; *Fritillaria cirrhosa*)	10 g
tai zi shen (Pseudostellariae Radix; *Pseudostellaria heterophylla*)	15 g
shan ci gu* (Cremastrae/Pleiones Pseudobulbus; *Cremastra/Pleione* pseudobulbs)	15 g

The therapeutic principle of this formula is to circulate liver qi, transform phlegm, detoxify or clear heat and toxin, and soften the hard mass. Chai hu, dang gui, and bai shao all smooth the liver qi. Yu jin is a liver- and blood-specific herb that moves the blood, and especially the liver blood. The liver channel and the flank area and axilla are liver and jueyin areas. Therefore, yu jin is a very beneficial herb in treating breast cancer where blood stasis is a component. Fu ling acts as an assistant with the cloying effects of the blood-nourishing herbs. It also combines with chuan bei mu and gua lou shi to act as a phlegm-transforming trio. Many cancers are forms of knotted qi, blood and phlegm. Tai zi shen helps promote the qi while also benefiting fluids and supporting spleen function. Shan ci gu is a primary antineoplastic herb used in many formulas to treat cancer.

Advanced stage formula base with deficiency heat symptoms[118]

jin yin hua (Lonicerae Flos; *Lonicera* flowers)	15 g
pu gong ying (Taraxaci Herba; *Taraxacum mongolicum*)	20 g
ban zhi lian (Scutellariae barbatae Herba; *Scutellaria barbata*)	15 g
shu di (Rehmanniae Radix preparata; *Rehmannia*)	12 g
mai dong (Ophiopogonis Radix; *Ophiopogon*)	15 g
shi hu (Dendrobii Herba; *Dendrobium*)	10 g
xuan shen (Scrophulariae Radix; *Scrophularia*)	10 g
fu ling (Poria; *Poria cocos*)	12 g
tai zi shen (Pseudostellariae Radix; *Pseudostellaria heterophylla*)	15 g
huang qi (Astragali Radix; *Astragalus membranaceus*)	20 g
jiao gu lan (Herba Gynostemmatis; *Gynostemma*)	15 g

Ba zhen tang can be added to this formula for later stage breast cancer. The therapeutic principles are to strongly detoxify by clearing toxic heat, resolve stasis, increase certain elements of immune function (NK and WBC cells and increase phagocytosis), and heal tissue. Frequently in later stage cancer necrosis occurs at the center of the tumor where the blood supply is low and the cells are least well oxygenated. This necrosis initiates an inflammatory response, which can manifest as low-grade fevers, pain, changes in the skin (as in IBC), and even bleeding as the tumor ulcerates internally. This is why there are so many clear-heat-and-toxin herbs in this formula.

Jin yin hua, pu gong ying, ban zhi lian, and jiao gu lan all act as clear-heat-and-toxin antineoplastic herbs. Some of them, especially ban zhi lian, potentiate the antineoplastic action of certain chemotherapeutic regimens (like Adriamycin). Shu di, mai dong, shi hu, and tai zi shen all generate fluids and are cooling. Heat is a major component of stasis and later stage cancers. Clearing heat and generating fluids helps alleviate pain, calms the spirit and helps to detoxify an advanced or large tumor burden. Huang qi improves immune function in various ways and is also the herb of choice in healing wounds whether they are visible or not.

Advanced stage with yang-deficient symptoms[118]

gua lou shi (Trichosanthis Fructus; *Trichosanthes* fruit)	15 g
ba yue zha (Akebiae Fructus; *Akebia*)	15 g
pu gong ying (Taraxaci Herba; *Taraxacum mongolicum*)	15 g
zi hua di ding (Violae Herba; *Viola yedoensis*)	15 g
xia ku cao (Prunellae Spica; *Prunella vulgaris*)	15 g
jin yin hua (Lonicerae Flos; *Lonicera* flowers)	30 g
dang gui (Angelicae sinensis Radix; *Angelica sinensis*)	12 g
huang qi (Astragali Radix; *Astragalus membranaceus*)	30 g
tian hua fen (Trichosanthis Radix; *Trichosanthes* root)	15 g
jie geng (Platycodi Radix; *Platycodon grandiflorus* root)	12 g
chi shao (Paeoniae Radix rubra; *Paeonia lactiflora* root)	12 g
xie bai (Allii macrostemi Bulbus; *Allium macrostemon*)	15 g
yi ren (Coicis Semen; *Coix lacryma-jobi*)	15 g
hai zao (Sargassum; *Sargassum*)	15 g
yuan zhi (Polygalae Radix; *Polygala*)	10 g
rou gui (Cinnamomi Cortex; *Cinnamomum cassia* cortex)	5 g
gan cao (Glycyrrhizae Radix; *Glycyrrhiza*; licorice root)	5 g

This formula is used when the tumor burden is large with metastatic spread and a large primary tumor. There may be swollen axillary lymph nodes and even an externally ulcerated mass. This is a late stage presentation that is no longer resectable. Accompanying the large mass and metastatic spread are fever and chills, severe fatigue, and signs and symptoms that help identify the areas and organs of involvement. Common sites for metastatic spread at this late stage are lungs, liver, bone, brain, and abdomen. There are heat signs present but these are accompanied by cold signs with yang deficiency. Therefore, the formula contains detoxifying heat-clearing herbs like pu gong ying, zi hua di ding, xia ku cao, jin yin hua, all of which are antineoplastic against breast cancer. The dose of jin yin hua is exceptionally high. The dose for huang qi is also very high, not only to improve immune function, but because it is a strong qi tonic herb that will work to improve appetite and digestion, and tonify the lungs to increase oxygenation of all tissues. It will help decrease fatigue.

Dang gui is a warming blood-nourishing and blood-invigorating herb that has mild analgesic and laxative properties. Constipation is often an issue in later stage cancer depending on the conventional interventions. Chi shao works with dang gui to move blood, nourish the blood in a possibly anemic patient, and reduce pain. Xie bai is warming and opens and warms the collaterals of the chest. Because of this it can treat pain. Yi ren helps transform damp and is also antineoplastic. Yi ren and hai zao work gently together to transform phlegm and act antineoplastically in a very deficient patient. Yuan zhi nourishes the heart to calm the spirit and promote a healthy sleep pattern. Sleep is very important in overall health and enables patients to endure pain and the psychoemotional impact of their condition. Rou gui leads the yang back to the source and warms the lower jiao. Some fevers and chills are due to neutropenia and are not caused by infection. These neutropenic fevers are partly yin deficient and partly yang deficient. when the yang is deficient this can manifest as floating yang which can look like yin deficiency. Rou gui helps to anchor the yang, reduce fevers, and eliminate cold in yang deficiency.

In late stage breast cancer there may be swollen lymph nodes, usually in the axilla and the cervical and supraclavicular chains. Hard swollen masses will be palpable. If the patient has swollen lymph nodes then mu li (Ostreae Concha; *Ostrea* shell) and xuan shen (Scrophulariae Radix; *Scrophularia*) can be added to the above formula. These two herbs combine to treat the main underlying problem in lymphadenopathy, i.e. phlegm and blood stasis. If there is an ulcerative tumor present, then the addition of zhi shi (Aurantii Fructus immaturus; *Citrus aurantium*) and qing pi (Citri reticulatae viride Pericarpium; *Citrus reticulata* green pericarp) can be added. These two strong qi regulating herbs help to reduce the pain caused by an ulcerating tumor.

Specific herbs can be added to a formula to help prevent metastatic spread. As discussed earlier, certain types of breast cancer have predictable sites to which they seem more likely to spread. Ductal carcinomas of the breast are more likely to spread to the lungs, bone, liver and brain. Lobular carcinomas are more likely to spread to the retroperitoneum and the other breast. Using this information, we can work prophylactically to help prevent this metastatic spread based on the type of cancer present as follows:

- bone: treat as a kidney yang-deficient pattern
- brain: treat as a fire poison and phlegm heat injuring the heart/kidney axis; heart = brain and mind, kidney = brain and yin
- liver: treat as liver qi and blood stasis
- lung: treat as qi and blood deficiency with strong qi tonic and blood nourishing herbs/formulas (Ba zhen tang).

Herb to direct the formula to a metastatic site:

- axillary lymph: pu yin gen (Wikstroemiae indicae Radix; *Wikstroemia indica* root).

HORMONAL THERAPY: POST-CHEMOTHERAPY AND/OR AS PREVENTION

Tamoxifen has become the treatment of choice in post-treatment premenopausal women with ER-positive breast cancer who are in the monitoring phase.[104,119] Many women become menopausal iatrogenically as a result of treatment for breast cancer. To some extent this depends on the therapies utilised for cytotoxic treatment (that ablate the ovarian function) and the age of the woman at the time of treatment. Many women under the age of 40 will re-establish a menstrual cycle even after chemotherapy. Some will even with tamoxifen therapy. Others over the age of 40, who were not menopausal before treatment, may never re-establish a menstrual cycle.

There are several second-generation antiestrogenic hormonal therapies that are off-shoots of tamoxifen, including raloxifene, anastrozole (Arimidex), megestrol, and letrozole (Femara). These are used for women who are post-menopausal. They have varying side effects. Other endocrine agents include progestins, antiadrenal drugs, and prednisone. The luteinising hormone-releasing hormone (LHRH) also allows for suppression of ovarian function. Please see the risk factor section for side effects of tamoxifen. Endocrine agents are used for up to 5 years.

Non-cross-resistant therapies are combinations of multiple non-cross-resistant drugs evolving out of the rationale that the presence of subsets of cells resistant to certain drugs require multipronged approaches. CMF is one of these. Sequential chemotherapy is also used in an effort to deal with the issue of cross-resistance. It is common to prescribe four courses of doxorubicin and cytoxan (AC) followed by eight courses of CMF or a combination thereof, equaling 12 courses. Chemohormonal regimens are also used. For example, CFP contains cyclophosphamide, 5-FU, and prednisone. Tamoxifen is added particularly in post-menopausal patients and ER-positive patients.

Herceptin is currently the only monoclonal antibody used in breast cancer treatment. It's primary side effect is cardiotoxicity, which occurs in a smaller percentage of women. Herceptin is sometimes used alongside Taxol to treat IBC and other breast cancers that express the *HER-2/neu* oncogene. Herceptin and Navelbine are also used together. The combined cardiotoxicity of Herceptin and Adriamycin make them a very poor combination. Cardiotoxic drugs will often require monitoring pre- and post- treatment. The tool of choice is a MUGA-scan, which measures the ejection fraction of the heart muscle. Since it is primarily the heart muscle itself that is injured by these chemotherapies, the ejection fraction is the best monitor.

Chinese medicine

Formula base for tamoxifen[120]

shu di (Rehmanniae Radix preparata; *Rehmannia*)	10 g
shan zhu yu (Corni Fructus; *Cornus officinalis* fruit)	10 g
shan yao (Dioscoreae Rhizoma; *Dioscorea opposita*)	10 g
ze xie (Alismatis Rhizoma; *Alisma*)	8 g
mu dan pi (Moutan Cortex; *Paeonia suffruticosa* root cortex)	8 g
fu ling (Poria; *Poria cocos*)	15 g
gui ban* (Testudinis Plastrum; *Chinemys reevesii* plastron)	15 g
jin ying zi (Rosae laevigatae Fructus; *Rosa laevigata* fruits)	12 g
fu pen zi (Rubi Fructus; *Rubus chingii*; Chinese raspberry)	10 g
shi di (Kaki Calyx; *Diospyros kaki* calyx)	10 g
wu wei zi (Schisandrae Fructus; *Schisandra*)	10 g
mu li (Ostreae Concha; *Ostrea* shell)	15 g
long gu (Fossilia Ossis Mastodi; fossilised bone)	15 g

As discussed above, tamoxifen is an antiestrogenic hormonal treatment that causes menopausal syndrome symptoms. These symptoms include flushing, night sweats, insomnia, vaginal dryness, digestive upset, and mood changes, especially anxiety and depression. There may be some patients, if not all, who are poor candidates for preventive prophylaxis with tamoxifen. These would be patients with a history of other primary cancers and breast cancer, patients with blood stasis syndrome manifesting as clotting disorders and coronary heart disease or DVT.

Shu di is a blood-nourishing herb that benefits the liver and kidney yin, the primary underlying diagnosis for menopausal syndrome. Shan zhu yu is an astringent herb that helps coalesce fluids and astringe qi. The astringent herbs seem to have a relationship with the lung and its ability to regulate the pores. The sweating that can result from flushing in menopausal syndrome is partly a yin deficiency heat problem and also a lung failing to regulate the pores problem. Shan yao strengthens the spleen, nourishes the kidneys and lungs, and astringes essence, all things vitally important in treating symptoms from menopause. Ze xie is a dampness-draining herb that also drains deficient kidney fire, a causal component in menopausal symptoms. Mu dan pi clears heat and cools the blood, clears deficiency fire, and also moves the blood and helps to prevent blood stasis. Fu ling is a drain damp herb that helps protect the spleen function from the cloying nature of the blood-nourishing herbs in the formula. It also benefits the spleen to help it transform fluids and improves digestive function in general by supporting the spleen. Fu ling is also a fungus that has properties that increase WBC counts and improves immune surveillance.

Gui ban strongly nourishes yin. By looking at the side effects of tamoxifen, we can make assumptions about its mechanism and resulting injuries in classical medical terms. Injury to the yin is apparent; tamoxifen lowers estrogen, a yin secretion, it also seems to act as a diuretic. And it causes blood stasis; perhaps this blood stasis evolves as a reaction to the yin-depleting aspects of the drug. Yin and blood are intimately connected and will draw fluids from one another in order to maintain homeostasis. If the yin becomes deficient, then it will draw fluid from the plasma (yin) portion of the blood causing blood dryness. Blood dryness leads to blood stasis and blood stasis leads to blood dryness. Over a period of 5 years, the usual time for tamoxifen treatment to prevent breast cancer recurrence, blood congealment can occur.

Jin ying zi is an astringent herb that stabilises the kidneys and consolidates the kidney qi. Fu pen zi is also a astringent that nourishes the liver and kidney yin; it tonifies the qi of the Ren and Chong. Shi di is a herb that regulates the qi and improves digestive function, especially of the stomach. Wu wei zi is an astringent that helps the lungs regulate the pores, nourishes the kidneys, calms the spirit and generates body fluids, and consolidates the Ren and Chong. Long gu and mu li help anchor ascending yang in yin deficient heat-rising syndromes like flushing.

METASTATIC BREAST CANCER

Fewer than 10% of newly diagnosed breast cancer patients will present with metastatic disease but nearly 50% of newly diagnosed patients will develop it.[121] Advanced breast cancer is considered incurable. There is a great deal we can do to help this fact. We can utilise and develop potential cytotoxic treatments within the context of Chinese medicine. We can help to improve overall general health in patients with advanced disease. We can use herbal means of addressing hormonal levels, means that have far fewer side effects.

Survival after relapse is directly related to the extent of the disease and not to the site of relapse, except for disease in the CNS, which implies very short survival. In metastatic disease the cancer cells must penetrate various basement membranes, degrade the underlying mesenchymal tissues, gain access to blood and lymph vessels, and enter the stroma of the target organ. Other events include stimulation of growth factor receptors, angiogenesis to support tumor growth, and evasion of host immune surveillance.[122]

Once metastatic disease is suspected a careful history and work-up must follow. This will include primary disease history, current symptoms, pre-existing comorbid disease, a review of the initial presentation, staging then and now, hormone-receptor status, pathology report, and treatments already employed. The disease-free interval and menopausal staus should be ascertained. Information on flushing, cyclic breast tenderness, premenstrual syndrome (PMS), follicle stimulating hormone (FSH) and luteinising hormone (LH) levels, and whether or not there has been a hysterectomy is important. Current symptoms can help ascertain the sites of potential metastatic spread and the current tumor burden. Pain, weight loss, activity constraints, nutritional status and the state of the spirit are very important.

The CEA, CA 15-3, and CA 27.29 levels are potentially helpful in detecting and monitoring metastatic disease and the effects of treatment. The CA 15-3 test is a combination of two reactive determinants expressed on mammary epithelial cells. It is much more sensitive than the CEA and is elevated in 70–85% of patients with metastatic disease. The CA 27.29 is the newest marker being utilised for detection of metastatic spread and efficacy of treatment.

Chest X-ray may be sufficient to assess the lungs. If not, a chest CT is done. In addition to the lungs, liver parenchymal involvement may be present, and there may be metastases to the periportal nodes with compression of the biliary tree or hepatic/portal vessels. When this happens ascites will result. A CT or ultrasound is necessary to detect these events. Jaundice may be present, and clay colored stools may indicate hepatic and biliary involvement. Hydroureter or hydronephrosis is the most common retroperitoneal metastasis in breast cancer. MRI and PET scans are also used to monitor advancement of metastatic disease.

Metastatic disease often follows one of two patterns.[123] The first is relatively asymptomatic and indolent. Patients whose disease follows this course are usually ER-positive with a disease-free interval of longer than 2 years, with metastases to the bone, soft tissue, or non-life-threatening visceral sites. If the tumor burden is small, then usually hormonal therapies are tried. Tamoxifen is used for the first 5 years, then megestrol or another generation antiestrogenic treatment is used depending on the reaction of the patient. A patient with this pattern will often live for several years with a fairly high functional quality of life.

The second pattern is highly symptomatic, ER-negative, aggressive, widely disseminated, with life-threatening visceral disease. In this case, cytotoxic therapy with sequential radiation is treatment. The patient's age usually does not influence the type of initial therapy. However, as stated before, there are contraindications in elderly patients such as diabetes, heart conditions, chronic liver disease, etc. One therapy is given at a time. Concurrent chemotherapy with radiation is rarely used. Combination hormonal therapy with chemotherapy is used. The risk of thromboembolic problems is increased using hormones and chemotherapy concurrently especially with CMF and prednisone. Renal insufficiency may impair the clearance of methotrexate. Biological response modifiers (BRMs) are not of use at this time in metastatic breast cancer. Herceptin (in patients with *HER-2/neu* overexpression), a monclonal antibody, and chemotherapy can be used together. Common combinations with Herceptin include vinorelbine (Navelbine), gemcitabine, gefitinib (Iressa), and others. Bone-marrow transplants have been studied and have not been found to increase survival.

The response rates of hormonal salvage therapy after induction chemotherapy are quite low. Paclitaxel (Taxol) is the newest agent to show activity in patients who have been heavily pre-treated or are doxorubicin refractory. The median response time is 9 months with a range of 3–19 months. Docetaxel is as active as Taxol and with a similar response duration. It is as active or more active as conventional chemotherapy for initial treatment or salvage treatment. Vinorelbine is a semisynthetic vinca alkaloid and has been approved for NSCLC and breast cancer. Neu-tropenia is a severe side effect, sometimes limiting the dose. However, it is active in patients who have received prior anthracyclines. The median response was found to be 12 months and the overall survival was 27.5 months. None of these salvage therapies are curative and only buy time for patients. This time can be amplified by using combined care.

Hormonal therapy in advanced disease is an appropriate first step if the disease is indolent, ER/PR-positive, with a disease-free interval longer than 2–5 years, postmenopausal, with metastases only to soft tissue (ie. nodes, chest wall, or skin). There are three clinical approaches to estrogen deprivation. One is to use antiestrogens like tamoxifen or androgens like fluoxymesterone (Halotestin). The second approach is to inhibit gonadotropin-induced estrogen production with LHRH inhibitory agents, which are less effective in postmenopausal patients. The third approach is to decrease estrogen biosynthesis by inhibiting aromatase enzyme, which catalyses the final step in estrogen production. This does not com-pletely block ovarian estrogen production in pre-menopausal women and there is concern that use of a single agent may cause a reflex increase in gonadotropin levels and result in ovarian hyperstimulation syndrome. Therefore, aromatase inhibitors like aminoglutethimide are used prima-rily in postmenopausal women.

There are fewer side effects in hormonal therapy than in chemotherapy. However, some unique complications occur. Flare is clinically defined as an abrupt, diffuse onset of muscu-loskeletal pain, increased size of skin lesions if present, erythema surrounding a skin lesion during the first month of endocrine therapy. The more serious complication of flare is hypercal-cemia, which is seen with all hormonal therapies except oophorectomy and aminoglutethimide. Serum calcium levels are monitored during the first weeks of hormonal therapy in treating metastatic disease. There is often weight gain, especially with progestins, only partially from water retention. Thromboembolism is a problem with progestins and often with tamoxifen. The main side effects of tamoxifen are hot flushes, mild nausea, transient thrombocytopenia and rarely leukopenia. See the risk factor section in this chapter.

The most commonly used progestin is mege-strol acetate (Megace). It also may cause mild nausea, flare, flushing, but it is also associated with more thromboembolic effects, weight gain, glucose intolerance, and increase in blood pres-sure. In patients with an intact uterus, vaginal bleeding will occur when progestins are discon-tinued. Megace is used as an appetite enhancer in AIDS patients and other patients where anorexia or cachexia is a complaint because one side effect is appetite enhancement.

Liver metastasis occurs in about 20% of patients either as an isolated metastasis or with other sites of metastatic disease. Chemotherapy is the standard of treatment. Hepatic artery infu-sion (intra-arterial infusion) with chemothera-peutic drugs may expose the tumor to higher levels of drug. This technique is used in China as a means of delivering a herbal sterilised formula to the liver, gallbladder or pancreas. The overall response rate with intra-arterial infusion of chemotherapy is 50%.[124] Currently there are studies under way to find out if garlic in supple-mental form can help protect the liver from metastatic spread in breast cancer. Similar studies could be done with Chinese herbs since many are found to be protective of liver function, includ-ing wu wei zi (Schisandrae Fructus; *Schisandra*), bai shao (Paeoniae Radix alba; *Paeonia lactiflora* root), nu zhen zi (Ligustri lucidi Fructus; *Ligus-trum lucidum* fruit), shi shang bai (Sellaginellae doederleinii Herba; *Selaginella doederleinii*), bai jiang cao (Thlaspi/Patriniae Herba; *Patrinia/Thlaspi*).

Breast cancer metastases to bone are lytic (48%), blastic, (13%), or mixed (38%), or a diffuse osteoporosis without bone destruction. After chemotherapy, a large number of women are found to be osteopenic. Whether this condition encourages bony metastases in recurrent disease is unknown. Bone metastases are the initial metastases in 29–46% of patients with breast cancer. Up to 70% of patients develop bone metastases during the course of the disease. Patients with bone-only or bone-predominant metastases often have prolonged survival offset by substantial clinical morbidity. Bone metastases manifest as pain, pathologic fracture, limited mobility, hypercalcemia, nerve-root or spinal cord compression, and compromised hematopoiesis. Localised complications are managed with orthopedic or neurosurgery with or without radiation. Bisphosphanates are also used. The most commonly used is pamidronate (Aredia). These substances are used to treat Paget's disease of bone, osteoporosis, hypercalcemia, and bone metastases from breast cancer. Prophylactic doses of pamidronate are given in patients with metastatic disease to reduce osseous complications, such as hypercalcemia, vertebral fractures, and bone pain. It also promotes healing of osteolytic lesions.[125]

In stage IV patients 50–80% of patients with no evidence of disease (NED) will develop systemic disease within 2 years despite curative local therapies. The 5-year survival rate ranges from 4 to 36%. The most common situation involves patients with a chest wall recurrence, and 50% have distant metastases upon further investigation. Only 25% have a single isolated lesion. Approximately 50% of these patients can be salvaged with surgery alone. There is some disagreement as to whether local or systemic treatment is more appropriate. Patients at a late stage have undergone many regimens and often are no longer responsive to the chemotherapeutic combinations available.

Please see the formulas utilised via the staging method. Also see Chapter 11 on concurrent issues in treatment. As the disease progresses more medical conditions evolve as a result of the cancerous spread itself and as a result of conventional treatment.

FORMULA BASES FOR CONSTITUTIONAL PATTERNS

KIDNEY YANG DEFICIENCY PATTERN

The main formula for this pattern presentation is You gui yin.[126] It can be modified according to the symptom presentation of the patient, the side effects of conventional treatment, and other parameters identified by the practitioner. In later stage breast cancer this is a common pattern.

Symptoms:

- cold and pain in the whole body and especially low back and extremities
- lower abdominal pain
- fatigue
- prolonged urination, incontinence
- menopausal hypertension
- can't lie down to rest, even though exhausted
- sweats easily
- may have loose stools.

Signs:

- frail pulse
- pale tongue
- tense abdomen around the navel.

KIDNEY YIN DEFICIENCY PATTERN

The main formula for this pattern presentation is Zuo gui yin.[127] Any of the constitutional formulas can be modified to fit the patient. It is recommended that they be modified to be more exacting and detailed. Conventional treatment interventions will sometimes drive the formula. Whenever possible, include constitutional elements in the overall formula.

Symptoms:

- sore and weak low back
- lightheadedness
- tinnitus
- chronic dry sore throat
- prone to urinary tract infection
- short and light menses or post-menopausal
- insomnia
- pale complexion with red hue above the paleness
- sore breasts from ovulation to the end of menses

- functional uterine bleeding
- patient complains of feeling hot.

Signs:

- rapid, thin, or irregular pulse
- red tongue with little coat and red points.

LIVER AND KIDNEY YIN DEFICIENCY PATTERN

The most commonly used formula for this pattern is Liu wei di huang wan.[127] This formula has been studied within the context of biomedical parameters. In premenopausal women it has been found to lower estrogen levels. This would be considered to be a positive in women with tumors that are estrogen sensitive (ER-positive). However, in post-menopausal women it raises estrogen levels slightly (by about 2%). In estrogen-sensitive breast tumors in a post-menopausal woman, this formula may not be the best choice. It is difficult at this point to understand the complexity of herbal combinations and how the components work together. The Chinese do not particularly worry about the concept of phytoestrogenicity. They use classical theory to treat breast cancers and other hormonally-responsive cancers. It is unknown if a 2% rise in circulating estrogen levels effects tumor cell growth. It is unknown if the effects of the other herbs in a formula, for example the antineoplastic herbs, offset this estrogenic effect. At the same time, herbs seem to act in different ways to fill estrogen/estradiol/estrone receptor sites, and some of them seem to lower those hormone levels. A separate section gives the most current information available on this subject.

Symptoms:

- dizziness
- tinnitus
- tidal fevers
- night sweats
- five-center heat
- thirst and/or dry mouth.

Signs:

- thready and rapid pulse
- red and dry tongue.

LIVER QI STASIS PATTERN WITH CONSTRAINT AS MAIN FEATURE

Liver yin deficiency can lead to liver qi stasis. Spleen deficiency can lead to blood failing to nourish the liver blood and liver qi stasis. Unresolved emotions and the resulting constraint can lead to liver qi stasis. All of these are vicious cycles. Sometimes they are difficult to differentiate. Liver qi stasis can present as a deficiency qi stasis or as an excess qi stasis. The excess liver qi stasis manifests with a wiry, forceful pulse. Typically Shu gan wan is the formula used to treat this type of constraint. Spleen deficiency leading to liver blood deficiency and then to liver qi stasis presents with a forceless and weak but wiry pulse. Typically Xiao yao san[128] is the formula used to treat this type of constraint. The signs, and mainly the pulse, are the key as to which type. The following formula is for a presentation due to constraint that has a wiry forceful pulse.

Symptoms:

- chronic stubborn headache (migraine-like)
- hiccough
- choking sensation when drinking fluids
- dry heaves
- depression
- palpitations
- restless sleep
- irritability
- mood swings
- dry skin
- sticky saliva
- dyspnea
- long cycle of premenstrual tension (10–14 days)
- cramping prior to menses
- deep aching in the breasts.

Signs:

- dark tongue with ecchymotic spots on the sides, dry thin yellow coat in rear only
- rapid, choppy, wiry, forceful, tight pulse.

Special formula

qing pi (Citri reticulatae viride Pericarpium; *Citrus reticulata* green pericarp) 10 g

chen pi (Citri reticulatae Pericarpium; *Citrus reticulata* pericarp) 10 g

mu li (Ostreae Concha; *Ostrea* shell)	10 g
si gua luo (Luffae Fructus Retinervus; *Luffa cylindrica*; loofah)	40 g
gua lou shi (Trichosanthis Fructus; *Trichosanthes* fruit)	40 g
pu gong ying (Taraxaci Herba; *Taraxacum mongolicum*)	40 g
mai ya (Hordei Fructus germinatus; *Hordeum vulgare*; barley sprouts; malt)	40 g
xuan shen (Scrophulariae Radix; *Scrophularia*)	15 g
chai hu (Bupleuri Radix; *Bupleurum*)	10 g
chuan bei mu (Fritillariae cirrhosae Bulbus; *Fritillaria cirrhosa*)	15 g
zhe bei mu (Fritillariae thunbergii Bulbus; *Fritillaria thunbergii*)	10 g

This formula is a strongly qi-regulating and mildly blood-moving formula. It also contains several herbs in very large dose to transform phlegm (si gua lou and gua lou shi, chuan bei mu, and zhe bei mu), detoxify (pu gong ying), and treat food stasis to transform phlegm and improve middle jiao function. A review of the basic constitutional patterns will show that middle jiao dysfunction is often implicated in breast cancer pathogenesis either starting with liver qi stasis or with spleen deficiency, and then leading to complications of these routes of pathogenesis. Chai hu and qing pi help regulate the function of the liver. And mu li helps to anchor the yang, which is flushing upwards due to constraint and latent liver heat, as exemplified by the symptoms of PMS, chronic headaches, hiccough, dry heaves, palpitations, insomnia, irritability, dyspnea. This formula can be modified for deficiency by adding middle jiao tonic herbs.

LIVER QI STASIS WITH SPLEEN DEFICIENCY PATTERN

This pattern is one in which pain due to stasis is present and qi and blood deficiency are the underlying causes of the stasis. It is really a combination of two formulas, one mainly to move the liver qi and the other to improve middle jiao function to tonify the qi and nourish the blood. The liver qi stasis formula is:

huang qi (Astragali Radix; *Astragalus membranaceus*)	20 g
dang gui (Angelicae sinensis Radix; *Angelica sinensis*)	10 g
tian hua fen (Trichosanthis Radix; *Trichosanthes* root)	10 g
bai zhi (Angelicae dahuricae Radix; *Angelica dahurica*)	6 g
jie geng (Platycodi Radix; *Platycodon grandiflorus* root)	10 g
chi shao (Paeoniae Radix rubra; *Paeonia lactiflora* root)	12 g
xie bai (Allii macrostemi Bulbus; *Allium macrostemon*)	10 g

The qi and blood deficient formula is:

bai ren shen (Ginseng Radix; *Panax ginseng*; white ginseng)	10 g
fu ling (Poria; *Poria cocos*)	10 g
bai zhu (Atractylodis macrocephalae Rhizoma; *Atractylodes macrocephala*)	10 g
chai hu (Bupleuri Radix; *Bupleurum*)	8 g
chuan xiong (Chuanxiong Rhizoma; *Ligusticum wallichii* root)	8 g
shan zha (Crataegi Fructus; *Crataegus*)	8 g
mu dan pi (Moutan Cortex; *Paeonia suffruticosa* root cortex)	8 g
shu di (Rehmanniae Radix preparata; *Rehmannia*)	30 g

These two formulas are combined and the following single herbs are added to detoxify and act antineoplastically:

pu gong ying (Taraxaci Herba; *Taraxacum mongolicum*)	20 g
zi hua di ding (Violae Herba; *Viola yedoensis*)	15 g
gua lou shi (Trichosanthis Fructus; *Trichosanthes* fruit)	20 g
jin yin hua (Lonicerae Flos; *Lonicera* flowers)	20 g
yan hu suo (Corydalis Rhizoma; *Corydalis yanhusuo*)	10 g

This pattern can lead to swollen and inflamed masses in the breast, everything from mastitis due to liver qi stasis to IBC. Thus there are mass-reducing herbs and also heat- and toxin-clearing herbs. It is designed to cool the tissue, alleviate pain, reduce swelling, move blood and act antineoplastically.

The liver qi stasis formula includes huang qi and dang gui in a 1:2 ratio, which is close to the formula Dang gui bu xue tang,[129] which is used to tonify qi and blood. Tian hua fen, bai zhi, and jie geng all work together to transform phlegm, direct the qi of the formula upwards to the chest, and detoxify. They are mildly antitumor and also circulate the qi. Chi shao nourishes the blood especially of the liver and it regulates the blood. Xie bai warms the channels and collaterals especially of the chest and opens the chest to circulate qi.

The qi and blood deficient formula contains Si jun zi tang,[128] the main qi tonic formula especially for the middle jiao. Chai hu smoothes the liver qi and helps raise the qi to help treat depression. Chuan xiong regulates the blood, especially the liver blood, and helps lift the qi to the head. Shan zha is a food stasis herb that helps to transform phlegm; phlegm stasis is often a secondary pattern in breast cancer. This is because any form of liver qi stasis can eventually harm the spleen; it is often difficult to know which came first, the spleen deficiency or the liver blood deficiency that can underlie liver qi stasis. Transform phlegm and move food stasis herbs help act prophylactically to prevent this occurence. Shu di is a strong blood-nourishing herb that also moves the blood.

The added herbs clear toxic heat and transform phlegm, especially relative to the breast. Yan hu suo is a blood-regulating herb that is especially good for treating the kind of pain caused by blood stasis and liver blood congealment.

LIVER QI STASIS WITH SPLEEN DEFICIENCY LEADING TO REBELLIOUS STOMACH QI PATTERN

The liver qi can traverse the ko cycle when depressed or constrained. It invades the spleen and causes damage to the middle jiao function. This is called a transverse rebellion. The spleen and stomach are intimately involved since they are the inner and outer, the yin and yang, aspects of the same functional unit. Liver invades the spleen and gallbladder invades the stomach. Liver and gallbladder are also coupled organs. When the gallbladder invades the stomach it causes the

stomach qi to flush upward. When the liver invades the spleen it causes the spleen qi to weaken and lose its transforming and transporting functions. These symptoms are generally lower jiao symptoms like loose stools, which are a manifestation of the loss of water metabolism tasks by the spleen. In other words, digestive symptoms above the navel are relative to stomach injury and symptoms below the navel are relative to spleen injury.

Symptoms:

- epigastric distention
- heaviness in the chest
- belching, nausea, vomiting
- acid regurgitation
- fatigue after eating
- wheezing on exhalation
- irritable bowel
- constipation prior to menses but diarrhea at onset
- obsessiveness.

Signs:

- large, pale tongue with a greasy and probably yellow coat and red points
- slippery and full pulse that is soft in the deeper levels.

This pattern requires a milder formula because the digestion is weak. The strongly detoxifying herbs from the previous formula are replaced with milder detoxifying herbs and many digestive tonic herbs are added.

hu lu ba (Trigonellae Semen; Trigonella)   10 g

bai zhi (Angelicae dahuricae Radix; Angelica dahurica)   8 g

san leng (Sparganii Rhizoma; Sparganium rhizome)   10 g

chuan xiong (Chuanxiong Rhizoma; Ligusticum wallichii root)   10 g

mo yao (Myrrha; Commiphora myrrha; myrrh)   10 g

zao jiao ci (Gleditsiae Spina; Gleditsia spines)   10 g

jie geng (Platycodi Radix; Platycodon grandiflorus root)   10 g

gui ban* (Testudinis Plastrum; Chinemys reevesii plastron)   10 g

gua lou shi (Trichosanthis Fructus;   15 g
  Trichosanthes fruit)
dang gui (Angelicae sinensis Radix;   12 g
  Angelica sinensis)
quan xie (Scorpio; *Buthus martensii*)   10 g
wu gong (Scolopendra; *Scolopendra*   3 g
  subspinipes)
mai ya (Hordei Fructus germinatus;   20 g
  Hordeum vulgare; barley sprouts;
  malt)
bai zhu (Atractylodis macrocephalae   10 g
  Rhizoma; *Atractylodes*
  macrocephala)

Trigonella is fenugreek seed and it warms and tonifies the kidney yang. This herb also helps alleviate the pain from cold that can manifest as irritable bowel and flank distention. Bai zhi is a warming herb that enters the lung and stomach. It helps reduce swellings and fevers due to infection, and is even antibiotic against some Gram-positive bacteria. In the case of IBC or more advanced cancer or when necrosis is present, this herb will help resolve the infection and reduce pain. San leng, chuan xiong, and mo yao all are blood-cracking herbs that reduce masses due to blood stasis. The liver qi when static can lead to blood stasis. Herbs that move blood and enter the liver channel can help resolve blood stasis due to liver qi stasis. These herbs also help reduce pain. Zao ci is the spine from the *Gleditsia* plant. It reduces inflammation and helps to resolve preulcerous sores where pus accumulates but hasn't yet opened outward. Although we can see this process in most cancers many go through a process by which they internally ulcerate and/or break through the basement membrane of the tissue in which they occur. Zao ci is a warming-transform-cold-phlegm herb.

Jie geng works with zao ci and gua lou shi to transform phlegm and direct the formula to the chest. Jie geng and gua lou shi are also antineoplastic. Gui ban nourishes the yin and the jin ye.

The warming nature and phlegm-transforming actions of most of the other herbs in the formula create the need to protect the normal fluids. Gui ban nourishes yin and also cools the blood and aids in the healing of ulcerative sores. Wu gong enters the liver, as is true of many pacify-wind herbs. It helps to reduce spasms when pain is present; it also reduces masses and nodules and is antitumor. Quan xie has similar properties and is used topically as an anticancer substance in pastes and local applications. Mai ya is added in the largest dose of any herb in the formula. It helps relieve food stagnation and harmonises the stomach/spleen function by stimulating the production of pepsin and gastric acid secretions. It also promotes the free flow of the liver qi and so it treats the two main injuries of this pattern. This formula is milder and far more tonifying than the previous formula.

LIVER QI STASIS LEADING TO LATENT LIVER HEAT PATTERN

When the liver is depressed or constrained over a long period of time or in the context of a liver constraint constitutional type it can lead to a transformation called depressive liver fire or latent liver heat. A common symptom in women is premenstrual headaches. The headaches occur as a result of liver constraint that becomes more pronounced during the premenstrual or follicular or yang phase of the menstrual cycle. If there is underlying constraint, it is more likely that liver yang rising will occur during that phase of the cycle when movement is the prime expression. Movement is primary during the yang part of the cycle as the body prepares for pregnancy. The liver qi is most active during this part of the cycle. The yin phase of the cycle is the rebuilding phase, especially for qi and blood, which become slightly deficient post-menses. The yin phase is quiet and deeper, cooler and less moving. Therefore, there are fewer symptoms and headaches do not occur. The heat of the yang phase, the underlying deficiencies, and the liver qi constraint and liver heat only become symptomatically visible during the yang phase of the cycle.

The main formula for this syndrome is Hei xiao yao san.[130] This formula in everyday circumstances is taken during the yang phase of the cycle and another qi-tonifying and blood-nourishing formula, like Ba zhen tang, is taken during the yin phase of the cycle. In breast cancer, this formula is utilised in various modified forms during the course of treatment and in a less modified form during treatment for prevention.

chai hu (Bupleuri Radix; *Bupleurum*)   10 g

qing pi (Citri reticulatae viride   10 g
Pericarpium; *Citrus reticulata* green
pericarp)

zhi zi (Gardeniae Fructus; *Gardenia*   10 g
fruit)

mu dan pi (Moutan Cortex; *Paeonia*   10 g
suffruticosa root cortex)

gua lou shi (Trichosanthis Fructus;   15 g
Trichosanthes fruit)

si gua luo (Luffae Fructus   15 g
Retinervus; *Luffa cylindrica*; loofah)

mai ya (Hordei Fructus germinatus;   15 g
Hordeum vulgare; barley sprouts;
malt)

pu gong ying (Taraxaci Herba;   15 g
Taraxacum mongolicum)

chen pi (Citri reticulatae Pericarpium;   6 g
Citrus reticulata pericarp)

This is a modification of Hei xiao yao san. The chai hu circulates the qi of the liver and also lifts the yang. This may seem contraindicated in a formula to treat headache but the addition of the other herbs in the formula help offset this action of chai hu which then also acts as an envoy. Qing pi is the immature green form of chen pi. It is a primary qi-regulating herb that is especially useful for liver qi constraint. It helps to reduce pain and also resolves phlegm. It is especially useful for treating breast pain because it enters the liver and gallbladder channels. Zhi zi is a clear heat herb that also cools the blood. It is analgesic and also antineoplastic. Mu dan pi clears heat at the blood level and is especially good at clearing liver fire rising, the cause of the main complaint. It is antitumor and reduces masses caused by blood stasis.

Gua lou shi is an anticancer herb that transforms phlegm, especially in the chest. Si gua lou is another breast herb that enters the lung, stomach, and liver. It helps resolve swellings in the breast and is mildly anticancer. Mai ya promotes the liver qi and harmonises the stomach. Pu gong ying is a clear heat and toxin herb that is almost like a breast antibiotic. This herb is used to treat many breast conditions. It is especially good at clearing liver heat and it reduces hard nodules. Chen pi regulates the qi and strengthens the spleen, dissolves damp and phlegm, redirects

upward flushing qi, and helps to prevent stagnation caused by the other harsher herbs in the formula. This is an important ameliorative action of this herb since stagnation and qi flushing up are strong causative factors in this pattern.

PREVENTION

Women who go into remission are monitored at first every 3 and then every 6 months for at least 2 years and up to 5 years. This becomes a time when the full force of Chinese medicine can be utilised without the need to address the side effects of pharmaceutical agents. Complete attention can be given to treating the underlying environment that was the substrate in which the cancer happened, and so it is very important to understand and identify the history of injury in a given patient. Treating the origin of the disease becomes most possible during prevention. There are also injuries created by conventional care that first need addressing. Many women enter the monitoring phase after conventional treatment for breast cancer with osteopenia, hypothyroidism, and various forms of anemia. Conventional providers do not generally conduct an 'exit interview' with the physical body; no common blood chemistries are done or panels that might provide information about the current status of the patient. The most common scans are a colonoscopy because women diagnosed with breast cancer are at higher risk for colorectal cancer, a MUGA scan if they were on therapies that were cardiotoxic, and a dual X-ray absorptiometry (DEXA) scan to determine bone density.

Many patients leave therapy anemic. Generally the blood will reconstitute itself within 2–3 months. But I have seen new patients who are still anemic as long as 1 year after therapy. This makes recovery and prevention of recurrence more problematic. Overall general health is an important component of prevention.

Osteopenia is also very common after cytotoxic therapy and requires intervention to prevent continued bone loss. A baseline DEXA scan is the tool of choice when determining bone loss. However, using urinalysis can help one understand if the kidneys are functioning well and not excreting calcium. Some feel that urinalysis is a more accurate test of knowing if bone loss continues. Antiestrogenic therapies can contribute to bone loss and so this makes management post-treatment an important part of prevention and general health promotion. Some hormonal therapies help prevent bone loss.

Many patients diagnosed with breast cancer are hypothyroid. This is often an underlying condition that existed before diagnosis. However, the condition can be made worse with cytotoxic therapies. Knowing and treating the correct diagnosis for hypothyroid according to Chinese medicine can help prevent recurrence. It is valuable to conduct various screens post-treatment:

- thyroid panel
- DEXA scan
- urinalysis to determine if calcium excretion is occuring
- hormone panel (FSH, LH , estradiol, etc.)
- toxic screen if not done before (for heavy metals, pesticides, PCBs, PBBs and other chemical toxins)
- CBC with differential
- Chem 23 blood test or equivalent to look at liver and kidney function.

If patients were diabetic prior to their diagnosis, then this condition needs continual treatment during conventional cytotoxic treatment and during prevention treatment. Glucose is the preferred substrate for cancer. Hyperinsulinemia is a condition that contributes to breast cancer and which must be managed as part of cure.

CHINESE MEDICINE

Prevention then becomes treatment:

- to resolve conditions that existed before the cancer
- for those conditions that occured as a result of cytotoxic treatment for the cancer
- of the constitution
- to have an antineoplastic effect.

If toxic exposure is defined or suspected as part of the pathogenesis of the cancer, then some means for clearing these toxins must be instituted. Chelation therapy is one way of clearing heavy metals. Please see Chapter 14 on prevention.

The first 2 years following the completion of the cytotoxic treatment for breast cancer is the most important period, since it is during this time that recurrence is most likely. Convince your patients that working to prevent recurrence is an extremely important and ongoing part of therapy and lifestyle. They must continue with Chinese medicine, dietary changes, and lifestyle changes.

Following are some preventive formulas. They can be partially included within a constitutional formula of choice and modified based on the presentation of the patient.

Taichung Medical College formula

ren shen (Ginseng Radix; *Panax ginseng*)	30 g
huang qi (Astragali Radix; *Astragalus membranaceus*)	30 g
ren dong teng (Lonicerae Caulis; *Lonicera japonica*)	30 g
bai zhu (Atractylodis macrocephalae Rhizoma; *Atractylodes macrocephala*)	60 g
qian cao gen (Rubiae Radix; *Rubia cordifolia* root)	10 g
bai jie zi (Sinapis Semen; *Sinapis*)	10 g
fu ling (Poria; *Poria cocos*)	15 g

I usually do not use ren shen or lu jiao (Cervi Cornu; deer antler) or other animal products that have a relationship to hormonal levels in formulas for women with breast or hormonally related cancers. Ren shen stimulates the pituitary and can initiate the estrogen cascade. Animal products like horn do contain estrogen and testosterone. Testosterone is stored in fat tissue and converted to estrogen.

Gua lou xiao yao tang

bai zhu (Atractylodis macrocephalae Rhizoma; *Atractylodes macrocephala*)	12 g
gua lou shi (Trichosanthis Fructus; *Trichosanthes* fruit)	30 g
fu ling (Poria; *Poria cocos*)	15 g
yu jin (Curcumae Radix; *Curcuma longa* rhizome)	15 g
bai shao (Paeoniae Radix alba; *Paeonia lactiflora* root)	15 g
chai hu (Bupleuri Radix; *Bupleurum*)	10 g
dang gui (Angelicae sinensis Radix; *Angelica sinensis*)	12 g

xiang fu (Cyperi Rhizoma; *Cyperus* 10 g
rotundus rhizome)

bo he (Menthae haplocalycis Herba; 15 g
Mentha haplocalyx)

lu jiao (Cervi Cornu; deer antler) 15 g

Lu jiao and some other herbs are substances that have an impact on circulating estrogen levels. The issue of phytoestrogenicity in herbs is a complex one both singly and in combination. Animal products in particular like lu jiao contain estrogens and testosterones and may be problematic in hormonally-sensitive cancers, usually glandular tissue cancers like breast, ovaries, uterus, kidneys, adrenals, prostate, testis. There are many other reasons to avoid animal products.

Qing zhi si wu tang

qing pi (Citri reticulatae viride 10 g
Pericarpium; *Citrus reticulata* green
pericarp)

zhi zi (Gardeniae Fructus; *Gardenia* 10 g
fruit)

dang gui (Angelicae sinensis Radix; 30 g
Angelica sinensis)

chuan xiong (Chuanxiong Rhizoma; 10 g
Ligusticum wallichii root)

bai shao (Paeoniae Radix alba; 15 g
Paeonia lactiflora root)

shu di (Rehmanniae Radix 15 g
preparata; *Rehmannia*)

xiang fu (Cyperi Rhizoma; *Cyperus* 10 g
rotundus rhizome)

fu ling (Poria; *Poria cocos*) 15 g

zhi ban xia (Pinelliae Rhizoma 15 g
preparatum; *Pinellia ternata*
rhizome)

zi cao (Arnebiae/Lithospermi Radix; 15 g
Arnebia/Lithospermum root)

ba yue zha (Akebiae Fructus; *Akebia*) 15 g

pu gong ying (Taraxaci Herba; 15 g
Taraxacum mongolicum)

shu yang quan (Solani lyrati Herba; 15 g
Solanum lyratum)

xia ku cao (Prunellae Spica; *Prunella* 30 g
vulgaris)

wang bu liu xing (Vaccariae Semen; 15 g
Vaccaria segetalis seeds)

chuan bei mu (Fritillariae cirrhosae 10 g
Bulbus; *Fritillaria cirrhosa*)

zhi ke (Aurantii Fructus; *Citrus* 10 g
aurantium)

shan ci gu* (Cremastrae/Pleiones 10 g
Pseudobulbus; *Cremastra/Pleione*
pseudobulbs)

Case study 4.1

This case involves a 42-year-old Japanese-American woman who was diagnosed in Japan at the age of 30 years. Her diagnosis was never made available but she was treated in Japan with various therapies and then with tamoxifen for 5 years. Therefore, it is assumed that she had an estrogen-receptor-positive breast cancer. This is all that is known about her markers. It was obvious that she had received radiation therapy to the left chest area; there was severe atrophy and deformity of the soft tissue and skeletal structure of the left shoulder and chest. She had a thoracic scoliosis of adolescent onset that had worsened as a result of radiation therapy. She had also had a radical left

mastectomy. She had no other pertinent medical history.

Her cancer recurred at the age of 39, 4 years after ending tamoxifen hormonal therapy for prevention of recurrence, while she was living in the United States. At the time of recurrence, metastatic spread was discovered to her left lung. There was no further spread but this finding placed the patient in the Stage IV category. Other studies were done at this time, particularly a bone scan, liver and kidney function tests (Chem 23) to rule out liver metastases, and chest CT to identify the status of the other lung, but all were clear.

Case study continues

The nature of the side effects of tamoxifen preclude its use for longer than 5 years. These side effects include uterine and liver cancer and clotting disorders like DVT. It was assumed that the tamoxifen had successfully staved off the disease for those years and so it was decided to use another type of antiestrogenic hormonal treatment: megestrol (Megace). The patient was placed on a tamoxifen-interface formula with the addition of herbs to protect the lungs and bones.

To the tamoxifen formula was added the formula Bai he gu jin tang. This formula was chosen because atrophy of the left lung was apparent from the radiation and it was assumed that yin deficiency was a primary injury. The combination of radiation injury and the fact that the lungs are a primary metastatic site for breast cancer made it important to treat to prevent any more metastatic spread in that lung or spread to the other lung. Also local spread to the bone is a common occurence and, therefore, bai hua she (Agkistrodon; *Agkistrodon acutus*) was added to act prophylactically. Herbs in the form of a kidney tonic formula were added at that time to protect the brain, which is also a predicted site for metastasis. Zuo gui yin was added to the tamoxifen formula with bai hua she added as a single herb. The doses for the tamoxifen formula were the same as those written earlier in the text and the Zui gui yin formula was added at similar doses. Bai hua she was added (20 g). The decision was made to focus on the hormonal treatment and the lungs and bone.

The patient did well on this combination of formulas alongside the megestrol for the next 4 years. She had no trouble eating a modified macrobiotic diet since it was so close to her native diet. She continued in a graduate program and did very well. She discontinued treatment with Chinese medicine in 2002 without explanation. In January 2004 she presented with brain metastasis and was treated with brain irradiation, which she apparently tolerated well. But then in April 2004 she presented with symptoms that looked very much like a stroke. There was mild paresthesia on the right side, temporary loss of orientation, a temporary dysphagia, and mild headache. She was taken to the emergency room and diagnosed with

a mild cerebrovascular accident (CVA). She was hospitalised and many studies were performed to determine the cause of the stroke. It was finally determined that there was a vegetative growth in one ventricle of the heart and on the mitral valve. Tiny pieces of this vegetative growth had broken off and clogged an artery (left cerebral artery) in her brain precipitating the stroke. The cause of the vegetative growth was considered secondary to the cancer. It is not known if the brain irradiation contributed to the stroke by weakening the cerebral arteries. It is not known if she was ever treated with Adriamycin, which could have injured the heart muscle. However, Adriamycin is and was the standard of care for earlier stage breast cancer.

She was also diagnosed with DIC (diffuse intra-arterial coagulopathy) and after being stabilised from the stroke placed on coumadin to treat this condition and to stave off a further stroke. Megestrol is associated with more thromboembolic effects and this probably contributed to the DIC and, therefore, the stroke. It is difficult to know for sure. Unfortunately, another stroke occured 3 months later and severe left-sided symptoms persisted as a result of this stroke. The patient has struggled, at the age of 44, to recover, and has regained a normal gait, normal swallowing, and is gradually able to read again. But the left arm and hand remain paralysed and speech is very difficult. The right arm is quite functional but weak. Her Japanese is far better than her English. Depression has been a large factor in treatment.

She has been placed on oral cyclophosphamide (Cytoxan) for 4 days running consecutively in each month. It was decided that some form of chemotherapy was called for at this time. Oral Cytoxan was chosen as the mildest agent that could be given orally in this case. The CA 27.29 has been a good monitoring marker and has lowered again into the normal range on this therapy. The natural history of this breast cancer over the past 14 years leads one to believe that this cancer is somewhat indolent and nonaggressive. It has taken its toll, but has been quite slow in its progression and fairly benign treatments have kept it in check. However, its path is relentless. This particular natural history of breast cancer is not uncommon and it is shared

Case study continues

here to demonstrate a typical progression. The earlier diagnosis is not as common, nor is the vegetative growth on the heart valve, but otherwise this progression is quite typical.

Treatment principles

The treatment principles at this time include interfacing with Cytoxan to potentiate its effectiveness, stop further spread to lung, bone and liver and brain, to treat the residual injuries from the stroke in an environment in which blood stasis (DIC and the strokes) is being treated with anticoagulants. Also the spirit needs strong support. And constipation has become an issue primarily due to lack of exercise. Following is the formula in use at this time:

he huan pi (Albiziae Cortex; *Albizia*)	25 g
zhi bai fu zi (Typhonii Rhizoma; *Typhonium giganteum*)	40 g
bai shao (Paeoniae Radix alba; *Paeonia lactiflora* root)	20 g
jing jie (Schizonepetae Herba; *Schizonepeta*)	25 g
da huang (Rhei Radix et Rhizoma; *Rheum*)	15 g
fang feng (Ledebouriellae Radix; *Ledebouriella* root)	25 g
bai zhi (Angelicae dahuricae Radix; *Angelica dahurica*)	25 g
hong hua (Carthami Flos; *Carthamnus tinctorius* flowers)	20 g
huang qi (Astragali Radix; *Astragalus membranaceus*)	30 g
bai ren shen (Ginseng Radix; *Panax ginseng*; white ginseng)	15 g
bai zhu (Atractylodis macrocephalae Rhizoma; *Atractylodes macrocephala*)	25 g
fu shen (Poriae Sclerotium pararadicis; *Poria cocos*)	25 g
di long (Pheretima; *Pheretima*; lumbricus)	25 g
bai zi ren (Biotae Semen; *Biota*)	20 g
tian nan xing (Arisaematis Rhizoma preparatum; *Arisaema erubescens* rhizome)	35 g

This formula is a modification of the formula Bu yang huan wu tang, Decoction for invigorating yang. The DIC and anticoagulants drive the changes in the base formula. The treatment principles of the base formula are to tonify the qi, promote blood circulation and dredge the channels. It is a formula used to treat symptoms of stroke sequelae like hemiplegia, facial deviation, and aphasia when the stroke is caused by yang deficiency and blood stasis. It was delivered at 6 g three times daily.

This patient was very petite and had lost weight since I had seen her a year and a half earlier, down from 125 to 90 lb. She was cold and had difficulty staying warm. She was very depressed and truly had given up on living. Although she had difficulty swallowing and drooled, wind phlegm was not part of her diagnosis. The conventional medical analysis of her stroke was taken into account. An infectious myocarditis was ruled out, her cholesterol was in the low range, she had no signs of cardiovascular disease. But an arteriogram showed vegetative growth on the mitral valve flap. This was considered to be secondary to cancer. Therefore, I considered this stroke to be due to a form of blood and phlegm stasis due to yang deficiency. But the principle of moving the blood by invigorating the blood had to be monitored very carefully because of the DIC, a form of more severe blood stasis syndrome, and the fact that her blood was being thinned by coumadin. Her prothrombin time and pulse were used as markers to determine the efficacy of the herbal formula.

Huang qi is the chief herb in the formula. It tonifies the zheng qi and, thereby, moves the blood. The symptoms of paralysis are attributable to internal wind. This wind is not due to liver yang rising but blood stasis in the head. The clot or material from the heart that occluded the vessel in the brain ended in stopping the blood flow to the brain tissue. The loss of blood flow generated a form of internal wind that resulted in paralysis. Because the second paralysis was quite severe herbs that eliminate wind were added. Bai fu zi expels wind and

Case study continues

phlegm and suppresses spasms; it is analgesic and tranquilising.

Jing jie relieves the surface and dispels wind. It is used to treat stroke and weakly inhibits cancerous swellings. It gently increases blood circulation and is an antispasmodic. Fang feng also relieves the surface and dispels wind. It is used to treat wind damp bi and is analgesic. Bai zhi expels wind from the yang ming channels and is analgesic. It reduces local swellings. Hong hua dispels congealed blood and relieves pain. It is an excellent post-stroke herb and is used for both brain and heart attacks. However, it also increases coronary blood flow and, therefore, this was the most problematic herb in the formula. Protime was watched very carefully while using this herb. No more pieces of the vegetative growth broke free of the heart valve as a result of blood thinning, blood moving or viscosity changes. It is hoped that the cytotoxic effect of the chemotherapeutic agent will be enough to stop the cancer progression and the vegetative progression on the valve flap. It is an unusual situation.

Bai ren shen strongly tonifies the source qi. It calms the spirit, is immunomodulating, and is one of the best cardiotonics. Although I consider ren shen to be contraindicated in breast cancer, I felt that the benefits in this case outweighed the negatives. Huang qi, ren shen, bai zhu, and fu shen all combine to form a modification of Si jun zi tang, the main formula to tonify the qi of the spleen. General tonification is important in this situation in order to support overall health. Tonification of the middle jiao function is especially important in a patient who has lost weight, has little appetite, and is suffering from general debility. Fu shen has the additional benefit of being a form of *Poria* that calms the spirit. The immunomodulating benefits of *Poria* are also found in this form of the herb.

Di long is a strange and remarkable herb that has many benefits in this case. It expels wind and clears the luo channels helping to re-establish blood circulation and resolve paralysis. It also helps to soothe fright and is used here because in some ways this patient was living in fright and with a lack of trust that another stroke was not around the corner. She was also very restless mentally and physically but could not express or discharge this feeling. Di long is an appropriate choice for all of these symptoms of post-stroke. It also alleviates the pain from chronic wind bi.

Bai zi ren is a calm-the-spirit herb that is a seed that moistens the stool and treats constipation. Da huang treats constipation and is also antineoplastic. When cooked longer it can move the blood. He huan pi relieves depression and calms the spirit; it vitalises the blood, calms irritability and restlessness, and helps patients to sleep when anxiety is present. Bai shao nourishes the blood and consolidates the yin, the mother of yang. It calms the liver and helps to relieve pain. In combination with the wind-expelling herbs it helps to repair the collaterals and re-establish blood circulation and normal qi flow in the channels. It is antispasmodic.

Tian nan xing is added here as a main antineoplastic herb where other stronger herbs would be contraindicated. It disperses phlegm and may be appropriate for the type of cancerous vegetative growth on the heart valve. It also dispels wind phlegm and stops spasms and relieves pain.

The patient has done well on this formula. The stroke sequelae continue to resolve, her spirits are much improved, weight has increased, constipation is no longer a problem helped to some extent by daily walks and minor changes in the diet. The main issues that persist are left-hand paralysis with slowness in speech, especially in English. As a result of terminating the hormonal treatment, a menstrual cycle has begun again after many years of dormancy. This implies that estrogen levels are sufficient to reinstitute a cycle and this, in turn, may mean that these same levels may be proliferative of the cancer. This patient situation is problemmatic from many points of view:

1. Rehabilitation and prevention of further stroke with the use of blood-thinning pharmaceuticals is difficult herbally; the DIC is a result of the cancer and is an environment in which cancer can proliferate – blood stasis; it and the stroke is being treated with blood-thinning drugs, which lower the circulating platelet levels

Case study continues

making the patient more susceptible to hemorrhage.

2. Prevention of spread of the cancer utilising chemotherapy because the hormonal treatment has failed creates a difficult choice that must be balanced with these other factors and the patient's overall ability to withstand the side effects of the chemotherapy regimen; chemotherapy can potentially cause myelosuppression and digestive insufficiency; many patients lose the battle with cancer partly as a result of malnutrition; therefore, maintaining the digestive fire, reducing constipation, and increasing absorption are all very important.

3. Making judgements about all of these issues in a frail patient who is still young becomes a juggling act in a complex case. One is led back to the primary concerns of classical medicine: maintain good sleep, regular stool, and the spirit of the patient as the foundation of health.

The manner in which these principles are delivered at this time is through the original formula. At some point, antineoplastics that potentiate the Cytoxan agent in oral form will be added to the formula. A large dose of ling zhi (Ganoderma; *Ganoderma*) will help ameliorate bone marrow suppression and the thrombocytopenia. A kidney yang tonic formula would help both the low platelet count (which is due to the DIC and coumadin therapy) and the fear of more brain metastases. Lu jiao jiao (Cervi Cornu; deer antler), e jiao (Asini Corii Colla; *Equus asinus*; donkey-hide gelatin) and other animal products like these may be too estrogenic for this case. For long-term use Liu wei di huang wan plus di yu (Sanguisorbae Radix; *Sanguisorba*) and higher dose huang qi (Astragali Radix; *Astragalus membranaceus*) might work well and work as a double agent to raise platelets and lower estrogen levels. In the case of more profound spleen deficiency, using Gui pi tang plus han lian cao (Ecliptae Herba; *Eclipta prostrata*) and san qi (Notoginseng Radix; *Panax notoginseng*) could be an approach.

There are other formulas that reduce the bioavailability of estrogen. Green tea inhibits the interaction between estrogen and estrogen receptors in ER-positive tumors. Dang gui xiao yao san suppresses estradiol secretion by the ovaries. Gui zhi fu ling wan acts as a weak antiestrogenic formula. These formulas could also be used to enhance the effect of the Cytoxan by working similarly to the megestrol and tamoxifen, which were used for so long to good effect. The results of tumor marker monitoring would drive the decision to use these formulas. And what remains uppermost is the prevention of spread of the disease, managing the thrombocytopenia without contributing to DIC and, therefore, the cancer, managing the stroke sequelae, and improving quality of life.

Case Study 4.2

This woman was diagnosed at age 50 years with a right breast cancer, ductal infiltrating, grade 2 out of 3 (intermediate grade), mitotic rate 1 out of 3, microcalcifications in all of the tissue, tubule formation is 3 out of 3, size 4.7 cm. The cancer was estrogen receptor positive, progesterone receptor positive, and *HER2-neu* negative – all of which carry a good prognosis. Ductal carcinoma in situ was also present. The DCIS was low nuclear grade, solid and cribiform types, without necrosis.

The CA 27.29 was 12 (in the normal range, with 38 being the upper border). The bone scan was negative. The stage was II with a Bloom–Richardson score of 6 out of 9. An MRI of both breasts showed no signs of disease in the left breast. A sentinel node biopsy was performed and micrometastatic carcinoma (<2 mm) was found in one axillary lymph node with no evidence of extracapsular extension (the lymph node confined the cancer and worked as it should). After partial

Case study continues

mastectomy, all of the margins were widely free of cancer except for one, which was 0.2 cm in depth. Because of the positive node and close margin, surgery was performed again to remove two more nodes and to enhance the margin of the lumpectomy. There was an effort to prevent lymphedema by limiting the number of nodes taken.

Pertinent history was a cholecystectomy at age 45 and fibroids with no bleeding. Her menstrual cycle had shortened to 23 days. Questioning the patient revealed that the gallstones and fibroids did represent high fat intake. The patient is somewhat overweight and sedentary in lifestyle. At the time of diagnosis, all of the blood chemistries in a CBC and Chem 23 were in the normal range.

Plan

The patient was offered two plans for treatment. One was Adriamycin with Cytoxan (AC) in a schedule of every 3 weeks for six courses followed by radiation and then hormonal treatment for 5 years. The other was cyclophosmamide, methotrexate, and fluorouracil (CMF) for 12 courses, then radiation for 6 weeks, then CMF for 12 courses followed by hormonal treatment for 5 years. The Cytoxan (cyclophosmamide) in the second choice would be administered in pill form. The patient was concerned about the toxicity of the AC regimen and chose the CMF, even though it lasted longer than the AC regimen.

At the time of the presentation, appetite was low normal, digestion was normal except for lower abdominal gas with some bloating, stools were regular and formed or loose. Sleep was good and eight hours per night but interrupted by recurrent nightmares on occasion. She had recently made changes in her diet from SAD to vegetarian. She was avoiding dairy, coffee, sugar, alcohol, and red meat. She had a history of acid regurgitation, which had resolved on her current diet. Green tea had been introduced, along with seaweeds, rice milk, more legumes and whole grains, and flax-seed oil. She was eating far more vegetables than previously. She ran slightly warm, was never thirsty, and had to remember to drink fluids. She was walking for half an hour daily and taking

lessons in yoga once weekly. She was also doing qi gong daily.

- Tongue: dark and slightly red, pale center area, a center line deep crack, light yellow greasy somewhat thick coat, red points on the anterior third of the tongue body, and +2 distention.
- Pulse: on the left the doyo or middle pulse was surrounded in hardness and somewhat hollow, overall it was a liver-deficient pulse with some kidney deficiency also. I called it a liver sho.
- Diagnosis: liver and kidney yin deficiency with damp heat due to spleen and stomach disharmony leading to stomach rebellion and fire poison disrupting the Chong and Ren.

Formula

I began seeing this patient right after diagnosis and surgery. The first formula was intended for use post-surgically. It was delivered in granulated form, three times daily at 6 g per dose.

Xiang sha liu jun zi tang	150 g
Liu wei di huang tang	100 g
plus the following herbs:	
jin yin hua (Lonicerae Flos; *Lonicera* flowers)	20 g
mu dan pi (Moutan Cortex; *Paeonia suffruticosa* root cortex)	15 g
lian qiao (Forsythiae fructus; *Forsythia*)	20 g
zao jiao ci (Gleditsiae Spina; *Gleditsia* spines)	15 g
huang qi (Astragali Radix; *Astragalus membranaceus*)	30 g
huang qin (Scutellariae Radix; *Scutellaria baicalensis*)	25 g

The intent was to address the underlying constitutional patterns for the cancer before chemotherapy began and pre-empted the direction of treatment. Xiang sha liu jun zi tang is a formula that addresses the stomach spleen disharmony and dampness. Liu wei di huang tang addresses another part of the diagnosis by nourishing the liver and kidney yin. In a premenopausal woman it lowers estrogen levels and, thereby, treats the constitution and the cancer. It is important to

Case study continues

address the constitutional environment of the patient and this is one time at which this can be done without concern for treating the side effects of chemotherapy or other cytotoxic therapies.

It is difficult to treat a spleen-deficient environment with damp heat and yin deficiency concurrently. The herbs added to this combination formula attempt to clear heat and act antineoplastically simultaneously. Jin yin hua is a clear heat and toxin herb that has action against breast cancer and also clears damp heat. It increases phagocytosis and is antibacterial. Preventing infection is one of the indications post-surgery. Preventing spread of the cancer is indicated; this herb is antineoplastic, especially against breast cancer.

Mu dan pi clears heat and cools the blood, it clears deficiency fire, moves congealed blood, reduces swelling and promotes the discharge of pus. It is antineoplastic, antipyretic, and is used to treat swollen painful breasts. It is also mildly analgesic. An excellent herb to prevent infection, prevent spread of the cancer, and promote healing of the surgical wound. Lian qiao clears heat and toxin and disperses swellings and drains pus. It is antibacterial and anti-inflammatory and is used to treat painful swollen breasts. It helps to prevent infection and to initiate the healing process. Zao jiao ci reduces inflammation and discharges pus and is used to treat swollen painful breasts. Huang qi is the empiric herb for wound healing. It also increases phagocytosis and WBC to prevent infection. It increases NK cells and activity to begin surveillance against spread. The clear heat herbs combine with the formula to treat the damp heat component of the diagnosis, hopefully not further injuring the spleen function. Huang qin adds to the treatment by clearing heat and drying dampness. It also lowers the liver yang, a potential in the liver and kidney yin deficient patient when under stress.

The patient remained on this formula for 3 weeks at which time she began chemotherapy in the form of CMF. The herbal orientation changed to meet the demands of the CMF regimen. Please see the section in this chapter on the CMF formula and the analysis of its construction. The main constitutional diagnosis was liver and kidney yin deficiency. Liu wei di huang wan is the primary formula of choice in this case and this formula also decreases estrogen levels in a perimenopausal or premenopausal patient. This was a positive in this case as the patient was still cycling and also had an estrogen-receptive tumor. If she had been menopausal, with or without an estrogen-receptive tumor, this formula would have been contraindicated.

Because there were stomach/spleen issues accompanying this diagnosis, the approach was to utilise the CMF formula without adjusting it to treat the liver and kidney yin deficiency. However, it was adjusted by adding herbs that would support the middle jiao and also mildly clear damp heat. Huang qin (Scutellariae Radix; *Scutellaria*) was added at a low dose of 12 g and the dose of fu ling (Poria; *Poria cocos*) was increased to 20 g. Zhu ru (Bambusae Caulis in taeniam; *Phyllostachys nigra*) was added to manage the stronger possibility of nausea in a stomach-deficient damp heat environment. The yin-nourishing herbs were lowered in dose. The patient was able to undergo chemotherapy with this regimen without high-dose antiemetics and eventually eliminated them from her regimen. She also dramatically lowered the dose of dexamethasone (a steroid) used to manage nausea and other more severe allergic reactions in patients undergoing chemotherapy. Her kidney function remained normal during treatment and she was only mildly anemic with her hematocrit never going below 34. The WBC count always remained in the normal range; she never had any acute infection like a cold or flu. Kidney function remained normal.

She underwent 12 infusions of CMF successfully and then switched to radiation of the tumor bed and scar midtreatment. Radiation therapy included 33 sessions of external beam field radiation and then five boost sessions to the tumor bed itself. During this time she was prescribed the radiation formula. She also used the Spring Wind Burn Creme applied before radiation and also twice daily during treatment. The main complaint during this phase of treatment was fatigue. The formula was modified slightly by adding huang qi (Astragali Radix; *Astragalus membranaceus*) at 20 g and Si jun zi tang at 100 g to the radiation formula.

Case study continues

Depression was a primary part of the fatigue. The therapy for this particular regimen was long and hard; it took its toll on the spirit and radiation was a daily commitment and constant reminder of the diagnosis. Therefore, he huan pi (Albiziae Cortex; *Albizia*) and ji xue cao (Centellae Herba; *Centella asiatica*; gotu kola) were added to lift the spirit. There was no burning from the radiation, the skin discoloration returned to normal pink 1 month after XRT ended. The spirit improved and energy returned even at session 20 of the XRT schedule. Except for shoulder pain and discoloration from XRT, the patient felt almost completely well when chemotherapy began again. The shoulder pain was due to chemotherapy agents persisting in the joints. It is a common symptom that often appears 2 months after stopping chemotherapy and lasts until 6 months post-chemotherapy. It is quite predictable and is the result of chemotherapeutic agents being cleared from the joints later than other tissue due to the lesser blood supply in synovial tissue. It is more common in the knees and hips but this patient was a flute player and repairer and had a pre-existing shoulder and postural pattern that precipitated 'chemotherapy arthritis' in the shoulder joint more than in the large joints of the lower extremity. 'Chemo arthritis' usually resolves on its own, but qi- and blood-moving herbs are of benefit, as well as acupuncture and moxibustion.

After a break in treatment of 3 weeks, the patient returned to the last phase of treatment, another 12 infusions of the CMF regimen every 2 weeks. This patient was able to travel cross-country midtreatment and play flute in an extended program of Bach. Although it was somewhat taxing physically, the inspiration of playing with others in this holiday Bach concert series was very uplifting. There was difficulty with her shoulder joints as a result of the 'chemo arthritis'. This had begun earlier during the break in treatment from the first round of chemotherapy. Because she was about to start radiation and then begin chemotherapy again it was decided not to treat this one symptom except with physical therapy. This worked well for her and she was able to hold her flute in position for 3-hour stints during the concert series.

She was switched back to the modified form of the CMF formula and did very well on this regimen. Her CA 27.29 had never gone out of the normal range, even prior to diagnosis, and so it was not considered a good marker for her in terms of monitoring the efficacy of chemotherapy. However, her level of wellness and her ability to go through the chemotherapy and radiation regimen were all considered good signs. At the end of treatment, a breast PET-scan was performed and found negative for any signs of active cancer. She was started on tamoxifen for 5 years.

At the end of cytotoxic treatment with conventional standard of care, this patient was iatrogenically menopausal. Because of her age and her pre-existing liver and kidney yin deficiency, it was assumed that her menopausal status was permanent. Tamoxifen enhanced the menopausal symptoms induced by the ovarian ablation from the chemotherapy. It was no longer appropriate to use Liu wei di huang, which would have raised her estrogen levels and acted against the effect of the hormonal anti-estrogenic treatment for recurrence with tamoxifen. The tamoxifen formula was used with some modifications. Dang shen (Codonopsis Radix; *Codonopsis pilosula* root) and nu zhen zi (Ligustri lucidi Fructus; *Ligustrum lucidum*) were added at a fairly high dose of 20 g each. Tian nan xing (Arisaematis Rhizoma preparatum; *Arisaema erubescens*) was added as an antineoplastic as well as chong lou (Paridis Rhizoma; *Paris*) and jin yin hua (Lonicerae Flos; *Lonicera*). These were added at a high dose of 40 g each.

To date the patient has been on this formula with varying modifications for 2 years now without difficulty. All of her monitoring screens have been negative. She has continued her dietary and lifestyle changes and has lost 45 lb. Her pulses are well balanced, her tongue is pink without scalloped edges, the coat is thin and white. She has no positive hara signs. The fibroids have resolved – probably as a result of dietary changes and her menopausal status. She sleeps well and her spirit is more positive than at any other time in her life. The side effects of tamoxifen are well-managed. She has no flushing, vaginal dryness, or other symptoms of menopausal syndrome. The plan is for her to remain on tamoxifen for the full 5 years, continue monitoring, return once monthly for monitoring and any necessary adjustments with Chinese medicine.

Case study 4.3

This case demonstrates the pathway of treating to prevent recurrence. This was a patient diagnosed with a right ductal infiltrating breast carcinoma at the age of 43 years. It was a papillary type with tubule formation at 2, grade 3, mitotic rate of 2, ER-negative, PR-negative, *HER2/neu* negative, node negative, T1cN0M0 and with a Bloom–Richardson score of 8/9. She was tested for *BR-CA 1* and *2* gene expression and found to be negative. The tumor size was 1.25 cm in diameter. The CA 27.29 was 14 at the time of diagnosis. The CEA was 0.75. Both are within normal ranges.

The Bloom–Richardson score is high and based on some rather difficult markers in this patient. The grade 3 indicates a tumor with rapid turnover. The ER and PR status indicate a poorer prognosis. These three pieces of information alone combine to drive a more difficult diagnosis in terms of treatment and outcome. The size, on the other hand, is small, and there are no positive nodes. The treatment options become somewhat open as a result. A small but aggressive tumor could indicate lumpectomy plus radiation and possibly chemotherapy. An antiestrogenic approach is not indicated because the cancer is ER negative.

Further non-traditional studies showed that DDT and DDE levels were high. DDT is a persistent pesticide that is xenoestrogenic and a known risk for breast cancer. DDE is a breakdown product of DDT and is also implicated in breast cancer. General history was of interest in that the patient had mastitis during her first pregnancy, which was 7 years prior to diagnosis of breast cancer. She also had a history of breast distention during premenses and her cycle was somewhat long at 30 days. These are all signs of liver qi stasis, possible blood stasis, and liver qi stasis leading to heat. These aspects of her history lay a foundation for the impact of xenoestrogenic exposure, which is carcinogenic. It is impossible to say when the carcinogenic hits occured and if they are ongoing. It is probable that the hits occured early in life and may have continued into adulthood when lifestyle changes occured that led to better eating habits and the institution of a vegetarian and organic foods lifestyle, including drinking filtered water.

It is not possible to say that the xenoestrogenic impact was greater because of liver qi stagnation and the history of mastitis. The main area of inflammation during the mastitis was the same area where the tumor was found. The history of breast distention implies a possible qi stasis pattern in the mastitis event, or it may be unrelated. Breast cancer is considered a multifactorial disease, and possibly these events and pattern combined in the presence of a carcinogenic hit (or hits) to initiate the cancerisation process. From the point of view of Chinese medicine, treating all of the above is part of the cure. She was diagnosed with polynephritis several years prior during a 5-month trip in China and was treated with antibiotics. This is probably not related to the diagnosis of breast cancer.

Her appetite was good and she experienced slight cramping around the navel on occasion. Stools were slightly loose and often quite odorous. As a health practitioner herself, this patient was sensitive to bodily odors and felt that her underarm odor was also stronger than normal. Urine had a marked odor, as well. Otherwise, stools and urination were normal. Thirst was quite high and she drank 3 L of water daily beyond other forms of fluids. She experienced heat at night without sweating. Sleep was normal.

- Tongue: reddish with a redder anterior area (upper jiao), red points on the tip, little coat, mild vein distention.
- Pulse: moderate (Nanjing); spleen sho (Japanese).
- Hara:
  - left lung: cool
  - kidney: cool
  - spleen area: flaccid
  - stomach area: tight
  - liver: slightly tight.
- Diagnosis: liver qi stasis with underlying spleen deficiency leading to Chong and Ren disharmony with fire poison.

Case study continues

This patient may have been heading into a slightly early menopause and liver/kidney yin deficiency. The red tongue, heat at night, and thirst all imply there may be yin deficiency. Neither the pulse nor the hara corroborated this. So it was decided to proceed with a liver qi stasis diagnosis with underlying spleen deficiency and to view the red tongue as a sign of fire poison.

Plan

The patient decided to be treated with a newer form of conventional treatment. She was advised to have a lumpectomy followed by radiation and possibly chemotherapy. She proceeded with the lumpectomy, which went very well and had already occured before she was seen for integrative treatment with Chinese medicine. The next phase of her treatment was with radiation but in a form rarely used in breast cancer. She travelled to the South-West and was treated for several days with brachytherapy. Tubes were strategically placed in the breast tissue around the tumor bed. Then for 12 minutes twice each day radioactive seeds were placed in the tubes and activated. This procedure took place for 5 days in a row. Then the tubes were removed and the patient sent home. For some time there was redness and discoloration from the tubes. Several months later there was no sign of the procedure.

The patient has decided not to seek further conventional treatment beyond monitoring. There is no stastistical evidence regarding brachytherapy in breast cancer. Her medical oncologist, however, approves of this path and sees the patient once every 3 months. It has been 1 year now and monitoring will be once every 6 months. A follow-up breast MRI has been performed with no signs of disease. This patient is now a part of the Marcia Rivkin Breast and Ovarian Cancer Study because of her Ashkenazi Jewish heritage and this diagnosis for breast cancer. She was screened for the *BR-CA 1* and *2* genes expression but found to be negative. However, because of her heritage she decided to become part of a monitoring study, partly for herself and partly in an effort to contribute something to the study of breast cancer.

Treatment principles

During the brachytherapy the patient was placed on the radiation formula and used Spring Wind Burn Creme with the blessings of the radiation oncologist. She remained on this formula for 6 months with the understanding that the effects of the XRT last for up to 6 months post-treatment. She went through this time period with very few side effects, only discoloration of the skin and slight tenderness in the rib below the primary site. At month four the formula was modified to begin to address the primary traditional diagnosis of liver qi stasis with underlying spleen deficiency. Xiao yao san is the primary formula for this presentation and it was added to the XRT formula in herb doses that approximated the doses in that formula. The patient took 6 g three times daily.

The patient also underwent another radical change in her lifestyle by adding several 3- to 5-day fasts to her daily regimen. These were water fasts and were used to clear toxins in the traditional sense of the word and also clear toxins (DDT and DDE) in the medical sense of the word (depuration; see Chapter 14 on prevention). Her sense of her body odors has changed dramatically. She has lost only 5 lb in the process but her stools have become formed (as opposed to loose in the past), she no longer has temperature discrepancies between daytime and evening, her energy has improved, there is no bodily odor and the DDT levels are no longer measurable. DDE continues to remain high but, because it is a breakdown product of DDT, it is assumed that this form of DDT is still clearing and she should continue with what she is currently doing.

As time progressed, it became clear that the underlying main pattern was spleen deficiency leading to liver qi stasis. This spleen deficiency could be traced back to early years and poor eating habits manifesting in many different digestive complaints including chronic constipation and then loose stools, poor appetite, weight loss, distention and bloating in both the upper and lower digestive tract. There was a long familial history for her, even as a child, of providing care for everyone except herself. Her ability to draw good boundaries around herself and her energy

Case study continues

was poor. She was literally being sucked dry and was malnourished on many levels for most of her life. These complaints were mildly present at the time of diagnosis, although a great deal had been done by the patient to change her diet and eating habits and work on self-esteem and personal boundaries prior to her diagnosis. She was on a good path and dedicated to remaining on this path. But the pulse, tongue, hara and symptom picture all corraborated spleen deficiency. This was reinforced as time progressed. So the approach changed in terms of her herbal formula.

Formula

The treatment principles evolved into treating the stomach/spleen axis and detoxification/depuration concurrently while preventing recurrence. The following formula is the current one in use for this patient one and one half years after completing conventional treatment. The treatment principles are: tonify the middle jiao and benefit the spleen, move qi and blood, regulate the menses, clear toxin, act antineoplastically to prevent recurrence.

hu lu ba (Trigonellae Semen; *Trigonella*)	15 g
bai zhi (Angelicae dahuricae Radix; *Angelica dahurica*)	12 g
san leng (Sparganii Rhizoma; *Sparganium* rhizome)	12 g
chuan xiong (Chuanxiong Rhizoma; *Ligusticum wallichii* root)	10 g
mo yao (Myrrha; *Commiphora myrrha*; myrrh)	10 g
zao jiao ci (Gleditsiae Spina; *Gleditsia* spines)	15 g
jie geng (Platycodi Radix; *Platycodon grandiflorus* root)	12 g
nu zhen zi (Ligustri lucidi Fructus; *Ligustrum lucidum* fruit)	15 g
gua lou shi (Trichosanthis Fructus; *Trichosanthes* fruit)	20 g
ba yue zha (Akebiae Fructus; *Akebia*)	25 g
mai ya (Hordei Fructus germinatus; *Hordeum vulgare*; barley sprouts; malt)	15 g
dang shen (Codonopsis Radix; *Codonopsis pilosula* root)	15 g
chen pi (Citri reticulatae Pericarpium; *Citrus reticulata* pericarp)	10 g
pu gong ying (Taraxaci Herba; *Taraxacum mongolicum*)	25 g
xia ku cao (Prunellae Spica; *Prunella vulgaris*)	25 g
chong lou (Paridis Rhizoma; *Paris*)	30 g

This formula moves blood and qi to treat the diagnosis of liver qi stasis secondary to spleen deficiency. Moving blood and qi has the added benefit of prevention of recurrence. The formula also tonifies the qi of the spleen and, in tandem with the blood and qi movers, helps to regulate the long menstrual cycle. The clear toxin herbs are specific to breast cancer and act antineoplastically to prevent recurrence.

Hu lu ba is fenugreek seed and may seem like an odd addition to the formula. It enters the kidney channel and warms Mingmen. This herb is used here to warm and awaken the middle jiao and because it is a breast-specific herb that can help lift the source qi to the breast. Under other circumstances, this herb can increase lactation. Bai zhi is a release-the-exterior herb that has anticancer activity. It is a spicy warming herb that also can treat swollen, painful breasts and breast abscesses. It is a detoxifying herb. San leng vitalises the blood and moves qi. It enters the spleen and liver channels addressing the two entities involved in this pattern. It is antineoplastic. Chuan xiong also vitalises the blood, entering the liver, pericardium and gallbladder channels. It helps dispel congealed blood, moves qi and blood in the hypochondrium, generally improves blood circulation, and serves as a protectant against radiation. Mo yao vitalises the blood, reduces swellings, promotes healing of chronic non-healing sores and is anticancer.

Zao jiao ci reduces inflammation and resolves swollen painful breasts due to abscess. It is used here as a detoxicant. Jie geng directs the effect of the other herbs in the formula upwards to the chest. It is bitter, spicy and neutral and helps to support the middle jiao and qi circulation without injuring the spleen. Nu zhen zi is a yin-nourishing herb that helps to protect the yin in this primarily warming formula. It is also antitumor and along

Case study continues

with dang shen increases WBC counts to increase surveillance post-radiation. Gua lou shi circulates static qi in the chest; it dissipates nodules and is antineoplastic. As an adjuvant, it supports the other antineoplastic breast cancer herbs. Ba yue zha is used as a blood-moving antineoplastic in the place of chuan shan jia, which is an animal product that is endangered.

Mai ya harmonises the stomach and promotes the flow of the liver qi. It enters the spleen and stomach channels, and works to treat the main pattern of spleen deficiency. It also treats the pre-menstrual symptom of breast distention caused by liver qi stasis. Dang shen is a main spleen qi tonic herb. Chen pi is a primary qi-regulating herb that serves to strengthen the spleen, treat liver qi stasis and chest qi stasis, and support the assimilation of the antineoplastics and blood moving herbs in a patient with spleen deficiency.

Pu gong ying, xia ku cao, and chong lou are all antineoplastics and clear toxin herbs that are bitter and cool or cold. These herbs are specific to breast cancer and are added to prevent recurrence in a younger patient diagnosed with an aggressive tumor who underwent a therapeutic approach that does not have statistical evidence of efficacy. She will remain on this formula for at least 2 years after the end of conventional treatment. She came in once per week for acupuncture treatment and monitoring during XRT. Then she came in every 2 weeks after the end of conventional treatment and now comes in once per month for monitoring and herbal formula adjustment.

Acknowledgement

I wish to acknowledge Michael Broffman and Isaac Cohen for information and organisational elements contained in this chapter. Because of the high incidence of breast cancer and the tremendous amount of study going on in this realm it is difficult to organise all of the information available on the subject. Both of these individuals have contributed to this realm of knowledge and their expertise is intertwined in this chapter in a way that is no longer separate from my own thinking. I am in debt to both.

References

1. National Cancer Institute. National Cancer Survey, 2000. Cancer Surveillance Epidemiology and End Results (SEER) Program; 2000.
2. Wingo PA. Cancer statistics, 1995. CA Cancer J Clin 1995; 45:8–30.
3. Love SM. Fibrocystic disease of the breast – a non-disease? N Engl J Med 1982; 307:1010–1014.
4. Nelson NJ. Cancer risk high, but lower than expected with breast cancer genes. New Engl J Med 1997; 89:680–681.
5. National Breast Center of Australia. Breast News; Spring 1995.
6. Kliewer EV. Breast cancer mortality among immigrants in Australia and Canada. JNCI 1995; 87:1154–1161.
7. National Cancer Institute. Science 1992; 259:618.
8. Marshall E. Epidemiology. Search for a killer: focus shift from fat to hormones. Science 1993; 259:618–620.
9. Dewailley E. Could the rising levels of estrogen receptor in breast cancer be due to estrogenic pollutants? JNCI 1997; 89:888.
10. Kelsey JL. Reproductive factors and breast cancer. Epidemiological Reviews 1993; 15:36–47.
11. Petrakis NL. Influence of pregnancy and lactation on serum and breast fluid estrogen levels: Implications for breast cancer risk. Intl J Cancer 1987; 40:587–591.
12. Frazier AL. Shifting the time frame of breast cancer prevention to youth. In: Stoll BA, ed. Reducing breast cancer risk in women. Durdecht, Netherlands: Kluwer Academic Publishers; 1995.
13. Wolfe SM. Women's health alert. Public Citizen Health Research Group; 1991:133.
14. Paffenbarger RS. Cancer risks as related to the use of oral contraceptives during fertile years. Cancer 1977; 39:1887–1891.
15. Pike MC. Oral contraceptive use and early abortion as risk factors for breast cancer in young women. Brit J Cancer 1981; 43:72–76.
16. Harris NV. Breast cancer in relation to patterns of contraceptive use. Am J Epid 1982; 116:643–651.

17. Meirik O. Oral contraceptive use and breast cancer in young women. A joint national case-control study in Sweden and Norway. Lancet 1986; 8508:650–654.

18. Lipnick RJ. Oral contraceptives and breast cancer. A prospective cohort study. JAMA 1986; 225:58–61.

19. Brinton LA. Oral contraceptives and breast cancer risk among younger women. JNCI 1995; 87:827–835.

20. Centers for Disease Control. Oral contraceptive use and the risk of breast cancer. N Engl J Med 1986; 315:405–411.

21. Norplant Update. Breast implants 1995; 3:1–3.

22. Lee NC. A case-control study of breast cancer and hormonal contraception in Costa Rica. J NCI 1987; 79:1247–1254.

23. WHO Collaborative Study. Breast cancer and depo-medroxy-progesterone acetate: a multinational study. Lancet 1991; 338:833–838.

24. Jordan VC. The estrogenic activity of synthetic progestins used in oral contraceptives. Cancer 1993; 71:1501–1505.

25. Stanford J. Exogenous progestins and breast cancer. Epidemiological Reviews 1993; 15:98–107.

26. Berrino F. Serum sex hormone levels after menopause and subsequent breast cancer risk. J NCI 1996; 88:291–296.

27. Colditz GA. Relationship between estrogen levels, using of hormone replacement therapy, and breast cancer. J NCI 1998; 90:814–823.

28. Bergkvist L. The risk of breast cancer after estrogen-progestin replacement. N Engl J Med 1989; 321:293–297.

29. Colditz GA. The use of estrogens and progestins and the risk of breast cancer in post-menopausal women. N Engl J Med, 1995; 332:1589–1593.

30. Schneider DL. Timing of post-menopausal estrogen for optimal bone mineral density. JAMA 1997; 227:543–547.

31. Potter JD. Hormones and colon cancer. J NCI 1996; 87:1039–1040.

32. Makinen JI. Transdermal estrogen for female stress urinary incontinence in post-menopause. Maturitas 1995; 25:233–235.

33. Gady D. Invited commentary: does post-menopausal HRT cause breast cancer? Am J Epidem 1991; 134:1396–1401.

34. Steinberg KK. A meta-analysis of the effect of estrogen replacement therapy on risk of breast cancer. JAMA 1991; 265:1985–1990.

35. Bergkvist L. The risk of breast cancer after estrogen-progestin replacement. N Engl J Med 1989; 321:293–297.

36. Rodriguez C. Estrogen replacement therapy and fatal ovarian cancer. Am J Epidem 1995; 141:828–835.

37. Fotsis T. Phytoestrogens and inhibition of angiogenesis. Baillière's Clin Endocrinol Metab 1998; 12:649–666.

38. Huang YT. Effects of luteolin and quercitin, inhibitors of tyrosine kinase, on cell growth and metastasis-associated properties in A 431 cells overexpressing epidermal growth factor receptor. Br J Pharmacol 1999; 128:999–1010.

39. Kawaai S. Antiproliferative activity of flavonoids on several cancer cell lines. Biosci Biotechnol Biochem 1999; 63:896–899.

40. Santell RC. Genistein inhibits growth of estrogen-independent human breast cancer cells in culture but not in athymic mice. J Nutr 2000; 130:1665–1669.

41. Wang TTY. Molecular effects of genistein on estrogen receptor mediated pathways. Carcinogenesis 1996; 17:271–275.

42. Zava DT. Estrogenic and antiproliferative properties of genistein and other flavonoids in human breast cancer cells in vitro. Nutr Ca 1997; 27:31–40.

43. Ryu SR. Antitumor activity of some phenolic compounds in plants. Arch Pharm Res 1994; 17:42–44.

44. Clark JW. Effects of tyrosine kinase inhibitors on the proliferation of human breast cancer cell lines and proteins important in the ras signaling pathway. Int J Cancer 1996; 65:186–191.

45. Demsey K. Screening mammography: what the cancer establishment never told you. Cambridge, MA: The Women's Community Cancer Project; 5 May 1992:9.

46. Fletcher SW. Report of the international workshop on screening for breast cancer. J NCI 1993; 85:1644–1656.

47. Wanebo CK. Breast cancer after the atomic bombings of Hiroshima and Nagasaki. N Engl J Med 1968; 279:667–671.

48. Modan B. Increased risk of breast cancer after low-dose radiation. Lancet 1989; 629–631.

49. Eddy DM. Screening for breast cancer. Ann Internal Med 1989; 11:389–399.

50. Wright CJ. Screening mammography and public health safety: the need for perspectives. Lancet 1995; 346:29–32.

51. Davis DL. Mammographic screening. JAMA 1994; 271:152–153.

52. Epstein S. Implants pose poorly recognized risks of breast cancer. Intl J Occup Med Toxicol 1995; 4:315–342.

53. Potter M. Induction of plasmocytomas with silicone gel in genetically susceptible strains of mice. J NCI 1994; 86:1958–1065.

54. Bryant H. Breast implants and breast cancer: reanalysis of a linkage study. N Engl J Med 1995; 332:1535–1539.

55. Marshall E. Reanalysis confirms results of 'tainted study'. Long-term tamoxifen study halted. Science 1995; 270:1562.

56. Fugh-Berman A. Tamoxifen: disease prevention or disease substitution. Lancet 1992; 340:1143–1145.

57. California Environmental Protection Agency. Evidence of the carcinogenicity of tamoxifen. Reproductive and Cancer Hazard Assessment Section, Office of Environmental Health Hazard Assessment; March 1995.

58. Smigel K. Next generation of SERMs being seen in clinic. J NCI 1997; 89:96.

59. Rutqvist LE. Contralateral primary tumors in breast cancer patients in a randomized trial of adjuvant tamoxifen therapy. J NCI 1991; 83:1299–1306.

60. Haraguchi S. Human prolactin regulates transfected MTV LTR-directed gene expression in human breast carcinoma cell line through synergistic interaction with steroidal hormones. Intl J Cancer 1992; 52:928–933.

61. Newman TB. Carcinogenicity of lipid-lowering drugs. JAMA 1996; 275:55–60.

62. Physician's Desk Reference. Spironolactone induces incidence of breast cancers in rodents and monkeys. Medical Economics Data Production Co., 1996; 2413–2416.

63. Shubik P. Experimental induction of hepatomas, mammary tumors, and other tumors with metronidazole in nobred Sas:MRC(WI)BR rats. J NCI 1979; 63:863–868.

64. Ertuak E. Transplantable rat mammary tumors induced by 5-nitro-2-furaldehyde semi-carbazine and by formic acid 2(4-(5-nitro-furyl)-2-thiazolyl)hydrazide. Cancer Research 1970; 30:1409–1412.

65. Brandes LJ. Stimulation of malignant growth in rodents by anti-depressant drugs at clinically relevant doses. Cancer Res 1992; 52:3796–3800.

66. Smedley HM. Malignant breast change in many given two drugs associated with breast hyperplasia. Lancet 1981; 2:638–639.

67. Hershcopf RJ. Obesity, diet, endogenous estrogens, and the risk of hormone-sensitive cancer. Am J Clin Nutr 1987; 45:283–289.

68. Seller TA. Effect of family history, body fat distribution, and reproductive factors on the risk of post-menopausal breast cancer. N Engl J Med 1992; 326:1323–1329.

69. den Tonkelaar I. A prospective study on obesity and subcutaneous fat patterning in relation to breast cancer in post-menopausal women participating in the DOM Project. Brit J Cancer 1994; 69:352–357.

70. Potischman N. Reversal of the relationship between body mass and endogenous estrogen concentrations with menopausal status. J NCI 1996; 88:756–758.

71. Hunter DJ. Cohort studies of fat intake and the risk of breast cancer – a pooled analysis. N Engl J Med 1996; 334:356–361.

72. Davis DL. Avoidable environmental links to breast cancer. Reducing breast cancer in women. Kluwer Publishers; 1995:231–235.

73. Wolff M. Blood level of organochlorine residues and the risk of breast cancer. J NCI 1993; 85:648–652.

74. Falck A. Pesticides and polychlorinated biphenyl residues in human breast lipids and their relationship to breast cancer. Arch Environ Health 1992; 47:143–146.

75. Hunter DJ. Plasma organochlorine levels and the risk of breast cancer. N Engl J Med 1997; 337:1253–1258.

76. Dewailley E. Could the rising levels of estrogen receptor in breast cancer be due to estrogenic pollutants? J NCI 1997; 89:888.

77. Hoy C. The truth about breast cancer. New York: Stoddart Publishing; 1995.

78. Raloff J. Menstrual cycles may affect cancer risk. Science News; 7 January 1995.

79. Dewailley E. High organochlorine body burden in women with estrogen receptor-positive breast cancer. J NCI 1994; 86:232–234.

80. Hunter DJ. Pesticide residues and breast cancer. The harvest of a silent spring? J NCI 1993; 85:598–599.

81. Sternglass EJ. Breast cancer: evidence for a relationship to fission products in the diet. Intl J of Health Services 1993; 23:783–804.

82. Smith-Warner SA, Spiegelman D, Yaun SS, et al. Alcohol and breast cancer in women: a pooled analysis of cohort studies. JAMA 1998; 279:535–540.

83. Colburn T. Developmental effects of endocrine-disrupting chemicals in wildlife and humans. Environmental Health Perspectives 1993; 101:378–384.

84. Salig J. Cancer mortality rates and drinking water in 346 counties of the Ohio River Basin. United States Environmental Protection Agency, PO-5-03-4528, 1977.

85. Cox C. Prevention is crucial. J Pesticide Reform 1996; 16:2–7.

86. Soto AM. P-nonyl-phenol: an estrogenic xenobiotic released from 'modified' polystyrene. Environ Health Perspect 1991; 92:167–173.

87. Steinman D. Diet for a poisoned planet. New York: Ballantine; 1992.

88. Environmental Working Group. Weed killers by the glass. Online. Available: www.ewg.org/reports/Weed_Killer/29_Cities.html.

89. Kelley RD. Pesticides in Iowa's drinking water. Pesticides and ground water: a health concern in the Midwest. Conference Proceedings. Navarre, MN: Freshwater Foundation; 16–17 October 1986

90. Pinter G. Long-term carcinogenicity bioassay of the herbicide Atrazine in F344 rats. Neoplasma 1990; 37:533–544.

91. Hiatt RA. Exogenous estrogen and breast cancer after bilateral oophorectomy. Cancer 1984; 54:139–144.

92. Dees C. Estrogenic-damaging activity of Red Dye No. 3 in human breast cancer cells. Environ Health Perspect 1997; 103(suppl 3):625–632.

93. Hertz R. The estrogen-cancer hypothesis with special emphasis on DES. In: Hiatt HH, Watson JD, eds. Origins of human cancer. Wisconsin: Cold Spring Harbor Laboratory; 1977:1665–1682.

94. Herrin A. FDA investigates 17 feedlots for improper hormone use. Food Chemical News; 28 July 1996:37–38.

95. Epstein S. Unlabeled milk from cows treated with biosynthetic growth hormones: a case of regulatory abdication. Intl J Health Sciences 1996; 26:1730–1785.

96. Hawkinson SE. Circulating concentrations of IGF-1 and the risk of breast cancer. Lancet 1998; 351:1393–1396.

97. Spiessl B. TNM atlas. Illustrated guide to TNM/pTNM classification of malignant tumors. UICCIntl Union Against Cancer; 1992:186–195.

98. Carter CL. Relation of tumor size, lymph node status, and survival in 24 740 breast cancer cases. Cancer 1989; 63:181–187.

99. Fisher B. Five-year results of a randomized clinical trial comparing total mastectomy and segmental mastectomy with or without radition therapy in the treatment of breast cancer. N Engl J Med 1995; 312:665–673.

100. Herrada J. Early-stage breast cancer and adjuvant therapy. In: Pazdur R, ed. Medical oncology, 2nd edn. New York: Huntington; 1995:303.

101. Zhu Dan Xi. Heart and Essence of Dan Xi's Methods of Treatment: 314.

102. Master Liu. Za Bin Zhi Li (Illustrations on the Treatment of Miscellaneous Diseases).

103. Nemato T. Management and survival of female breast cancer: results of a national survey by the American College of Surgeons. Cancer 1980; 45:2917–2924.

104. Early Breast Cancer Trialists Collaborative Group. Systemic treatment of early breast cancer by hormonal, cytotoxic, or immune therapy: 133 randomized trials involving 31 000 recurrences and 24 000 deaths among 75 000 women. Lancet 1992; 339:1–15,71–85.

105. Paik S. Pathological findings from the National Surgical Adjuvant Breast and Bowel Project: prognostic significance of erbB-2 protein overexpression in primary breast cancer. J Clin Oncol 1990; 8:103–112.

106. Haguley CM. Breast self-examination and survival from breast cancer. Cancer 1988; 62:1389–1396.

107. O'Malley MS. Screening for breast cancer with breast self-examination. JAMA 1987; 257:2197–2203.

108. Gao Bingjun. Yang Ke Xin De Ji (A collection of experiences in the treatment of sores). 1805ACE.

109. Zhu Dan Xi. Ge Zhi Yu Lun (On inquiring into the properties of things). 1347ACE.

110. Li Gao. Pi Wei Lun (A treatise on the stomach and spleen). 1240ACE.

111. Epstein AH. The predictors of distant relapse following conservative surgery and radiation therapy for early breast cancer are similar to those following mastectomy. Intl J Radiat Oncol Biol Phys 1989; 17:755–760.

112. Zhang Dai Zhao. From notes in training at the Sino-Japanese Friendship Hospital, 1995–1996. Beijing, PRC.

113. Fletcher GH. Long-range results for breast cancer patients treated by radical mastectomy and postoperative radiation therapy without adjuvant chemotherapy: an update. Intl J Radiat Oncol Biol Phys 1989; 17:11–14.

114. Zhang Dai Zhao. Fu zheng zeng xiao fang dui fei ai fang liao zeng jin zuo yong de lin chuang guang cha (Clinical observation of fu zheng zeng xiao fang (Synergistic formula for supporting vital qi) in increasing the efficacy of radiotherapy for lung cancer).

115. Zhong Guo Zhong Xi Yi Jie He Wai Ke Za Zhi (Integrative TCM and Western Med J of Surgery) 1998; 20:75–77.

116. Zhang Dai Zhao. Zhong yi yao yu fang she xiang jie he de zhe liao (Treatment with a combination of Chinese materia medica and radiotherapy). Zhong

Guo Zhong Liu (Chinese Oncology Journal) 1993; 2:15.

117. Lang Wei Jun. Kang Ai Zhong Yao Yi Rian Fang (One thousand anti-cancer prescriptions). Beijing: TCM and Materia Medica Science and Technology Publishing House, 1992.

118. Baltzer L. Oncology: pocket guide to chemotherapy. St Louis: Mosby; 1994:49–51,68–69.

119. Wang Yu Sheng. Zhong Yao Yao Ci Yu Ming Yong (Pharmacology and application of Chinese materia medica), 2nd edn. Beijing: People's Medical Publishing House; 1998.

120. Zhang Dai Zhao. Zhang Dai Zhao Zhi Ai Jing Yan Ji Yao (A collection of Zhang Dai Zhao's experiences in the treatment of cancer). Beijing: China Medical and Pharmaceutical Publishing House; 2001.

121. Rivkin S. Adjuvant combination chemotherapy (CMFVP) versus tamoxifen (TAM) versus CMPVP plus TAM for postmenopausal women with ER positive operable breast cancer and positive axillary lymph nodes: an intergroup study. Proc Am Soc Clin Oncol 1990; 9:24.

122. Bloom HJG. Natural history of untreated breast cancer. Br Med J 1962; 1:213–221.

123. Liotta LA. Cancer invasion and metastasis. JAMA 1990; 263:1123–1126.

124. Tormey DC. Comparison of induction chemotherapies for metastatic breast cancer. Cancer 1982; 50:1235–1244.

125. Zinser JW. Clinical course of breast cancer patients with liver metastasis. J Clin Oncol 1987; 5:773–782.

126. Glover D. Intravenous pamidronate disodium treatment of bone metastasis in patients with breast cancer. Cancer 1994; 74:2949–2955.

127. Zhang Jing Yue. Jing Yue Quan Shu (Collected treatises of Zhang Jing Yue), 1624 ACE. Shanghai Science and Technology Press; 1959.

128. Qian Yi. Xiao Er Yao Zheng Zhi Jue (Craft of medicinal treatment for childhood disease patterns). 1119 ACE.

129. Chen Shi Wen. Tai Ping Hui Min He Ji Ju Fang (Imperial grace formulary of the Tai Ping era). 1107–1110 ACE.

130. Li Dong Yuan. Nei Wai Shang Bian Huo Lun (Clarifying doubts about injury from internal and external causes). 1231 ACE. Jiangsu Science and Technology Press; 1982.

Further reading

Asbell B. The pill: a biography of the drug that changed the world. Random House; 1995.

Carson R. Silent spring. Houghton Mifflin; 1994.

Lamson D, Brignall M. Antioxidants in cancer therapy; their actions and interactions with oncologic therapies. Altern Med Rev 1999; 4:304–329.

Chapter 5

Prostate Cancer

CHAPTER CONTENTS

Epidemiology   156

Etiology   156

Anatomy   157
  Chinese medicine   158

Pathogenesis   158
  Chinese medicine   159

Pathology and natural history   160
  Chinese medicine   161

Diagnosis   161

Screening   162

Staging   163

Treatment   163
  Watchful waiting   163
  Surgery versus radiation   164
  Radical prostatectomy   164
  Radiation therapy   164
  Stage C prostate cancer   165
  Metastatic prostate cancer   165
  Hormone-refractory prostate cancer   166

Chinese medicine diagnostic categories and
    treatment   166
  Spleen qi deficiency   166
  Damp heat accumulation   167
  Early stage kidney deficiency in an older
      man   168

Liver qi stasis   169
Advanced stage with yin and qi
    deficiency   170
PC-SPES   171
Treatment principles   171

The Yellow Emperor asks,
I have heard that in ancient times the people lived to be over a hundred years, and yet they remained active and did not become decrepit in their activities. But nowadays people reach only half that age and yet become decrepit and failing. Is it because the world changes from generation to generation? Or is it that mankind is becoming negligent of the laws of nature?

Qibo answers,
In ancient times those people who understood the way of self-cultivation patterned themselves upon the yin and the yang, the principles of nature, and they lived in harmony with the art of the divine.

The opening lines of the Nei Jing Su Wen. First published 100 BCE

EPIDEMIOLOGY

Prostate cancer accounts for 40% of all cancers in men.[1] The incidence and mortality of prostate cancer continues to rise and pose a major health problem especially in the West. It is the most common newly diagnosed cancer in American men, possibly because of mass screening of asymptomatic individuals. In 2000, about 350 000 men in the US were diagnosed with prostate cancer and 50 000 died from it. This cancer mortality rate in men is second only to lung cancer. The increase in incidence is mainly in patients with localised disease. Local therapy is commonly sufficient to cure this level of disease. However, fundamental questions still remain about the etiology, prevention, and treatment of prostate cancer. Treatment for metastatic disease is strictly palliative and there is still no treatment for hormone-refractory disease.

The lifetime probability for developing prostate cancer in the US is 20% (for developing breast cancer it is 24%). The lifetime probability of dying from prostate cancer is 3.5% (breast cancer is 3.6%).[2] The highest global death rate from prostate cancer is in Switzerland. The lowest death rates are in China. Prostate cancer incidence is related to age, geographic and racial factors. The rates of incidence in Shanghai are 0.8 per 100 000 but 100.2 per 100 000 in blacks in Alameda County, California.[3] Rates are increasing more rapidly among males over the age of 74.[4] The prevalence of latent prostate cancers is similar across ethnic groups. Therefore, identification of progression factors has obvious therapeutic value. Environmental factors must play a role because men who emigrate from countries of low incidence have an increased incidence after immigration to countries with higher incidence, and especially the US.[5,6]

ETIOLOGY

Studies have not linked prostate cancer with sexually transmitted disease or sexual habits. However, studies are underway that implicate family history, dietary fats, low ultraviolet light exposure, and smoking. The role of benign prostatic hypertrophy (BPH) remains unclear but appears not to be a link.[7] It is believed that benign hypertrophic prostatic cells do not directly transform into malignant cells. Vasectomy is not a definite risk factor for future development of the disease.[8] Elevated serum testosterone concentrations probably have a link. Afro-American black men have serum testosterone levels 15% higher than American caucasians[9] and this is one of many reasons given for higher rates in Afro-American men. Detectable prostate cancer in eunuchs, who have lower levels or neglible levels of testosterone, and vegetarians, is very low.[10] Men with lower levels of sex-hormone-binding globulin (SHBG) seem to be at higher risk. Men with higher levels of estradiol seem to be at lower risk. The role of the hormone dihydrotestosterone (DHT), which was thought to increase prostate cancer risk, is undefined.

Studies still underway show a more definitive link with diet, especially a diet high in animal fat. In fact, there is a great deal of evidence that the diet responsible for cardiovascular disease is also responsible for prostate cancer. Asians tend to eat less fat and larger quantities of fish (a good source of vitamin D). Vitamin D allows better absorption of vitamin A and vitamin A may play a role in decreased incidence because African, Dravidian and Aryan blacks living in southern climates with higher ultraviolet light exposure (vitamin A) do not have a high incidence of prostate cancer. This may link diet, ultraviolet light exposure, and lower testosterone levels to prevention. No studies have assessed the role of societal stress and race in combination with higher testosterone levels and prostate cancer.

Beta-carotene has not been shown to reduce risk but lycopene, found in tomato pigment, has been found to lower the risk of many cancers, including prostate cancer. The risk of getting prostate cancer rises with the amount of alcohol consumed. Hyperinsulinemia and prediabetic conditions may contribute to the cancer environment and promoting factors in many cancers, including prostate cancer.

People who work in industries such as water treatment, aircraft manufacturing, power, gas, and water utilities, farming, fishing and forestry have a higher risk of prostate cancer. It is thought that chemical exposures are at fault but these exposures, unfortunately, have not been specifically

> **Box 5.1 Factors that increase risk for prostate cancer[14]**
>
> - Alcohol.
> - Arsenic levels in well water.
> - Decreased levels of sex-hormone-binding globulin.
> - Decreased ultraviolet light exposure or decreased amounts of vitamin D.
> - Diet high in saturated fat and low in fiber, especially vegetable (versus grain) fiber.
> - Family history of prostate cancer.
> - Increasing age.
> - Increased levels of testosterone.
> - Race (Afro-American).
> - Some occupations.

> **Box 5.2 Factors that may decrease risk for prostate cancer[14]**
>
> - Diet low in saturated fat, high in vegetable fiber.
> - Exercise.
> - Increased levels of estradiol.
> - Increased ultraviolet exposure or increased vitamin D.
> - Selenium.
> - Soy products.
> - Tomatoes or lycopene.
> - Black and green tea.

studied. Environmental exposures are often the last area of pathogenesis to be researched.

Every decade of ageing nearly doubles the incidence of microscopic prostate cancer from 10% for men in their 50s to 70% for men in their 80s.[11,12]

There appears to be significant clustering of prostate cancer within families, along with breast and central nervous system tumors.[13] This suggests a role for genetic factors. Men in families in which two or more first-degree relatives have prostate cancer may have as high as eight times greater risk for prostate cancer than the average male. This inherited susceptability may lead to much earlier onset, and earlier onset usually means a more aggressive form of prostate cancer.

Some occupational exposures include metallic dust, liquid fuel combustion products, lubricating oils, polyaromatic hydrocarbons from coal, rare elements like tritium, ^{51}Cr, ^{59}Fe, ^{60}Co, ^{65}Zn, or large amounts of herbicides and pesticides.

Box 5.1 lists risk factors for prostate cancer; Box 5.2 lists factors that decrease risk for prostate cancer.

Foods that are beneficial with regards to prostate cancer include soy, green tea, seafood, and especially deep water fish with high omega-3 fatty acid content, olive oil, tomato, vegetables, especially broccoli sprouts and pumpkin seeds, legumes and whole grains. Soy contains high levels of genistein, which inhibits the growth of prostate cancer. A survey of 42 countries found that soy provided more protection against prostate cancer than any other food.

ANATOMY

The prostate is located deep within the pelvis and below the bladder and next to the rectum. Tunneling through the prostate is the urethra, which carries urine and semen from the body. The urethra is about 8 in long, beginning at the bottom of the bladder and ending at the tip of the penis. The prostate surrounds only about the first inch of the urethra. There are four zones of the prostate:

1. The peripheral zone: the gland's largest zone and can be palpated during the digital rectal examination (DRE), and this is where most prostate cancers begin to grow.
2. The transition zone: BPH occurs here and a small number of prostate cancers begin here.
3. The central zone: an even smaller number of prostate cancers grow here.
4. The periurethral zone: a tiny area where virtually no malignancies originate.

The prostate is surrounded by the blood vessels and nerves responsible for erection. The external sphincter is located here and is the primary muscle needed for urinary control. Androgen hormonal activity regulates the activity of the prostate gland. Testosterone is the major hormone involved and DHT is another stronger androgen. Testosterone is secreted primarily by the testes and secondarily by the adrenals.

CHINESE MEDICINE

The channels involved with the prostate gland are the:

- Du
- Ren
- Chong
- kidney
- bladder
- liver
- small intestine
- large intestine.

The liver channel wraps the testes. The kidney channel and qi governs water and controls the water transformative mechanism and the jing relating to the lower orifices. Qi transformation in the kidneys regulates the opening and closing function of the urethra and ureters and this puts it in relationship to the prostate gland. The kidneys also have a relationship to the testes, and by extension, the prostate gland, through the jing. The kidneys are also the floodgate of the stomach. If the floodgate cannot move smoothly, the water will accumulate and gather with its kind.

The large intestine regulates the qi of the lower jiao. Therefore, problems with either the channel or the organ can be reflected in pathology in the lower jiao, even reproductive pathology. The small intestine regulates the flow of urine and separates the turbid. It has an internal trajectory straight to the bladder. Problems with the qi transformation mechanism in the small intestine channel or organ that result in a build up of turbid fluids can result in damp accumulation in the lower jiao. Damp accumulations, in this case, can refer to urine or damp accumulation in the prostate. In other words, the overall environment is one of dampness. Atherosclerosis, BPH, colon polyps, urinary dysfunction, and prostate cancer are all examples of damp accumulation. The last four refer to the lower jiao specifically.

The seminal fluid is the energetic part of male reproduction. There is a mechanical valve that opens the urethra and seminal duct and that helps to control blood flow to the penis. Retention or irregular flow or a start/stop stream to this urinary flow is most commonly related to small intestine function. It may also be related to liver.

Ejaculation is regulated by the liver and kidneys and requires smooth flow of qi via the liver's charge and stable yang to support the driving force via the kidney yang. Semen relates to the kidneys and is a form of jing. Bone marrow (kidney) irrigates the marrow (jing) and marrow irrigates the semen (the fluid that carries the sperm). Orgasm relates to the liver and, therefore, to the hun (the liver shen). External stimulation is initiated by the heart via the liver, which supplies blood. The heart and liver move the blood to the penis and the kidneys maintain this blood flow thus creating an erection.

PATHOGENESIS

The Western knowledge of the molecular and cellular biology of prostatic adenocarcinoma (the most common type) is small when the incidence rates are taken into account. Those cancers that are not hormone-refractory and that have a development of hormone-independent growth may have a distinct genetic basis.[15] Several oncogenes are expressed with a higher frequency in prostatic cell lines. Also loss of expression of tumor-suppressor genes appears to play a role. The abnormal expression of peptide growth factors and their receptors may contribute to growth and development in both local and metastatic prostate cancer. Several other growth factors have been implicated as well. The tyrosine kinase growth factor receptor family related to epidermal growth factor receptor (EGFR) includes the Her-2/neu oncogene.[16] This oncogene has a relationship to some breast cancers as well. The increased expression of this gene has been demonstrated in prostatic intraepithelial neoplasia.[17]

Tumor-induced angiogenesis is an essential step in the progression of malignant neoplasms and the development of metastases. The microvessel count in the invasive primary prostate tumor is significantly higher for patients with metastatic disease than that for patients without metastases.[18]

Recognition of premalignant lesions in the prostate may permit identification of high-risk populations that may benefit from early screening. Prostatic intraepithelial neoplasia is much more common in prostate glands with invasive carcinoma than in those without. This lesion has been designated a premalignant lesion, and is not unlike a cervical intraepithelial neoplasm (CIN) in cervical dysplasia. Another example is atypical adenomatous hyperplasia, or prostatic adenosis.

Foods to avoid in prostate and many other cancers include sugar, alcohol, fried foods, dairy products (probably), high doses of calcium, and red meats, especially those high in animal fats. There seems to be a relationship between arachidonic acid and prostate cancer. The cancerous cells convert arachidonic acid to prostaglandin2 (PGE2) at a rate 10 times higher than even BPH cells. Oleic acid is the best inhibitor of PGE2 synthesis by prostate cancer cells. Inhibition of 5 HETE induces massive apoptosis in prostate cancer cells. Eliminating red meat from the diet reduces intake of animal fats from the diet. Since meats are also high in arachidonic acid, lowering or eliminating meat, especially red meats, can help reduce the incidence of prostate cancer from two important causes. Perhaps it is correct to say that uric acid build up and high testosterone levels are a form of yin-deficient heat and hyperactive yang. These functional injuries also lend themselves to an environment in which a carcinogenic hit becomes more problematic and can lead to malignancy because yin deficiency, dampness, and liver qi stasis are the main environments in which a latent pathogenic factor can sink deeper into the body. These injuries may, in fact, be carcinogenic themselves.

CHINESE MEDICINE

Kidney qi and yang deficiency lead to a malfunction in water metabolism. In the case of prostate cancer, this includes water metabolism and hormonal dysfunction (testosterone). This aspect of pathogenesis probably relates to aging, but may also relate to stress factors. Chronic high-level stress, survival stress, depletes the yin. Yin is the mother of yang. The adrenals, or Mingmen, are fire within water. Adrenal exhaustion from chronic stress is a form of yang deficiency.

Another factor in pathogenesis is spleen deficiency that evolves out of poor dietary habits. Dampness pouring downward is a manifestation of sinking spleen qi. The spleen governs transportation and transformation, and when this is impaired, it cannot generate the clear and bear the turbid downward. The turbid refers to urinary retention and to damp toxins that come through the diet. A high animal fat diet leads to obstructive diseases caused by damp accumulation – anything from atherosclerotic plaques to damp phlegm masses like polyps and BPH and prostate masses that are malignant. The foundation for these manifestations is spleen deficiency.

Poor diet leads to internal heat over a lifetime. Spleen deficiency fails to nourish the liver blood leading to liver qi stasis. Liver qi stasis leads to internal heat. Spleen deficiency also can result in dampness, which causes stasis in the middle jiao. This stasis can traverse the Ko cycle leading to liver qi stasis and heat. Therefore, in two ways, spleen deficiency can contribute to internal and pathogenic heat. If kidney deficiency is a contributing factor, then from several directions heat and dampness evolve. All of the above discussions on risk factors and food contribute to this path of injury.

Beer and phosphated fizzy drinks compete with the kidneys for zinc and leach out zinc. Zinc is essential for prostate health. Perhaps we could say that zinc is energetically a yang substance that nourishes the qi and yang of the kidney.

There is a relationship between the spleen and the San Jiao and the small intestine. All are related to water metabolism and also with the Taiyang urinary bladder. These interactions, when dysfunctional, lead to urinary retention, to sinking spleen qi and resultant dampness pouring down. Dampness is a magnet for latent pathogenic factors. When these problems are combined with kidney yang deficiency through aging or heredity, then the environment is in place for a lower jiao malignancy.

Liver qi depression can impede qi transformation and movement in the San Jiao and this can lead to urinary retention, as well. The liver channel wraps the testes and when there is constraint or blockage in the channel, then the blood does not move smoothly, leading to blood and phlegm stasis. Prostatic tumors are very much manifestations of blood and phlegm stasis bound with toxin. The toxin is most likely hormonal in nature, but not all is known about the pathology of this cancer. There may be other chemical toxins that are linked.

The last aspect is more difficult to describe. The pericardium is the ministerial fire and the heart and pericardium have an internal/external relationship, which is essential for normal sexual and reproductive health. Just as the pericardium/heart has a relationship with the uterus and sexuality in women, this same relationship exists in men with the testes and prostate. Issues of power and control stemming from lack of self-esteem, earlier psychic injuries, war, post-traumatic stress disorder, fear, and paranoia all injure liver and kidney function leading to heart qi constraint and energetic or physical or psychic impotence. This forces the spiritual and psychic mechanism of intimacy back onto itself. Living from the heart becomes taboo. Men are pressured into splitting in this way just as women are forced to split from their powerful and yang selves. What is common to both, and the dilemma in which we all find ourselves now, is the damaged energetic reality of the liver and spleen, Chong and Ren, and heart and kidneys, which are central axes to our humanity, and to love and intimacy.

Another way to describe this potential conflict is through the hun aspect of the liver or wood. The hun is composed of the jing, which is associated with the kidneys and is the storehouse of all of life's varied manifestations, the shen of the heart, which is the creative spark that must illuminate potential in order for it to manifest, and the qi that the liver regulates. If the liver cannot smoothly foster the connection between the two poles of the heart and kidney, water and fire, then we become stuck in the duality of life and never find the heaven within, the wholeness of our spiritual inheritance. I thank Lonnie Jarrett for this deeper view into the meaning of life as seen through the window of Chinese medicine. It is interesting that the primary cancers of modern men and women are of those glands that foster new life and are permeated with such intense meaning and false ideals.

Lack of exercise may also play a role in pathogenesis. Not exercising leads to poor qi and blood circulation and thus stasis. It eliminates a pathway for normal discharge of emotional constraint and internal heat. It leads to fatigue and often poor dietary habits and low esteem. Exercise helps to regulate endocrine functions including hormonal balance. The physical, psychoemotional and spiritual bodies are all one. Exercise is important in the prevention of cancer because it circulates qi and fluids, raises the yang, prevents blood and phlegm stasis, and discharges toxins (material and immaterial).

Internal complex processes are often magnets for latent pathogenic factors. It is unknown currently what the whole terrain is for the pathogenesis of prostate cancer. Because prostate cancer can remain indolent and asymptomatic for many years, it seems feasible that a latent pathogen, like a chemical exposure, could be a trigger for malignancy.

The combination of these primary and secondary factors with a carcinogenic exposure can lead to prostate cancer. They all can lead to congestion of fluids, hormonal and otherwise, in one way or another. Congestion leads to obstructive disease, poor flow of body fluids, congealment of blood, knotted blood and phlegm, and finally (when these occur) act as a magnet for toxins or are toxins themselves that initiate a malignancy. When treating any cancer, we are striving to reverse this evolution and change the underlying environment that caused the cancer. We are also striving to improve the overall health of the patient even while going through cytotoxic treatment to treat the end event of this process; that is the cancer. This approach means that the patient must be actively and deeply involved in changing this environment and reversing this evolution to cancer.

PATHOLOGY AND NATURAL HISTORY

Almost all prostate cancers are adenocarcinomas, but the rarer types have different clinical behaviors and require different therapy. For example, patients with unusual sites of metastasis and low or normal prostate-specific antigen (PSA) values probably do not have an adenocarcinoma. They may, in fact, have small cell anaplastic pathology. There is also a transitional cell type and squamous cell type of prostate cancer. It is important to know the type because it changes treatment options and, therefore, side effects. Most prostatic cancers are treated according to staging and with surgery, surgery and radiation, radiation alone, and hormonal therapy.

The Gleason score is a measuring range for biopsy specimens that describes the level of differentiation of cells.[19] The poorer the differentiation the poorer the prognosis. Well-differentiated cells with scores of 2–4 usually indicate early-stage disease and a better prognosis. Gleason scores of 8–10 correlate with other prognostic factors such as tumor size (the bigger the tumor, the worse the prognosis), presence of pelvic lymph node metastasis, and the PSA level. PSA is a protein in the blood produced by prostate tissue that serves as a tumor marker. It is not an ideal marker because it can be present in higher levels in patients with BPH and other prostate problems. Therefore, it is used in combination with a DRE, ultrasound, biopsy, and cytology from the biopsy. When the prostate has been removed (radical prostatectomy), PSA testing may then be more sensitive than a bone scan when monitoring for recurrence. The S-phase fraction and DNA ploidy of prostatic tumors provide additional information.[20] Diploid tumors are associated with improved survival. High S-phase in a primary tumor may indicate lack of hormonal responsiveness and, thus, a poorer prognosis.

Low-grade tumors can grow very slowly and remain localised. They can remain clinically undetectable. Clinically significant tumors arise 80% of the time in the peripheral zone of the gland, 15% in the transitional zone, and 5% in the central zone. Only tumors in the peripheral zone are detectable by DRE.

Prostate cancers typically grow peripherally through the capsule along perineural sheaths that perforate the capsule at the upper outer corner and at the apex. These tumors can invade the seminal vesicles and the neck of the urinary bladder. Some prostate tumors may invade into the rectal wall.

Spread is both lymphatic and via blood circulation. Lymphatic spread usually affects first the obturator lymph nodes, and then advances into the external iliac and the hypogastric nodes, and finally into the common iliac and the periaortic nodes. Hematogenous spread is also orderly. The axial skeleton is usually the first site of metastasis. This is followed by the proximal appendicular skeleton and then the lungs and liver. Metastases to either the lung or liver alerts to the possibility of small-cell carcinoma of the prostate and, there-fore, to a different strategy for treatment. Brain metastases are very rare. Bone metastases are osteoblastic and easily detectable by bone scan. Metastatic bone disease is almost always present when the pelvic lymph nodes are involved but can occur without lymph node involvement. Spinal metastases may extend into the epidural space and cause compression of the spinal cord and progression to paraplegia. Evaluation of back pain is important.

Paraneoplastic syndromes can be associated with disseminated disease and include DIC and neuromuscular abnormalities. DIC is common in mucin-secreting adenocarcinomas of the pancreas and the prostate and some forms of leukemia. DIC is associated with thromboembolic complications of hypercoagulability including venous thrombosis, heart valve thrombotic vegetations, and arterial emboli. This form does not cause abnormal bleeding but in acute DIC abnormal bleeding may be serious. This can occur in a prostatectomy where tissue factor activity enters the main blood supply as a complication of surgery. Acute DIC may cause fibrin to be deposited in multiple small blood vessels causing hemorrhagic tissue necrosis. The most vulnerable organ is the kidney where fibrin depositions in the glomerular capillary bed may lead to acute renal failure. Hypercalcemia is very rare in prostate cancer, and is usually caused by some other factor and not bone loss due to metastatic disease.

CHINESE MEDICINE

Please refer back to Huo xue qu yu section in Chapter 1 for a further discussion of DIC and hypercoagulability syndrome.

DIAGNOSIS

Transrectal ultrasonography (TRUS) can detect lesions as small as 5 mm. Since most lesions are adenocarcinomas in the apex of the prostate, TRUS and TRUS-guided biopsy permits a very precise sampling of hypoechoic areas suggestive of cancer.[21] This procedure is usually performed on an outpatient basis. Usually only 20% of hypoechoic areas are malignant because nonmalignant tissue effects by inflammtion will appear similarly to highly dense cancerous tissue. Up to 30% of lesions are palpable during DRE but can be missed on ultrasound because they are isoechoic rather then hypoechoic. Cancers arising in the transition zone, an area that is also the site of BPH, cannot be detected as hypoechoic tumors because of the heterogeneous texture of this region of the gland.

The PSA is a glycoprotein produced by both normal and malignant prostate cells.[22] The PSA is expressed in other cancers, such as breast and ovarian but at much lower levels. An enlarged prostate caused by BPH in older males accounts for the majority of borderline PSA elevations. Levels above 10 are unlikely to be due to BPH alone and require a urologic evaluation. Serum PSA will increase more rapidly in prostate cancer than in BPH. A comparative rise is relation to previous measurements may be highly predictive of cancer. The normal ranges are adjusted for age with 2.5 being considered normal in a 45-year-old man and 6.5 being considered normal in a 75-year-old man.[23]

Ongoing research is working to find a better prostate tumor marker or one that can be used in addition to the PSA test. Men who have a PSA in the so-called 'gray zone' (between 3 and 10) could have BPH or they could have cancer. The 'percent-free' PSA is helping to distinguish men with early prostate cancer from those with BPH. This looks at types of PSA. There are at least six types, and two of these are found in large quantities in the blood. There is a free form of PSA and a complexed form. Current tests measure the total amount of free and complexed PSA to give a single PSA value. The newer test measures the quantity of free PSA and compares it to the total amount of both free and complexed PSA. Scandinavian researchers have shown that measuring the proportion of free to total PSA gives a better idea of whether a patient has BPH or prostate cancer. Men with BPH have higher amounts of free PSA, whereas men with prostate cancer have higher amounts of the complexed form. With the new percent free PSA test, the lower the value, the greater the chance of having prostate cancer. This is slightly confusing since it is the opposite of the old total PSA test measurement. It is, therefore, important to know which test is being used.[24]

After trauma that involves any medical procedures, the PSA can rise up to fifty times over baseline and remain so for several weeks. Bacterial prostatitis can also raise PSA levels. It is important to read PSA levels prior to any other evaluation, including DRE. These levels should be re-evaluated after resolution of any inflammation. Serum PSA levels are lowered in patients taking finasteride (Proscar) used to treat BPH. Starting patients on finasteride requires ruling out prostate cancer prior to beginning the drug. If PSA levels remain elevated while on this drug, a further workup for prostate cancer must take place. The age-adjusted reference range of normal PSA levels is reduced by 50% for patients taking finasteride.

SCREENING

To date no study has shown a reduction in mortality attributable to annual prostate screening. (The same is true for breast cancer and mammographic screening. The only screen for cancer that has reduced mortality is the PAP smear, which has reduced the incidence of cervical cancer in the West.) This is in no way a recommendation to forego screening. Because prostate is usually a fairly indolent cancer and the doubling time of a primary tumor is slow, screening has traditionally been confined to men with a life expectancy greater than 10 years.[25] On the other hand, there are no long-term studies that show that early detection and treatment do not save lives. There is some controversy on the subject. The PIVOT (Prostate Cancer Intervention vs Observation Trial) and the PLCO (Prostate, Lung, Colon, Ovarian Cancer) studies are seeking to determine the impact of screening on life expectancy. PIVOT is evaluating a comparison between watchful waiting and radical prostatectomy among men with early, localised, prostate cancer. Some doctors leave the rate of screening up to the individual. Some results from the studies should be available in May 2006.

The following factors can affect PSA level:

- acute urinary retention due to BPH; an emergent condition

- ejaculation; levels rise up to 40% within an hour and return to normal within 48 hours
- procedures like TRUS, high-intensity focused ultrasound (HIFU), transurethal incision of the prostate (TUIP), transurethral microwave therapy (TUMT), transurethral needle ablation (TUNA), transurethral resection of the prostate (TURP), very late antigens (VLA), and balloon dilation
- medications like finasteride; doxazosin and terazosin do not affect PSA levels.

STAGING

The TNM system is used, and a combination of TNM plus the Jewett ABCD system. Stage A disease has a less than 2% mortality rate. The tumor is not palpable and is not usually found incidentally. Stage B tumors are palpable, are confined to the prostate, and have not penetrated the capsule. Stage C disease indicates that the tumor has penetrated the capsule and has invaded local tissues. In patients with Stage B and C tumors a quarter will die within 15 years. About 70% of patients will present with Stage C or D prostate cancer. Stage D prostate cancer indicates the tumor has spread to lymph nodes, bones or other distant sites. The 5-year survival rate for patients with Stage D disease is less than 20%.

Angiogenesis refers to the ability of a cancer to grow new blood vessels in order to obtain a blood supply. As a prostate cancer moves from one stage to the next, the number of new blood vessels feeding the tumor usually increases dramatically. Analysing the degree of angiogenesis is being tested as a way to stage a prostate cancer. Beyond staging, the use of angiogenesis is also being used in terms of strategising treatment. Possible antiangiogenic treatments include anticancer drugs like retinoids, antiestrogens, interferon, methotrexate, and interleukin-12. Anticancer treatments that may act antiangiogenically are hyperthermia and radiation therapy.

Antibiotics in this realm include penicillin and suramine. Aspirin, thalidomide, vitamin-D derivatives, angiostatin, endostatin, TNP-470, BB-216, platelet factor 4, and carboxyaminotriazole are all possible antiangiogenic treatments to prevent the growth of blood vessels in prostate tumors.

The disease is investigated according to locoregional disease and metastases. Bone scans are performed in most patients. High PSA values with positive bone scans correlates with D2 disease. Therefore, local therapy is not possible. CT scans are used to look for involvement of pelvic lymph nodes. TRUS mat be used to clarify the extent of local disease. Tumor volume in advanced disease influences response to therapy. A system to stratify patients with metastatic disease further categorises according to O1 (osseus 1), which is metastatic axial skeletal involvement only, and O2 (osseus 2), or axial involvement plus extremity-skeletal involvement. Visceral 1 denotes pulmonary metastases and visceral 2 denotes metastases in other viscera.

TREATMENT

Early stage or stages A and B treatment for prostate cancer remains somewhat controversial. Evaluating interventions is difficult because early detection may increase the interval between diagnosis and death, regardless of the effectiveness of the treatment. This is called lead-time bias. Also diagnosis and treatment of latent rather than clinical prostate cancer may seemingly achieve therapeutic results when, in fact, these tumors were intrinsically innocuous anyway. Valid comparisons between radiation therapy, radical prostatectomy, and watch-and-wait approaches are lacking. This means that no final consensus is available for early-stage prostate cancer.

WATCHFUL WAITING

Difficulties arise in identifying patients in whom deferred treatment can be employed without jeopardising survival or adversely effecting quality of life. Patients with well-differentiated tumors of low volume usually have the option of deferring treatment. Problems with radiation and with surgery make this a preferred choice, as impotence and urinary difficulties commonly arise from treatment. Generally men who have been judged to have a life expectancy of 10 years or more are offered curative treatments, although there is no compelling evidence that a watch-and-wait policy in this group is inferior.[26,27]

It might be better to think of this option in terms of a broader intervention with complementary medicine. This option then becomes an integrated management strategy to prevent spread of disease, through dietary and herbal medicine, regular DRE and PSA monitoring, and lifestyle changes. The improvement of overall health is a primary factor in positively changing the outcome. Watchful waiting that is proactive can give the patient time to evaluate treatment options. On the negative side, watchful waiting can delay treatment until some options are no longer appropriate. The best candidates for watchful waiting are men:

- whose life expectancy is no more than 10 years due to age, illness, or genetic history
- over the age of 70 with a well-differentiated, very small, cancer (Gleason score of 2–4)
- whose cancer is confined to the prostate and who want to take the time to consider options
- who have advanced prostate cancer and have not experienced symptoms.

SURGERY VERSUS RADIATION

In localised disease, surgery seems to have a lower recurrence rate than radiation therapy. On the other hand, a retrospective study comparing long-term outcomes of radiation therapy and surgery showed neither treatment to be statistically superior. This shows the dilemma regarding choices and outcomes versus side effects. Usually patients with a 10- to 15-year life expectancy, good performance status, localised cancer with a low Gleason score, and a PSA ≤ 15 are considered ideal candidates for prostatectomy.[28,29]

RADICAL PROSTATECTOMY

This involves the removal of the entire prostate, including the capsule, a layer of surrounding connective tissue, and the attached seminal vesicles. Newer techniques have significantly reduced impotence and hemorrhage, but urinary incontinence still occurs in some patients. A nerve-sparing technique pioneered by Walsh limits impotence, and potency returns in 50–80% of patients after 1 year. However, only patients whose tumors do not involve the neurovascular bundle in the pelvic plexus and branches inner-vating the corpus cavernosa lateral to the prostate gland are eligible for this modified surgery. Detectable PSA levels post-surgery indicate residual prostate cancer cells. Survival rates at 10 years are 90% and at 15 years are 83%.[30]

Radical prostatectomy has the potential to be curative. However, there are multiple side effects and frequent treatment failures. Early complications from prostatectomy are rectal injury, thromboembolism, myocardial infarction, sepsis, anastomotic urinary leakage, and potential spread of cancerous cells. The advantages include potential cure and none of the side effects seen in radiation or hormonal therapy. Late complications include incontinence, impotence (erectile dysfunction – ED), and disease recurrence.

RADIATION THERAPY

Radiation therapy is delivered in various ways. External beam radiation is used in localised tumors.[31] Delayed impotence (ED) may occur in up to 40% of patients. Rectal damage due to radiation may also be a side effect. The presence of residual tumor after radiation can be present in 35–91% of patients who have been treated with radiation. This is a predictor for metastatic disease in the future. PSA levels fall to within normal limits within 6–12 months after radiation therapy. Three-dimensional conformal radiation therapy (3D-CRT) is used when local tumor failure occurs after prior radiation.

In brachytherapy, radioactive seeds are implanted within the prostate tissue.[32] Between 70 and 150 seeds are implanted throughout the prostate via thin needles passed through the perineum. An ultrasound probe is inserted into the rectum and is used to aid the surgeon in determining placement. There are several types of seeds: ^{125}I, which has a half-life of 60 days, ^{103}Pd, which has a half-life of 17 days, ^{198}Au, which has a half-life of 2.7 days, and ^{169}Yb, which has a half-life of 32 days. These are all permanent implants. A temporary implant is ^{192}Ir, which has a half-life of 70 days. For the first several months patients are instructed to stay away from children and pregnant women, who are the most sensitive to radiation.[32]

The best candidates for this type of radiation treatment are:

- those who have localised prostate cancer
- older men with local prostate cancer who are not candidates for surgery
- some men with locally advanced cancer (T3 or C).

The advantages to treatment with radiation include less incontinence and impotence, no anesthesia or other surgical risks. Radiation therapy can be a regional treatment. The side effects can vary with the type of radiation used. These side effects can include radiation enteritis, radiation cystitis, ED, incontinence, a possible lower cure rate, and the necessity (with external beam radiation) of daily treatment for 6–8 weeks. Radiation treatment makes surgery at a later date a more difficult option.

STAGE C PROSTATE CANCER

Over 50% of patients with stage C prostate cancer will already have pelvic lymph node involvment. The chances of leaving residual tumor behind are great. Radiation has been the primary mode of treatment. Hormonal therapy is also used with the aim of local tumor control and/or downstaging of a tumor to allow for resection. Survival rates are identical in patients who are treated initially with hormonal therapy and in those treated first with radiation and then hormonal therapy.[33,34]

METASTATIC PROSTATE CANCER

Antiandrogen therapy, or hormonal therapy, is the primary therapy. Androgen ablation is not curative but is usually associated with significant disease control. The duration of response is variable. Usually most patients respond for up to 2 years and then develop hormone-refractory prostate cancer.[35]

There are two sources of androgens in humans; the testes produce most of the testosterone, which is converted in the target cells by 5-alpha-reductase to DHT; the adrenal cortex produces androstenedione and dehydroepiandrosterone, which constitue about 5% of all circulating androgens. Bilateral orchiectomy is the definitive antitestosterone treatment. Estrogenic preparations have also been used. They inhibit pituitary luteinising hormone through a negative feedback loop. These effectively suppress testosterone

levels to castrate levels in only 70% of patients. Gynecomastia may be prevented by superficial irradiation of the breast tissue before the start of therapy.

Flutamide is one of the most common antiandrogens.[36] The most commonly used approach involves the use of hypothalamic luteinising hormone-releasing hormone (LHRH) analogs. These are synthetic peptides and are administered via parenteral injection. Leuprolide, buserelin, and goserelin are examples. Depot preparations are now available that require only monthly injections to achieve castrate levels of testosterone. These substances allow for potentially reversible testicular suppression. These drugs are contraindicated in patients with spinal column involvement because they can exacerbate spinal compression. They are quite expensive and therefore, combined therapy with androgen blockade and antiandrogens are used and show modestly longer survival times than do antiandrogen therapies alone.[37]

Newer ways of delivering hormonal therapies include intermittent androgen-deprivation. In advanced prostate cancer, treatment with hormonal therapy usually works for about 3 years. Intermittent hormonal treatment 'tricks' the cancer cells into remaining vulnerable to the drug's effects, thus widening the window of survival. Intermittent therapy involves taking an LHRH agonist and an antiandrogen until the PSA level decreases, and then taking a break from the medication, forcing the body into so-called 'hormonal withdrawal'. When the PSA starts to rise again, treatment is resumed. This on-again, off-again drug regimen appears to delay the cancer's ability to start growing again, which increases the length of survival.

In summary, the LHRH analogs include lupron and goserelin (Zoladex). The antiandrogens include flutamide (Eulexin), bicalutamide (Casodex), and megestrol. Finasteride (Proscar) is another type of hormonal treatment. Tamoxifen is sometimes used as a hormonal treatment in prostate cancer, and certain aromatase inhibitors, like anastrozole (Arimidex), are also used. Orchiectomy, or castration, remains an option. The benefits of hormonal therapy include their usefulness in advanced disease; they work by starving the tumor of promoting factors, and are a reasonable option if the patient refuses surgery or radiation.[38] Hormonal therapy is a systemic treatment, having multiple side effects, especially a triple hormone blockade. The disadvantage is that eventual resistance is common. Side effects include hot flushes, impotence or reduced sexual drive, gynecomastia, accelerated bone loss, weakness, and muscle wasting. There may be possible liver damage, nausea, diarrhea, alcohol intolerance, and reduced night vision.

The newest approaches include:

- aromatase inhibitors, which convert androgens to estrogens
- lovastatin
- selenium plus vitamin E
- paclitaxel (Taxol)
- retinoids
- TIMP-2 treatments to block metastasis
- TGF-beta stimulators to inhibit cancer growth
- tyrosine kinase blockers.

HORMONE-REFRACTORY PROSTATE CANCER

Hormone-refractory cancer is defined as disease progression in the presence of castrate level of testosterone. Median survival is 1 year. Patients whose disease progresses despite hormonal therapy are paradoxically sensitive to additional stimulation of tumor growth by androgens. Therefore, they must continue therapy with estrogen or LHRH analogs.[39]

Flutamide withdrawal or discontinuation in patients who have been in remission for a longer period of time is commonly done with lowered PSA levels of 50–80%. Ketoconazole is an antifungal commonly used in HIV/AIDS treatment, but when used in higher doses inhibits the adrenal and testicular synthesis of androgens. There are more severe side effects with this treatment, including gastric intolerance and adrenal suppression requiring supplemental hydrocortisone.

Chemotherapy is rarely used. The combination of doxorubicin and ketoconazole has produced some good responses based on tumor size reduction. Oral etoposide and estramustine have had some good effect.[40] Combinations of cytotoxic drugs with antiandrogens have also been studied. Strontium-89 is a β-emitting radionuclide used for bone metastasis. Strontium-89 is similar chemically to calcium and is preferentially localised to bone as a result. Thrombocytopenia is the major side effect. Local-field radiotherapy plus strontium-89 have been used together to reduce the progression of new painful bony metastases.[41]

Novantrone is used to reduce pain and is delivered intravenously once every 3 weeks, along with oral prednisone taken daily.[42] Estrogen therapy in the form of DES, estramustine phosphate, ethinyl estradiol, polyestradiol phosphate (Estradurin), and diethylstilbestrol (Stilphostrol) are all used singly for stages C, T3, or T4, or stage D, T3, T4, N+, and M+ prostate cancers.

Provenge is a new vaccine-like therapy that is still in trial and is showing good results.

CHINESE MEDICINE DIAGNOSTIC CATEGORIES AND TREATMENT

SPLEEN QI DEFICIENCY

This leads to dampness and dampness pouring down due to sinking spleen qi, a form of prolapse. It is caused by overwork, dietary irregularities, prolonged illness, and weak constitution. Turbid yin cannot be born downward and out of the body and this leads to a damp phlegm accumulation in the lower jiao, specifically in the bladder/prostate.

Tongue

Pale, possibly swollen with teethmarks, white coat that may be thin or thick.

Pulse

Thready, moderate, soggy, or slippery.

Treatment principles

Tonify the spleen qi, lift the qi and yang, transform dampness and phlegm, antineoplasm.

Formula

Bu zhong yi qi wan jia jian[43]

shan zha (Crataegi Fructus;   20 g
Crataegus)

mai ya (Hordei Fructus germinatus;   20 g
  Hordeum vulgare; barley sprouts;
  malt)
wang bu liu xing (Vaccariae Semen;   20 g
  Vaccaria segetalis seeds)

Bu zhong yi qi wan is the primary formula to tonify the spleen and raise the sunken yang. In this case the inability of the pure yang to rise allows for prolapse, which manifests as dampness and phlegm in the lower jiao caused by spleen deficiency. In a woman this same formula slightly modified could be used to treat leukorrhea caused by dampness pouring down due to spleen deficiency. Prostate cancer is a form of dampness and phlegm; in this case, in a mass.

Shan zha relieves food stagnation and is used here as a phlegm-transforming herb that also disperses blood stasis and reduces masses. Shan zha is used to reduce gynecological and some male urogenital tumors. It is valuable here because it not only helps to dissolve phlegm masses but also breaks up congealed blood, both of which are the very essence of prostate masses. Mai ya enters the spleen and stomach and tonifies their function to enable the transformation of dampness and phlegm. It also promotes the circulation of the liver qi. This action enables the herb to act as a messenger herb to deliver the phytochemical action of the other herbs in the formula since the liver channel wraps the testes and prostate gland. Wang bu liu xing is a blood-moving herb that also reduces swellings, relieves pain and promotes healing by increasing blood circulation. It enters the stomach and liver channels, has a propensity for the testes and is antineoplastic. Pharmaceutical studies show that it has activity against HSV2. It is the primary antineoplastic herb in the formula.

If the diagnosis is appropriate then this formula can be used during watchful waiting in order to begin work on the underlying environment for the cancer and to prevent spread while conventional cytotoxic options are considered.

DAMP HEAT ACCUMULATION

This is usually caused by spleen or kidney deficiency that leads to dampness; dampness causes an obstruction that causes heat. This pattern manifests as a start–stop urinary stream, lower abdominal bloating, chronic constipation, a bitter taste in the mouth.

Tongue

Redder with a thin or thick yellow greasy coat.

Pulse

Soggy or slippery and rapid.

Treatment principles

Drain dampness, clear heat, resolve heat, antineoplasm, diuresis.

Formula

Special formula

yi ren (Coicis Semen; *Coix lacryma-jobi*)	30 g
yin chen hao (Artemisiae scopariae Herba; *Artemisia scoparia/A. capillaris*)	15 g
qu mai (Dianthi Herba; *Dianthus*)	15 g
hai jin sha (Lygodii Spora; *Lygodium japonicum* spores)	15 g
san leng (Sparganii Rhizoma; *Sparganium* rhizome)	15 g
yu jin (Curcumae Radix; *Curcuma longa* rhizome)	15 g
dan shen (Salviae miltiorrhizae Radix; *Salvia miltiorhiza* root)	20 g
dang gui (Angelicae sinensis Radix; *Angelica sinensis*)	10 g
chi shao (Paeoniae Radix rubra; *Paeonia lactiflora* root)	10 g
tao ren (Persicae Semen; *Prunus* ssp. seed)	10 g
ba yue zha (Akebiae Fructus; *Akebia*)	15 g
fu ling (Poria; *Poria cocos*)	15 g
zhu ling (Polyporus; *Polyporus – Grifola*)	15 g
bai zhu (Atractylodis macrocephalae Rhizoma; *Atractylodes macrocephala*)	10 g
tai zi shen (Pseudostellariae Radix; *Pseudostellaria heterophylla*)	20 g

The formula is divided into three combinations of herbs. One combination works to drain dampness and clear heat. This group includes yi ren, yin chen hao, qu mai, hai jin sha, fu ling and zhu ling.

The second group includes blood-regulating herbs that act antineoplastically and, at the same time, as messenger herbs to improve circulation to the prostate tissue. These herbs are san leng, yu jin, dan shen, chi shao, tao ren, and ba yue zha. Many of the herbs in both groups are antineoplastic in various ways; by draining dampness they treat symptomatically and also enter the 'scene of the crime'; by cracking blood they allow for better circulation of antineoplastic actions of other herbs and of cytotoxic treatment. Ba yue zha has been found to be antineoplastic against many blood-stasis-type masses.

The third group tonifies the spleen to enable it to utilise the drain damp herbs and the blood-cracking herbs. Fu ling, zhu ling, bai zhu, and tai zi shen all support the spleen to transform and transport dampness. The spleen also has a relationship with blood. Tonifying the spleen to nourish the blood helps the blood-cracking herbs, which are often cloying, to avoid damaging the spleen and to enter the target tissue. Increasing the blood volume by tonifying the spleen is also a means of helping to move blood in order to crack blood. The blood-stasis and drain-damp herbs work together to resolve heat.

EARLY STAGE KIDNEY DEFICIENCY IN AN OLDER MAN

Polyuria, low back weakness, aversion to cold, dry mouth but doesn't drink, general weakness.

Tongue

Pale or dark with thin white coat.

Pulse

Thready or sunken.

Treatment principles

Tonify the qi, tonify the kidney qi, strengthen yang, move blood, resolve phlegm, antineoplasm.

Formula

Special formula

huang qi (Astragali Radix; *Astragalus membranaceus*)	20 g
bu gu zhi (Psoraleae Fructus; *Psoralea*)	15 g
yi zhi ren (Alpiniae oxyphyllae Fructus; *Alpinia oxyphylla* fruit)	15 g
mu dan pi (Moutan Cortex; *Paeonia suffruticosa* root cortex)	15 g
fu ling (Poria; *Poria cocos*)	15 g
gou qi zi (Lycii Fructus; *Lycium chinensis* fruit)	15 g
nu zhen zi (Ligustri lucidi Fructus; *Ligustrum lucidum* fruit)	15 g
yin yang huo (Epimedii Herba; *Epimedium grandiflorum*)	15 g
yu zhu (Polygonati odorati Rhizoma; *Polygonatum odoratum*)	15 g
dang shen (Codonopsis Radix; *Codonopsis pilosula* root)	15 g
ze xie (Alismatis Rhizoma; *Alisma*)	10 g
shan yao (Dioscoreae Rhizoma; *Dioscorea opposita*)	15 g
shu di (Rehmanniae Radix preparata; *Rehmannia*)	20 g
tai zi shen (Pseudostellariae Radix; *Pseudostellaria heterophylla*)	20 g
mai dong (Ophiopogonis Radix; *Ophiopogon*)	10 g
bai zhu (Atractylodis macrocephalae Rhizoma; *Atractylodes macrocephala*)	10 g
gan cao (Glycyrrhizae Radix; *Glycyrrhiza*; licorice root)	10 g

Dang shen, fu ling, bai zhu and gan cao form the basic qi tonic formula Si jun zi tang. Bu gu zhi, yi zhi ren, yin yang huo, shan yao all tonify the kidney qi. Bu gu zhi is very high in genistein, which is an anticancer substance and prevents the promotion of prostate cancer cells. Gou qi zi, shu di, yu zhu, nu zhen zi and mai dong all act synergistically to nourish the blood and yin and, thereby, gently move the blood. The yin-nourishing herbs help to protect the yin in a formula that is warming and drying. Tai zi shen benefits fluids while tonifying the qi. The yang tonics in the formula are warming. Tai zi shen helps to support the tonifying action without being warming, and therefore, drying. Huang qi is an antineoplastic herb that lifts the yang, increases white blood cells (WBCs) and natural killer (NK) cells. Dong ling cao (Rabdosiae rubescentis Herba; *Rabdosia*) could be added to this formula to help regulate testosterone levels in a prostate cancer that will probably be treated hormonally.

LIVER QI STASIS

The liver channel runs through the genital region and wraps the testes. Unresolved emotional material binds the circulating function of the liver. This constraint affects the San Jiao's function of qi transformation and transport and transformation of water, and fluids become obstructed leading to mass in the lower jiao. Frequently this presentation will be combined with another. Constrained, irritable, 'type A personality', stressed with poor coping mechanisms, possibly hypertensive, jueyin headaches, possible signs of spleen deficiency if the pulse is wiry but forceless, possible signs of kidney deficiency if the pulse is wiry forceful – these are all signs of liver qi stasis.

Tongue

Either dark or pale, thin white coat.

Pulse

Wiry forceless (deficiency type of constraint), or wiry forceful (excess type of constraint).

Treatment principles

Deficiency type – benefit the spleen to nourish the liver blood, mildly move the liver qi, antineoplasm. (Xiao yao san); excess type – circulate the liver qi, antineoplasm (Shu gan wan).

Formula

Chen xiang san jia jian

(Can add elements of the above two possible formulas depending on excess or deficiency)

chen xiang (Aquilariae Lignum resinatum; *Aquilaria*)	10 g
chen pi (Citri reticulatae Pericarpium; *Citrus reticulata* pericarp)	10 g
dang gui (Angelicae sinensis Radix; *Angelica sinensis*)	10 g
wang bu liu xing (Vaccariae Semen; *Vaccaria segetalis* seeds)	10 g
shi wei (Pyrrosiae Folium; *Pyrrosia* leaves)	10 g
tian kui zi (Semiaquilegiae Radix; *Semiaquilegia adoxoides* root)	10 g

Liver qi stagnation can cause urinary obstruction. The San Jiao fluid pathways can become obstructed, or the qi transformative process of the urinary bladder can become obstructed. Liver qi blockage will lead to either heat or damp, or both. When the liver qi is blocked then there are symptoms of tension and constraint. Middle jiao dampness occurs alongside these symptoms but not combined as in damp heat. The tongue here is dark whereas in damp heat the tongue will probably be red and have a yellow greasy coat. So the damp heat pattern is not the same as the liver qi stasis pattern where damp can occur. Chen xiang san is a formula from the Jin Gui Yi (Supplement to the Golden Cabinet, 1768). It promotes the smooth flow of liver qi, promotes urination, and is antineoplastic in the modified form above. Dong kui zi has been substituted with tian kui zi, which is the anticancer herb. This formula can be added to other formulas in this pattern list when liver qi stasis is a strong component of the constitution of the patient. Chai hu shu gan san could be substituted and modified to have a similar effect. The task is to understand if the stasis is due to excess or deficiency.

Internal stasis of toxins

The toxins in this presentation are possible chemical contaminants, high testosterone, phlegm, blood stasis and the cancer itself, which has spread to the bone and the pelvic lymph nodes. The symptom picture is bone pain, bradyuria, lower abdominal pain and fullness, possibly ascites due to metastatic spread, dry mouth, fever, restlessness, constipation or frequent stool with tenesmus. This is a late-stage presentation without yang deficiency.

Tongue

Crimson, little coat or greasy coat, dry.

Pulse

Thready and rapid or thin and taut.

Treatment principles

Crack blood, move stasis, resolve toxin, confine the cancer and stop spread, protect yin and strengthen the qi.

Formula

Special formula

yi ren (Coicis Semen; *Coix lacryma-jobi*)	30 g
jiao gu lan (Herba Gynostemmatis; *Gynostemma*)	20 g
hai jin sha (Lygodii Spora; *Lygodium japonicum* spores)	15 g
zhu ling (Polyporus; *Polyporus – Grifola*)	20 g
fu ling (Poria; *Poria cocos*)	15 g
bai zhu (Atractylodis macrocephalae Rhizoma; *Atractylodes macrocephala*)	15 g
dan shen (Salviae miltiorrhizae Radix; *Salvia miltiorhiza* root)	15 g
yu jin (Curcumae Radix; *Curcuma longa* rhizome)	15 g
tai zi shen (Pseudostellariae Radix; *Pseudostellaria heterophylla*)	20 g
mai dong (Ophiopogonis Radix; *Ophiopogon*)	10 g
xi yang shen (Panacis quinquefolii Radix; *Panax quinquefolium*)	10 g
bai mao teng (Solani lyrati Herba; *Solanum lyratum*)	20 g
bei sha shen (Glehniae Radix; *Glehnia*)	10 g

Resolving toxin is a major intent in this pattern. There are, therefore, several antineoplastic herbs including yi ren, qi ye dan, hai jin sha, bai mao teng, fu ling and zhu ling. The qi tonic herbs are bai zhu and tai zi shen which are both neutral in temperature, an important feature of the herbs' use in a formula where the heat from toxin is unavoidable. Xi yang shen also tonifies qi while nourishing yin. Although it is cooling it also tonifies the qi, and the combination of the tonic herbs with the antineoplastics helps to prevent spread of the cancer. Dan shen and yu jin break the blood stasis and enable cytotoxic therapies, including the antineoplastics in this formula, to have better access to the tumor.

ADVANCED STAGE WITH YIN AND QI DEFICIENCY

Cachexia, symptoms of lung metastasis, bone symptoms, aggressive cancer, fatigue, weakness, anemias, emaciation, dypsnea on exertion, bradyuria, anorexia, dry mouth but cannot drink.

Tongue

Crimson and purple, small short shrivelled tongue body, no coat, dry.

Pulse

Deep, thready, or thready and taut.

Treatment principles

Tonify the qi and nourish the blood, adjust the digestive function to move stool and improve appetite, nourish yin and jin ye, reduce pain, antineoplasm.

Formula

Special formula

tai zi shen (Pseudostellariae Radix; *Pseudostellaria heterophylla*)	20 g
bei sha shen (Glehniae Radix; *Glehnia*)	15 g
fu ling (Poria; *Poria cocos*)	15 g
mai dong (Ophiopogonis Radix; *Ophiopogon*)	10 g
gou qi zi (Lycii Fructus; *Lycium chinensis* fruit)	15 g
huang qi (Astragali Radix; *Astragalus membranaceus*)	20 g
mu dan pi (Moutan Cortex; *Paeonia suffruticosa* root cortex)	10 g
gui ban* (Testudinis Plastrum; *Chinemys reevesii* plastron)	15 g
yu zhu (Polygonati odorati Rhizoma; *Polygonatum odoratum*)	15 g
ji nei jin (Gigeriae galli Endothelium corneum; *Gallus gallus domesticus* chicken gizzard lining)	15 g
shen qu (Massa medicata fermentata; medicated leaven)	15 g
bai zhu (Atractylodis macrocephalae Rhizoma; *Atractylodes macrocephala*)	15 g
bai ren shen (Ginseng Radix; *Panax ginseng*; white ginseng)	10 g

This is a palliative formula used as salvage therapy in a patient who has advanced disease. There are several qi-tonic herbs combined with yin-nourishing herbs, middle jiao tonics to improve appetite and digestive fire. The yin- and blood-nourishing herbs are synergistic and help generate blood to treat various kinds of anemia. Huang qi increases the WBCs. Gou qi zi, bai ren shen and the yin-nourishing herbs increase RBCs. The short and shrivelled tongue body implies there is dehydration and an inability to absorb fluids digestively. Gui ban is especially helpful in nourishing the yin in this case. This formula can be modified in many ways in order to help the patient be comfortable, calm the spirit, improve sleep, and maintain whole body health as much as possible. A patient with this presentation will probably be treated with hormonal therapy. The side effects of hormonal treatment are bound to further injure the yin. Therefore, the modification of this formula to more strongly protect yin would be necessary and appropriate.

PC–SPES

PC-SPES[44–46] is a proprietary product of International Medical Research, Inc. The name means prostate cancer (PC)/hope (spes is the Latin for hope). This formula was also studied at the Cancer Research Institute at New York Medical College in Valhalla, New York. The extract from these herbs was found to exert potent cytotoxic and cytostatic activity on prostate cancer cell lines. It arrested tumor cells in the G1 phase of the reproductive cycle and actively induced apoptosis. The *bcl-2* gene was downregulated in the presence of this formula, which may indicate that cells treated with this formula may be more sensitive to other antitumor agents. This formula is especially appropriate for treatment with hormone therapies. It potentiates the androgen-antagonist effect.

The formula has been taken off the market because of issues of contamination from the producer/distributor Botaniclab. It was found to have levels of DES and other contaminants. Following is a list of the herbs in the formula without dose. Using these herbs in their uncontaminated form as whole or granulated high quality assayed herbs poses no risk to patients.

ling zhi (Ganoderma; *Ganoderma*)

dong ling cao (Rabdosiae rubescentis Herba; *Rabdosia*)

huang qin (Scutellariae Radix; *Scutellaria baicalensis*)

ban lan gen (Isatidis/Baphicacanthis Radix; *Isatis/Baphicacanthus* root)

ju hua (Chrysanthemi Flos; *Chrysanthemum/ Dendranthema morifolium*)

ju ye zong (Serenoae repens Fructus extractum; *Serenoa repens*; saw palmetto)

ren shen (Ginseng Radix; *Panax ginseng*)

gan cao (Glycyrrhizae Radix; *Glycyrrhiza*; licorice root)

TREATMENT PRINCIPLES

All of these formulas are designed to treat the main Chinese diagnosis for prostate cancer. It is important to incorporate the correct formula or a portion of the formula with a larger formula that is intended to treat the side effects of the conventional treatment. For example, if a patient is receiving radiation therapy in some form, there is a set of symptoms that can be predicted to arise. Radiation in the form of external beam irradiation has strong and specific side effects that it is important to address. Because these side effects can persist for months and possibly even longer, addressing them during the radiation therapy can help stave off the harder and more oppressive long-term problems, like radiation enteritis and cystitis.

Sometimes it may be necessary to treat only the side effects and to potentiate the conventional treatment, completely leaving off the constitutional approach. When possible during conventional treatment it is important to address the foundational constitution according to the prior list of pathogenic patterns. However, the conventional cytotoxic treatment is the primary treatment around which everything else revolves. After radiation therapy, then, the fuller force of Chinese medicine can be utilised. In other words, you may have to draw from radiosensitising formulas and herbs during radiation without adding the constitutional formula to your approach. It is best to prioritise the approach rather than use a 'shotgun' approach.

Another example of where you might have to draw from a conventional medicine-driven approach is hormonal therapy. Hormonal therapies are antiandrogenic in nature and can cause symptoms of testosterone deficiency, which often look like menopausal syndrome. There is no reason not to treat these symptoms as though they were menopausal syndrome. Therefore, combining a formula for these symptoms with the constitutional diagnosis will work well. Because hormonal therapies are most frequently used in the context of more advanced disease, they are not considered curative, therefore, the object becomes to design a formula that will allow a patient to live as long as possible and as comfortably as possible. Addressing the overall environment is important, whereas during radiation therapy, addressing the side effects of radiation, potentiating the radiation, and fitting in the constitution, if there is room, is most important.

Case study 5.1

This patient was a 53-year-old white male with a rising PSA level and a suspicious hypoechoic area in the right lobe of his prostate which had been monitored for several years. He had been diagnosed with BPH and prostatitis, and his PSA was never in a range that would cause alert. However, he had multiple biopsies over 6 years, which all had normal results. Then a recent biopsy showed that 40% of the tissue from the right lobe was involved with adenocarcinoma. His Gleason score was 5. Several cores were taken from the right and left lobes. All of the right cores were positive and all of the left cores were negative for adenocarcinoma.

- Bone: negative.
- Pelvic and abdominal CT scan: negative.
- Nodes: negative.
- PSA: 4.7.
- Staging: early (A) or T1N0M0.
- History: BPH and prostatitis.

General

- Appetite: good.
- Digestion:
  - upper: slight acid reflux on occasion
  - lower: gas and bloating.
- Stools: regular and loose (unformed).
- Temperature: normal; Raynaud's syndrome.
- Thirst: normal.
- Sleep: good; does not dream.
- Pain: none.
- Eyes: cataracts, mild.

- Headaches: occasional jueyin-type (not hypertensive).
- Skin: rash on back and flank, worse in warm weather; red, raised, dry, itchy for 3 years now; no known allergies.
- Toenail fungus: for years.
- Fevers: none.
- Spirits: very positive and hopeful regarding diagnosis; job is very stressful due to boss' style (constant control).

Tongue
Pale, wet, quivering, with a slightly greasy coat, no vein distention.

Pulse
Liver sho (lowest); slight tight at liver heart positions; spleen also low.

Diagnosis
Deficiency liver/heart qi constraint with underlying spleen qi deficiency leading to dampness pouring down with toxin.

Plan

The patient was offered several options including radical prostatectomy (unilateral nerve-sparing procedure), brachytherapy with or without external beam radiation, or just external beam radiation. The patient decided to take some time, seek second opinions, see the providers who would be doing the procedures, and then make a decision.

Case study continues

The following formula was given while information was compiled in order to make a decision:

huang qi (Astragali Radix; *Astragalus membranaceus*)	15 g
bu gu zhi (Psoraleae Fructus; *Psoralea*)	15 g
yi zhi ren (Alpiniae oxyphyllae Fructus; *Alpinia oxyphylla* fruit)	10 g
mu dan pi (Moutan Cortex; *Paeonia suffruticosa* root cortex)	10 g
fu ling (Poria; *Poria cocos*)	10 g
nu zhen zi (Ligustri lucidi Fructus; *Ligustrum lucidum* fruit)	10 g
yin yang huo (Epimedii Herba; *Epimedium grandiflorum*)	10 g
yu zhu (Polygonati odorati Rhizoma; *Polygonatum odoratum*)	10 g
chai hu (Bupleuri Radix; *Bupleurum*)	10 g
sheng di huang (Rehmanniae Radix; *Rehmannia*)	10 g
dang shen (Codonopsis Radix; *Codonopsis pilosula* root)	10 g
ze xie (Alismatis Rhizoma; *Alisma*)	10 g
yi ren (Coicis Semen; *Coix lacryma-jobi*)	20 g
yin chen hao (Artemisiae scopariae Herba; *Artemisia scoparia/A. capillaris*)	20 g
qu mai (Dianthi Herba; *Dianthus*)	15 g
yu jin (Curcumae Radix; *Curcuma longa* rhizome)	10 g
hai jin sha (Lygodii Spora; *Lygodium japonicum* spores)	10 g
san leng (Sparganii Rhizoma; *Sparganium* rhizome)	10 g
ba yue zha (Akebiae Fructus; *Akebia*)	20 g
dan shen (Salviae miltiorrhizae Radix; *Salvia miltiorhiza* root)	10 g
dong ling cao (Rabdosiae rubescentis Herba; *Rabdosia*)	20 g

Dose: 6 g three times daily.

The purpose of this formula is to prevent spread and to begin treatment of the constitution and the diagnosis for the cancer while awaiting the onset of conventional treatment. There are several parts of the formula:

1. To address spleen and kidney yang deficiency.
2. To transform dampness and act as prophylactic against damp heat.
3. To prevent blood stasis and improve overall circulation in the local area of the cancer.
4. To act antineoplastically and treat the symptom of frequent and unsmooth urination.

Huang qi, bu gu zhi, fu ling, chai hu, and dang shen all tonify the spleen qi to lift the yang. Since part of the diagnosis is sinking spleen qi leading to dampness pouring down, this part of the formula begins to address a main aspect of injury. Yi zhi ren also helps to lift the yang and treats a primary symptom, frequent urination. It is astringent and helps to regulate and hold in the urine. Fu ling, yi ren, yin chen hao, qu mai, and hai jin sha all drain dampness. Fu ling, yin chen hao, and yi ren all have antineoplastic properties, as well. Hai jin sha enters the small intestine and bladder channels and helps to regulate urination. Yu jin, san leng, ba yue zha and dan shen are all blood-regulating herbs that help to eliminate blood stasis, a component of the cancerisation process. Ba yue zha, dong ling cao, fu ling, yi ren, yin chen hao, huang qi, bu gu zhi are all antineoplastic in various ways. Ze xie, mu dan pi, and sheng di clear heat and yu zhu and yin yang huo help to protect the yin in a clear heat and drain dampness formula. Chai hu not only lifts the yang qi but also circulates the liver qi. In fact, elements of Bu zhong yi qi tang are in this formula.

The patient continued on this formula for 4 months while he interviewed various practitioners regarding options and their expertise in those options. He decided that radiation was not a comfortable treatment form to him because of the toxicity of radiation. He was very sensitive to the possible ongoing effects of radiation and opted for a radical prostatectomy.

He was given the following formula post-surgery at 6 g three times daily:

zhi huang qi (Astragali Radix; *Astragalus membranaceus*)	20 g
dang gui (Angelicae sinensis Radix; *Angelica sinensis*)	15 g

Case study continues

jin yin hua (Lonicerae Flos; *Lonicera* flowers)	15 g
mu dan pi (Moutan Cortex; *Paeonia suffruticosa* root cortex)	10 g
lian qiao (Forsythiae fructus; *Forsythia*)	15 g
zao jiao ci (Gleditsiae Spina; *Gleditsia* spines)	15 g
dang shen (Codonopsis Radix; *Codonopsis pilosula* root)	20 g
nu zhen zi (Ligustri lucidi Fructus; *Ligustrum lucidum* fruit)	20 g
zhu ling (Polyporus; *Polyporus – Grifola*)	15 g
tai zi shen (Pseudostellariae Radix; *Pseudostellaria heterophylla*)	15 g
tian dong (Asparagi Radix; *Asparagus*)	15 g
xian he cao (Agrimoniae Herba; *Agrimonia pilosa* var. *japonica*; agrimony)	15 g
dong ling cao (Rabdosiae rubescentis Herba; *Rabdosia*)	20 g

Fried (zhi) huang qi and dang gui make up Dang gui bu xue tang. They work together to heal wounds and replenish blood lost in surgery. Jin yin hua, mu dan pi and lian qiao all clear heat to reduce inflammation and help to promote healing and establish normal function. Zao jiao ci also reduces inflammation and helps to prevent infection along with the clear-heat herbs. Ziao jiao ci is a warming herb whereas the heat-clearing herbs are cooling or cold. It helps to protect a deficient spleen, which is part of the underlying diagnosis for this patient. Dang shen and nu zhen zi are an excellent combination to increase WBC and RBC counts. They are synergistic in this respect.

Zhu ling is antineoplastic and also drains damp. Draining damp helps to reduce inflammation and swelling from the surgical trauma. Zhu ling also increases the WBC count and increases phagocytosis to prevent infection. It is mildly analgesic. Tai zi shen and tian dong benefit fluids. Tai zi shen tonifies the qi of the spleen; tian dong nourishes the yin. Xian he cao stops bleeding and is also antineoplastic. Dong ling cao is a primary antineoplastic herb against prostate cancer.

The surgery went well and resulted in the best possible prognosis. There were no surprises or complications. Post-surgery there was hematuria and incontinence. His sleep was normal, stools were regular and formed, there was no pain. The pulse was a spleen sho or moderate. The tongue was slightly dark in the center area, reddish body, with right vein distention that was moderate. Over the next months, the patient remained on modifications of this formula. The xian he cao was removed because the bleeding stopped early on. Then the heat-clearing herbs were eliminated. The tongue was then slightly pale with a thin white coat. The pulse was a spleen sho with deficient kidney pulses on both sides. Incontinence and erectile dysfunction persisted. The patient wore Attends incontinence products, first six per day and then three per day and finally none. The erectile function was slower to return, but in 1 year had returned to normal function.

At 6 months post-surgery, the following formula was given at 6 g three times daily:

You gui wan	150 g[47]
Add:	
zhu ling (Polyporus; *Polyporus – Grifola*)	50 g
san qi (Notoginseng Radix; *Panax notoginseng*)	15 g
huang qi (Astragali Radix; *Astragalus membranaceus*)	40 g
tai zi shen (Pseudostellariae Radix; *Pseudostellaria heterophylla*)	40 g
gua lou ren (Trichosanthis Semen; *Trichosanthes* seed)	40 g
yi ren (Coicis Semen; *Coix lacryma-jobi*)	40 g
shan ci gu* (Cremastrae/Pleiones Pseudobulbus; *Cremastra/Pleione pseudobulbs*)	25 g
chong lou (Paridis Rhizoma; *Paris*)	25 g
bai shao (Paeoniae Radix alba; *Paeonia lactiflora* root)	30 g
bai hua she she cao (Hedyotis diffusae Herba; *Oldenlandia*)	50 g

There are many antineoplastic herbs in this formula, which is meant to treat erectile dysfunction and to prevent recurrence. You gui

Case study continues

wan treats kidney yang deficiency with insufficient fire at the gate of vitality. Kidney yang warms the lower burner, is the primary motivator in the functional transformation of water, including urination and testosterone. The fire of kidney yang is partially responsible for erection. This formula is essentially Liu wei di huang wan plus fu zi (Aconiti Radix preparata; *Aconitum carmichaelii*) and gui zhi (Cinnamomi Ramulus; *Cinnamomum cassia* branches), two warming herbs that draw the fire back to the kidneys.

Several of the herbs in the formula are antineoplastic in order to prevent recurrence. The first 2 years post-treatment are usually the most critical in terms of recurrence. It is best to convince patients to continue treatment to prevent recurrence. This includes persisting in dietary changes and all other lifestyle changes that have been made. In fact, these changes should become a permanent part of one's life. The antineoplastics include zhu ling, huang qi, gua lou ren, yi ren, shan ci gu*, chong lou, and bai hua she she cao. San qi is added to regulate the blood and to act as an antineoplastic. If this patient had decided to be treated with radioactive seed implants, then the following formula would have been appropriate:

Fu zheng zeng xiao fang:[48]

huang qi (Astragali Radix; *Astragalus membranaceus*)	30 g
ji xue teng (Spatholobi Caulis; *Spatholobus suberectus*)	15 g
tai zi shen (Pseudostellariae Radix; *Pseudostellaria heterophylla*)	15 g
bai zhu (Atractylodis macrocephalae Rhizoma; *Atractylodes macrocephala*)	15 g
tian dong (Asparagi Radix; *Asparagus*)	15 g
tian hua fen (Trichosanthis Radix; *Trichosanthes* root)	15 g
gou qi zi (Lycii Fructus; *Lycium chinensis* fruit)	15 g
nu zhen zi (Ligustri lucidi Fructus; *Ligustrum lucidum* fruit)	15 g
hong hua (Carthami Flos; *Carthamnus tinctorius* flowers)	15 g
su mu (Sappan Lignum; *Caesalpinia sappan*; lignum sappan)	15 g

References

1. Parker SL, Tong T, Bolden S, et al. Cancer statistics, 1996. CA Cancer J Clin 1996; 46:5–27.
2. American Foundation for Urologic Disease; 1996.
3. Ross RK. Epidemiology of prostate cancer. In: Skinner DE, ed. Diagnosis and management of genitourinary cancer. Philadelphia: WB Saunders; 1988:40–45.
4. Hsing AW. Prostate cancer mortality in the United States by cohort year of birth, 1865–1990. Cancer Epidemiol Biomarkers Prev 1994; 3:527–530.
5. Haenzel W. Studies of Japanese migrants: I. Mortality from cancer and other diseases among Japanese in the United States. J Natl Cancer Inst 1968; 40:43–68.
6. Staszenski J. Cancer mortality among the foreign born in the United States. J Natl Cancer Inst 1961; 26:37–132.
7. Carter HB. The prostate: an increasing medical problem. Prostate 1990; 16:39–48.
8. Healy B. From the NIH: does vasectomy cause prostate cancer? JAMA 1993; 269:2620.
9. Ross RK. Serum testosterone levels in young healthy black and white men. J Natl Cancer Inst 1986; 76:45–48.
10. Hill PB. Effect of a vegetarian diet and dexamethasone on plasma prolactin, testosterone and dehydroepiandrosterone in men and women. Cancer Lett 1979; 7:273–282.
11. Gittes RF. Carcinoma of the prostate. N Engl J Med 1991; 324:236–245.
12. Steinberg GD. The familial aggregation of prostate cancer: a case control study (abstract). J Urol 1990; 143:313A.
13. Cannon L. Genetic epidemiology of prostate cancer in the Mormon genealogy. Cancer Surv 1982; 1:47.
14. Aronson KJ, Siemiatycki J, Dewar R, et al. Occupational risk factors for prostate cancer: results from a case-control study in Montreal, Quebec, Canada. Am J Epidemiol 1996; 143:363–373.
15. Visakorpi T. Genetic changes in primary and recurrent prostate cancer by comparative genomic hybridization. Cancer Res 1995; 55:342–347.

16. Peehl DM. Oncogenes in prostate cancer. Cancer 1993; 71:1159–1164.
17. Sadasivan R. Overexpression of HER-2/neu may be an indicator of poor prognosis in prostate cancer. J Urol 1993; 150:126–131.
18. Weidner N. Tumor angiogenesis correlates with metastasis in invasive prostate carcinoma. Am J Pathol 1993; 143:401–408.
19. Brawn PN. Histologic grading study of prostate carcinoma: the development of a new system and comparison with other methods – a preliminary study. Cancer 1982; 49:525–532.
20. Visakorpi T. Review of new prognostic factors in prostate carcinoma. Eur Urol 1993; 24:438–449.
21. Terris MK. Prediction of prostate cancer volume using prostate-specific antigen levels, transrectal ultrasound, and systematic sextant biopsies in patients with prostate cancer. Urology 1995; 45:75–80.
22. Hudson MA. Clinical use of prostate-specific antigen in patients with prostate cancer. J Urol 1989; 142:1011–1017.
23. Oesterling JE. Serum PSA in a community-based population of healthy men. Establishment of age-specific reference ranges. N Engl J Med 1993; 270:860–864.
24. Catalina WJ. Evaluation of percentage of free serum PSA to immune specificity of prostate cancer screening. JAMA 1995; 274:1214–1220.
25. Stenman U. Serum concentrations of PSA and its complex with alpha1-antichymotrypsin before diagnosis of prostate cancer. Lancet 1994; 344:1594–1598.
26. Adolfsson J. Recent results of management of palpable clinically localised prostate cancer. Cancer 1993; 72:310–322.
27. Chodak GW. Results of conservative management of clinically localized prostate cancer. N Engl J Med 1994; 330:242–248.
28. Bagshan MA. Status of radiation treatment of prostate cancer at Stanford University (NIH Publ 88 – 3005). Natl Cancer Inst Monogr 1988; 7:47–60.
29. Middleton RD. Prostate Cancer Clinical Guidelines Panel summary report on management of clinically localized prostate cancer. J Urol 1995; 154:2144–2148.
30. Zincke H. Long-term (15 years) results after radical prostatectomy for clinically localized (Stage T2c or lower) prostate cancer. J Urol 1994; 152:1850–1857.
31. Hawks GE. External beam radiation therapy for prostate cancer: still the gold standard. Oncology 1992; 6:79–94.
32. Porter AT. Brachytherapy for prostate cancer. CA Cancer J Clin 1995;45:65–178.
33. Zincke H. Bilateral pelvic lymphadenoma and radical prostatectomy for clinical Stage C prostatic cancer: role of adjuvant therapy for residual cancer and in disease progresion. J Urol 1986; 135:1199–1205.
34. Frydenberg M. Therapeutic strategies for clinical Stage C prostate cancer. Problems in Urology 1993; 7:166–179.
35. Hsieh WS. Systemic therapy for prostate cancer. New concepts from prostate cancer tumor biology. Cancer Treat Rev 1993; 19:229–260.
36. McLeod DG. The use of flutamide in hormone refractory metastatic prostate cancer. Cancer 1993; 72:3870–3873.
37. Goldenberg SL. Intermittent androgen suppression in treatment of prostate cancer: a preliminary report. Urology 1996; 45:839–844.
38. Denis, L.J. Gosarelin acetate and flutamide versus bilateral orchiectomy: a phase III EORTC Trial (30853). Urology 1993; 42:119–130.
39. Taylor CD. Importance of continued testicular suppression in hormone-refractory prostate cancer. J Clin Oncol 1993; 11:2167–2172.
40. Pienta KJ. Phase II evaluation of oral estramustine and oral etoposide in hormone-refractory adenocarcinoma of the prostate. J Clin Oncol 1994; 12:2005–2012.
41. Porter AT. Results of a randomized Phase III trial to evaluate the eefficacy of strontium-89 adjuvant to local field external beam irradiation in the management of endocrine resistant metastatic prostate cancer. Int J Radiat Oncol Biol Phys 1993; 25:805–813.
42. Payne R. Pain management in the patient with prostate cancer. Cancer 1993; 71:1131–1137.
43. Liu Wan Su. Su Wen Xuan Ji Yuan Bing Shi (Examination of the original patterns of disease from the mysterious mechanisms of the Su Wen (Chapter 61)). 1182 ACE. Zhejiang Science and Technology Press; 1984.
44. Di Paola RS. Clinical and biologic activity of an estrogenic herbal combination (PC – SPES) in prostate cancer. N Engl J Med 1998; 339:785–791.
45. Darzynkiewicz Z. Chinese herbal mixture PC – SPES in treatment of prostate cancer (review). Int J Oncol 2000; 17:729–736.
46. Oh WK. Activity of the herbal combination, PC–SPES, in the treatment of patients with androgen-independent prostate cancer. Urology 2001; 57:122–126.
47. Zhang Jing Yue. Jing Yue Quan Shu (Complete works of Jing Yue). 1624 ACE. Shanghai Science and Technology Press; 1959.
48. Zhang Dai Zhao. Zhong yi yao yu fang she xiang jie he de zhi liao (Treatment with a combination of Chinese materia medica and radiation therapy). Zhong huo Zhong liu (Chinese Oncology Journal) 1993; 2:15.

Chapter 6

Cervical and Uterine Cancers

CHAPTER CONTENTS

Cervical cancer   177
  Epidemiology   177
  Pathology   178
  Etiology   178
  Natural history   179
  Invasive cervical carcinoma   179
  Screening and diagnosis   180
  Management of abnormal smears and
      preinvasive lesions   180
  Staging   181
  Prognosis   181
  Treatment   182

Uterine cancer   188
  Diagnosis   189
  Clinical presentation   189
  Staging and prognosis   189
  Treatment   190

*Yet there is mystery here and it is not one I under-
    stand.
Without this sting of otherness, of – even – the
    vicious,
without the terrible energies of the underside of
    health, sanity,
sense, then nothing works or can work. I tell you
    that goodness:
the ordinary, the decent –
these are nothing without the hidden powers
that pour forth continually from their
shadow sides.*

by Doris Lessing, *The Marriages
Between Zones Three, Four and Five.*

CERVICAL CANCER

EPIDEMIOLOGY

The incidence and mortality rates of cervical cancer have decreased in the US by as much as 75% in the last 40 years.[1] This change is the largest seen in any cancer site and is attributed to cytological screening in the form of the Papanicolaou smear.[2] The Pap smear allows for the detection of early disease at the preinvasive stage. About 65 000 cases of carcinoma in situ are found in this way annually.[3] However, cervical cancer remains the most common female cancer in developing countries.[4] In the US it is the seventh most common cancer in women. In 1995, 15 800 cases were diagnosed and there were 4800 deaths.[3]

PATHOLOGY

Most cervical cancers are squamous-cell carcinomas.[5] Adenocarcinomas of the cervix arise from endocervical cells and account for 14% of these cancers.[6] The percentage of adenocarcinomas has risen over the years. This is possibly due to the fact that they are more difficult to detect than squamous-cell carcinomas at the preinvasive stage. The long-term survival for both types is not significantly different.

Adenosquamous carcinomas are a mixed type and are associated with a higher risk of pelvic lymph node metastasis.[7] Glassy-cell carcinoma is a poorly-differentiated form of adenosquamous carcinoma that responds poorly to surgery and radiation therapy.[8] Verrucous carcinoma is an extremely well-differentiated form of squamous-cell carcinoma. This tumor may invade the vagina and the endometrium but does not usually metastasise to lymph nodes. Small-cell carcinomas are distinctive and usually have a very poor prognosis. The most aggressive tumors are those with neuroendocrine differentiation. Other cervical malignancies include sarcomas, malignant melanomas, lymphomas, mixed mullerian tumors, germ-cell tumors, and trophoblastic tumors.

ETIOLOGY

There is a well-established association between sexual activity and cervical neoplasia.[9] Human papilloma virus (HPV) is the most important factor in this association. Factors that were thought to be responsible for cervical intraepithelial neoplasia (CIN) include increased number of sex partners, earlier age at first intercourse, lower level of education, and lower income, which can be translate into poorer screening, and smoking. These factors have all now been reduced to one factor; HPV.[10]

Many types of HPV have been isolated in the human genital tract; types 16, 18, 45, and 56 all have a high correlation with cervical cancer.[11] These high-risk types of HPV have been found in 74% of cases of invasive cervical cancer and in 53% of those with moderate to severe dysplasia. HPV-16 is the most prevalent. HPV 16 and 18 can combine with the p53 protein and cause the same functional consequence as a *p53* gene mutation.

An increased risk of cervical neoplasia also results from immunosuppression.[12] This immunosuppression is associated with an increased rate of HPV infection. Women with HIV infection have an increased incidence and recurrence rates of CIN. Also women who are HIV positive who developed invasive cervical cancer were found to have more advanced disease at the time of presentation.[13] A direct molecular relationship exists between HIV, herpes simplex virus (HSV), and HPV. HIV gene products cause a transactivation of HPV proteins.[14] (This relationship also exists in men with HIV infection and manifests as anal condyloma.)

Smoking has also been reported to increase HPV infection.[15] Conflicting data have been reported regarding the implication of oral contraceptives but estrogen exposure seems to have a direct relationship with many reproductive cancers, male and female. Women who use the oral contraceptive pill have dryer and more delicate vaginal tissues. This makes them more susceptible to abrasion during sexual activity and, therefore, more susceptible to sexually transmitted diseases, including HPV. Estrogen exposure can also increase through xenoestrogenic exposures. Xenoestrogenic exposures are most highly implicated coming through the food chain and via water. Xenoestrogens activate and also increase the number of certain estrogen receptors in all responsive tissues, including the transition zone of the cervix. It is probable that the combination of many factors, including increased estrogen exposure from many sources can contribute to carcinogenicity. Prenatal exposure to DES is also implicated.

Talc is a substance used as a delivery mechanism for fragrance in many feminine hygiene products including powders, sanitary pads, and tampons. Talc is a known carcinogen; it occurs naturally in the presence of asbestos, which is often found in cosmetic talc. It has not been studied as a causative factor in cervical cancer. The political lobby to keep talc on the market has made accessing this information difficult and, as a result, most of the population is unaware of the carcinogenic effects of talc, whether or not it contains asbestos. Using pure cotton tampons and other feminine products is essential. Talc is also found in facial cosmetics and should be eliminated from use.

Chinese medicine

Cervical cancer is almost always associated with a latent pathogenic factor (LPF): HPV and possibly HSV infection. HPV is considered a damp phlegm pathogen, which can occur as a result of sexually transmitted disease exposure. This exposure can occur in an internal environment of sinking spleen qi, which is especially common in women who are HIV positive. Any chronic pathogen that has a local hold on tissue will cause several levels of persistent and ongoing stasis. Women with spleen deficiency, yin deficiency, a damp constitution, or liver qi constraint are more susceptible to LPFs. See Chapter 11 on leukemias, which goes more deeply into the concept of latent pathogens.

If HPV is left untreated it will move from a damp phlegm stasis to blood level stasis and then blood heat with toxin. This progression is apparent when looking at the progression of asymptomatic presentations with an early abnormal Pap result to later presentations with abnormal bleeding and then obstructive symptoms and pain.

The procedures utilised by conventional medicine in diagnosis, that is cone biopsy and other surgical procedures, also cause blood stasis. This is not a recommendation to avoid those procedures, which can be curative. But it is important to treat the underlying environment and to prevent recurrence of the LPF after these procedures, whether they are considered curative or not.

Clinical manifestations

- Post-coital bleeding.
- Vaginal bleeding or profuse or prolonged menstruation and a shortened menstrual cycle.
- Irregular post-menopausal bleeding.
- Vaginal discharge.
- Distention and dull pain in the low back and abdomen.
- Fever.

NATURAL HISTORY

The development of invasive cervical cancer has traditionally been viewed as a continuum that begins with mild dysplasia. Mild dysplasia has been designated as CIN-1, moderate as CIN-2, and severe dysplasia and carcinoma in situ as CIN-3.

Cervical lesions with histologic features of HPV infection are also referred to as flat condylomas.

The current understanding of the pathogenesis of cervical squamous-cell neoplasia has modified the terminology for the histopathologic classification of CIN. CIN-2 and CIN-3 lesions are now grouped together as high-grade CIN because they both have a high probability of transforming into invasive carcinoma if left untreated. They are associated with aneuploidy and infection with just one of the high-risk HPV types. Flat condylomas and CIN-1 are both associated with multiple infections from a heterogeneous group of HPV types and are grouped as low-grade CIN. This group has uncertain oncogenic potential. These lesions usually do not have any histological features that will progress to carcinoma and they generally either remain stable or regress. This classification reflects the fact that these lesions may involve two separate disease processes rather than a continuum as previously thought.

CIN-1 lesions have a spontaneous remission rate. Progression to CIN-3 or invasive carcinoma occurs in only 16% of cases. The average time to progression is 48 months. Because biopsy can eradicate the lesion, it is sometimes difficult to study. In CIN-3, it is generally agreed that patients will progress to invasive cancer. A range of 3–10 years has been reported for this to occur.

Preinvasive lesions are usually confined to the transformation zone of the cervix. This is a region in the cervical mucosa originally composed of columnar epithelial cells that are being replaced by squamous epithelium through the normal physiologic process of metaplasia. This change occurs most actively during fetal development, adolescence, and during the first pregnancy.

INVASIVE CERVICAL CARCINOMA

Invasive carcinoma develops when malignant epithelial cells break through the basement membrane and spread to the cervical stroma. As the malignancy grows it can produce a visible ulceration or an exophytic mass, or it may extensively infiltrate the endocervix, causing the cervix to expand and harden. The tumor usually presents as vaginal bleeding, frequently post-coital. A malodorous vaginal discharge becomes pronounced. The tumor then extends into the paracervical tissue, vagina, and endometrium. Inflammatory changes or tumor necrosis may produce a dull pain in the pelvic region.

Lateral extension of the disease to the pelvic wall often results in severe pain, and the lumbrosacral nerve and nerve root involvement causes pain resembling that of sciatica. Anterior tumor growth results in bladder involvement and symptoms of urinary frequency, hematuria, a vesicovaginal fistula, or obstructive uropathy. Posterior tumor growth causes rectal extension, which leads to tenesmus, rectal bleeding, or a rectovaginal fistula. Lymphatic spread occurs with sequential involvement of pelvic, para-aortic, mediastinal, and supraclavicular nodes. Hematogenous dissemination usually occurs late and most commonly involves the lungs, bones, and liver.[16]

SCREENING AND DIAGNOSIS

The Pap smear as a screening tool has been endorsed since 1945. The recommendation is to begin yearly screens as soon as sexually active or at the age of 18. After three normal Paps have occurred sequentially in 3 years then the frequency of the Pap and pelvic examination can be less, at the discretion of the physician. Most doctors recommend every other year.[17] The false-negative rate with the Pap has been reported to be 20%.[18] These errors are due to laboratory errors or inadequate sampling. The samples obtained are from the cervical surface with an Ayre spatula or from the endocervical canal using a cytobrush. These cells must undergo rapid fixation. The Pap is a screening tool and not a diagnostic procedure. A biopsy should be done on any visible lesion.

There are five groups within the cytologic classification system with a Pap smear. There are further CIN-based classification systems as well. The National Cancer Institute (NCI), the International Federation of Gynecology and Obstetrics (FIGO), and Bethesda systems have all made changes to the way Pap smears are reported.[19] The term squamous intraepithelial lesion (SIL) is used to refer to precursor lesions of invasive squamous-cell carcinoma. Low-grade SIL includes CIN-1 and cellular changes associated with HPV. High-grade SIL combines CIN-2 and CIN-3. This categorisa-

tion is based on the similarity in etiology, behavior, and treatment of the lesions within each group. Atypical squamous cells of undetermined significance (ASCUS) is a term used strictly for inflammatory or atrophic changes that truly are of unknown significance.

MANAGEMENT OF ABNORMAL SMEARS AND PREINVASIVE LESIONS

The main objective in the evaluation of Pap smears that are abnormal is to rule out invasive carcinoma and to determine the extent of noninvasive lesions. A colposcopy is usually performed first when further evaluation is required. This procedure involves the use of a stereotaxic microscope to examine the cervix. A 3% acetic acid solution applied to the cervix prior to the examination will cause epithelial lesions to turn white. The epithelial vascular distribution is also closely examined because it may be abnormal in the presence of CIN. This examination is considered adequate only if the entire transformation zone and any lesions that may be present are seen in their entirety. Otherwise, the presence of invasive cancer cannot be ruled out. Punch biopsies are done on areas with significant colposcopic abnormalities, and an endocervical curettage (ECC) is performed to evaluate the endocervical canal.

Some patients may require a cone biopsy (conisation), which involves the removal of a cone- or wedge-shaped section of the cervix. This is done using either a cold knife, electrosurgery, or laser surgery. Indications for conisation are:

- an inadequate colposcopic examination
- a positive ECC
- biopsy results showing microinvasive carcinoma or possible invasive carcinoma
- findings of a lesion on a Pap smear with a higher grade than that found in colposcopy.

Complications with this procedure include hemorrhage, cervical stenosis, or cervical incontinence. Laser conisation is a technically more difficult procedure but commonly results in fewer complications than a cold knife conisation. Laser conisation, however, may cause thermal damage to the margins of the specimen, making it difficult to know if the tumor is involved with the margins.

Fewer than 5% of patients with ASCUS have high-grade SIL on colposcopy. It is, therefore, common to defer this procedure initially and repeat a Pap in 4–6 months. If the atypical findings persist, then a colposcopy is needed.

Patients with a Pap smear showing low-grade SIL usually undergo a colposcopy. Some physicians will opt to manage these patients by repeating the Pap in 4 months.

Patients with high-grade SIL require a colposcopy. If the colposcopy confirms a high-grade lesion, then immediate treatment is necessary.

SIL can be treated with either ablative therapy with laser or cryotherapy or by excisional methods, which include shallow laser conisation or loop electrosurgical excision procedure (LEEP). LEEP uses thin wire loop electrodes to excise the entire transformation zone and any lesions it may contain.

Chinese medicine

These procedures cause blood stasis and it is therefore necessary to begin treatment for the pre-cancerous condition by preventing blood stasis and by working to expel the pathogen, which is stuck in either the qi level or the blood level.

STAGING

Staging is done according to the FIGO system. Staging occurs using findings from physical examination, colposcopy, biopsies, ECC, computerised tomography (CT), magnetic resonance imaging (MRI), intravenous pyelography (IVP), cystoscopy, and proctosigmoidoscopy.

Preinvasive carcinoma

- Stage 0: carcinoma in situ, intraepithelial carcinoma.

Invasive carcinoma

- Stage I: carcinoma is strictly confined to the cervix
  - Ia: invasive cancer identified only microscopically; all gross lesions, even with superficial invasion, are stage Ia
  - Ib cancers: invasion is limited to measured stromal invasion with a maximum depth of 5 mm and no wider than 7 mm

- Ia1: measured invasion of stroma no greater than 3 mm in depth and no wider than 7 mm
  - Ia2: measured invasion of stroma greater than 3 mm in depth and no greater than 5 mm in depth and no wider than 7 mm
  - Ib: clinical lesions confined to the cervix or preclinical lesions greater than Ia
  - Ib1: clinical lesions no greater than 4 mm in size
  - Ib2: clinical lesions greater than 4 mm in size.
- Stage II: carcinoma extends beyond the cervix but has not extended on to the pelvic wall; the carcinoma involves the vagina, but not as far as the lower third.
  - IIa: no obvious parametrial involvement
  - IIb: obvious parametrial involvement.
- Stage III: carcinoma has extended to the pelvic wall; on rectal examination, there is no cancer-free space between the tumor and the pelvic wall; the tumor involves the lower third of the vagina; all cases with a hydronephrosis or nonfunctioning kidney should be included, unless they are known to be due to another cause
  - IIIa: no extension onto the pelvic wall, but involvement of the lower third of the vagina
  - IIIb: extension onto the pelvic wall or hydronephrosis or nonfunctioning kidney.
- Stage IV: carcinoma has extended beyond the true pelvis or has clinically involved the mucosa of the bladder or rectum
  - IVa: spread of the growth to adjacent organs
  - IVb: spread to distant organs.

PROGNOSIS

The disease stage is an important factor, which affects long-term survival. Clinical stage correlates with tumor burden as well as the risk for lymph node and distant metastases.[20] Tumor size and volume, endometrial extension, and bilateral parametrial involvement are all prognostic factors.

Five-year survival ranges from 91% in patients with tumors <2.5 cm to 48% in patients with tumors >50 cm.[3] The histologic cell type helps determine prognosis as stated earlier. And the presence of periaortic and pelvic lymph node involvement also results in lower survival rates. A higher rate of recurrence is seen in patients with an S-phase fraction greater than or equal to 20%. The overexpression of *HER-2/neu* and *c-myc* oncogenes has been found to be associated with a poor prognosis.[21] In patients treated with radiation therapy, both anemia and thrombocytopenia have been associated with decreased survival rates.

Chinese medicine

Prognosis can be improved by working to clear the pathogen, preventing further blood stasis caused by conventional procedures, and by potentiation of radiation therapy with radiosensitising formulas.

TREATMENT

Surgery can be curative for patients with stage I and IIA disease. Pelvic exenteration is an option in some patients who develop central disease recurrence following radiation therapy. This includes removing the vagina, cervix, uterus, fallopian tubes, ovaries, bladder, and rectum. An anterior exenteration spares the rectum and may be used when disease recurrence is confined to the anterior vagina, cervix, or bladder.

Radiation is used as a primary treatment for all stages of cervical cancer. External and intracavitary irradiation is used for most stages except for stage IA, in which intracavitary radiation is adequate. External pelvic radiation is delivered by a linear accelerator. Brachytherapy is also used in various forms. An intrauterine tandem together with vaginal ovoids placed beside the cervix deliver radioactive isotopes via two separate brachytherapy insertions, which are given 1–3 weeks apart. Interstitial implants can also be used.

In patients with carcinoma in situ the treatment involves cryotherapy, LEEP, laser therapy, or conisation. A total abdominal or vaginal hysterectomy is the treatment of choice for women past the reproductive age, especially if the lesion involves the inner cone margin. In patients who have gone through these procedures, are free of signs in the cervix itself, but have evidence of spread to the vaginal wall, a topical chemotherapy called Efudex (fluorouracil) is applied to the affected areas once a week for 10 weeks.

In patients with stage IA disease the treatment is surgery. In stage IB and IIA some patients can be managed with radical hysterectomy or radiation therapy. In premenopausal or sexually active patients, surgery may be preferred because ovarian function and vaginal pliability can be preserved. Patients having stage IB disease and a tumor size >3 cm have lower recurrence rates when treated with radiation therapy than with surgery. Patients with IIA disease and extensive extracervical involvement should be treated with radiation therapy.

Stages IIB, III, and IV require radiation therapy. Concomitant use of hydroxyurea as a radiosensitiser results in an improved complete response, a longer progression-free interval, and a better survival rate in patients with stage IIIB and IVA.[22]

Patients with recurrent disease are generally treated with radiation therapy. Chemotherapy is also used for palliative therapy. Management during pregnancy varies according to the staging of the disease and the gestational age of the fetus. First trimester disease is treated as it would be without pregnancy and will result in termination of the pregnancy. Patients in the second trimester of pregnancy can delay treatment until fetal maturity is reached. Women with more advanced cancer should undergo immediate treatment.

When invasive carcinoma is found upon a simple hysterectomy, treatment depends on the extent of the disease.

Chemotherapy is sometimes used for cervical cancer. Because many patients who would ordinarily be considered candidates for chemotherapy present with impaired renal function, the use of some regimens is limited. Single agents used for more advanced disease are cisplatin and ifosfamide. Bleomycin, ifosfamide, and cisplatin are used together in patients with tumors located in tissue that was previously irradiated. Theoretically, toxic effects from neoadjuvant chemotherapy may prevent the delivery of adequate doses of radiation, and the issue of cross-resistance between these two modalities is problematic. Chemotherapy is considered more suitable when used with surgery and when other treatments have failed.

Intra-arterial chemotherapy should be possible and offer an advantage. However, response rates have not been shown to be superior to systemic chemotherapy.

Tumor regression continues for up to 6 months after a patient completes radiation therapy. The majority of recurrences occur in the first 2 years after treatment. Patients are evaluated every 3 months. Low-dose estrogen is used indefinitely if no contraindications are present. Sexual activity can be resumed after completion of radiation therapy. If the vagina has been irradiated, expanders must be used for a period of time to reduce atrophy from radiation. A vaginal dilator may be used to help in maintaining vaginal patency. This is important whether or not the patient intends to resume sexual activity. The atrophy and dryness can be severe enough to make walking difficult. Progesterone is omitted in patients who have had a hysterectomy. Estrogen-containing creams are used vaginally for patients who still have vaginal dryness and dyspareunia secondary to radiation therapy and loss of ovarian function.

Chinese medicine

The following herbs are commonly used as part of a formula to treat HPV infection specifically:

ren dong teng (Lonicerae Caulis; *Lonicera japonica*)
jin yin hua (Lonicerae Flos; *Lonicera* flowers)
lian qiao (Forsythiae fructus; *Forsythia*)
da suan (Allii sativi Bulbus; *Allium sativum*; garlic)
huang lian (Coptidis Rhizoma; *Coptis*)
huang qin (Scutellariae Radix; *Scutellaria baicalensis*)
ban lan gen (Isatidis/Baphicacanthis Radix; *Isatis/Baphicacanthus* root)
huang bai (Phellodendri Cortex; *Phellodendron* cortex)
ku shen (Sophorae flavescentis Radix; *Sophora flavescens*)
huo tan mu (Polygoni chinensis Herba; *Polygonum chinense*)
pu gong ying (Taraxaci Herba; *Taraxacum mongolicum*)
long kui (Solani nigri Herba; *Solanum nigrum*)
zi cao (Arnebiae/Lithospermi Radix; *Arnebia/Lithospermum* root)

bai hua she she cao (Hedyotis diffusae Herba; *Oldenlandia*)
ban mao (Mylabris; *Mylabris*)
bing lang (Arecae Semen; *Areca catechu*; betel nut)
tu bie chong (Eupolyphaga; *Eupolyphaga sinensis*)

These herbs are detoxifying, clear heat, transform phlegm, and are antineoplastic.

Combinations of these herbs are added to a formula that addresses the constitutional presentation and the Chinese diagnosis for the cancer of the patient. Obviously it is important to treat chronic viral infections and especially HPV and HSV in women. The powdered formula given later in this chapter is appropriate to use in a modified form as a vaginal suppository or on the end of a tampon to locally treat an HPV infection.

Formula for use during radiation therapy

The main injuries during radiation therapy are local tissue damage resulting in severe yin deficiency and blood stasis. The burning of tissue causes scarring, which is a form of blood stasis. These two factors can, in themselves, lead to the formation of malignancy. It is important to treat these side effects to prevent recurrence. It is also important to potentiate the radiation therapy, whether it be external beam, intraoperative, or brachytherapy. Radiation works best in the presence of highly oxygenated tissue. Most cancer cells are poorly oxygenated and live in a low-oxygen environment. Blood-regulating herbs increase circulation generally and also locally by breaking down the fibrinogen coating around some tumors, by 'cracking' the coagulation of blood in and around tumors, and by changing the viscosity of blood. These changes increase the oxygen supply to the tumor tissue and, in doing so, increase the oxygenation of the cancer cells making them more susceptible to radiation. The increase in oxygenation to local healthy tissue increases immunity and helps protect that tissue from the carcinogenic effect of the radiation.

The following formula clears heat at the qi and blood level, increases WBC counts to protect against abnormal cells and helps to flush tissue debris from cell die-off. It reduces swelling, generates fluids, and has a moderate antineoplastic effect.

jin yin hua (Lonicerae Flos; *Lonicera japonira*)	15 g
huang qi (Astragali Radix; *Astragalus membranaceus*)	15 g
bai hua she she cao (Hedyotis diffusae Herba; *Oldenlandia*)	30 g
tai zi shen (Pseudostellariae Radix; *Pseudostellaria heterophylla*)	15 g
zi cao (Arnebiae/Lithospermi Radix; *Arnebia/Lithospermum* root)	20 g
yi ren (Coicis Semen; *Coix lacryma-jobi*)	20 g
zhu ling (Polyporus; *Polyporus – Grifola*)	20 g
dan shen (Salviae miltiorrhizae Radix; *Salvia miltiorhiza* root)	15 g
fu ling (Poria; *Poria cocos*)	15 g
gou qi zi (Lycii Fructus; *Lycium chinensis* fruit)	15 g
bai zhu (Atractylodis macrocephalae Rhizoma; *Atractylodes macrocephala*)	15 g
jiao gu lan (Herba Gynostemmatis; *Gynostemma*)	15 g
bei sha shen (Glehniae Radix; *Glehnia*)	15 g
huang qin (Scutellariae Radix; *Scutellaria baicalensis*)	10 g

Several herbs in this formula clear heat and are antineoplastic. Jin yin hua, bai hua she she cao, qi ye dan, and huang qin, are all in this category of detoxifying and clear-heat herbs. Yi ren, dan shen, zhu ling, and huang qi potentiate radiation therapy. The rest of the herbs protect spleen function and nourish the yin and blood. Zi cao clears heat and cools the blood. It is an antifungal and is specific to vaginitis and cervicitis. It is also antineoplastic.

Radiation vaginitis

Radiation treatment can cause vaginal atrophy, which results in painful intercourse and ambulation. This can be persistent as sometimes radiation side effects can persist for several months and even years.

Vaginal douche

yi zhi huang hua (Solidaginis virgaureae Herba; *Solidago*; golden rod)

250 g decocted in 2000 ml water reduced to 1000 ml.

Oral decoction

yi ren (Coicis Semen; *Coix lacryma-jobi*)	30 g
bai zhu (Atractylodis macrocephalae Rhizoma; *Atractylodes macrocephala*)	15 g
yu zhu (Polygonati odorati Rhizoma; *Polygonatum odoratum*)	10 g
jin yin hua (Lonicerae Flos; *Lonicera*)	15 g
huang qin (Scutellariae Radix; *Scutellaria baicalensis*)	10 g
tai zi shen (Pseudostellariae Radix; *Pseudostellaria heterophylla*)	15 g

Yi zhi huang hua contains salicylic acid and quercitin and many polysaccharides. It is used in botanical medicine to treat many conditions including skin conditions. It promotes tissue repair, reduces inflammation, and is a radioprotective herb. It should not be used during radiation treatment but can be used afterwards. Yi ren enhances the effect of radiation while also repairing the inflammation and swelling that occurs as a result of radiation. It increases WBCs and NK cells and their activity in order to reduce the risk of infection and improve outcomes from this kind of treatment. Jin yin hua clears heat and reduces infection as does huang qin. Tai zi shen tonifies the qi and generates fluids. Yu zhu also generates fluids.

Accumulation of damp heat

Symptoms: odorous leukorrhea, lower abdominal pain, dark urine, possibly constipation, bitter taste, foul breath.

Tongue: dark red with possible greasy yellow coat.

Pulse: fast and wiry/slippery.

Treatment principle: clear heat, drain dampness, clear toxin, antineoplasm.

Formula:[23]

chong lou (Paridis Rhizoma; *Paris*)	15 g
bai hua she she cao (Hedyotis diffusae Herba; *Oldenlandia*)	25 g
ban zhi lian (Scutellariae barbatae Herba; *Scutellaria barbata*)	30 g
tu fu ling (Smilacis glabrae Rhizoma; *Smilax glabra*)	25 g
yi ren (Coicis Semen; *Coix lacryma-jobi*)	25 g

jiao gu lan (Herba Gynostemmatis;   20 g
   Gynostemma)

zhu ling (Polyporus; *Polyporus –*   15 g
   Grifola)

fu ling (Poria; *Poria cocos*)   15 g

bai zhu (Atractylodis macrocephalae   15 g
   Rhizoma; *Atractylodes*
   macrocephala)

huang qin (Scutellariae Radix;   10 g
   Scutellaria baicalensis)

jin yin hua (Lonicerae Flos; *Lonicera*)   15 g

tai zi shen (Pseudostellariae Radix;   15 g
   Pseudostellaria heterophylla)

shan yao (Dioscoreae Rhizoma;   15 g
   Dioscorea opposita)

yu jin (Curcumae Radix; *Curcuma*   15 g
   longa rhizome)

gan cao (Glycyrrhizae Radix;   5 g
   Glycyrrhiza; licorice root)

This is a strong formula for an aggressive tumor at a later stage. There are several antineoplastic herbs, including chong lou, bai hau she she cao, ban zhi lian, jiao gu lan, huang qin, jin yin hua. They all clear heat and toxin. The herbs that drain damp are yi ren, zhu ling and fu ling. These herbs are also antineoplastic by improving NK cell activity, increasing WBCs and phagocytosis, and they are also radiosensitising herbs. Tu fu ling reduces inflammation, clears damp heat toxins and is also antineoplastic. Tai zi shen tonifies qi while generating fluids, which is important in draining dampness and clearing heat. Shan yao tonifies the qi of the spleen and kidneys. Yu jin moves blood and circulates the liver qi in order to provide better access to the tumor for the herbs in the formula and cytotoxic agents like radiation or chemotherapy.

Toxin accumulation in the lower jiao due to damp heat in the liver channel

Symptoms: fishy smelling thick and sticky red vaginal discharge, profuse menstruation, lower abdominal pain, low back pain, frequent urination with urgency, constipation. This presentation has a stronger element of heat and the dampness has been congealed to some extent. This combination has led to bleeding, which is not present in the last presentation.
Tongue: crimson with yellow dry coat.

Pulse: wiry and rapid.
Treatment principle: drain damp, clear heat from the qi and blood levels, clear toxin, stop bleeding, antineoplasm.

Formula: Qing gan zhi li tang[24] with Long dan xie gan tang[25] jia jian

bai shao (Paeoniae Radix alba;   20 g
   Paeonia lactiflora root)

huang bai (Phellodendri Cortex;   10 g
   Phellodendron cortex)

mu dan pi (Moutan Cortex; *Paeonia*   20 g
   suffruticosa root cortex)

huai niu xi (Achyranthis bidentatae   15 g
   Radix; *Achyranthes* bidentata)

tong cao (Tetrapanacis Medulla;   10 g
   Tetrapanax papyriferus)

che qian zi (Plantaginis Semen;   20 g
   Plantago)

qu mai (Dianthi Herba; *Dianthus*)   10 g

zhi zi (Gardeniae Fructus; *Gardenia*   10 g
   fruit)

xian he cao (Agrimoniae Herba;   30 g
   Agrimonia pilosa var. *japonica*;
   agrimony)

tu fu ling (Smilacis glabrae   20 g
   Rhizoma; *Smilax glabra*)

chong lou (Paridis Rhizoma; *Paris*)   20 g

long dan cao (Gentianae Radix;   10 g
   Gentiana)

ze xie (Alismatis Rhizoma; *Alisma*)   10 g

dang gui (Angelicae sinensis Radix;   10 g
   Angelica sinensis)

e zhu (Curcumae Rhizoma; *Curcuma*   15 g
   zedoaria; zedoary)

Huang bai clears heat and dries dampness, especially lower jiao dampness. It works in consort with mu dan pi, which clears heat and cools the blood. This herb is antineoplastic, especially for blood stasis tumors and, by moving the blood, the herb helps the clearing and detoxifying herbs to enter the tumor. Huai niu xi is a blood-regulating herb that has many other useful properties in this case. It promotes urination and drains damp heat in the lower jiao and it conducts the downward movement of blood. It is especially useful in gynecological tumors. There are several drain-damp herbs that promote urination; tong cao, che qian zi, ze xie, and qu mai – which is also antineoplastic – all help to clear heat through urination. Zhi zi clears heat, drains dampness, cools the blood to stop bleeding, and is antineoplastic, especially for tumors where ascites is present. Tu fu ling clears damp heat toxins and is antineoplastic; it enters the liver channel, which is useful in cervical cancer. Xian he cao cools the blood to stop bleeding and is antineoplastic. Long dan cao also clears heat and dries dampness but cannot be used in the long term because of its especially cold nature. Dang gui and e zhu complement one another by nourishing and moving the blood. E zhu is especially antineoplastic for cervical cancer. Chong lou is the main primary antineoplastic in the formula and is potentiated by the heat-clearing and toxin-clearing herbs surrounding it. This is a strong formula that would need to be adjusted in a patient with spleen deficiency or yang deficiency. The herbs in this formula can potentiate radiation therapy or chemotherapy with moderate modification.

Spleen and kidney deficiency due to residual damp toxin

Symptoms: fishy smelling clear and thin vaginal discharge, cold and aching low back and abdomen, night sweats, low-grade afternoon fever, five center heat, dizziness and insomnia, loose stools, frequent urination and nocturia. This is a mixed presentation with spleen and kidney yang deficiency with kidney yin deficiency. In later-stage disease it is common to see these mixed signs.

Tongue: red with little coat.

Pulse: deep, thready and forceless and rapid.

Treatment principles: tonify spleen and kidney yang, nourish the yin and blood, clear heat from the blood, drain damp, clear heat and antineoplasm.

Formula: Gui pi tang[26] plus Liang di tang ji nei bu wan[27] jia jian

huang qi (Astragali Radix; *Astragalus membranaceus*)	30 g
dang shen (Codonopsis Radix; *Codonopsis pilosula* root)	20 g
bai zhu (Atractylodis macrocephalae Rhizoma; *Atractylodes macrocephala*)	10 g
nu zhen zi (Ligustri lucidi Fructus; *Ligustrum lucidum* fruit)	10 g
han lian cao (Ecliptae Herba; *Eclipta prostrata*)	10 g
e jiao (Asini Corii Colla; *Equus asinus*; donkey-hide gelatin)	10 g
dang gui (Angelicae sinensis Radix; *Angelica sinensis*)	10 g
he shou wu (Polygoni multiflori Radix preparata; *Polygonum multiflorum* root)	20 g
sheng di huang (Rehmanniae Radix; *Rehmannia*)	20 g
di gu pi (Lycii Cortex; *Lycium*)	30 g
xuan shen (Scrophulariae Radix; *Scrophularia*)	10 g
bai shao (Paeoniae Radix alba; *Paeonia lactiflora* root)	20 g
mai dong (Ophiopogonis Radix; *Ophiopogon*)	10 g
tu si zi (Cuscutae Semen; *Cuscuta* seeds)	20 g
rou cong rong (Cistanches Herba; *Cistanche*)	20 g
rou gui (Cinnamomi Cortex; *Cinnamomum cassia* cortex)	5 g
e zhu (Curcumae Rhizoma; *Curcuma zedoaria*; zedoary)	10 g
bai hua she she cao (Hedyotis diffusae Herba; *Oldenlandia*)	20 g
zhu ling (Polyporus; *Polyporus – Grifola*)	30 g

Huang qi, dang shen, and bai zhu are modified components of Si jun zi tang to tonify the qi. This provides a good basis to drain dampness. Nu zhen zi, han lian cao, and mai dong nourish the yin to potentiate the blood that has been injured. E jiao, dang gui, he shou wu, bai shao, and sheng di huang all nourish the blood to potentiate the yin that has been injured. Xuan shen and sheng di huang also clear heat from the blood. Di gu pi also clears heat from the blood and is antifungal (HPV). Tu si zi and rou cong rong are warming-kidney-yang-tonic herbs. Rou cong rong also nourishes the blood and tu si zi also warms the kidneys and spleen to treat loose stools due to spleen and kidney yang deficiency and to aid in reducing fluid loss through urination. Rou gui generates qi and blood and leads the fire back to Mingmen. It is a very warming herb that is useful in reducing blood stasis swellings. E zhu vitalises the blood and is especially antineoplastic against cervical cancer. Bai hua she she cao is a clear-heat and clear-toxin herb that is also antineoplastic. Zhu ling not only drains damp but also increases immunity. Since this cancer is often treated with radiation, zhu ling is a vital herb to add since it potentiates radiation therapy.

Liver kidney yin deficiency

Symptoms: stage II to IV; dizziness, bitter taste, dry throat, more severe pain in pelvic area, low back pain, five center heat, constipation due to radiation and obstructive disease, leukorrhea, vaginal bleeding.
Tongue: crimson without coat.
Pulse: thready rapid, may be taut from pain.
Treatment principle: nourish the yin of the liver and kidney, clear toxic heat, antineoplasm.

Formula

mai dong (Ophiopogonis Radix; *Ophiopogon*)	15 g
bei sha shen (Glehniae Radix; *Glehnia*)	15 g
shu di (Rehmanniae Radix preparata; *Rehmannia*)	15 g
mu dan pi (Moutan Cortex; *Paeonia suffruticosa* root cortex)	10 g
ze xie (Alismatis Rhizoma; *Alisma*)	15 g
fu ling (Poria; *Poria cocos*)	15 g
zhi mu (Anemarrhenae Rhizoma; *Anemarrhena*)	15 g
huang bai (Phellodendri Cortex; *Phellodendron* cortex)	10 g
jiao gu lan (Herba Gynostemmatis; *Gynostemma*)	15 g
gou qi zi (Lycii Fructus; *Lycium chinensis* fruit)	10 g
tai zi shen (Pseudostellariae Radix; *Pseudostellaria heterophylla*)	15 g
shi hu (Dendrobii Herba; *Dendrobium*)	10 g
yu zhu (Polygonati odorati Rhizoma; *Polygonatum odoratum*)	15 g
bai hua she she cao (Hedyotis diffusae Herba; *Oldenlandia*)	30 g
long kui (Solani nigri Herba; *Solanum nigrum*)	25 g

This formula includes Liu wei di huang wan, which nourishes the liver and kidney yin. Additional herbs have been added that also nourish the yin, reduce thirst, tonify the qi, while benefiting the fluids and act against the neoplasm. Long kui is especially antineoplastic against cervical cancer. It can be used as an application on a tampon to be used several times per week for several weeks.

Spleen and kidney yang deficiency

Symptoms: late-stage presentation, weakness, cachexia, anemia, pale, pain, aversion to cold, tenesmus, bloody leukorrhea, changes in stool, ascites and lower extremity edema may be severe.
Tongue: swollen and pale, may have thick white slimy coat that may be candidiasis.
Pulse: deep, thready, slow.
Treatment principle: warm the kidneys, transform fluids if necessary, tonify the spleen, antineoplasm.

Formula

huang qi (Astragali Radix; *Astragalus membranaceus*)	20 g
dang shen (Codonopsis Radix; *Codonopsis pilosula* root)	15 g
bai zhu (Atractylodis macrocephalae Rhizoma; *Atractylodes macrocephala*)	15 g
fu ling (Poria; *Poria cocos*)	15 g
bu gu zhi (Psoraleae Fructus; *Psoralea*)	15 g
sheng ma (Cimicifugae Rhizoma; *Cimicifuga*)	15 g
suan zao ren (Ziziphi spinosae Semen; *Ziziphus spinosa* seed)	10 g
ji xue teng (Spatholobi Caulis; *Spatholobus suberectus*)	30 g
gou qi zi (Lycii Fructus; *Lycium chinensis* fruit)	15 g
shu di (Rehmanniae Radix preparata; *Rehmannia*)	15 g
dang gui (Angelicae sinensis Radix; *Angelica sinensis*)	10 g
fu zi (Aconiti Radix preparata; *Aconitum carmichaelii*)	6 g
long yan rou (Longan Arillus; *Dimocarpus longan* aril)	15 g
gan cao (Glycyrrhizae Radix; *Glycyrrhiza*; licorice root)	6 g

The first four herbs are Si jun zi tang, the main qi tonic formula for the spleen. Bu gu zhi, and long yan rou are both kidney yang tonic herbs that warm the source and help reduce diarrhea and increase the kidneys' ability to transform and move fluids. This supports fluid metabolism and reduces ascites and edema. Sheng ma lifts the yang and helps support spleen qi to transport and transform fluids. Spleen support is important to treat cachexia, a condition in which the body begins to metabolise its muscle mass for organ support. Many patients with advanced disease do not die of cancer but rather from malnourishment. Suan zao ren calms the spirit and reinforces the yin and blood. It should be used carefully as it also moistens the stool and can exacerbate diarrhea or loose stool caused by spleen and kidney yang deficiency. Here it also protects the yin in a formula that is very warming. Ji xue teng, gou qi zi, shu di, and dang gui all nourish the blood to contain the blood in bloody leukorrhea and to treat the anemias present from malnutrtion. Fu zi rescues the yang to draw back the kidney fire, the source. It is especially good for alleviating diarrhea, warming the channels and relieving pain. Gan cao is a harmonising herb but can also work with rou gui (*Cinnamomum* bark) to enter the channels and relieve pain.

Local application

This formula is powdered and applied either on the end of a dampened tampon or made into a cocoa butter suppository to be applied directly against the cervical carcinoma after conisation or colposcopy. It is meant to prevent exfoliation and necrosis after the procedure and has been studied in China. After using this technique in 220 women and following these women for 10 years there was no recurrence of cervical dysplasia or HPV infection. It is important to use a tampon that is made from pure cotton and without contamination from talc.

It is suggested that a powered form of e zhu (*Curcuma zedoaria*) plus long kui (*Solanum nigrum*) be used. The amounts should be equal. The powder should be as fine as possible.

A similar application contains:

zi cao (Arnebiae/Lithospermi Radix; *Arnebia/Lithospermum* root)	30 g
zi hua di ding (Violae Herba; *Viola yedoensis*)	30 g
cao he che (Bistortae Rhizoma; *Polygonum bistorta*)	30 g
huang bai (Phellodendri Cortex; *Phellodendron* cortex)	30 g
han lian cao (Ecliptae Herba; *Eclipta prostrata*)	30 g
bing pian (Borneolum; *Dryobalanops aromatica*; borneol)	3 g

All of the above are ground into a fine powder, placed in a fine wrapper and autoclaved. This material is then applied on a tampon as described above. An alternative form of topical application is the infusion of these same herbs in cocoa butter at a very low heat for 1 hour. This is then refrigerated in a form mold to stiffen the product into suppositories. These are applied at night-time while the patient is in recumbent.

Another mode of delivery applicable for cervical cancer that is more advanced in stage is that of a retention enema. The Shuangzi powder can be used and delivered via this method. Any of the above formulas can be used in this manner with the net effect of a larger amount of phytochemical material delivered more locally by using the bowel wall. This highly vascularised surface allows for the transference of more active ingredients into the lower abdominal cavity. The effectiveness of this method involves not only higher levels of herbal drugs but also the localised anti-neoplastic function of the herbs and the immune enhancement capacities of herbs to help prevent metastatic spread. The formula utilised for an individual patient must, therefore, be written specifically for the presentation and staging of the patient.

UTERINE CANCER

Endometrial cancer is the most common pelvic cancer in women. The mortality is low primarily because the cancer is found when it is still confined to the uterus. This cancer occurs 75% of the time in postmenopausal women. Only 4% of women who are diagnosed with this cancer are younger than 40 years at the time of diagnosis. Tumors of the uterus include adenocarcinomas and their variants, and sarcomas.

There seem to be two types of endometrial cancer: type I, which is estrogen related, and type II, which is estrogen independent. The estrogen-related tumors are better differentiated and are usually grade 1 and stage 1. The estrogen-independent tumors are often poorly differentiated, present at an advanced stage, and occur in patients who are older (mean age is 66). There are some unfavorable subtypes, such as serous carcinoma, adenosquamous carcinoma, and clear cell carcinoma. These are all estrogen-independent.

Conditions resulting from hyperestrinism predispose patients to endometrial carcinoma. Obesity increases the risk 3- to 10-fold depending on the weight excess. Adipose tissue contains aromatase enzymes that convert adrenal-derived androstenedione to estrone, which can then be converted to estradiole, which is a more potent estrogen. This results in endometrial proliferation, hyperplasia, and possibly carcinoma. Polycystic ovarian syndrome (POS), which is characterised by obesity, anovulation, abnormal bleeding or amenorrhea, hirsutism, and polycystic ovaries, increases the risk of endometrial cancer. Anovulation results in prolonged periods of estrogen exposure unopposed by a progestational agent. Infertility is also associated with this carcinoma. Unopposed contraceptives are recognised as another predisposing factor. Please see Chapter 4 on breast cancer for an in-depth discussion of estrogenic and xenoestrogenic exposures and cancer of glandular tissues.

Hyperplasia is an important characteristic that correlates with low tumor grade and lack of myometrial (muscle) invasion. Hyperplasia is divided into simple – which rarely progresses to carcinoma; complex – which also rarely progresses to malignancy; and atypical – which carries a higher risk of 10–30% for malignant transformation. Tamoxifen is a known causative factor in uterine cancer.[28]

Chinese medicine

Obesity contributes to uterine cancer because fat cells are repositories for estrogen or xenoestrogenic molecules. Therefore, the bottom line in terms of pathogenesis is an inverted fire toxin. It is very much the same as in breast cancer. The sources of the exposures are also the same.

DIAGNOSIS

Screening of high-risk groups for uterine cancer is appropriate. High-risk groups include women who are postmenopausal and are being treated with exogenous estrogens, particularly if they are obese and began menopause after the age of 50 years, or have polycystic ovarian disease, or a family history of breast, endometrial, or ovarian cancer. Women with a family history of hereditary nonpolyposis colorectal cancer are also at higher risk. In families with this syndrome, uterine cancer is the most common extracolonic malignancy.[29]

About 50% of women with endometrial cancer have a positive Pap smear. Endometrial tissue in a Pap implies endometrial pathology. Dilatation and curettage (D&C) will provide enough tissue to analyse for cancer, and this technique is 90% accurate.

CLINICAL PRESENTATION

Abnormal vaginal bleeding will be present in 90% of patients. In more advanced cases, pelvic pain and leukorrhea may occur. Patients are frequently obese, hypertensive, and postmenopausal. An enlarged uterus and ascites may occur.

Adenocarcinomas are the most common uterine cancer. These are classified into three grades from well-differentiated in 75% of cases, to poorly differentiated, in which the glandular structure is overgrown by epithelium.

There are variants of adenocarcinoma. Uterine papillary serous carcinoma is similar in clinical behavior to ovarian papillary serous carcinoma. More than 50% of patients with stage 1 uterine papillary serous carcinoma have a relapse outside the pelvis and in the abdomen. This type of uterine cancer is a virulent subtype of adenocarcinoma. It carries a poor prognosis, a high relapse rate, a propensity for transperitoneal seeding, and usually more advanced disease at the time of diagnosis. This type is treated with surgery, careful staging and adjuvant therapy, including radiation and chemotherapy.[30]

STAGING AND PROGNOSIS

Staging, including the grade, is the most important prognostic factor. Other factors can include age and vascular space invasion. Pelvic lymph node metastasis is increased many-fold if the vascular space has been invaded with tumor. Estrogen and progesterone receptor status is inversely proportional to tumor stage, grade, and depth of invasion. Tumor grade and stage and invasiveness correlate with expression of several oncogenes, including *fms, neu, fos, myb, erb-B,* and *myc.* Some growth factors are also implicated.[31]

The FIGO system of staging is as follows:

- Ia: tumor limited to endometrium.
- Ib: invasion to 50% or less of myometrium.
- Ic: invasion to more than 50% of myometrium.
- IIa: endocerical glandular involvement only.
- IIb: cervical stroma invasion.
- IIIa: tumor invasion of serosa and/or adnexa, and/or positive peritoneal cytology.
- IIIb: vaginal metastases.
- IIIc: metastases to pelvic and/or para-aortic lymph nodes.
- IVa: tumor invasion of bladder and/or bowel mucosa.
- IVb: distant metastases, including intra-abdominal and/or inguinal lymph node.

TREATMENT

In stage I and II disease, all patients should undergo a total abdominal hysterectomy and bilateral salpingo-oophorectomy. Peritoneal washings are taken from the pelvis, the paracolic gutters (running alongside the large bowel), and subdiaphragmatic region. The uterus is examined for depth of invasion. Pelvic and para-aortic lymph nodes are examined if there is grade 3 lesion, adenosquamous, clear cell, or serous tumor, if the myometrial invasion is more than 50%, or if there is cervical extension of the tumor. Disease will have spread to pelvic or para-aortic lymph nodes in fewer than 1% of patients with disease limited to the endometrium.

Patients with this stage disease and a grade 2 tumor may receive intravaginal radiation, which reduces the vaginal recurrence rate from 14% to 1.7%. Patients with grade 3 disease and invasion into the myometrium, with cervical extension and positive lymph nodes, usually receive external beam pelvis irradiation.

Stage II disease can be confused with stage Ib disease of the cervix. Differentiating factors are that endometrial cancer typically occurs in an elderly woman with a bulky uterus, whereas cervical cancer occurs in a younger woman with a normal-sized uterus but a bulky cervix. Seed implants are often used in this stage of disease.

Stage III disease is less common, and treatment is often individualised. Parametrial involvement is determined surgically and has a 5-year survival rate of 40%. Abdominal recurrence occurs in 80% of patients but is not confined to the abdomen and so whole abdominal radiation is rare.

Stage IV treatment is designed only for palliation, and includes irradiation and brachytherapy. Often in cases of endometrial cancer following a hysterectomy, the hysterectomy is performed for reasons other than cancer, the uterus is not opened, and proper staging following positive findings does not occur. If this is the case, then surgery is performed again to remove any residual reproductive tissues and any other gross disease. Then external beam radiation is carried out to the whole pelvis, or treatment is based on the surgical findings.

In recurrent disease, treatment can be based in hormonal therapy. Lupron, goserelin (Zoladex), and medroxyprogesterone acetate are progestational agents used as antitumor treatments. In patients with negative receptor status, with an undifferentiated tumor, and who are in poor condition with a rapidly advancing tumor where there is no time to await the results of hormonal manipulation, then chemotherapy is used palliatively. Cisplatin, doxorubicin, carboplatin, paclitaxel (Taxol), cyclophosphamide, and altretamine (Hexalen) are all possibilities. Response rates are between 20% and 50%.[32]

Uterine sarcomas are rare heterogeneous tumors that account for only 3% of all uterine neoplasms in White women and 10% in Black women. They are treated with various chemotherapeutic regimens. The primary treatment is total surgical excision. Frequently used chemotherapy agents for this type are dacarbazine, dactinomycin, vincristine, or ifosfamide; in other words, those chemotherapies commonly used to treat soft-tissue sarcomas.

Chinese medicine

Endometrial cancers are phlegm damp tumors with blood stasis. The nature of the uterus is phlegm and dampness. Ovarian, cervical and uterine malignancies all occur in similar fast-turnover tissues. These organs have epithelial and secretory components. Organs that have epithelial tissues tend to slough off tissue almost continuously. There is a cycle built into the tissue that has a sloughing nature. Glandular tissues like these are emblematic of this fact of nature. The nature of these tissues can be easily altered by several influences including external exposures that interrupt their natural cycles and internal exposures that contribute to a promoting environment. The uterus also has a strong relationship with blood and is a very highly vascularised tissue. Since phlegm and dampness have a relationship with obesity, women who are overweight or obese have a propensity to sinking spleen qi behaviors and the end results of these behaviors. Fatty tissue stores estrogen and xenoestrogens. A diet high in animal fat, in the form of red meats and dairy products, contributes to estrogenic exposures that are proliferative in these glandular phlegm damp tissues that already turnover rapidly. Obesity provides a medium of sinking spleen qi, which is damp in nature; the uterus can become bulky,

fatty, and also a storage site for estrogen that then releases and increases systemic estrogen.

The uterus can also become exposed to several of the same factors that have been implicated in ovarian and cervical cancer. There do not appear to be links with viral factors, but there may be links with talc and asbestos entering through the dilated cervical canal. It is currently unknown if and how multiple external hits may link with the internal environment to create a latent pathogenic factor that requires both external and internal components in order to evolve.

The treatment for uterine cancer is not unlike that for cervical cancer, except that the emphasis is not on clearing a viral pathogen but rather on transforming phlegm and dampness with anti-neoplastic herbs, lifting the spleen qi, interfacing with conventional treatment, and supporting the patient to exercise, change the diet, lose weight, and make general lifestyle changes.

Case study 6.1

This case involves a patient who was diagnosed with stage IIIb squamous cell carcinoma of the cervix. She had one child from a previous marriage, and for 14 years had partnered with a woman. Because of this change in her life she had erroneously thought that Pap screening was no longer necessary because she had no male sexual partner. She had not had a Pap smear for 15 years when she was diagnosed. However, prior to discontinuing gynecological screening, she had a history of 8 years of abnormal Pap smears with a history of HPV. Unfortunately, she was not adequately informed by past healthcare providers that close monitoring was necessary, given the HPV status.

At the time she presented she was 47 years of age. She was otherwise in good health. She had a large necrotic tumor involving the entire cervix and the right vaginal fornix. The pelvic side-wall had adhesions and was very tender to palpation. There was a moderate amount of bleeding that began with very gentle examination. She originally presented with pelvic and low back pain with

irregular menstrual bleeding. The first time she was seen in my office, she began hemorrhaging spontaneously without any palpation. Her vagina was packed with gauze and with a compression bandage and she was immediately sent to the emergency room.

General signs and symptoms

- Appetite: poor, nothing is interesting, trying to change diet but tired of eating well, craves sugar.
- Digestion
  - above the navel: belching
  - below the navel: bloating, cramping, pain.
- Stools: intermittent diarrhea and constipation, hot type diarrhea, frequent, dark color even with vegetarian diet.
- Thirst: constant.
- Sweats: mild night sweats on occasion.
- Temperature: running cold even with heat signs.
- Cough: none.

Case study continues

- Fevers: yes; neutropenic fevers; no infection; fevers that are intermittent, especially in the late afternoon.
- Headaches: none.
- Sleep: poor due to pain and anxious thoughts about her daughter, who is still young.
- Pain: lower abdominal and low back pain with sciatica-like symptoms down both legs.
- Skin color: yellow/green.
- Skin: very dry and 'thin'.
- Extremities: there is pitting edema on both lower extremities up to the knee.
- Hair: fallen out due to chemotherapy.
- Energy: 3/10 for her; very poor in the late afternoon.
- Tongue: red and dry with no coat; not swollen; vein distention gross +4 and very dark, venules running off main vein.
- Pulse: thready on the surface caving in to soft and then flat; the yang pulses are thready, the doyo is almost gone, the yin pulses are non-existent; the lowest pulse is the spleen.
- Hara spleen reflex: very hot to touch.
- Liver reflex on right: very tender and tight.
- Palpable lumps across the abdomen, especially over the bladder in the kidney reflex area, which is hot and hard.
- Stomach reflex area is flaccid and caved in, it is neither hot nor cold.
- WBCs: 1.2.
- RBCs: 2.9.
- Haematocrit: 24.
- Platelets: 138 000.
- Liver and kidney functions: close to normal.
- LDH: high.

Diagnosis

This was spleen and kidney yin and yang deficiency. It was exacerbated by the fact that the patient was already undergoing treatment. Many of the above signs and symptoms were the result of current and past treatment. She had undergone external beam pelvic irradiation. The tumor was pressing on the right ureter and a stent had been placed to relieve hydronephrosis. A fentanyl patch was placed over the site of worst pain on the right St 25. Radioisotopes were implanted

(brachytherapy) after three courses of cisplatin and 5-FU were given to act as radiosensitising agents for the seed implants. The hope was for at least a 50% response rate, but the 5-year survival rate for this stage of disease is very low.

Treatment principles

The patient was unable to eat well; she was showing signs of exhaustion. Her sleep was disturbed by pain and anxiety. The doyo, or middle pulse, was barely palpable, which is a very poor sign. She had a large and necrotic tumor that had invaded her abdomen. She was very anemic and approaching the transfusable range. Pain was a major problem and not well controlled. Treatment for this cancer now rested on the effectiveness of the brachytherapy. In such cases, the question becomes one of how strong a treatment can be given to this patient without undermining her body's ability to survive and to metabolise herbal medicine and utilise it to potentiate the radiation. Regarding all of the possible elements to be addressed in this case, which are the most crucial? Should the focus be one of palliation or aiming for cure?

Besides the struggle for life, so many different considerations come into play in an individual diagnosed with a later stage cancer, especially a younger patient. This is one reason why this case was included. In younger women with children, often the primary goal is to survive for one's children, and the sense of responsibility to live for one's children cannot be put into words. The responsibility to one's children commonly outweighs the struggle for life for oneself. This patient wanted to live to be there for her daughter at all of the landmarks of life. She felt an immense responsibility to be alive to care for her child. And so this drove the decision to do whatever it took to potentiate the radiation. She became even more strongly dedicated to lifestyle changes, and made a trip to the Chipsa Hospital in Tijuana to undergo Gerson treatment there. This included daily coffee enemas, juice fasting, vegetarian diet, protein restriction, and some supplementation.[33] This treatment was very time- and energy-intensive

Case study continues

and proved to be very exhausting for this patient with late-stage disease.

At the same time as the patient was undergoing Gerson therapy, she was also taking a modified version of the radiation formula. Portions of the spleen and kidney yin and yang pattern formula were added. There was concern that this pattern, already present in a patient with advanced disease, would be exacerbated by the strict dietary regimen of the Gerson treatment. She had been through several rounds of a chemotherapeutic regimen known for its toxicity, the seed implants were still in place and manifesting an ongoing cytotoxic effect. The edema was worsening and demonstrated a level of spleen and kidney deficiency that warranted extreme caution regarding the nutritional status of the patient. The raw foods diet may have been more than this patient could metabolise and assimilate. The herbs added to the radiation potentiating formula were:

huang qi (Astragali Radix; *Astragalus membranaceus*)	20 g
dang shen (Codonopsis Radix; *Codonopsis pilosula* root)	15 g
nu zhen zi (Ligustri lucidi Fructus; *Ligustrum lucidum* fruit)	15 g
ji xue teng (Spatholobi Caulis; *Spatholobus suberectus*)	20 g
di gu pi (Lycii Cortex; *Lycium*)	10 g
dong chong xia cao (Cordyceps; *Cordyceps*)	10 g
e zhu (Curcumae Rhizoma; *Curcuma zedoaria*; zedoary)	15 g
bai hua she she cao (Hedyotis diffusae Herba; *Oldenlandia*)	20 g
zhu ling (Polyporus; *Polyporus – Grifola*)	25 g

Huang qi and dang shen tonify the qi of the spleen and the zheng qi. This supports one aspect of fluid metabolism. It improves appetite and helps the spleen function to metabolise and assimilate nutrition. The raw food diet drives the need to support the spleen, which prefers a warm and mildly cooked food diet. Dang shen and nu zhen zi are synergistic and work together to improve WBC and RBC counts. Ji xue teng is a blood-regulating herb that is especially good in treating anemias by nourishing and harmonising the blood while moving the blood. It is also mildly analgesic. Di gu

pi clears heat and cools the blood. It helps to reduce fevers, is antibacterial and antifungal, and helps to increase weight. Neutropenic fevers are often a result of yin and qi deficiency. Huang qi and dang shen treat the qi deficient aspect of the fevers and nu zhen zi treats the yin deficient aspect. Dong chong xia cao enters the kidneys and strengthens the source qi. It is antineoplastic and is commonly used to rehabilitate normal function after serious illness. It is used to stop bleeding, is antibiotic and antifungal. E zhu and bai hua she she cao are the antineoplastics in the formula. E zhu is especially antitumor for cervical cancer. Zhu ling is a mushroom that strongly potentiates radiation therapy and increases WBCs, phagocytosis, and is mildly analgesic. It drains damp and supports the spleen and kidneys to control the accumulation of fluids in the form of lower extremity edema.

This patient also retained the services of a psychic during the end of her treatment. The patient was informed by the psychic that she had a parasitic infection in her large bowel and that this was the cause of her cancer. A theory of cancer pathogenesis regarding parasitic overgrowth and toxicity does exist. The patient was placed on a herbal regimen to kill and flush the parasites from her body. While doing so she continued on her Chinese herbal formula but the course of treatment had shifted away from Chinese medicine and the patient rarely came for follow-up. After the course of treatment from the psychic, which took 3 months, the patient was told she no longer had cancer. As a result, she discontinued all treatment. However, the lower extremity edema worsened, the pain worsened, the masses in her abdomen enlarged and spread.

With extreme edema, abdominal ascites, and precipitous organ failure beginning with kidney failure, the patient died 3 months later. She weighed 100 lb over her average weight; most of the weight was confined to her legs, which were grossly edemic due to obstructive disease caused by loss of venous return and because of severe kidney failure. The many difficult challenges from the beginning of this case made this a terribly problematic case for treatment. The path for her providers was less one of treatment and more one of compassion.

References

1. Devesa SS. Cancer incidence and mortality trends among whites in the United States, 1947–84. J Natl Cancer Inst 1994; 79:701–770.
2. Guzick DS. Efficacy of screening for cervical cancer: a review. Am J Public Health 1978; 68:125–134.
3. Wingo PA. Cancer statistics, 1995. CA Cancer J Clin 1995; 45:8–30.
4. Parkin DM. Cancer incidence in five continents, volume VI. Lyon: International Agency for Research on Cancer; 1992.
5. Zaino RJ. Histopathologic predictors of the behaviour of surgically treated stage IB squamous cell carcinoma of the cervix: a Gynecologic Oncology Study Group study. Cancer 1992; 69:1750–1758.
6. Greer BE. Stage IB adenocarcinoma treated by radical hysterectomy and pelvic lymph node dissection. Am J Obstet Gynecol 1989; 160:1509–1514.
7. Hale RJ. Prognostic factors in uterine cervical carcinoma: a clinicpathological analysis. Int J Gynecol Cancer 1991; 1:19–23.
8. Maier RC. Glassy cell carcinoma of the cervix. Obstet Gynecol 1982; 60:219–224.
9. Harris RWC. Characteristics of women with dysplasia or carcinoma in situ of the cervix uteri. Br J Cancer 1980; 42:359–369.
10. Schiffman MH. Epidemiologic evidence showing that human papillomavirus infection causes most cervical intraepithelial neoplasia. J Natl Cancer Inst 1993; 85:958–964.
11. Lorincz AT. Human papillomavirus infection of the cervix: relative risk associations of 15 common anogenital types. Obstet Gynecol 1992; 79:328–337.
12. Schneider V. Immunosupression as a high-risk factor in the development of condyloma acuminatum and squamous neoplasia of the cervix. Acta Cytol 1983; 27:220–224.
13. Maiman M. Human immunodeficiency virus infection and invasive cervical carcinoma. Cancer 1993; 71:401–406.
14. Verson SD. The HIV-1 tat protein enhances E2-dependent human papillomavirus 16 transcription. Virus Res 1993; 27:133–145.
15. Burger MPM. Cigarette smoking and human papillomavirus in patients with reported cervical cytological abnormality. Br Med J 1993; 306:749–752.
16. Carlson V. Distant metastasis in squamous-cell carcinoma of the uterine cervix. Radiology 1967; 88:961–966.
17. Fink DJ. Change in the American Cancer Society checkup guidelines for detection of cervical cancer. Cancer 1988; 38:127.
18. Gay JD. False-negative results in cervical cytologic studies. Acta Cytol 1985; 29:1043–1046.
19. Ismail SM. Reporting cervical intraepithelial neoplasia (CIN): intra- and interpathologist variation and factors associated with disagreement. Histopathology 1990; 16:371–376.
20. Fagundes H. Distant metastases after irradiation alone in carcinoma of the uterine cervix. Int J Radiat Oncol Biol Phys 1992; 24:197–204.
21. Berchuk A. Expression of epidermal growth factor receptor and HER-2/neu in normal and neoplastic cervix, vulva and vagina. Obstet Gynecol 1990; 76:381–387.
22. Stehman FR. A randomized trial of hydroxyurea versus misonidazole adjunct to radiation therapy in carcinoma of the cervix: a preliminary report. A Gynecologic Oncology study. Am J Obstet Gynecol 1988; 159:87–94.
23. Sun, Gui Zhi. Kang Ai Zhong Yao Fang xuan (Treatment of cancer with Chinese herbal medicine); 1992.
24. Lang, Weijian. Kang Ai Zhong Yao Yi Qian Fang (One thousand anti-cancer formulas). Beijing: China TCM Publishing house; 1996.
25. Wang Ang. Yi Fang Ji Jie (Analytic collection of formulas); 1682 ACE.
26. Yan, Yong He. Ji Sheng Fang (Formulas to aid the living); 1253 ACE.
27. Li, Peiwen. Ai Zhong De Zhong Xi Yi Zui Xin Dui Ce (New cancer strategies in Chinese and Western medicine). Beijing: China TCM Publishing House; 1995.
28. Seachrist L. Restating the risks of tamoxifen. Science 1994; 263:910–911.
29. Watson P. The risk of endometrial cancer in hereditary nonpolyposis colorectal cancer. Am J Med 1994; 96:516–520.
30. Mallipeddi P. Long-term survival with adjuvant whole abdominopelvic irradiation for uterine papillary serous carcinoma. Cancer 1993; 71:3076–3081.
31. Frank AH. Adjuvant whole abdominal radiation therapy in uterine papillary serous carcinoma. Cancer 1991; 68:1516–1519.
32. Burke TW. Treatment of advanced or recurrent endometrial carcinoma with single agent carboplatin. Gynecol Oncol 1993; 51:397–400.
33. James N. Mexico: juices, coffee enemas, and cancer. Lancet 1990; 336:677–678.

Chapter 7

Ovarian Cancer

CHAPTER CONTENTS

Epidemiology   195

Etiology   195

Screening   196

Biology, tumor markers and
    pathogenesis   196

Pathology   197

Staging   197

Treatment   198
    Biological therapies   199

Ovarian cancer in pregnancy   200

Chinese medicine   200
    Anatomy and physiology   200
    Pathology   201
    Patterns for ovarian cancer   202
    Prevention   207

> Hope is the thing with feathers
> that perches in the soul
> and sings the tune without words
> and never stops at all.
>
> Emily Dickinson

EPIDEMIOLOGY

Ovarian cancer is one of the most common gynecologic malignancies and the fourth most common cause of cancer-related death in American women. The median age at diagnosis is 62 years, and the incidence rises rapidly after age 60.[1] In a large number of cases it is entirely curable when found early. However, it is commonly asymptomatic in the earlier stages and most women will present with widespread disease at the time of diagnosis. Partly because of this the death rate from ovarian cancer exceeds that for all other gynecologic malignancies combined. Of approximately 30 000 cases diagnosed in any year 15 000 will not survive. In the United States the lifetime risk for ovarian cancer is 1 in 70 and 1 in 100 women will die from it. Sweden has the highest international incidence of ovarian cancer. Japan has the lowest incidence.[2]

ETIOLOGY

The etiology for this cancer is unknown. Many studies have looked at dietary factors, environmental links, endocrine links, viruses, and hereditary factors. But no clear conclusions have been made. Lynch II syndrome (see Chapter 3 on colorectal cancer) may be present in some patients, and there does appear to be a pattern of family history in ovarian cancer.[3] In women with *BRCA1* oncogene expression the rate of either breast or ovarian cancer is very high.[4]

The factor that consistently reduces risk for ovarian cancer is increased number of pregnancies.[5] This factor reduces estrogen exposure and many ovarian tumor specimens show the presence of estrogen receptors. There are no studies looking at the role of exogenous estrogen exposures or xenoestrogenic exposures and their link to ovarian cancer. Both talc, used in female hygiene products, including tampons, sanitary pads and even cosmetics, and asbestos have been linked to ovarian cancer.[6,7] A slightly increased risk for ovarian cancer is found in women with type A blood.

SCREENING

Screening could be incredibly valuable in increasing survival by allowing an earlier diagnosis while disease is still localised. Physical examination of the pelvis is of limited value in women who are asymptomatic; locating adnexal masses through physical examination is not dependable. Abdominal/transvaginal ultrasound (TVUS) is of greater value and screening studies have shown diagnostic specificities as high as 97% with TVUS and 76% with abdominal ultrasound. However, these screens are done routinely only in those women who are at high risk, and this accounts for less than 3% of all ovarian cancer cases.

CA125 is an antigenic determinant on a glycoprotein shed into the bloodstream by malignant cells derived from coelomic epithelium.[8] CA125 is elevated in about 80% of patients with epithelial ovarian cancers. These levels are also increased in patients with endometrial and pancreatic cancer. CA125 may also be increased in patients with some benign conditions, including endometriosis, uterine leiomyoma, pelvic inflammatory disease (PID), in early pregnancy, with benign ovarian cysts, and in patients with cirrhosis and pericarditis.

The serum level of CA125 fluctuates with the menstrual cycle and, therefore, screening with CA125 in premenopausal women has not been studied. The sensitivity of this marker for clinically diagnosed ovarian cancer ranges from 61 to 96%. In about one-third of women who ultimately develop ovarian cancer, CA125 levels rise above 35 units/mL 18 months before the disease is detected clinically.[9]

Other potential serum tumor markers include alpha fetoprotein (AFP), human chorionic gonadotropin (HCG), lactate dehydrogenase (LDH), carcinoembryonic antigen (CEA), lipid-associated sialic acid protein, and NB-70K. Because there are so few options with ovarian cancer screening, there are several ongoing trials that are monitoring and following women who have not been diagnosed with ovarian cancer but are at high risk, usually because of family history. Multiple vaccine trials are ongoing.

BIOLOGY, TUMOR MARKERS AND PATHOGENESIS

Many ovarian cancers have histologic characteristics similar to endocrine-responsive tissues. This suggests a role for hormones in the etiology of these cancers.[10] Estrogen receptors are present in a large number of ovarian tumor specimens and estrogen stimulates growth of ovarian cell lines. Progesterone and androgen receptors are also present in some tumor specimens. There may also be a role for peptide hormones in the regulation of growth or function of either normal or neoplastic ovarian epithelial cells.

Ovarian cancer localises to the peritoneal cavity and is, therefore, amenable to immunotherapy. This intraperitoneal growth may, in fact, be related to the local deficiency of antitumor immune effector mechanisms. Several cytokines and growth factors have been studied in this respect. IL-10 and IL-6 are elevated in ovarian cancer ascites. Endogenously produced IL-6 can protect tumor cells from natural killer (NK) cell-mediated killing, and IL-10 may play a role in immune responsiveness and the promotion of tumor growth.

Oncogenes also may be related to ovarian cancer. *HER-2/neu* is the most studied.[11] Normal ovarian epithelium expresses low to moderate levels of *HER-2/neu*, but overexpression of this oncogene may impart a biological advantage to tumor cells by enhancing their resistance to cytotoxicity.[12] *HER-2/neu* is overexpressed in about 30% of ovarian malignancies and indicates poor clinical prognosis and survival. It may be useful as a clinical marker and as a potential therapeutic target.

The *p53* tumor suppressor gene has also been studied and appears to be mutated and knocked out in 30–50% of ovarian cancers.[13] TNF-alpha has been shown to upregulate p53mRNA and to induce apoptosis in some ovarian cell lines.

DNA ploidy, which is the expression of a cell's nuclear DNA content, is also important in prognosis. Aneuploidy increases with age, stage, histology other than serous or mucinous, and degree of atypia in the presence of pseudomyxoma peritonei. In patients with invasive cancer most tumors are aneuploid. The 5-year disease-free survival for patients with diploid tumors is 90% vs 64% for those with aneuploid tumors.

PATHOLOGY

Ovarian cancer most commonly arises from epithelial cells. There are five major types in this category: serous, mucinous, endometrioid, clear cell, transitional, and undifferentiated. Clear cell and undifferentiated carcinomas have the poorest prognosis. Two other major types of ovarian cancers are germ cell tumors, which arise from the eggs, and ovarian stromal tumors, which arise from supportive tissue. These last two types account for 10% of all ovarian malignancies.

The epithelial cell types are potentially hormone-producing. Serous cells represent 50% of epithelial tumors, and 50% of these occur before the age of 40. Mucinous tumors make up 10% of epithelial tumors and can reach an enormous size, filling the entire abdominal cavity. These tumors are bilateral in 10% of cases and are usually intraovarian rather than on the surface. Pseudomyxoma peritonei is common secondary to this carcinoma and refers to the presence in the peritoneal cavity of mucoid material from a ruptured ovarian cyst.

Endometrioid tumors resemble endometrial carcinoma and these cancers occur simultaneously in 30% of patients. It is important to identify multifocal disease. This type of tumor can be result from metastatic spread from the uterus; the 5-year survival rate is 30%. Concurrent endometriosis is present in 10% of cases. The malignant potential of endometriosis is low but transitions from benign to malignant epithelium have been seen.

Adenocarcinoma with benign-appearing squamous metaplasia has an excellent prognosis, but adenosquamous carcinoma with glandular tissue and squamous epithelial involvement has a very poor prognosis.

Clear-cell carcinoma occurs in 5% of cases and may also be associated with endometrial cancer or endometriosis. It can coexist with other types and can also be associated with hypercalcemia from metastatic disease. This type has a worse prognosis than all others.

Small-cell carcinomas are rare and can have neuroendocrine features and a poor prognosis. Brenner tumors are very rare and can be malignant, borderline or benign. Transitional-cell tumors can resemble transitional-cell carcinoma of the bladder. Ovarian tumors that are more than 50% transitional-cell are more sensitive to chemotherapy and have a good prognosis. Undifferentiated types make up 17% of epithelial types and have a poor prognosis. Peritoneal mesotheliomas are located on the peritoneal epithelium. The ovaries are not involved or only their surfaces have tumor cells. Some women with this tumor have a history of oophorectomy. The connection is not clear.

STAGING

Ovarian cancer spreads via intraperitoneal, lymphatic, and locally invasive pathways. Intraperitoneal pathways show a predilection for the omentum and diaphragm, but no organ is spared, and concomitant ascites are frequent. The incidence of lymph-node involvement at the time of the original surgical exploration is 25% in stage I, 50% in stage II, and 74% in stages III and IV.

Surgical staging entails a midline incision, evacuation and analysis of any ascites fluid present, pelvic washings to provide cytologic specimens, inspection and palpation of all sites within the abdomen, removal of the mass and both ovaries to be frozen. If carcinoma is present, then a complete hysterectomy is performed with bilateral salpingo-oophorectomy. The omentum is also removed with a debulking of all remaining tumor. If the colon is involved then any intestinal obstruction is resected and a colostomy may be put in place. If the disease is limited to the ovaries, multiple biopsies are taken from multiple areas in the abdomen including subdiaphragmatic sites and various lymph nodes. This is called cytoreductive surgery. Unfortunately, there are no current studies showing that this kind of surgery increases survival.[14]

The International Federation of Gynecology and Obstetrics (FIGO) system is used for staging according to surgical findings.

TREATMENT

Surgery is indicated in ovarian cancer. Cytoreductive surgery leads to a better response to chemotherapy and palliates abdominal and intestinal obstructive complications. There is no proof as to longevity with this type of surgery, however, even though debulking enhances the effect of chemotherapy. In the early stages one or both ovaries may be removed with or without a hysterectomy. Meticulous surgical staging is done involving washings from the abdominal cavity, selective sampling of pelvic and aortic lymph nodes, careful inspection of abdominal cavity surfaces with biopsy of any suspicious lesions, removal of fatty tissue attached to the stomach and large intestine, plus possible omenectomy. Random biopsies are taken of the lining of the abdominal cavity, including the surface of the diaphragm.

In advanced cancer, tumor debulking is the intention of surgery. It is possible that 25–35% of all patients will require intestinal or urologic surgery to obtain optimal debulking; no tumor implant greater than 2 cm is left behind after surgery.

Second-look surgery is primarily diagnostic and is often performed after six cycles of chemotherapy in women without evidence of persistent disease. This is determined by physical examination, the serum CA125 level and pelvic and abdominal CT scans. It is the most reliable way of determining whether any cancer remains. At this time peritoneal washings and biopsies from as many as 20–30 random adhesions are taken. These include the surfaces of the bladder, pelvis, pelvic sidewalls, diaphragm, and pelvic and aortic lymph nodes. If any omentum remains it is commonly removed at this point. Second-look surgery can be done laparoscopically.

Chemotherapy is begun 2–3 weeks after surgery. The standard regimen includes cisplatin or carboplatin plus cyclophosphamide (Cytoxan), or cisplatin/carboplatin plus paclitaxel (Taxol) given i.v. every 3 weeks for at least six cycles. A dose-dense cycle of every 2 weeks can also be given in the interest of maintaining an ongoing cytotoxic effect. The response rate depends to a large degree on the amount of cancer remaining after surgery and, thus, optimal debulking is important for this reason. It is important to remember that response rate does not equal survival time. Paclitaxel (Taxol) has also been used as a single agent in advanced disease; survival rates in patients on a paclitaxel/carboplatin combination were significantly higher.[15]

Intraperitoneal chemotherapy is based on the rationale of spread patterns in ovarian cancer. Intraperitoneal platinum appears moderately efficacious in patients with small-volume residual cancer. The survival of patients treated with platinum was increased from 41 months to 49 months compared to patients treated with i.v. regimens of standard chemotherapeutic choices. Paclitaxel in intraperitoneal treatment is now being studied. Intraperitoneal chemotherapy is generally given monthly for 6 months.

A recent addition to the armamentarium for advanced ovarian cancer in patients in whom carboplatin/taxol has failed is gemcitabine (Gemzar). The use of this single agent shows efficacy in many patients. Altretamine (Hexalen) is another single agent sometimes used in platinum-resistant ovarian cancer. Topotecan shows some response. Hormonal therapies are also being used. Tamoxifen (Nolvadex), progestational agents, antiandrogens, and gonadotropin agonists have all shown some efficacy in stabilising patients in whom other therapies have failed.[16]

The spread of ovarian cancer begins early, with the shedding of malignant cells into the abdominal cavity. The cells implant on the peritoneum and can grow on the surface of the liver, the fatty tissue attached to the stomach and intestine, the omentum, the bladder, and the diaphragm. Disease on the diaphragm can result in impaired fluid drainage from the abdominal cavity resulting in ascites. Cancer cells can occasionally cross the diaphragm and spread to the surface of the lungs and the pleura and the mediastinum, resulting in pleural effusion.

Radiation therapy is used in two situations:

- as adjuvant therapy for stages I–III disease without residual tumor after surgery
- as consolidation after chemotherapy in advanced disease with minimal residual tumor at second-look laparotomy.

Whole abdominal radiation (WAR) and intraperitoneal isotopes have been used. WAR can help to prolong disease-free survival in early-stage ovarian cancer. This therapy has not been compared to cisplatin. Complications in WAR are considerable, including diarrhea, nausea and vomiting, rectal bleeding, hematuria, vaginal scarring, intestinal obstruction, and urinary or intestinal tract fistulas. These complications are cumulative and may appear after treatment. Complications can also be frequent with isotope implantation. The complications from radiation are significant and it is rarely used today in either of the above situations.

Drug resistance that is either intrinsic or acquired is common in ovarian cancer. The natural history of the disease after relapse is characterised by the eventual development of broad cross-resistance to various regimens. Patients who have a relapse within 6 months of a complete response (CR) have only a 10–20% chance of responding to platinum retreatment. Patients with longer treatment-free intervals of 20 months or longer have a 90% response rate to the same drugs.[17] Drug resistance may result from alterations in host drug metabolism, from the spread of tumor cells to sites poorly accessible to chemotherapy, or biochemical changes at the cellular level.

Glutathione transferases are being explored as enzymatic detoxifiers. Many such interfacers are being studied in an effort to repair damage so that the cytotoxicity of chemotherapeutic regimens can be enhanced in refractory disease. Autologous bone marrow transplantation (ABMT) and peripheral blood stem cells (PBSC) are also being researched for patients with drug-sensitive small-volume disease. The response rate appears high but is not durable.

This single intense course is inadequate because of the low-growth fraction of tumor cells; this fact implies that a significant number of clonogenic tumor cells are unaffected by most chemotherapeutic agents. An alternative is to use PBSC with repeated courses of dose-intensified chemotherapy. The final answer has not yet been reached on these kinds of therapies for ovarian cancer.

BIOLOGICAL THERAPIES

In the realm of biological therapies, interferon is the most studied. It is commonly administered intraperitoneally and has demonstrated good response rates. MoAb-directed therapy might be possible with the use of immunotoxins like *Pseudomonas* and diphtheria. Plant toxins like ricin and abrin have also been used. These studies have been problematic so far. Tumor-infiltrating lymphocytes that have been expanded from malignant tissue and then reinfused intraperitoneally with IL-2 have been used to reduce ascites secondary to portal vein obstruction or diaphragmatic lesions.

Gene therapy involving the *MDR* gene may prove to be a powerful approach. The rationale behind *MDR* gene transduction into hematopoietic stem cells is to protect against the toxic effects of high-intensity chemotherapy and to overcome drug resistance. These *MDR* genes are introduced into the bone marrow cells to protect them from paclitaxel. Once the marrow is returned to the patient, continued intensive therapy can be given cyclically. With each cycle, the marrow should become increasingly enriched with chemotherapy-resistant stem cells. As the old stem cells die they are replaced with the chemotherapy-resistant stem cells.[18] This kind of therapy is a cross between typical biologic therapy and vaccines. There is a lot of work being done in this realm of research for ovarian cancer.

OVARIAN CANCER IN PREGNANCY

Ovarian cancer during pregnancy is rare and occurs in one in every 25000 pregnancies. Detection during pregnancy is very difficult. Exploratory laparotomy is deferred until the second trimester. Surgical resection during pregnancy is possible in early stages. Chemotherapy is sometimes used without harm to the fetus but the long-term effects of chemotherapy are unknown.

CHINESE MEDICINE

ANATOMY AND PHYSIOLOGY

The uterus and the ovaries are rarely spoken of separately in Chinese medicine. They are considered a unit called zigong or nu zi bao or bao gong. This unit is directly related to the Chong, Ren and Dai channels. It is also connected with the zang fu and the 12 regular channels. There are internal channels directly linking the uterus (and ovaries) with the heart and the kidney. The collateral of the uterus and ovaries is related to the kidney, pertains to the heart, and connects with the uterus/ovaries itself. The heart dominates blood and the kidneys store essence. Normal functioning of the heart and kidney ensures that the ovaries will be supplied with blood and essence.[19]

The ovaries are the repository of the yuan qi and essence in females. The yuan qi is the purest energy in the body and is, therefore, the rarest. This genetic energy constitutes the basis for all somatic organisations. It is a part of periodic tissue structure and contains embryonic qualities that are constantly evolving or turning over. It is because of this nature, a kind of hyper-yang within yin, that it is possible for unrestrained activity of this type of tissue to evade immune surveillance. Injuries to jing can result in injuries to the ovaries and vice versa.

The estrogen receptors found on many ovarian tumor tissues can be infiltrated with xenoestrogenic herbicides and pesticides and chemical contaminants like talc. Talc is commonly found in nature alongside asbestos. Either separate or together, both of these compounds are carcinogenic and injure the jing, the DNA, of a highly sensitive tissue. The xenoestrogenic influences increase the number of receptors on responsive tissue and this increases the estrogenic exposure over a lifetime. Perhaps the sensitivity of those carrying the BRCA1 or 2 genes explains the link between ovarian and breast cancers in these people. In Chinese medicine, these exposures and injuries correlate with latent pathogens. Injuries to the jing are the deepest injuries possible and happen as a result of latent pathogenic factors or as a direct insult to the essence. Xenoestrogenic influences are cumulative. Chemical exposures are more direct.

The essence stored in ovaries is responsible for the development of the nervous system, reproductive system, the bone and bone marrow, and the five singular organs. The yuan qi as it relates specifically to the yuan qi has its own unique circulatory pattern through the Eight Extraordinary Channels. These meridians are connected to the essence via the ovaries and the adrenals. Yuan qi flows in these meridians to the surface of the body and to the singular organs and then back to the kidney fire. The singular organs contain an exceptional amount of essence and also rely heavily on essence for their nourishment.[20] When these organs are impacted by xenoestrogenic exposures their functional activity is impaired usually by creating an excess.

A relationship exists between the essence and the ying and wei. The essence catalyses ying and wei in order to activate their functions; and just as essence catalyses the function of ying and wei they in turn reinforce the essence. Wei qi is also reinforced by the essence, and the Eight Extra Meridians bring the essence to the outer surface of the body where it circulates and eventually some of it joins or enters the principal meridians, the rest going back to the adrenals. Injuries at this level can lead to poorer surveillance and, therefore, later diagnosis.[20] When the essence is damaged the wei and ying can be damaged. The dynamic interplay of all of these circulatory units demonstrates the profound reality that cancer is a systemic disease and not just a local phenomenon. Biologic therapies in conventional medicine are being analysed according to their ability to improve surveillance in the pelvis and abdomen in order to prevent ovarian cancer and also to improve treatment outcomes.

The Ren channel is referred to as the sea of all the yin channels, the Chong as the sea of blood. The Ren is considered the director of energy and particularly yin energy. According to Stephen Birch, the Ren channel in Eight Extra Meridian theory has a character 'congested with dampness and phlegm'. Lu 7 (Lieque), as a master point in this theory, relates to lung conditions where congested qi and fluids manifest. K6 is often used as a key point in treating menstrual and menopausal symptoms. It has a direct relationship with the mucous membranes. Many of the Ren channel pelvic region points treat issues of water metabolism whether they relate to the urinary bladder, the small intestine, yin deficiency, edema, or reproductive hormones. All of these issues become prominent in ovarian cancer where the water metabolism of the pelvic area is highly specialised, where the jing is constantly turning over and replenishing, where blood and yin is essential to the proper functioning of reproductive tissues, and where ascites is a common outcome of injury to these deeper structures.[21]

The Chong channel, according to some people, arises in the uterus/ovaries with a posterior branch ascending to the kidneys and an anterior branch passing to CV1. It is known as the sea of blood because of its governing effect on the menses. The Chong is also known as the sea of the 12 meridians because it has numerous connections linking with the tendinomuscular meridians, especially in the chest and the abdomen. Perhaps we could say that the Chong is the energetic material mechanism or pathway by which the pericardium and uterus are connected. It regulates the sinews and meridians of the whole body, and the lower part of its pathway is connected to all of the yin meridians and the upper pathway to all of the yang meridians. This meridian also regulates the placenta.[22]

Other aspects of reproductive function include:

- kidney: yang, qi, yin, jing, channel
  - qi: warms and restrains, holds things in place
  - yin: root of all yin, which nourishes, cools, moistens, subdues, and is the basis of blood
  - jing: basis of all material substance
  - meridian: passes through the uterus and ovaries and supplies jing

- spleen: qi wraps the blood
  - transforms the gu qi into blood and milk
  - raises the qi by its ascending action
  - transforms dampness
- liver: stores the blood
  - maintains flow of qi, especially of the uterus (including the ovaries) and breast
- stomach: root of the postnatal qi
  - the meridian irrigates the pelvis
- large intestine: regulates the flow of qi in the lower burner.

PATHOLOGY

All of the above mechanisms, when dysfunctional, can contribute to ovarian cancer pathogenesis. In some patients the following causes may combine to cause qi and blood and phlegm stasis. These factors then act as magnets for a latent pathogenic factor:

- Laparoscopy, abortions via D&C, colposcopy; when these procedures are done during the menses the injury is greater – some of these procedures cause backflow of menstrual blood, adhesions, injury to the channels, all of which can lead to blood stasis, and blood stasis creates an environment in which chemical exposures have even greater impact.
- Using hemostatics to stop abnormal uterine bleeding also causes blood stasis, and this again leads to phlegm stasis and an environment in which other pathogens have a larger impact; regulating the cycle with oral contraceptive hormones may be in this arena.
- Sex during the menses also causes backflow because the cervix is slightly dilated during the menses and this allows access to the uterus and beyond. The whole direction of movement during the menses is downward and out; backflow causes stasis as above; it also allows entry of pathogenic substances including the products of sexual activity, which need to flush downward and out, not upward and in. The menses is an energetic mechanism by which material and immaterial toxins can leave the female body, which is more open and receptive than the male body.
- Blood stagnation that is left untreated; blood stasis is generally not a condition that automatically resolves itself.

- Tampon use causes backflow and stasis and this is counteractive to the downward and out stream of the menses, which then has no place to go or is stored materially inside the vagina and thus acts like a plug for the menstrual fluids.
- A retroverted uterus can cause blood and qi stasis, and is commonly a sign of kidney or jing deficiency.
- Clomifene citrate (Clomid) and other fertility drugs cause yin injury and blood stasis.
- Phlegm stasis is most commonly related to diet and spleen deficiency, which causes dampness, damp heat, and phlegm; at the same time, phlegm and dampness are the nature of this type of epithelial tissue and, therefore, this propensity acts like a magnet for a latent pathogenic factor. Avoiding pathogens is therefore important; all of the above factors may act as pathogenic influences.

The following pathologies contribute to an environment in which immunity and the energetic mechanisms necessary for normal function are undermined. Over time these untreated and/or chronic injuries can lead to malignancy. These injuries are:

- stagnant qi and blood
- stagnant qi
- stagnant blood
- cold stasis
- heat and toxin accumulation
- spleen qi deficiency and kidney jing deficiency.

All of these injuries should be identified and treated early along with eliminating exposures for prevention.

1. Stagnant qi

Abdominal distention more than pain, moody, irritable, men (the Chinese means gate or, when connected to the emotions, stifling sensation in the chest that makes one sigh and try to expand the chest), breast distention, excess or diminished menses.

Pulse: wiry.
Treatment principle: disperse the liver, regulate the menses.
Formula: Xiao yao with blood movers.

2. Blood stasis

Dark blood with clots, nausea and vomiting with menses, cold extremities.

Tongue: purple.
Pulse: wiry or choppy.
Treatment principle: vitalise the blood, move stasis, stop pain.
Formula: Xue fu zhu yu tang.

3. Qi and blood stasis

Abdominal distention with pain, breast distention, combinations of the above.

Formula: Ge xia zhu yu tang.

4. Cold blood stasis

Pain better with warmth, general cold sensation, dark, even black, blood, pale.

Tongue: pale and dark hue.
Pulse: deep, slow choppy.
Treatment principle: warm the meridians, vitalise the blood, disperse the cold, stop pain.
Formula: Wen jing tang.

5. Heat and toxin accumulation

Fever, thirst, restlessness, insomnia, constipation, dark urine.

Tongue: red/purple.
Pulse: fast and choppy.
Treatment principle: clear heat, vitalise the blood, nourish yin while clearing heat or damp heat.
Formula: Yin qiao hong jiang jie du tang.

These are commonly used formulas for gynecological presentations.[23] Because of the insidious nature of ovarian cancer it is important to treat these possible precancerous conditions because they can contribute to an environment in which ovarian cancer is more likely to evolve, and oftentimes the symptoms associated with these patterns are, in fact, the very symptoms that may be attributable to early stage ovarian cancer. Therefore, a gynecological referral is also important.

PATTERNS FOR OVARIAN CANCER

If a patient presents with a diagnosis of ovarian cancer, the common patterns include Ren and

Chong channel disharmony with stasis, blood and damp stasis with knotted toxin, liver and kidney yin deficiency with stomach/spleen disharmony, and deficient qi and blood with knotted toxin. These diagnoses and formulas also comply with pattern according to staging.[24] Treatment for ovarian cancer includes diagnosis and treatment for the correct pattern alongside potentiation and amelioration of conventional treatment, which is primarily surgery and chemotherapy or hormonal therapy.

1. Ren and Chong channel stasis of blood and toxin

Symptoms: Stage I or IIa, may be asymptomatic except for abdominal mass or irregular menstruation. A movable palpable mass, delayed menstruation, abnormal uterine bleeding after menopause, metorrhagia, fatigue, slight weight loss. Possible elevation of the CA125 level. Blood levels look normal and liver and renal function tests (LFTs and RFTs). Although the cancer is material, it does not yet mean that it cannot be reversed; hence the idea that the channel is involved and not yet the organ. Logically this is not true as there is a mass, but adjusting the Chong and Ren is a major part of cure, whereas it is not as primary in later-stage presentations.

Tongue: may look normal or be dark with petechiae. See above.

Treatment principle: adjust the Chong and Ren, resolve stasis, soften hardness, antineoplasm.

Special formula:

tu bie chong (Eupolyphaga; *Eupolyphaga sinensis*)	12 g
san leng (Sparganii Rhizoma; *Sparganium* rhizome)	12 g
dang gui (Angelicae sinensis Radix; *Angelica sinensis*)	9 g
chi shao (Paeoniae Radix rubra; *Paeonia lactiflora* root)	10 g
fu ling (Poria; *Poria cocos*)	12 g
gan cao (Glycyrrhizae Radix; *Glycyrrhiza*; licorice root)	3 g
dang shen (Codonopsis Radix; *Codonopsis* pilosula root)	10 g
shan yao (Dioscoreae Rhizoma; *Dioscorea opposita*)	10 g
huang qi (Astragali Radix; *Astragalus membranaceus*)	15 g
chai hu (Bupleuri Radix; *Bupleurum*)	12 g
dan shen (Salviae miltiorrhizae Radix; *Salvia miltiorhiza* root)	8 g
bai zhu (Atractylodis macrocephalae Rhizoma; *Atractylodes macrocephala*)	10 g
shan ci gu* (Cremastrae/Pleiones Pseudobulbus; *Cremastra/Pleione* pseudobulbs)	12 g

This formula contains Si jun zi tang, a common qi tonic formula that increases immunity, tonifies the spleen to enable it to metabolise the cloying blood-regulating herbs and antineoplastics. The spleen is also related to the Chong and Ren channels through its relationship to blood. These embryonic channels are adjusted in many ways by this formula, including through nourishing and moving of the blood through tonification of the spleen. The blood nourishing and regulating herbs also contribute to this balancing because they have a propensity for the 'seas of yin and blood'.

The blood-regulating herbs contained in the formula nourish and move blood to change the environment in which the cancer has occurred. These herbs also act as messenger herbs to enable the antineoplastics to gain access to the target tissue. This includes the antineoplastic herbs in the formula and also conventional cytotoxic agents. The better the response in early-stage ovarian cancer to chemotherapeutic regimens and the longer the remission, the better the outcome for patients. The antineoplastic herbs in this formula are tu bie chong, san leng, fu ling, dan shen, huang qi, and shan ci gu* (the main cytotoxic antineoplastic herb along with tu bie chong). This formula is a potentiating formula for platinum-based regimens. Minor adjustments also treat the side effects of this regimen. For example, increasing the dosage of huang qi ameliorates the side effect of myelosuppression, which can be quite severe with platinum drugs. Adding bai hua she she cao (Hedyotis diffusae Herba; *Oldenlandia*) and ren shen (Ginseng Radix; *Panax ginseng*) can help protect heart muscle function, which is damaged by cisplatin or carboplatin. If paclitaxel (Taxol) is combined with carboplatin, as is common in a first round of chemotherapy for ovarian cancer, then further protection of the marrow is important. Granulocytopenia is severe with this drug. Adding herbs to protect against peripheral neuropathy is also important. These herbs are generally used: gu sui bu (Drynariae Rhizoma; *Drynaria*), chuan xiong (Chuanxiong Rhizoma; *Ligusticum wallichii* root), dan shen (Salviae miltiorrhizae Radix; *Salvia miltiorhiza* root), and bu gu zhi (Psoraleae Fructus; *Psoralea*).

It is important to remember that, even in early-stage ovarian cancer (which is rarely found), surgery is not considered curative. And, therefore, chemotherapy is almost always used. The shedding of cells into the peritoneal cavity is emblematic of this cancer and the removal of micrometastatic disease is impossible. Adjunctive chemotherapy becomes necessary.

2. Blood and damp stasis with knotted toxin

Symptoms: Stage IIb and IIc and III, complicated by ascites and lower-extremity edema with possible compression symptoms. Lower abdominal mass, hard mass, frequent urination with dark urine due to compression on the bladder, constipation due to involvement of the colon, sallow complexion may be due to jaundice caused by common bile duct obstruction, emaciation and/or weight loss, fatigue, dry mouth but unable to drink. Lower-extremity edema may be due to renal deficiency caused by metastatic disease, obstruction of lymph nodes in the pelvis, which then obstruct the return of blood and fluids, or the cumulative effect of cytotoxic agents in an elderly patient. This kind of lymphedema can lead to local infection and is considered an urgent but not emergent condition. This is a very common presentation. Blood and dampness or phlegm frequently become knotted in epithelial ovarian cancer.

Dampness is also a digestive manifestation causing anorexia and, therefore, weight loss. The middle jiao begins to literally and energetically swim in fluids and this causes the stomach qi to flush upwards causing nausea, queasiness, frothy sputum, acid reflux, lack of thirst but low-level dehydration. These same conditions can interrupt sleep.

Tongue: red or purple with petechiae.

Pulse: thready and uneven/choppy.

Treatment principle: resolve qi and blood stasis, transform damp, soften the hardness, antineoplasm.

Formula:

tu bie chong (Eupolyphaga; *Eupolyphaga sinensis*)	12 g
hai zao (Sargassum; *Sargassum*)	12 g
yu jin (Curcumae Radix; *Curcuma longa* rhizome)	12 g
dan shen (Salviae miltiorrhizae Radix; *Salvia miltiorhiza* root)	12 g
chi shao (Paeoniae Radix rubra; *Paeonia lactiflora* root)	10 g
bai hua she she cao (Hedyotis diffusae Herba; *Oldenlandia*)	20 g
ze xie (Alismatis Rhizoma; *Alisma*)	15 g
che qian zi (Plantaginis Semen; *Plantago*)	15 g
zhu ling (Polyporus; *Polyporus – Grifola*)	15 g
wei ling xian (Clematidis Radix; *Clematis chinensis*)	12 g
yi ren (Coicis Semen; *Coix lacryma-jobi*)	20 g
gua lou ren (Trichosanthis Semen; *Trichosanthes* seed)	20 g
huo ma ren* (Cannabis Semen; *Cannabis sativa* [sterilised] seeds)	9 g
tai zi shen (Pseudostellariae Radix; *Pseudostellaria heterophylla*)	15 g
mai dong (Ophiopogonis Radix; *Ophiopogon*)	12 g
bei sha shen (Glehniae Radix; *Glehnia*)	10 g
bai zhu (Atractylodis macrocephalae Rhizoma; *Atractylodes macrocephala*)	12 g
gan cao (Glycyrrhizae Radix; *Glycyrrhiza*; licorice root)	6 g

This is knotted blood and phlegm with toxin. Therefore, there are several herbs in the formula that are heat-clearing and toxin-resolving in action. These include tu bie chong, hai zao, bai hua she she cao, wei ling xian, gua lou ren, yi ren and chi shao. These work together to crack blood and phlegm and reduce toxin. Yu jin, dan shen, chi shao all move blood to open a mass and allow cytotoxic drugs and toxin-clearing herbs into the center of the mass. Some of the phlegm-transforming herbs also contribute to immune function. These are zhu ling, yi ren, hai zao, and gua lou ren.

The herbs ze xie, che qian zi, and zhu ling aid in promoting urination and, thereby, provide a means for the clearing of toxin and phlegm via urination. Mai dong and sha shen protect the yin in a dampness-draining and phlegm-transforming formula that could be drying. Huo ma ren acts as a mild laxative to provide another route, the stool, for elimination of toxins. Tai zi shen, bai zhu, and gan cao combine to almost form Si jun zi tang. This provides support to the spleen to utilise the transforming and draining herbs without loss of qi.

This is a stronger formula than the last, and is for a later stage or more aggressive ovarian cancer. It can also be combined with chemotherapy to potentiate the cytotoxic effect. When using more toxin-resolving herbs with chemotherapy, more attention needs to be paid the spleen and overall digestive function. The same issues regarding chemotherapeutic side effects need to be attended to as in the last formula. Using cytotoxic therapies and antineoplastic herbs requires a stronger effort to protect the middle jiao function, which must metabolise and clear these medications. In other words, if the spleen is more than the pancreas and includes the whole digestive mucosa, its job is intensely important and stressed while undergoing conventional cytotoxic therapy and herbal antineoplastic therapy. Supporting the middle, the nutritive and zheng qi, is metaphorically central to good outcomes in combined care. This supportive action of herbal medicine is one reason why outcomes in patients who combine care are better than in those who do not. If nothing else, patients who combine care usually have a better nutritional status.

Adding herbs that protect marrow, prevent nausea and lower gastrointestinal tract changes, prevent peripheral neuropathy, increase energy, prevent insomnia and other yin-deficient or heart/kidney axis symptoms is very important. To a large extent, the primary goal in treating ovarian cancer is quality and quantity of life, and not cure.

3. Liver and kidney yin deficiency with stomach/spleen disharmony

Symptoms: stage III and IV, following surgery, chemotherapy, and radiation, bone marrow suppression, possible infection.

Nausea and vomiting, anorexia, diarrhea, dry mouth, wu xin re (five-center heat), dizziness, restlessness, low back pain, ascites, liver metastasis with symptoms like acute pain due to obstruction of the common bile duct or jaundice, large palpable masses in the abdomen, constipation, dehydration, weakness.

Tongue: crimson with no coat, or dark with a greasy coat.

Pulse: thready rapid.

Treatment principle: nourish the yin of the liver and kidney, strengthen the stomach/spleen function, antineoplasm.

Formula:

dang shen (Codonopsis Radix; *Codonopsis pilosula* root)	15 g
bai zhu (Atractylodis macrocephalae Rhizoma; *Atractylodes macrocephala*)	15 g
fu ling (Poria; *Poria cocos*)	15 g
gan cao (Glycyrrhizae Radix; *Glycyrrhiza*; licorice root)	6 g
shen qu (Massa medicata fermentata; medicated leaven)	10 g
mai ya (Hordei Fructus germinatus; *Hordeum vulgare*; barley sprouts; malt)	15 g
ji nei jin (Gigeriae galli Endothelium corneum; *Gallus gallus domesticus*; chicken gizzard lining)	15 g
shan yao (Dioscoreae Rhizoma; *Dioscorea opposita*)	15 g
jiao gu lan (Herba Gynostemmatis; *Gynostemma*)	20 g
zhi ban xia (Pinelliae Rhizoma preparatum; *Pinellia ternata* rhizome)	10–15 g
mai dong (Ophiopogonis Radix; *Ophiopogon*)	15 g
bei sha shen (Glehniae Radix; *Glehnia*)	15 g

shi hu (Dendrobii Herba; *Dendrobium*)	10 g
huang qi (Astragali Radix; *Astragalus membranaceus*)	20 g
huang jing (Polygonati Rhizoma; *Polygonatum*)	15 g
tai zi shen (Pseudostellariae Radix; *Pseudostellaria heterophylla*)	15 g

The first four herbs in this formula make up Si jun zi tang. There is a stomach and spleen disharmony, which is often due to spleen deficiency and stomach yin deficiency from chronic illness and drug therapies that are cold in nature injuring the spleen qi and yang while simultaneously injuring the stomach yin. The next four herbs help the stomach/spleen injury and increase appetite. This enables the patient to find nourishment and fluids through food, which also helps to maintain liver and kidney yin. Ban xia contributes to redirecting the stomach qi by transforming phlegm.

Mai dong, sha shen, and shi hu protect the yin and fluids in a patient who is dehydrated. Shi hu is also an empiric herb for dry mouth, which can be very uncomfortable. The diarrhea or constipation can fluctuate according to the level of stomach/spleen disharmony and the level of dehydration. Dealing with these symptoms will help the patient to be more comfortable. When constipation occurs it contributes to stomach qi flushing up, or nausea. This stops the patient from eating or drinking and so a vicious cycle begins. Constipation is often a symptom of obstructive abdominal cancers; it is also a symptom of treatment with antiemetic drugs like ondasentron (Zofran). If patients are on steroids like dexamethasone that enable them to tolerate chemotherapeutic drugs, then these drugs also contribute to constipation. If diarrhea is dominant, then adding herbs that are spleen and kidney yang tonics may be helpful. Jiao gu lan is the primary antineoplastic herb in a formula that is designed primarily to be palliative. Tai zi shen helps to tonify qi of the middle jiao while benefiting fluids. Huang qi is here in a high dose to tonify the middle jiao function, increase blood counts, and improve energy. Adjusting this formula to meet the particular needs of a given patient is important. This is later-stage disease and advanced disease presentations require fine adjustment based on patient issues.

4. Qi and blood deficiency with knotted toxin

Symptoms: stage IIc through IV with metastatic disease, cachexia, fatigue, weakness, vertigo, shortness of breath, sallow complexion, spontaneous day and night sweats, dry mouth but cannot drink, anorexia, nausea, abdominal fullness, edema of lower extremities, abdominal pain and muscle contractions, large mass in lower abdomen.
Tongue: red with no coat.
Pulse: sunken, rapid, weak.
Treatment principle: nourish the blood, tonify the qi, antineoplasm.

Formula:

huang qi (Pseudostellariae Radix; *Astragalus membranaceus*)	20 g
dang shen (Codonopsis Radix; *Codonopsis pilosula* root)	15 g
bai zhu (Atractylodis macrocephalae Rhizoma; *Atractylodes macrocephala*)	10 g
gan cao (Glycyrrhizae Radix; *Glycyrrhiza*; licorice root)	5 g
fu ling (Poria; *Poria cocos*)	15 g
shu di (Rehmanniae Radix preparata; *Rehmannia*)	15 g
gou qi zi (Lycii Fructus; *Lycium chinensis* fruit)	15 g
tai zi shen (Pseudostellariae Radix; *Pseudostellaria heterophylla*)	15 g
mai dong (Ophiopogonis Radix; *Ophiopogon*)	10 g
huang jing (Polygonati Rhizoma; *Polygonatum*)	15 g
nu zhen zi (Ligustri lucidi Fructus; *Ligustrum lucidum* fruit)	15 g
san qi (Notoginseng Radix; *Panax notoginseng*)	1.5 g
zhu ling (Polyporus; *Polyporus – Grifola*)	20 g
shi hu (Dendrobii Herba; *Dendrobium*)	15 g

This is a palliative formula which begins with Si jun zi tang to tonify the qi of the spleen. This will improve digestive function and appetite and increase energy. The abnormal sweating is partly due to qi deficiency and partly due to yin deficiency. Si jun zi tang will address the qi deficient aspect of which spontaneous sweating is only one manifestation. Tonifying the spleen is one way to not only tonify qi but also to nourish blood. Shu di and gou qi zi are the blood-nourishing herbs, which are potentiated by the yin-nourishing herbs including mai dong, huang jing, nu zhen zi, shi hu. Blood is nourished through the spleen qi (white and red blood cells) and the kidney essence (platelets). Tai zi shen tonifies the spleen and lung qi while benefiting fluids. Zhu ling is a drain-damp herb that acts to enhance immunity and act antineoplastically. Zhu ling is a mushroom in the family Polyporaceae called *Grifola*. *Grifola* protects the bone marrow, is synergistic with many chemotherapeutic agents, is antibiotic and also acts as a diuretic to reduce edema. It is also mildly analgesic. Huang qi also tonifies the qi of the spleen and lungs and enhances immunity by increasing the white blood cells and NK cells; in this way it is antineoplastic. San qi is a stop-bleeding herb that vitalises the blood, reduces swelling, and relieves pain. It is antineoplastic, especially for blood stasis tumors. It also protects the heart from damage from cardiotoxic chemotherapy like the platinum drugs.

PREVENTION

Although there may be periods of remission after treatment for ovarian cancer, the key characteristic of this cancer is recurrence. The vast majority of patients will have recurrences and, therefore, it is immensely important to realise that ongoing treatment is necessary. It is a delicate matter to drive home this point to patients without creating deep discouragement. Even in times of remission, it is mandatory that patients and providers remain vigilant and dedicated to those strategies that will prolong life.

In Chinese medicine, this means treating the constitution of the patient and the identified pattern for the cancer itself. To this complex are added herbs that have been found to act antineoplastically against ovarian cancer. The injuries caused by the cancer itself and conventional treatment must also be addressed. Insomnia, depression and anxiety are expressions of a profound transition that many patients go through as they find their way between life and possible death. Giving patients time to express this process is extremely valuable. And treating to keep patients well enough to live through this process is a great gift. Patients get tired not so much from fatigue but from hanging on and continuing the struggle to live. In conventional medicine, the processing that happens regarding these deeper life experiences is usually referred out of the treatment room, but in Chinese medicine, it is integrated in the medicine itself. Knowledge gained from listening can help us to better understand how to treat our patients. Listening is often the treatment itself. Patients cope differently and manifest their true spirit in this process. This, in turn, helps us to understand the root of the being across from us and how to help that being walk their path. The healer and the healed become one.

 Case study 7.1

This woman, now aged 71, was diagnosed with a right ovarian cancer, stage IIIc at the age of 68. She underwent an exploratory laparotomy, then total abdominal hysterectomy, bilateral salpingo-oophorectomy, debulking, and rectosigmoid resection. The cancer was a papillary serous type that had metastasised to the omentum, cecum, rectum, and periaortic nodes. Peritoneal washings were positive. Her CA125 was not considered a useful marker.

She had an optimal cytoreduction and was started on a protocol including paclitaxel (Taxol), carboplatin, and IM8262-302, which was an antiangiogenesis agent in trial. A second-look surgery was done 6 months later and found to be negative. She was due to receive consolidation

Case study continues

therapy with the antiangiogenesis drug, but the company went bankrupt, and therefore she received tamoxifen. While on tamoxifen, she complained of leg swelling and nausea. The leg swelling was due to thromboembolic side effects and the nausea was also a side effect. After 3 months of this therapy she elected to discontinue the treatment.

A computerised tomography (CT) scan 2 years later began to show some small calcifications in her liver. These had previously been stable but now started to change and increase in size. A repeat scan 5 months later revealed significant progression of disease. The largest lesion in her liver was 31 × 36 mm. A small lesion in her pelvis, which had been followed post-treatment the first time was thought to possibly represent an area of recurrence. However, since it had not changed in size over the 2-year period, it was decided that it was probably scar tissue from previous surgery. The patient underwent a CT-guided liver biopsy, which was positive for papillary serous carcinoma.

Because the patient was 2 years out from original treatment, she was considered a platinum-sensitive patient. The patient and her family were offered several options. Docetaxel (Taxotere) and carboplatin with PSOC 1702, a sensitising agent, was one option. Another was treatment with weekly (dose-intense) paclitaxel (Taxol) or single-agent carboplatin. She decided to proceed with the Taxotere/carboplatin regimen with PSOC 1702, three courses every 3 weeks. The supporting medications were ondansentron (Zofran) and lorazepam (Ativan), Colace to maintain stool, and ranitidine (Zantac) to treat gastroesophageal reflux (GERD) caused primarily by a hiatal hernia.

Current general presentation

- Nausea.
- Rectal itching, probably from thrush.
- Constipation.
- Appetite: poor; cannot eat or drink comfortably.
- Diet: reasonably good, but hard to find energy to prepare food.
- Thirst: none; trying to drink.

- Digestion:
  - upper: acid reflux, burping, queasy, frothy expectoration, history of hiatal hernia leading to GERD
  - lower: cramping with no or little stool.
- Stools: can go 3 days without stool.
- Sleep: gets to sleep easily but wakes hot at night; mind is restless with worry.
- Temperature: can get fevers and then chills post-chemotherapy; 'shake and bake syndrome'.
- Sweats: only at night post-chemotherapy; no daytime sweating.
- Energy: 4 out of 10.
- Exercise: walking three times weekly; otherwise quite sedentary.
- Skin: rash around anus (candidiasis).
- DEXA-scan prior to first chemotherapy courses: good.
- DEXA-scan prior to this course: osteopenia.
- WBC: 4.0
- RBC: 3.2
- Haematocrit: 35
- Platelets: 187 000
- CA125: 14
- Tongue: dark purple, little coat, horizontal cracks all over stomach/spleen area, swollen.
- Pulse: kidney sho, thready and rapid.

Medications

- Ondasentron (Zofran): 5 days starting day 1 of chemotherapy infusion.
- Lorazepam (Ativan): daily as part of GERD management and for general queasiness.
- Colace: daily to move stool.
- Ranitidine (Zantac): antacid to manage GERD.
- Dexamethasone (Decadron): preinfusion as a steroidal drug to manage side effects.

Diagnosis

The patient has mixed signs and symptoms that are generated less by her diagnosis regarding the cancer pattern and more by chemotherapy. It is not uncommon to initiate treatment with Chinese medicine in the middle of cytotoxic treatment. This makes it very difficult to know the underlying environment for the cancerisation process. Because of this, all that can be done is to treat the current

Case study continues

presentation and try through time to gain views of the constitution and the environment. There are signs of stomach qi flushing up as expressed by the GERD, with concomitant spleen deficiency. However, the GERD is primarily due to the hiatal hernia caused by many childbirths – this patient had seven children. Therefore, this is more a sign of spleen deficiency and sinking spleen qi than stomach disharmony. It is a prolapse syndrome. The horizontal cracks across the stomach and spleen area of the tongue are a strong sign of spleen deficiency, as are the swelling and lack of coat. Inability to drink and anorexia are also symptoms of spleen deficiency leading to dampness.

There are also signs of blood stasis as reflected by the purple tongue. Blood stasis is a manifestation of cancer and the patient has been diagnosed, at this point, with stage IV ovarian cancer because of the liver metastasis. Is it important to the concept of blood stasis that the metastasis is to the liver and the liver has a strong relationship with the circulation of qi and blood? It is hard to know. There are few clear signs of liver and kidney yin deficiency. Her 'shake and bake' syndrome is confined to post-chemotherapy and lasts for about 3 days. It is no worse at night. There are no five center heat signs. The patient does run warmer than she used to; at the same time, her basal body temperature is about 1 °C lower than normal. This may be her norm or it may be due to hypothyroid. We could call this a kidney qi or yang-deficient symptom.

Given her tongue and pulse and symptom presentation, the diagnosis appeared to be spleen deficiency with sinking spleen qi, stomach/spleen disharmony, and knotted toxin with dampness and blood stasis.

The side effects of carboplatin[25] are myleosuppression with a platelet nadir at 14–21 days and a leukocyte nadir at days 21–28. Thrombocytopenia may be severe and colony-stimulating factors (CSFs) are used in the form of abdominal injections of Epo or another CSF. Some doctors do this as part of the standard of care and others only as needed. Leukocyte injury is usually managed as needed with filgrastim (Neupogen) or Pegfilgrastim (Neulasta). Nausea and vomiting can be severe with anorexia, diarrhea or constipation,

and liver toxicity. Renal and cardiac toxicities are important to monitor and blood chemistries in the form of a complete blood count (CBC) with differential and Chem 23 (liver and kidney function tests) are used. A MUGA-scan was given prechemotherapy and will be repeated every 6 months as long as chemotherapy of this kind continues.

Taxol carries similar side effects, including quite severe granulocytopenia. Additionally there are peripheral neuropathies that almost always occur with this drug. Preventing these neuropathies at the start of treatment is much easier to manage than beginning treatment for them after they are already present.

Treatment principles

Although good management dictated including treatment for these side effects in a larger formula that also addressed the constitution and the diagnosis according to Chinese medicine, the digestive complaints of the patient precluded a larger approach. She had lost 30 lb since the recurrence of the cancer, mainly as a result of chemotherapy and nausea and anorexia. Anorexia and nausea combined with fairly severe constipation were primary problems that needed to be addressed immediately. Her blood levels were good enough to continue treatment and, therefore, the focus was on symptoms and not overall environment. It was very important to keep the stool moving in order to treat the lower jiao stasis. When constipation is present, the upper jiao qi mechanism also becomes involved and nausea is worsened. Some of the antiemetic drugs also contributed to constipation. Maintaining appetite and nutritional status through normal digestion would help to maintain energy, blood levels, and general health allowing the patient more strength to work antineoplastically from the inside out.

Having never treated the patient before, the approach was cautious, especially given the long-term treatment she had undergone and her age and compromised digestive status. The following formula was used to treat the presentation and also as a test to gain knowledge of how she would respond. The dose was 5 g three times daily.

Case study continues

xuan fu hua (Inulae Flos; *Inula* flowers [wrapped])	15 g
zhi ban xia (Pinelliae Rhizoma preparatum; *Pinellia ternata* rhizome)	15 g
sheng jiang (Zingiberis Rhizoma recens; *Zingiber officinale* fresh rhizome)	10 g
huang lian (Coptidis Rhizoma; *Coptis*)	10 g
wu zhu yu (Evodiae Fructus; *Evodia*)	10 g
dang gui (Angelicae sinensis Radix; *Angelica sinensis*)	15 g
huang qi (Astragali Radix; *Astragalus membranaceus*)	20 g
fo shou (Citri sarcodactylis Fructus; *Citrus sarcodactylis*)	15 g
bai bian dou (Lablab Semen album; *Dolichos lablab* seeds)	15 g
da huang (Rhei Radix et Rhizoma; *Rheum*)	15 g
sha ren (Amomi Fructus; *Amomum*)	15 g
fu ling (Poria; *Poria cocos*)	15 g
lai fu zi (Raphani Semen; *Raphanus sativus*)	15 g
mai ya (Hordei Fructus germinatus; *Hordeum vulgare*; barley sprouts; malt)	15 g
lu gen (Phragmitis Rhizoma; *Phragmitis communis*)	15 g
xi yang shen (Panacis quinquefolii Radix; *Panax quinquefolium*)	5 g

Very few heat symptoms were visible and so the overall digestive environment was considered to be one of spleen deficiency with damp phlegm stasis. The constipation was primarily due to side effects of Zofran and Ativan. The steroid Decadron (dexamethasone) was given as an i.v. bolus premedication during chemotherapy infusion and continued for 3 days after the infusion. Steroids in general contribute to yin deficiency. In this case it was intermittent but the intermittency may have added another causative factor to the constipation. Xuan fu hua is a slightly warming herb that redirects the qi downwards and stops vomiting. It is especially good for water retention in the middle jiao, and it increases peristalsis to help the other herbs move stool out.

Ban xia is the empiric herb for nausea. It dries dampness and transforms phlegm and has the added benefit of breaking up phlegm nodules like ovarian cysts and cancer. It is antineoplastic, especially for cervical and ovarian cancer. Sheng jiang warms the middle jiao and controls vomiting and harmonises the ying and wei, which is disturbed in an injury to the essence. Huang lian clears heat and dries dampness, especially of the stomach. It is a cooling herb that is also antineoplastic. It was added here for its empiric ability to control nausea and also to prevent mucositis, which could be predicted with this chemotherapeutic regimen. It also promotes peristalsis and is mildly antibiotic to clear the candidiasis, which was in the gut. Because it was surrounded by warming herbs, it was felt that the empiric uses of this herb could be used safely in this patient. This use was weighed against the use of diflucan to treat the candidiasis and the herbal approach appeared better given the spleen deficient damp environment of the patient. This middle jiao injury was probably caused by pharmaceutical drugs in the first place (especially chemotherapy); adding diflucan could have cleared the yeast but, at the same time, exacerbated the environment in which the yeast occurred, setting up the patient for another episode later after more chemotherapy.

Wu zhu yu warms the middle jiao to stop vomiting and acid regurgitation due to spleen deficiency and cold stasis. It helps to prevent oral ulcers. In combination with the ginger (shen jiang) it is a strong antiemetic. All of the digestive herbs in the formula work together to redirect the qi, transform phlegm and dampness in the middle jiao, move stool, and tonify the spleen. Fo shou regulates the qi of the middle jiao, harmonises the stomach and spleen by making the spleen qi go up and the stomach qi go down, stops nausea, and improves appetite. Bai bian dou tonifies the spleen and resolves dampness. Lai fu zi and mai ya help to redirect the stomach qi and treat acid regurgitation, a longstanding condition in this patient that contributed to the nausea. Sha ren is a fragrant herb that warms and awakens the spleen to improve appetite, stop nausea, and transform dampness. Fu ling supports the spleen to

Case study continues

enable it to transform and transport fluids and eliminate dampness.

Da huang moves the stool, and vitalises and cracks the blood when prepared correctly; it drains dampness via the stool, clears fire toxins, and acts as an antineoplastic in this formula. Huang qi tonifies the spleen and stomach complex and harmonises the two by lifting the spleen qi and descending the stomach qi, as needed in this patient. It is an excellent herb for maintaining and raising WBCs and RBCs. It is cardiotonic, which is important when using platinum-based drugs. Lu gen clears heat and generates fluids. It also treats acid reflux. It was used in this case to protect the fluids in a patient who was not necessarily yin deficient but who was suffering from mild dehydration because she was not eating or drinking. Xi yang shen was added to tonify the qi and increase body fluids and protect the yin in a formula that is draining damp and is mostly warming, and therefore drying.

The patient did exceptionally well in metabolising and assimilating this formula. She had no side effects, which is the first thing to analyse when treating a new patient. Beyond the lack of negatives with this formula, there were also positives. The nausea resolved and appetite improved and the patient was able to eat normally. She was able to stop using the antiemetics and this meant that the side effect of constipation began to resolve. This resolution occurred partly because she also began to change her diet based on recommendations made during weekly treatment.

The patient began eating a diet that included at least four servings of vegetables daily. This improved the bulk in her stool and also added fluids to her intake; eventually she was able to stop taking the antiemetic drugs that were partially responsible for the constipation. Therefore, a combination of approaches resolved the constipation. Maintaining bowel movements is immensely important in treating any disease, but especially so in treating cancer and more especially in treating a lower jiao cancer. The large intestine channel regulates the qi of the lower jiao. Stasis in the channel means stasis in the lower jiao. Stasis is part of the overall picture in cancer.

The candidiasis resolved and no yeast was found in her stool after that. She gained 10 lb in one month and was able to drink more fluids which eliminated the need for her to receive i.v. fluids once every other week. Her weight gain was probably in the form of fluids, and demonstrates how serious the dehydration may have been. Even with i.v. fluids and a very damp jiao middle environment, this patient was moderately dehydrated because the spleen was so weakened it could not absorb and transform fluids. In Western physiology, the small intestine absorbs the largest portion of water from food and drink. Therefore, it must be anatomically part of the orb of function that Chinese medicine attributes to spleen function. Tonifying the spleen is one way of tonifying the small intestine's capacity to absorb fluids. Chemotherapy consistently damages the mucosal lining of the entire gastrointestinal tract, including those embedded structures in the wall of the gut that have to do with absorption. Continually rebuilding this structure and qi transformative mechanism is very important in maintaining overall health.

The dampness took away her thirst, and the loss of appetite left her with no means by which to take in fluids. To a large degree, all of her fluids were being received intravenously. As an aside, her blood levels may not have been quite as low as they appeared because her blood was diluted by the fluid volume she received intravenously. Receiving fluids intravenously probably took some of the pressure off of her spleen but also promoted the spleen function to shut down slightly. This meant that she was less nourished from two points of view, although both had their source in spleen deficiency. All of these issues contributed to the constipation and the constipation contributed to her nausea, a vicious cycle.

As is emblematic of ovarian cancer, a recurrence was found again during the second rounds of carboplatin and Taxol. This occurred approximately 9 months after the first recurrence. Signs appeared that the cancer was moving again. The CA125 was not a very useful marker for the patient, as sometimes is true, but the level was rising slightly. Repeat CT scans of the abdomen and pelvis showed that the area that was suspicious previously had grown slightly, and the spots in the

Case study continues

liver were significantly larger. Because of these findings, it was assumed that the carboplatin/Taxol regimen was no longer keeping the cancer in check. A new plan had to be implemented.

The next chemotherapy regimen consisted of a single agent, gemcitabine (Gemzar). During those 9 months of treatment the pulse remained a kidney-deficient pulse, the tongue lost its dark hue and became paler, and many of the initial digestive complaints were resolved; nevertheless, the cancer marched on. Gemzar is considered salvage therapy for advanced ovarian cancer. Its side effects are generally less severe than carboplatin and Taxol.

The patient experienced some nausea, changes in stool fluctuating between loose and constipation, mild thrombocytopenia, and neutropenia. Mild signs of lower extremity lymphedema were manifesting. The formula was changed to help maintain normal blood levels, especially platelets (essence) and RBCs (yang). In a patient of this age with kidney deficiency, it is possible for lower extremity lymphedema to become complicated by infection. It was important to treat this and prevent a possible life-threatening problem. Lymph drainage techniques were instituted and pressure stockings were worn to reduce swelling. The following formula was begun:

You gui yin jia jian[26]
add:

bu gu zhi (Psoraleae Fructus; *Psoralea*)	30 g
nu zhen zi (Ligustri lucidi Fructus; *Ligustrum lucidum* fruit)	40 g
dang shen (Codonopsis Radix; *Codonopsis pilosula* root)	40 g
huang qi (Astragali Radix; *Astragalus membranaceus*)	60 g
ji xue teng (Spatholobi Caulis; *Spatholobus suberectus*)	60 g
dan shen (Salviae miltiorrhizae Radix; *Salvia miltiorhiza* root)	40 g
bai ren shen (Ginseng Radix; *Panax ginseng*; white ginseng)	25 g
fu ling (Poria; *Poria cocos*)	30 g
zhu ling (Polyporus; *Polyporus – Grifola*)	30 g
ling zhi (Ganoderma; *Ganoderma*)	30 g
zhi ban xia (Pinelliae Rhizoma preparatum; *Pinellia ternata* rhizome)	30 g
shen qu (Massa medicata fermentata; medicated leaven)	30 g
chen pi (Citri reticulatae Pericarpium; *Citrus reticulata* pericarp)	30 g
zhi shi (Aurantii Fructus immaturus; *Citrus aurantium*)	20 g
xiao hui xiang (Foeniculi Fructus; *Foeniculum vulgare*; fennel seed)	20 g
tu bie chong (Eupolyphaga; *Eupolyphaga sinensis*)	50 g
chong lou (Paridis Rhizoma; *Paris*)	50 g

The dose was 7 g three times daily.

You gui yin is a classical formula for treating exhaustion from long-term illness with signs and symptoms of kidney yang deficiency. This patient suffered from many kidney yang deficient symptoms: incontinence, loose stools, cool extremities, low back pain, low energy not caused by anemia, floating edema. The chronic illness and, more importantly, long-term treatment with cytotoxic drugs had taken their toll. The ginseng was added to potentiate the effect of You gui yin. Bu gu zhi was added as a yang tonic and also as a biological response modifier because it has very high levels of the anticancer substance, genistein. Nu zhen zi, dang shen, huang qi, and ling zhi are synergistic and increase WBCs, RBCs and phagocytosis. These same herbs work together to repair prolapse. The patient was treated with visceral manipulation to reduce and repair the hiatal hernia, which was responsible for the acid reflux disease. This is a difficult repair to make while undergoing chemotherapy. But the maintenance of normal digestive function had been central for some time.

Ji xue teng and dan shen worked together to improve blood flow to the liver metastases while also increasing the overall blood counts. Fu ling and zhu ling increased immune function in various ways and helped to drain dampness from the middle jiao and also from kidney-deficient lower extremity edema. The digestive phlegm-transforming herbs and qi-regulating herbs all helped to regulate the middle jiao and prevent

Case study continues

nausea and stomach qi flushing upwards symptoms.

Tu bie chong and chong lou were the primary antineoplastic herbs in the formula. Tu bie chong is used especially in treating pelvic and abdominal tumors. Chong lou is especially useful in treating gynecological tumors. These antineoplastic herbs work in conjunction with the biological response modifiers to change the overall environment that promotes the cancer. The patient is elderly and has digestive dysfunctions, which makes delivering

strong herbal formulas complex. It is a blessing that her heart function is strong, she does not have diabetes or hypertension, or any other long-term chronic disease that would make treatment for cancer even more complex.

This formula has been used for the past 6 months with minor modifications. The Gemzar is keeping the cancer at bay with no new signs of progression. It will be used as a maintenance drug for as long as it works. When its efficacy fails a new drug will replace this last one, and so on.

References

1. National Center for Health Statistics. Vital statistics of the United States, 1999. Washington, DC, Public Health Service; 1999.
2. World Health Organization. World health statistics annuals: 1987–1998. Geneva, Switzerland: World Health Organization; 1987–1998.
3. Schildkraut JJ. Familial ovarian cancer: a population-based control study. Am J Epidemiol 1998; 128:456–466.
4. Kerlikowske K. Should women with familial ovarian cancer undergo oophorectomy? Obstet Gynecol 1992; 80:700–707.
5. Whittemore AS. Characteristics relating to ovarian cancer risk: collaborative analysis of twelve US case-control studies. II. Invasive epithelial ovarian cancers in white women. Am J Epidemiol 1992; 136:1184–1203.
6. Cramer DW. Ovarian cancer and talc: a case-control study. Cancer 1982; 50:372.
7. Whittemore AS. Personal and environmental characteristics related to epithelial ovarian cancer: II. Exposure to talcum powder, alcohol and coffee. Am J Epidemiol 1988; 128:1228.
8. Jacobs F. The CA-125 tumor associated antigen: a review of the literature. Hum Reprod 1989; 4:1–12.
9. Carlson KJ. Screening for ovarian cancer. Ann Intern Med 1994; 121:124–132.
10 Berek JS. Molecular and biological factors in the pathogenesis of ovarian cancer. Semin Oncol 1993; 4(suppl):S3–16.
11. Berchuck A. Expression of the epidermal growth factor receptor, HER-2/neu, and p53 in ovarian cancer. In: Sharp F. Ovarian cancer 2: biology, diagnosis, and management. London: Chapman & Hall Medical; 1992:53–59.
12. Lichtenstein A. Resistance of human ovarian cancer cells to tumor necrosis factor and lymphokine-activated killer cells: correlation with expression of HER-2/neu oncogenes. Cancer Res 1990; 50:7364–7370.
13. Marks JR. Overexpression and mutation of p53 in epithelial ovarian cancer. Cancer Res 1991; 51:2979–2984.
14. Ozols RF. Treatment of ovarian cancer: current status. Semin Oncol 1994; 21(suppl. 2):1–9.
15. Alberts DS. Improved therapeutic index of carboplatin and cyclophosmamide versus cisplatin and cyclophosmamide: final report of the Southwest Oncology Group of a phase III randomized trial in stages III and IV ovarian cancer. J Clin Oncol 1992; 10:718–726.
16. Ahlgren JD. Hormonal palliation of chemoresistant ovarian cancer: three consecutive phase II trials of the Mid-Atlantic Oncology Program. J Clin Oncol 1996; 11:1957–1968.
17. Blackledge G. Response of patients in phase II studies of chemotherapy in ovarian cancer: Implications for patient treatment and the design of phase II trials. Br J Cancer 1989; 59:650–653.
18. Hanania E. Serial transplantation shows that early hematopoietic precursor cells are transduced by MDR-1 retroviral vector in a mouse gene therapy model. Cancer Gene Therapy 1994; 1:21–25.
19. Fu Shan. Fu Qing Zhu Nu Ke (Fu Qing Zhu's obstetrics and gynecology). 1127 ACE.
20. Wu Zhi Wang. Ji yin gang mu (Compendium of therapy for women's diseases) 1620 ACE.
21. Zhang Yin An. Huang Di Nei Jing Su Wen Ji Zhu (Collected annotations to the Su Wen). 670 ACE. Shanghai Science and Technology Press; 1980.
22. Zhang jing Yue. Fu Ren Gui (Standards of gynecology). 1636 ACE. Guangdong Science and Technology Press; 1984.

23. Zhejiang College of TCM (compilers). Zhong Yi Fu Ke Shou CE (A handbook of traditional Chinese gynecology). 1987 ACE.

24. Sun Gui Zhi. Kang Ai Zhong Yao Fang Xuan (The treatment of cancer with Chinese herbal medicine);1992.

25. Baltzer L. Oncology pocket guide to chemotherapy. Mosby Year Book; 1994.

26. Zhang Jing Yue. Jing Yue Quan Shu (The complete works of Jing Yue). 1624 ACE. Shanghai Science and Technology Press; 1959.

Chapter 8

Bladder and Renal Cancer

CHAPTER CONTENTS

Bladder cancer   215
   Epidemiology   215
   Biology   216
   Pathology   216
   Diagnosis and staging   216
   Treatment   217

Renal–cell carcinoma   218
   Epidemiology   218
   Pathology   218
   Clinical presentation   218
   Diagnosis and staging   218
   Treatment   219

Chinese medicine   219
   Bladder and renal–cell carcinoma   219
   Differential diagnosis   222

> *What is at equilibrium is easy to maintain;*
> *What has not emerged is easy to plan;*
> *What is fragile is easy to dissolve;*
> *What is minute is easy to disperse.*
> *Act when there is yet nothing to do.*
> *Govern when there is yet no disorder.*
>   *Dao De Jing,* by Chuang Tzu; Chapter 64.

BLADDER CANCER

EPIDEMIOLOGY

In 2000, 50 500 new cases of bladder cancer were diagnosed in the USA. Annually, 11 200 patients die of this disease. Bladder cancer accounts for 6.5% of all cancers in the United States. It is the most common cancer among American men, and two-thirds of all cases occur in men.[1]

Seventy-five percent of bladder cancers are superficial and confined within the lamina propria at diagnosis. About 50–80% of superficial bladder cancers recur, but only 15–20% progress to invasive disease. Despite very aggressive surgery or radiation, 50% of those patients with muscle-invasive disease will die of this cancer.[2] Cytotoxic chemotherapy is the only option for patients with metastatic disease, and long-term survival is rare.

Bladder cancer is primarily a disease of older men and the peak incidence is at the age of 70. The incidence is higher in American Whites than in American Blacks, and lower in African and Asian nations than in the Western industrialised world.[3] Chemical carcinogens are linked to bladder cancer and include 2-naphthylamine, benzidine, auramine, and 4-aminibiphenyl among others.[4] Workers in the rubber, textile dyeing, paint manufacturing, leather processing, and hairdressing industries are at higher risk.[3] Chlorinated water and the trihalomethane (THM) by-products of chlorination are considered risk factors for bladder cancer. Any THMs above 10 ppm (parts per million) make water unusable for drinking, cooking, and bathing.

Saccharin is considered a causative factor for bladder cancer. A Canadian study from the 1970s was considered definitive, but the politics of the sugar and sugar-substitute industry suppressed the study.[5–8] Saccharin should be avoided because of the carcinogenic link to bladder cancer.

Cigarette smoking is the most widely acknowledged risk factor for bladder cancer.[9–13] Smokers have a risk of bladder cancer twice that of non-smokers. The risk is dose-related. Chewing tobacco does not predispose to bladder cancer. Phenacetin-containing analgesics have been implicated, and the effect of analgesics is cumulative. Women who have been taking a derivative for 20 years or longer have increased risk. Chronic bladder infections or irritations, and conditions requiring chronic indwelling catheterisation are associated with squamous cell carcinoma of the bladder. Studies looking at coffee and other artificial sweeteners have been inconclusive. Milk and vitamin A have been associated with lowered risk.[14]

BIOLOGY

The *p53* tumor suppressor gene is the most frequently altered gene in bladder cancer.[15] The role of oncogenes is less prevalent in this cancer than in others. Overexpression of *HER-2/neu*, however, is one of the highest among all human malignancies.[16]

PATHOLOGY

The majority of bladder cancers originate in the transitional-cell epithelial lining of the urinary tract; 95% of bladder cancers are transitional-cell carcinomas. Some mixed tumors are found, which contain squamous-cell and adeno-carcinomas. The grading of transitional-cell carcinoma is based on cellular atypia, nuclear abnormalities, and the number of mitoses. Grading is from 1 to 3 from low to high with solidity and invasiveness. The staging of bladder cancer is specific to transitional cell bladder cancer and not to the other very rare types of this cancer.

Carcinoma in situ (CIS) is found in the bladder. This tumor is, by definition, superficial, non-papillary, noninfiltrating and flat. Brunn's nests – outpocketings of epithelium into the lamina propria – are characteristic of this type.[17] Carcinoma in situ frequently occurs in patients with other types of bladder tumors. Primary tumors with CIS have a high frequency of recurrence and progression. 40% of patients with CIS develop invasive disease within 5 years. Diffuse CIS can involve 50–85% of the mucosa of the bladder. As a distinct subset of CIS it will yield positive results on cystoscopy because anaplastic cells shed easily into the lumen of the bladder and urinary tract due to the lost adhesion molecule in CIS.[18]

DIAGNOSIS AND STAGING

There are no symptoms or signs of bladder cancer. Presentation is usually due to intermittent and painless hematuria. In invasive disease or CIS, irritative symptoms such as dysuria or urinary frequency may be present. Bimanual examination under anaesthesia (EUA) and cystoscopy are the standard procedures for diagnosis. All visible tumors are removed and biopsied. The biopsy should extend deep into the muscle layer. EUA is done immediately after cystoscopy to assess the extent and movability and thickness of the tumor.

Urine cytologic analysis and flow cytometry are tools used to screen higher risk populations and for follow-up after tumor resection. X-rays are done according to the clinical presentation. Computerised tomography (CT) helps to evaluate the extent of tumor invasion and metatstatic disease. Intravenous pyelography can detect concurrent tumors higher up in the urinary tract. There are no markers specific to bladder cancer, although the carcinoembryonic antigen (CEA) level is commonly elevated.

There are two staging systems for bladder cancer; the TNM and the Jewett–Marshall. The TNM is most commonly used:

- T0: no definitive tumor.
- Tis: carcinoma in situ.
- Ta: papillary tumor without invasion.
- T1: lamina propria invasion.
- T2: superficial muscle invasion.
- T3a: deep muscle invasion.
- T3b: perivesical fat invasion.
- T4: prostate, vagina, uterus, or pelvic side wall invasion.
- N1–3: pelvic lymph node metastasis.
- M: lymph node metastasis beyond pelvis; distant metastasis.

There is no serologic marker specific to bladder cancer.

TREATMENT

The goals of treatment in patients with superficial disease are to reduce recurrence and to prevent progression. Transurethral bladder resection is the treatment of choice for superficial disease. This staging includes Ta, T1, and Tis. More than 80% of lesions can be controlled locally by surgery alone. However, 30–80% of these will recur. Patients with high-grade tumor, multiple primaries, cellular atypia, three previous recurrences, and residual tumor have the highest tendency to recur.[19] The highest rate of recurrence happens within 3 months of the first resection.[20]

CIS

Local CIS can be controlled by surgery alone. This procedure can be done endoscopically. When the lesions are not controlled, or when the bladder becomes severely contracted or there is evidence of persistent CIS of the prostatic duct then cysto-prostatectomy is indicated.

Intravesical therapy is the administration of cytotoxic agents or immunomodulators through a catheter into the bladder. The indications are a T1 tumor, multiple Ta tumors, a high-grade Ta tumor, or CIS. Complete removal of all gross tumor is necessary before intravesical therapy. Agents for this procedure are doxorubicin, mitomycin, and BCG (bacillus Calmette–Guerin). BCG is a tuber-culin bacillus used to induce an immune response, and is the agent of choice at this time with a 78% response rate. A 6-week course of consecutive therapy is commonly administered.[21]

The toxic effects of intravesical therapy include myelosuppression, local irritative symptoms, and some systemic toxic effects. BCG induces local granulomatous inflammation over the bladder wall and results in irritative symptoms. Patients will typically have hematuria for 1–3 weeks post-infusion. Fever occurs in about one-third of patients, and other systemic side effects include pneumonitis, hepatitis, arthritis, arthralgia, skin rash, and sepsis, which occur in about 5% of patients. Patients who live with others must be careful to treat their urine with chlorine bleach before flushing the toilet, as their urine contains active bacillus after each infusion. Since BCG is a multi-step process that lasts for up to 6 months it is necessary to manage the infectious nature of this treatment for some time.

Invasive disease

For muscle-invasive disease the treatment of choice is radical cystectomy with bilateral pelvic lymph-node dissection. Radiotherapy as the primary treatment is another option. Local disease recurrence with radiation is a major problem. Neoadjuvant and adjuvant chemotherapy is utilised because the recurrences of locally advanced disease are in the form of distant metas-tases. Commonly used agents include cisplatin alone and MVAC (methotrexate, vinblastine, dox-orubicin, and cyclophosphamide) for preoperative chemotherapy. Also, CISCA (containing cisplatin, cyclophosphamide, and doxorubicin) is used with good results in changing the survival rates for high-risk patients to those for low-risk patients.

Metastatic bladder cancer can be treated only with systemic chemotherapy. To date, the most active agents are cisplatin, methotrexate, and taxol. MVAC is the most popular regimen. When compared to cisplatin alone, the MVAC regimen showed response rates of 65% compared to 46% with cisplatin. Patients with liver metastasis did the most poorly. About 15% of patients with metastatic disease achieve a long-term remission with any form of chemotherapy. The toxic effects of MVAC are significant; myelosuppression, sepsis, mucositis, nephrotoxicity, and neuropathies are common.

RENAL-CELL CARCINOMA

Renal-cell carcinoma (RCC) is curable only in patients who present with early-stage disease. Advanced local or metastatic disease has a 15% 5-year survival rate. The natural history of metastatic RCC in heterogeneous and therefore, aggressive palliative treatment is recommended especially for patients with a solitary metastatic process and good performance status. Response rates for cytotoxic treatments are quite low, usually less than 25%, and complete response is rare. Combinations of chemotherapeutic agents and biologic agents are currently being studied. Gene modulation is currently being researched as a treatment for RCC.

EPIDEMIOLOGY

The incidence of RCC is on the rise in the US with 30 000 cases in the year 2000.[22] Females have a higher occurence.[22] It occurs most commonly in adults over the age of 40, but familial clustering with younger ages at presentation have been reported.[23]

Renal-cell carcinoma is relatively rare and associations with RCC are not commonly significant because of the low rates of the disease. The most prominent risk factor to date from epidemiological meta-analysis is tobacco use.[24] Dietary fat, alcohol, and obesity have also been evaluated, with inconsistent results.[24] Cadmium, asbestos, and petroleum products have been implicated but the link has not been proven.[25] Some RCC has been reported in association with various kidney diseases. RCC is known to develop in 40–70% of patients with von Hippel–Lindau (VHL) disease.[26]

PATHOLOGY

Renal-cell carcinoma, on gross examination, is characteristically a solid hemorrhagic and necrotic mass. There are three histological cell types; clear, granular, and sarcomatoid.[27] Clear-cell is the most common type and is present in 90% of tumors. The cells are characterised by unusually clear cells with a cytoplasm rich in lipids and glycogen. A further differentiation is made according to cellular arrangement; solid and papillary tumors. A grading scale for RCC based on nuclear size and shape is frequently used. The system for grading commonly used is that of Furhman, which classifies cells from grades 1 to 4.[28] Nuclear grade appears to provide prognostic information, especially for tumors that are grade 1 and 4.

CLINICAL PRESENTATION

Common symptoms at presentation include hematuria, abdominal mass, weight loss, anorexia, or symptoms arising from metastatic sites. Flank pain, hematuria, and a palpable mass is a classic triad and suggests advanced disease.[29] A unique characteristic of RCC is the frequent occurrence of various paraneoplastic syndromes including hypercalcemia, polycythemia, fever, cachexia, hypertension and hepatic dysfunction.[30] Metastatic disease is detectable in up to 30% of patients at presentation. Lung, bone, lymph, liver, and adrenal glands are common sites of metastasis, and occur in this order of frequency.[30]

DIAGNOSIS AND STAGING

Computerised tomography is the most useful tool; the accuracy of CT in staging RCC is 95%. Renal arteriograms are occasionally used. Chest X-ray is used to determine lung or chest metastases. Bone scan is not always useful because bone metastases from RCC are purely lytic and may produce a weak signal or no signal on bone scan, leading to a false-negative reading.

There are two staging systems commonly used: the TNM and the Robson's.

- T1: tumor less than 2.5 cm and confined to the kidney.
- T2: tumor greater than 2.5 cm and confined to the kidney.
- T3: extension into the renal vein, infradiaphragmatic vena cava, adrenal gland, or perinephric fat.
- T4: extension beyond Gerota's fascia.
- N1: single node less than 2 cm.

- N2: single node greater than 2 cm and less than 5 cm, or multiple nodes less than 5 cm.
- N3: any node greater than 5 cm.
- M1: distant metastasis.

TREATMENT

Radical nephrectomy is used in local RCC. This surgery includes the kidney, Gerota's fascia, and the ipsilateral adrenal gland. Regional lymphadenectomy may be included in the surgery. The benefit of removing the adrenals and local nodes is debated and some surgeons will omit their removal.[31] Partial nephrectomy or tumor enucleation is performed when RCC occurs in a patient with only one kidney or in the case of renal insufficiency.[32]

Metastatic disease

Palliative nephrectomy can be offered to patients with intractable hematuria, severe pain, or compressive symptoms. This procedure does not improve survival but improves quality of life.[33] Prior nephrectomy is an entry criteria for trials underway on biologic agents.

Renal cancer is generally radioresistant, and radiotherapy is not used.[34]

The vascular nature of RCC, lends itself to angio-infarction.[35] There are two general applications. First, preoperative infarction of the primary or metastatic focus may be performed. Second, embolisation may be performed for palliation in an unresectable tumor. Embolisation of a large renal mass frequently produces postinfarction syndrome consisting of pain, fever and gastrointestinal disturbances. These resolve after several days.

Hormonal therapy, usually progestins like Depo-Provera, has been used to very little effect. RCC is refractory to most chemotherapy. Vinblastine and floxuridine have been shown to have some effect.[36]

Immunotherapy in the form of alpha interferon, interleukin-2, aldesleukin (Proleukin), and gamma interferon is used. The highest response rate for any of these agents is 15%. Combination biochemotherapy is an experimental model of antitumor synergy induced by combined IFN-α and IL-2 alongside 5-FU or floxuridine.[37]

CHINESE MEDICINE

BLADDER AND RENAL-CELL CARCINOMA

Syndrome differentiation for urinary bladder and renal cancers are almost the same. The bladder, however, is the yang aspect of the kidney function. The urinary bladder is the lowest organ in the body. All fluids flow naturally downhill to the urinary bladder. Fluids held in the urinary bladder are eventually acted upon by the steaming action of the kidney yang. This is a form of qi transformation where reusable fluid qi is separated from the rest of fluids, and this clear fluid qi is carried back up to the lungs through the San jiao and via the kidney channel itself. The turbid fluids are excreted.

Turbid fluids in modern life carry substances that may not be entirely recognisable by the human body. Chemicals that were developed during and since the 1940s are foreign, and the body is unable to adjust to these chemicals in the same way it does to other, naturally occurring, turbidities. The bladder, at the lowest point in the body, acts as a swamp and a dredge for all substances. Swamps are, in fact, immensely valuable places where unclear and murky waters are cleaned for recirculation. Modern living has produced unclean substances that cannot be cleared. These chemicals cause constant irritation and inflammation leading to malignancy.

There are three sources of the fluids flowing into the urinary bladder. The middle jiao, and anatomically the small intestine where the majority of water absorption occurs, is one source. Turbid fluids are separated out as a result of qi transformation by the spleen function and are carried downward by the action of the descending and dispersing irrigation of the lung qi through the San Jiao to the urinary bladder. Part of this action is potentiated by the pumping action of the diaphragm, which moves the lung qi, disperses heat of the upper jiao, and moves fluids downward. The second source is the lung's qi transformation in the upper jiao, which again irrigates the upper and middle jiaos. The third is the small intestine, which separates reusable fluid qi from the dross carried downward from the stomach. The small intestine absorbs the reusable as part of a feedback loop between the kidney qi and the small intestine. The rest is sent downward via the San Jiao to the urinary bladder.[38] In terms of water metabolism, the San Jiao acts as the great communicator. In a sense, it is the feedback loop communicating body needs throughout the three jiao. When unclearable chemicals are present in the water stream not only is the bladder injured but also the functional activities of the San Jiao in terms of both water metabolism and immune function.

The ability of the urinary bladder to excrete fluids depends upon kidney yang energy supporting the qi transformation of the San Jiao.[39] Qi transformation has its source in the Dan Tian or the lower sea of qi. Qi transformation is the primary activity of the zang fu. Yuan qi, or source qi, is what activates this transformation. The water pathways remain open when the yuan qi and the transformative process are sufficient. The yuan qi is like a pilot light that sits in the base of the triangle of the body. This pilot light provides fire to light all of the functions of the zang fu. The direct relationship of the kidney source qi to San Jiao is impaired when the San Jiao cannot perform its function.

The kidneys control water and this refers to jing and to water metabolism. The jing stored in the kidneys is of two types: constitutional and acquired. Constitutional kidney jing is the basic inherited root qi. It is our genetic substance from which our original body forms, our gene pool and our DNA; it is material and subtle. Perhaps we could even say that it is our karma, if the concept of reincarnation is accepted. It is also our hormonal and reproductive root. Acquired jing is derived from the essential qi transformed from food and fluids and then distributed through the zang fu. If a person is healthy, the kidneys continually receive this essence from the five zang and six fu to be stored. Imbalances can result for many reasons but most of them are related to lifestyle imbalances. Preserving yuan qi preserves the balance of all kidney function, which, in turn, preserves the vast array of total body health. These basic concepts in Chinese philosophy are what drive Daoism, many meditational practices, internal/external exercises, martial arts, medicine and the whole concept of health in Chinese medicine.

Various hormonal imbalances can be early signs of renal malignancy or premalignancy.

Potassium, calcium, sodium and other basic imbalances disturb blood and fluid balance and these disturbances lead to physical signs and symptoms of disease. Adrenal exhaustion may lead to hormonal imbalances that set the stage for various cancers in terms of acting as promoting factors.

The kidney yang produces yuan qi, or original qi, through its steaming action on the jing of the kidneys. Perhaps if we think of this steaming action producing the hormones of reproduction and the adrenals (Mingmen), hormones like corticosteroids and testosterone, for example, these Western analogs may help us to understand better the idea of qi transformation, which is ultimately a major driving force in the body. All of these qi transformative mechanisms have feedback loops that relate to the jing or essence and the kidney yang. Since the kidney yang and essence also relate to the sea of marrow via the San Jiao this can help to explain not only hormonal balances but also the modern science of neurotransmitters.[40]

Stephen Birch has postulated the idea that the San Jiao is ultimately the fascial system, which is ubiquitous in the body surrounding every type of tissue. His idea is that the San Jiao is the feedback loop, the communication mechanism by which all body balances are communicated to and from the source qi, the kidney yang and jing.[41] The San Jiao becomes the ancient form of neurotransmitter, or at least a stream that is ubiquitous and in which neurotransmitters flow. Perhaps the San Jiao is the fluid and tissue channel through which neurotransmitters travel and communicate. This is not intended to be a theoretical text, but the concepts of kidney yang and jing have no correlates in Western medicine. And yet, according to Chinese medicine, the kidney yang and jing and the source qi provide the base of the triangle of all human activity. Therefore, it seems fair to at least try and put a modern face on these highly sophisticated concepts. Perhaps not all cancers have an immediate relationship with the kidney yang and source but if they progress into a later stage cancer, then the relationship becomes imminent and obvious.

The yuan qi moves into the San Jiao where one of its functions is to ensure the continuous and free movement of jin and ye fluids. The interstitial fluids thereby carry yuan qi and within this cycle the jing is transformed into yuan qi, which in turn powers the qi transformation process through which the acquired jing can be obtained by the kidneys and stored to provide fuel for future yuan qi. This cycle is present in all fluids and in the trillions of cells of the body, all of which carry the essence of the yin and the yang qi. All are driven by the sodium/potassium pump to drive body function through cyclic ATP and to maintain homeostasis. Part of the substance for acquired jing is made up of jin and ye fluids.

The nature of the kidneys corresponds to the energetic qualities of water, and fluids have a natural affinity for the kidneys. There is a saying: 'The source of fluids is in the lungs, the root of qi is in the kidneys'. The polarity of the kidney and lung axis is expressed in this saying. Fluid metabolism is central to the kidneys and qi generation is central to the lungs. One cannot exist without the other. There are many feedback loops like this that have the source qi, the kidneys, as the base. For example, the warmth of kidney yang supports spleen yang and so the middle jiao transformation of fluids. The kidneys and liver are intimately related through the kidney yin, which is the mother of yang. The kidneys, via the urinary bladder, also provide a draining function for the rest of the body. This is especially true in the case of excess fluid build-up into pathogenic water. The Su Wen (chapter 61) says: 'The kidneys are the floodgate of the stomach, if the floodgate cannot move smoothly, the water will accumulate and gather with its kind'. And so these two concepts provide an energetic relationship between diet and bladder cancer and also smoking and the lungs with bladder cancer.

As discussed above, the urinary bladder's ability to excrete is directly related to the kidneys, to spleen transformation and transportation (diet), the regular spread and descent of the lung qi (smoking), and the maintenance of open fluid pathways by the San Jiao. Urination reflects the state of fluids in the entire body.

Mingmen is the place where the warming yuan qi issues from the kidneys to be spread by the San Jiao. As yin enters the water phase it carries a seed of yang. This is Mingmen fire or the fire contained within the water. It is not unlike a place in the ocean from where volcanic fire issues. This same process is emblematic of yuan qi moving out of Mingmen through the urinary bladder.

Mingmen has a doorway, which is the gate of consolidation for the whole body. Primary and potent body hormones are secreted by the adrenals, which are probably the anatomical equivalent of Mingmen. These hormones are fire within water. The governing command of the kidneys is Mingmen. Mingmen is the axis and holds control ultimately over yin and yang. If yin and yang are in harmony then 'exiting and entering' are in order, if yin and yang are diseased then opening and closing are in disarray. From Zhang Jing-Yue:

> Thus there are those with urinary obstruction from exhaustion of yin and parched water [for example, the heat of smoking injures not only the lungs but all of the Taiyang organs]; there are those with unstoppable leakage and draining from yang deficiency and failed fire [adrenal exhaustion]. Once jing is exhausted, without strengthening water it will be unable to flow; once yang is deficient, without assisting fire it will not be able to consolidate. Jing without qi cannot move, just as qi without water cannot transform, and in this there is also the subtle employment of 'separable' and 'inseparable' which is within the ken of the wise, but which cannot be completely expressed with paper and ink.[42]

Kidney qi is derived from the steaming action of kidney yang on the kidney yin. Therefore, kidney qi deficiency is based on deficiency of either kidney yang or yin. Lack of kidney qi consolidation is based on kidney qi deficiency. The urinary bladder's qi consolidation, or ability to hold in urine, depends primarily on the kidney qi. If the kidney qi becomes weak, the urinary bladder consolidation will lack support. Thus, it seems possible that finally kidney qi is also weakened by either bladder or renal cell carcinoma.

The wei qi also moves from the moving qi between the kidneys. Its movement circulates throughout the body, has a direct relationship with the San Jiao and the lung. The combination of kidney qi deficiency and wei qi deficiency is associated. Lung qi deficiency from smoking has a direct relationship with the kidneys, the San Jiao, the bladder, and many other organs. Lung cancer is potentiated through combinations of exposures with smoking. It may be that smoking also potentiates exposures that are causative factors for bladder cancer. There is not enough known to say without doubt that this is true. However, logic would dictate that this is true.

Wei qi deficiency also provides another connection between the Taiyang organs. Conventional medical studies of immune function, such as levels of antioxidant activity and natural killer (NK) cells and others, are not commonly done in bladder cancer. It is somewhat common in patients with chronic illness to urinate very little during the day and to cycle fluids primarily at night. Frequent night-time urination interrupts the circadian cycle and the wei qi cycle. At the same time, it may be a symptom that is caused by wei qi deficiency. Dumping fluids at night may be a cause and a symptom of wei qi deficiency caused by deficiency in the whole fluid physiology of the body. The basis for most of the above discussion comes from Steven Clavey's book *Fluid Physiology and Pathology in Traditional Chinese Medicine*. It is with immense gratitude that I cite this reference. Although bladder cancer is generally very treatable, renal cancer is not. And in either case, the mechanism of injury is deep and complex.

Differentiation of urinary symptoms in Chinese medicine can be complex. The following are possible diagnoses for urinary symptoms:[43]

- pent-up heat in the heart channel
- excess heat in the stomach and intestines
- damp heat in the liver/gallbladder
- obstructed cold/damp
- urinary bladder damp heat
- yin-deficient internal heat
- summer exterior pernicious influence (EPI) damp heat
- EPI wind heat invading the lung.

The formulas used to treat all of these conditions are quite different.

DIFFERENTIAL DIAGNOSIS

Toxic heat or toxic damp heat accumulating in the bladder or kidney

Symptoms: painless hematuria, intermittent hematuria over several months, possible low back pain, low fever that is intermittent, fatigue, possible mild anorexia, no palpable mass, sagging feeling in the lower abdomen, especially when urinating.

Comments: probable smoker at one time, occupational exposures.

Tongue: red with possible greasy coat or yellow dry coat.

Pulse: rapid and slippery or thready.

Treatment principle: clear heat, drain damp, clear toxin, resolve blood stasis, antineoplastic.

Formula:[44]

bai mao teng (Solani lyrati Herba; *Solanum lyratum*)	30 g
she mei (Herba Duchesneae indicae; *Duchesnea indica*)	30 g
long kui (Solani nigri Herba; *Solanum nigrum*)	20 g
bai mao gen (Imperatae Rhizoma; *Imperata cylindrica* rhizome)	20 g
xian he cao (Agrimoniae Herba; *Agrimonia pilosa* var. *japonica*; agrimony)	20 g
zhu ling (Polyporus; *Polyporus – Grifola*)	20 g
fu ling (Poria; *Poria cocos*)	20 g
bian xu (Polygoni avicularis Herba; *Polygonum aviculare*)	20 g
shan dou gen (Sophorae tonkinensis Radix; *Sophora tonkinensis*)	30 g
dan shen (Salviae miltiorrhizae Radix; *Salvia miltiorhiza* root)	30 g
jin qian cao (Lysimachiae Herba; *Lysimachia*)	20 g
san qi (Notoginseng Radix; *Panax notoginseng*)	6 g
dang gui (Angelicae sinensis Radix; *Angelica sinensis*)	15 g
tong cao (Tetrapanacis Medulla; *Tetrapanax papyriferus*)	10 g

This is a modified formula that contains parts of Ba Zheng San (Eight Corrections Powder) with elements of Bai She Liu Wei Wan (White Snake Six Ingredient Pill). Tong cao and bian xu clear heat to promote urination and move out dampness. Shan dou gen, jin qian cao, fu ling and zhu ling clear heat, promote urination, and have antineoplastic properties. Moving blood is important in treating this cancer because blood stasis is part of the presentation as manifested in hematuria. The herbs that act in this way are long kui, she mei, bai mao teng, and xian he cao. Dang gui, dan shen and san qi all act to regulate the blood.

Qi failing to contain the blood with underlying spleen and kidney deficiency

Symptoms: frequent or persistent hematuria, waist pain, abdominal mass, tumor recurrence, loose stools, cold lower extremities, fatigue or gradual weakness, sagging pain in lower abdomen, a pale white coloring to face.
Tongue: pale and swollen with teethmarks and white slightly greasy coat.
Pulse: deep and thready or soft.
Treatment principle: tonify the kidneys to support the spleen, transform dampness, move blood to resolve stasis, antineoplasm.

Formula:[44]

sheng di huang (Rehmanniae Radix; *Rehmannia*)	20 g
shan zhu yu (Corni Fructus; *Cornus officinalis* fruit)	15 g
tu fu ling (Smilacis glabrae Rhizoma; *Smilax glabra*)	30 g
mu dan pi (Moutan Cortex; *Paeonia suffruticosa* root cortex)	30 g
bai mao gen (Imperatae Rhizoma; *Imperata cylindrica* rhizome)	30 g
xian he cao (Agrimoniae Herba; *Agrimonia pilosa* var. *japonica*; agrimony)	30 g
shan dou gen (Sophorae tonkinensis Radix; *Sophora tonkinensis*)	20 g
bai mao teng (Solani lyrati Herba; *Solanum lyratum*)	20 g
long kui (Solani nigri Herba; *Solanum nigrum*)	20 g
she mei (Herba Duchesneae indicae; *Duchesnea indica*)	20 g
dan shen (Salviae miltiorrhizae Radix; *Salvia miltiorhiza* root)	20 g
dang gui (Angelicae sinensis Radix; *Angelica sinensis*)	10 g
jiang huang (Curcumae longae Rhizoma; *Curcuma longa*)	10 g
nu zhen zi (Ligustri lucidi Fructus; *Ligustrum lucidum* fruit)	30 g
han lian cao (Ecliptae Herba; *Eclipta prostrata*)	20 g
yi ren (Coicis Semen; *Coix lacryma-jobi*)	30 g
huang qi (Astragali Radix; *Astragalus membranaceus*)	20 g
sheng ma (Cimicifugae Rhizoma; *Cimicifuga*)	15 g

Even though the principles of this treatment plan state differently, this formula is a combination of Liu wei di huang wan to nourish the yin of the liver and kidneys and Bai she liu wei wan, or White Snake Six Ingredient Pill. Nourishing the kidney yin is a way to tonify the yang of the kidneys, which in turn supports the spleen qi. Supporting the spleen qi helps the spleen to transform fluids and to lift the spleen qi to hold the blood in its place. Huang qi and sheng ma are added to these other formulas in order to support the spleen to metabolise and absorb the yin nourishing herbs and to lift the spleen qi.

Sheng di, nu zhen zi, and shan zhu yu supplement the kidneys and nourish the yin to nourish the blood. Yin and blood nourishing herbs are synergistic. There is an underlying assumption here that heat is a primary aspect of the presentation even though the treatment principles do not indicate that clearing heat is necessary. Enriching the blood helps to stop bleeding. Tu fu ling and shan dou gen clear heat, reduce inflammation, and clear toxins. This makes them somewhat antineoplastic. Bai mao gen, xian he cao, and han lian cao all clear heat and nourish the yin to stop bleeding. These herbs are also antineoplastic. Long kui, shi mei and bai mao teng all have various antineoplastic properties through their blood-regulating effects. Dan shen, dang gui, jiang huang and mu dan pi move or crack the blood to resolve blood stasis and break up the mass. Yi ren supports the spleen to filter dampness and promote urination. It is also an antineoplastic herb.

Metastatic renal cancer with spleen/kidney yang deficiency and blood stasis

Symptoms: fatigue, abnormal sweating, hematuria, low back pain from obstructive masses and possible bone metastasis, anemia, cachexia, low-grade fever, cough, shortness of breath from lung metastasis, abdominal pain, and other symptoms relative to where the spread has occurred.

Tongue: pale or dark with dark petechiae.

Pulse: weak, feeble or wide and rapid.

Treatment principle: nourish qi and blood, antineoplastic.

Formula:[44]

huang qi (Astragali Radix; *Astragalus membranaceus*)	30 g
tai zi shen (Pseudostellariae Radix; *Pseudostellaria heterophylla*)	20 g
dang shen (Codonopsis Radix; *Codonopsis pilosula* root)	15 g
fu ling (Poria; *Poria cocos*)	15 g
mai dong (Ophiopogonis Radix; *Ophiopogon*)	15 g
gou qi zi (Lycii Fructus; *Lycium chinensis* fruit)	15 g
xi yang shen (Panacis quinquefolii Radix; *Panax quinquefolium*)	10 g
da ji (Cirsii japonici Herba sive Radix; *Cirsium japonicum*)	20 g
e zhu (Curcumae Rhizoma; *Curcuma zedoaria*; zedoary)	10 g
shui niu jiao (Bubali Cornu; *Bubalus* horn)	20 g
san leng (Sparganii Rhizoma; *Sparganium* rhizome)	10 g
wu ling zhi (Trogopterori Faeces; *Trogopterus xanthipes* excrement)	10 g
pu huang (Typhae Pollen; *Typha* pollen)	10 g
san qi (Notoginseng Radix; *Panax notoginseng*)	10 g
yu jin (Curcumae Radix; *Curcuma longa* rhizome)	20 g
lu feng fang (Vespae Nidus; *Vespa*; wasp/hornet nest)	10 g
yan hu suo (Corydalis Rhizoma; *Corydalis yanhusuo*)	15 g
zhu ling (Polyporus; *Polyporus – Grifola*)	60 g
bai shao (Paeoniae Radix alba; *Paeonia lactiflora* root)	15 g
yi ren (Coicis Semen; *Coix lacryma-jobi*)	30 g
long kui (Solani nigri Herba; *Solanum nigrum*)	30 g

This formula tonifies the qi, supports the spleen to transform dampness, clears heat and toxin, clears heat from the qi and blood level, moves blood, stops pain, and acts antineoplastically. Huang qi, tai zi shen, dang shen, and fu ling all work together to act as a form of Si jun zi tang, the main qi tonic formula for the spleen. Mai dong and gou qi zi nourish the yin and blood to protect the fluids and build the blood to move the blood. There are several herbs that detoxify and clear heat like da ji, shui niu jiao, pu huang, and lu fang feng. These herbs are diuretic, clear heat, antineoplastic and mildly analgesic. They also help to stop bleeding. San leng, wu ling zhi, e zhu, yu jin, yan hu suo combine to stop pain. Yi ren promotes urination along with zhu ling. Together they are antineoplastic and immunomodulating. Long kui is also antineoplastic.

Formula for use during BCG intravesical therapy

Symptoms: frequent urination with blood clots and sometimes tissue, lower abdominal pain and sagging pain on urination, possible fever, flu-like symptoms and general discomfort, whole body aching.

Tongue: red with thin coat.

Pulse: rapid and possible floating or deep and rapid wiry.

Treatment principles: potentiate the BCG intravesical therapy, treat pain, prevent infection.

Formula:[45]

sheng di huang (Rehmanniae Radix; *Rehmannia*)	15 g
mu dan pi (Moutan Cortex; *Paeonia suffruticosa* root cortex)	10 g
da ji (Cirsii japonici Herba sive Radix; *Cirsium japonicum*)	20 g
xiao ji (Cirsii Herba; *Cirsium*)	20 g
tong cao (Tetrapanacis Medulla; *Tetrapanax papyriferus*)	15 g
pu huang tan (Typhae Pollen; *Typha* carbonated pollen)	10 g
ou jie (Nelumbinis Nodus rhizomatis; *Nelumbo nucifera* rhizome node)	10 g
bai mao gen (Imperatae Rhizoma; *Imperata cylindrica* rhizome)	30 g

dan zhu ye (Lophatheri Herba;   10 g
   Lophatherum gracile)

zhi zi (Gardeniae Fructus; *Gardenia*   10 g
   fruit)

qu mai (Dianthi Herba; *Dianthus*)   10 g

che qian zi (Plantaginis Semen;   10 g
   Plantago)

ze xie (Alismatis Rhizoma; *Alisma*)   15 g

wei ling xian (Clematidis Radix;   10 g
   Clematis chinensis)

huai niu xi (Achyranthis bidentatae   10 g
   Radix; *Achyranthes bidentata*)

Several of the herbs in this formula clear heat and cool the blood. Sheng di clears ying stage heat and cools the blood to stop bleeding. It stops hemorrhaging and helps to lower fevers. Mu dan pi acts similarly and also removes congealed blood, which helps to flush tumor tissue from the bladder. It also reduces swelling, lowers fevers, and it is antineoplastic. Da ji cools the blood to stop bleeding and is an antineoplastic when used topically. It is a topical agent, as it washes through the bladder. Tong cao promotes urination and drains heat and is useful in treating urinary symptoms like painful urination, hematuria and urinary retention. Pu huang tan stops bleeding, relieves pain, moves blood and promotes urination. It is antineoplastic for blood stasis tumors. Ou jie also stops bleeding through its astringing effect. It will not cause blood stasis in the process of stopping bleeding.

Bai mao gen, qu mai, and wei ling xian all act as antineoplastics. They help to potentiate the effect of the BCG. Bai mao gen cools the blood to stop bleeding, clears heat and promotes urination. It enters the lung, stomach, small intestine and bladder channels, all of which have to do with water metabolism and separation of the pure from the turbid fluids (except for lung). Qu mai is a drain-damp herb that promotes urination and clears heat while cracking the blood. It is antineoplastic and is an empiric herb for bladder conditions including gravel, cystitis, hematuria, retention. Wei ling xian regulates urination and is analgesic besides being antineoplastic.

Dan zhu ye clears heat, promotes urination, reduces fevers, helps to clear Taiyang-stage disease (BCG can cause a systemic reaction which is the cause of the general malaise and aching), is especially good for urinary tract infections, hematuria. It is also antineoplastic. Zhi zi clears heat, drains damp heat, cools the blood to stop bleeding, lowers fevers, and is antineoplastic. Che qian zi promotes urination and clears heat, stops hematuria. Ze xie acts similarly. And huai niu xi acts as a messenger herb in the formula. It also vitalises the blood, conducts the movement of blood downward, promotes urination and clears damp heat from the lower jiao. It is antineoplastic for pelvic tumors.

Herbs that are particularly useful in treating bladder symptoms and bladder cancer are:

- shi wei (Pyrrosiae Folium; *Pyrrosia* leaves): clears stones from the bladder and kidney
- qu mai (Dianthi Herba; *Dianthus*)
- chi xiao dou (Phaseoli Semen; *Phaseolus calcaratus*): clears damp heat, breaks blood and anticancer
- dan zhu ye (Lophatheri Herba; *Lophatherum gracile*): clears heat, specific for urinary tract
- che qian zi (Plantaginis Semen; *Plantago*)
- huang bai (Phellodendri Cortex; *Phellodendron* cortex)
- deng xin cao (Junci Medulla; *Juncus effusus*).

Case study 8.1

This case involves a 44-year-old man who had been diagnosed with transitional cell carcinoma (TCC) of the bladder. He was seeking options for integrated care. He had sought medical help because he had a 6-month history of gross hematuria. He had a 20-pack-year smoking history. The history was also pertinent for asthma, depression, and genital herpes. Cystoscopy revealed several tumors on the wall of his bladder.

Findings from transurethral bladder resection (TURBT) procedure:

- normal urethra
- normal prostate
- frondular posterior wall tumor, 1 cm, which was resected during the procedure
- large nodular 3.5 cm right latter wall tumor, also resected
- ~6 cm tumor, carpeting the posterior right lateral wall fulgurated using a rollerball. The urine cytology was positive for TCC Grade 3. Staging was TaG3.

Treatment plan

6 weeks of BCG intravesical infusion once weekly.

General information

- Appetite: up-and-down relative to emotional status.
- Digestion
  - upper: heartburn on occasion
  - lower: gas on occasion; both based on diet.
- Stools: regular once daily, slightly loose.
- Hemorrhoids: occasionally and without bleeding.
- Thirst: moderate; drinks a lot, but not during the workday because of frequent urination and the fact that he works outside without adequate access to a bathroom.
- Sweats: night sweats, sometimes drenching for the last 2 months.
- Lungs: bronchial constriction requires the intermittent use of an albuterol inhaler; no wheezing or shortness of breath for 5 years now; considering quitting smoking now.

- Sleep: night sweats can awaken; frequent night-time urination; up at 3 am thinking and worrying.
- Temperature: feels comfortable.
- Pain: slight pain on urination with a sagging kind of pain on the right groin.
- Chronic earaches: even as adult; usually is prescribed antibiotics, perhaps twice per year.
- Headaches: temporal from alcohol 'hangover' six times per year.
- Teeth: healthy.
- Tonsils: removed as a child.
- Spirits: moderately good; still recovering from death of his child from leukemia 1 year before.
- Fingernails: white.
- Tongue: red, stripped tip, red points all over, yellow sticky coat, red below but no distention.
- Pulse: liver sho, strong doyo, lung secondary.

Diagnosis

1. Heat toxin pouring down.
2. Liver constraint due to spleen deficiency.
3. Lung qi deficiency with early signs of lung yin deficiency.

Treatment plan

1. Interface with BCG treatment to potentiate BCG.
2. Post-BCG treat the constitution and primary diagnosis for the bladder cancer to prevent recurrence and to support the patient to make primary lifesaving lifestyle changes by quitting smoking and alcohol, change diet, work on issues causing depression and other behaviors.

Outcome

The patient was motivated to make several changes in his life as a result of this diagnosis. He quit smoking and was able to maintain this change even 3 years later. Because he quit smoking during treatment some changes were made in the supplement protocol he was given. These protocols are included as part of Chapter 12

Case study continues

on concurrent issues. In this case, the antioxidant part of a typical protocol was removed. One reason is because the biological therapy BCG requires an acute immune response as part of its mechanism. The bacillus provokes an immune response in the bladder and this ongoing stimulation scavenges cancer cells to eradicate the tumor. The rate of complete response to this technique for early stage bladder cancers is 70%. This technique reduces recurrence and progression of the cancer. Theoretically, using antioxidants during the infusion period may be contraindicated, as it could interfere with the intended immune and inflammatory reaction.

Secondly, using higher doses of antioxidants while trying to quit smoking may clear the receptor sites for nicotine in a sweeping event each time the antioxidants are taken. When the receptor sites are cleared the craving increases. Therefore, while quitting smoking it may be best to initiate a gradual rather than a sweeping cleansing process. This makes the withdrawal period more comfortable, stable and potentially shorter.

This patient also stopped drinking alcohol. Alcohol and smoking go together; it is difficult to stop smoking and drinking simultaneously. Mainly he drank beer almost on a daily basis but occasionally he used harder alcoholic drinks. Either way, alcohol of any kind contributed to a damp heat environment and also to a lifestyle that contributed to the promotion of cancer. The diagnosis of bladder cancer theoretically put him at higher risk for other cancers. As a man he was at risk for prostate cancer, and as a smoker he was at risk for lung cancer, and it was suggested that he have a chest CT. Having been diagnosed with bladder cancer he was at risk for recurrence. One might even go so far as to say that the diagnosis of early bladder cancer may have saved his life because it is treatable, whereas later-stage lung cancer is not. This diagnosis encouraged the patient to make a huge life change that probably rescued him from more dire diagnoses later.

This patient also moved from a meat-and-potatoes diet to one of no red meat (risk factor for prostate cancer), organic foods, large vegetable portions, low-glycemic-index foods with complex carbohydrates. He lost 40 lb. His body odor changed dramatically because he was not smoking and was clean from the inside out. He smelled sweet and looked 15 years younger. His spirit shined and the depression from which he had suffered for so long began to lift. He stopped seeking out others to give his life meaning and began to meditate and find peace within himself.

After the intravesical treatment, the patient was switched to a modified version of the formula for his diagnosis. To formula number one were added several herbs that tonified the spleen to nourish liver blood and move the liver qi. A modification of Xiao yao san. He remained on this formula for 1 year. The support from this formula helped him to maintain his lifestyle changes including no smoking or drinking. He stabilised into this new life and remains well and happy.

References

1. Wingo PA. Cancer statistics, 2000. CA J Clin 2000; 45:8–30.
2. Fair WR. Cancer of the bladder. In: Devita VT, ed. Cancer: principles and practices of oncology. Philadelphia: JB Lippincott; 1993: 1052–1072.
3. Jones G. From cancer to cholesterol. New Scientist, 21 November 1992.
4. Forman D. Cancer near nuclear installations. Nature 1987; 329:499–505.
5. Howe GR. Artificial sweeteners and human bladder cancer. Lancet 1977; 2:578–581.
6. Hicks RM, Wakefield JJ. Co-carcinogenic action of saccharin in the chemical induction of bladder cancer. Nature 1973; 243:347–349.
7. Batzinger RP, Ou S-Y, Bueding E. Saccharin and other sweeteners: mutagenic properties. Science 1977; 198:944–946.
8. Burbank F, Fraumeni JF. Synthetic sweetener consumption and bladder cancer trends in the US. Nature 1970; 227:296–297.
9. Berkson J. Smoking and lung cancer: some observations on two reports. American Statistical Association Journal 1958; 53: 28–38.
10. Aronow WS. Carbon monoxide and cardiovascular disease. In: Wynder JL, Hoffman, Gori G, eds. Smoking and health: a report of the Surgeon General. Government Printing Office; 1979:321–328.

11. Gori G. Towards less hazardous cigarettes. JAMA 1978; 240:1255–1259.
12. Luce BR. Smoking and alcohol abuse: a comparison of their economic consequences. N Engl J Med 1978; 298:569–571.
13. Gould JM. Deadly deceit; a low level radiation high-level cover up. New York: Four Walls Eight Windows; 1991.
14. Silverman DT. Epidemiology of bladder cancer. Hematol Oncol Clin North Am 1992; 6:1–30.
15. Sidransky D. Identification of p53 gene mutations in bladder cancers and urine samples. Science 1991; 252:706–709.
16. Coombs LM. Amplification and overexpression of c-erbB-2 in transitional cell carcinoma of the urinary bladder. Br J Cancer 1991; 63:601–608.
17. Friedell GH. Summary of workshop on carcinoma in situ of the bladder. J Urol 1986; 136:1047–1048.
18. Farrow GM. Clinical observation on sixty-nine cases of in situ carcinoma of the urinary bladder. Cancer Res 1977 37:2794–2798.
19. Heney NM. Superficial bladder cancer: progression and recurrence. J Urol 1996; 130:1083–1086.
20. Fitzpatrick JM. Superficial bladder tumors (stage pTa, Grade 1 and 2): the importance of recurrence pattern following initial resection. J Urol 1996; 135:920–922.
21. Herr HW. Bacillus Calmette–Guerin therapy for superficial bladder cancer: a 10-year follow up. J Urol 1992; 147:1020–1023.
22. National Center for Health Statistics. Vital Statistics of the United States, 2001. Washington, DC: Public Health Service; 2004.
23. Lynch HT. Genetics in urologic cancer. Urol Clin North Am 1990; 7:815–829.
24. Dayal H. Epidemiology of kidney cancer. Semin Oncol 2003; 10:366–377.
25. Thomas TL. Mortality among workers employed in petroleum refining and petrochemical plants. J Occup Med 1997; 22:97–103.
26. Maher ER. Familial renal cell carcinoma: clinical and molecular genetic aspects. Br J Cancer 1991; 63:176–179.
27. Foster K. Molecular genetic investigation of sporadic renal cell carcinoma: analysis of allele loss on chromosomes 3p, 5q, 11p, 17 and 22. Br J Cancer 1994; 69:230–234.
28. Fuhrman SA. Prognostic significance of morphologic parameters in renal cell carcinoma. Am J Surg Pathol 1982; 6:655–663.
29. Sene P. Renal cell carcinoma in patients undergoing nephrectomy: analysis of survival and prognostic factors. Br J Urol 1992; 70:125–134.
30. Altaffer LF. Paraneoplastic endocrinopathies associated with renal tumors. J Urol 1979; 122:573–577.
31. Pizzocaro G. Pros and cons of retroperitoneal lymphadenectomy in operable renal cell carcinoma. Eur Urol 1990; 18:22–23.
32. Licht MR. Nephron sparing surgery for renal cell carcinoma. J Urol 1993; 129:1–7.
33. Golimbu M. Aggressive treatment of metastatic renal cancer. J Urol 1986; 136:805–807.
34. Kjaer M. Radiotherapy versus observation in stage II and III renal adenocarcinoma. Scan J Urol Nephrol 1997; 21:285–289.
35. Bracken RB. Percutaneous transfemoral artery occlusion in patients with renal carcinoma. Urology 1995; 6:6–10.
36. Yagoda A. Cytotoxic chemotherapy for advanced renal cell carcinoma. Urol Clin North Am 1993; 20:303–321.
37. Sella A. Interleukin-2 with interferon-alpha and 5-FU in patients with metastatic renal cell carcinoma. Proc Am Soc Clin Oncol 1994; 13:237.
38. Clavey S. Fluid physiology and pathology in Chinese medicine. Edinburgh: Churchill Livingstone; 1995:10–11.
39. Cao X, ed. Sheng Ji Zong Lu (Comprehensive recording of the sage's benefits), compiled by the Song Dynasty Tai Yi Medical College, c. 1111–1117 ACE. Beijing: People's Health Publishing; 1984.
40. Pert C. Molecules of emotion. New York: Scribner; 1997.
41. Birch S. Hara diagnosis: reflections on the sea. Brookline, Ma: Paradigm; 1988:160–201.
42. Zhang JY. Jing yue Quan Shu (The complete works of Jing Yue), 1624 ACE. Shanghai Science and Technology Press; 1959.
43. Clavey S. Fluid physiology and pathology. Edinburgh: Churchill Livingstone; 1995:73–116.
44. Li P. Notes from studies at the Sino-Japanese Friendship Hospital, Beijing; 1996.
45. Zhang Dai Zhao. Notes from studies at the Sino-Japanese Friendship hospital, Beijing; 1997.

Further reading

Clavey S. Fluid physiology and pathology. Edinburgh: Churchill Livingstone; 1995:73–116.

Chapter 9

Pancreatic and Hepatic Cancers

CHAPTER CONTENTS

Pancreatic cancer   229
   Epidemiology and etiology   229
   Pathology   230
   Clinical features   230
   Diagnosis   230
   Markers   231
   Staging   231
   Treatment   231

Hepatocellular cancer   232
   Pathology   232
   Clinical features   232
   Diagnosis   233
   Staging   233
   Treatment   233

Gall bladder carcinoma   234
   Pathology   234
   Natural history   234
   Clinical features   234
   Diagnosis   235
   Staging   235
   Treatment   235

Chinese medicine   235
   Pancreatic cancer   235
   Liver cancer   240
   Treatment for hepatitis C virus   244

'The center in the midst of the conditions' is a very subtle expression. The center is omnipresent; everything is contained in it; it is connected with the release of the whole process of creation.

From the *Tai I Chin hua Tsung Chih*
(Secret of the Golden Flower) attributed
to Lu Tung Pin, 796 ACE.

PANCREATIC CANCER

This is the second most common gastrointestinal cancer, and the fourth leading cause of cancer death in the USA. Its incidence is exceeded only by that of lung, colorectal, skin, prostate, and breast cancers. Approximately 25 000 new cases are diagnosed each year.[1] The median survival is 3–4 months and the 5-year survival rate is 3%.[2] One reason for this is that the initial symptoms are very nonspecific and the disease is advanced when a diagnosis is made.

EPIDEMIOLOGY AND ETIOLOGY

Incidence increases with age. Most cases occur between the ages of 65 and 79, although this cancer has been reported in younger adults and occasionally in children. A slight male predominance exists in both Whites and non-Whites in the younger age group. But this cancer is more common in Hispanic and African-American populations. The incidence in Blacks is 14.9 per

100 000 and in Whites is 8.7 per 100 000.[2] There is also an increased incidence in Jews living in New York City and in Israel than in non-Jews, and a lower incidence among Mormons. The rate in first-generation immigrants increases to the rate of US Whites.

The cause is uncertain but cigarette smoking has been associated with increased risk;[3] the rate among heavy smokers is twice that of non-smokers. Dietary factors also seem to play a role. Dietary fat increases the risk for development of pancreatic cancer.[4] Coffee consumption has been believed to play a role, but recent studies have failed to support this observation. Alcohol has also not been conclusively linked to pancreatic cancer, but alcohol is a primary causative factor in pancreatitis, and chronic pancreatitis is linked to pancreatic cancer. Prior gastrectomy for benign conditions may increase the risk two- to fivefold.[5] The thought is that the post-gastrectomy achlorhydric environment favors the colonisation of bacteria that reduce nitrate-containing compounds to N-nitroso- compounds, which are believed to be carcinogenic.[6]

Chronic pancreatitis and diabetes mellitus have also been associated with pancreatic cancer. Calcifications associated with chronic pancreatitis are found in some patients. About 15% of pancreatic cancer patients are diabetics. The onset of clinical diabetes will precede that of cancer in 50% of patients.[7] There appears to be a familial or genetic component in pancreatic cancer, and several cohort studies are ongoing in families where this cancer occurs more frequently.

Occupational exposure to solvents, petroleum compounds, beta-naphthylamine, and benzidine is also associated with pancreatic cancer. Nitrosamines and azaserine have produced pancreatic cancers in laboratory animals.[8]

PATHOLOGY

Pancreatic cancer arises from both exocrine and endocrine parenchyma. About 95% occur within the exocrine portion and may arise from the ductal epithelium, acinar cells, connective tissue, or lymphatic deposits. The most common type is ductal adenocarcinoma, which accounts for 80% of all pancreatic cancers. Most arise in the proximal portion of the pancreas, which includes the head

and neck and uncinate process. Only 20% arise in the body, and only 5% in the tail.[9]

The great majority of patients present with advanced disease. Nearly 85% will have clinically obvious metastases. At the time of diagnosis only 20% of patients will have disease confined to the pancreas; 40% will have locally advanced disease; and 40% will have visceral metastases. Common metastatic sites are the liver, peritoneum, lymph nodes, and lung.

CLINICAL FEATURES

Anorexia, weight loss, abdominal pain, and jaundice are common initial symptoms. These symptoms commonly do not begin until as late as 2 months before diagnosis. However, patients often report a long history with various digestive complaints. Weight loss is often gradual and unappreciated, happening over a period of 6 months or more. A typical patient will have lost 10% of their total body weight by the time of diagnosis; a 30 lb loss in weight is common. Abdominal pain is the most common symptom and is due to local tumor infiltration into the retroperitoneum and the splanchnic nerve plexus. Severe pain is considered a sign that the tumor is unresectable.

Jaundice secondary to biliary obstruction can be present at any time in the cancer. Associated symptoms are dark urine and pale stools. Gastric outlet obstruction and duodenal obstruction can occur in cancers of the pancreatic head. Sometimes a palpable gall bladder (Courvoisier's sign), splenomegaly, venous thrombus and migratory thrombophlebitis (Trousseau's sign) are present.

DIAGNOSIS

Computerised tomography (CT), ultrasound, endoscopic cholangiopancreatography, and fine-needle aspiration are used to confirm diagnosis.[10] Abdominal CT is the most useful procedure for diagnosis and staging.[11] It is not limited by stomach or bowel gas, it can show liver metastases as small as 2 cm, will show peripancreatic nodal involvement, perivascular invasion, and lymphadenopathy. It can also reveal dilation of the pancreatic duct and the site of obstruction in almost 95% of cases. In patients with jaundice, ultrasonography is more accurate than CT in distinguishing obstructive from non-obstructive jaundice.[11] Its usefulness, however, will decrease with obesity and excessive bowel gas.

The other procedures are invasive but offer some advantages. Endoscopic retrograde cholangiopancreatography (ERCP) has high sensitivity in diagnosing pancreatic cancer (94%). It can localise the tumor and detect the site of ductal obstruction, and it permits the aspiration of pancreatic secretions for cytologic examination. Access to bile can also allow measurement of cancer-derived factors like the K-*ras* oncogene. ERCP has a false negative rate of only 3%. All of the above procedures are used in diagnosing and staging.

MARKERS

Carcinoembryonic antigen (CEA) is elevated in only 40–50% of patients with pancreatic cancer. CA 19-9 is a mucinous glycoprotein associated with pancreatic, colorectal, liver and gastric cancers.[12] Its level will increase with more advanced disease. Also the ratio of testosterone to dihydrotestosterone is commonly lower in men with pancreatic cancer. DU-PAN-2 and SPAN-1 are antibodies that have been screened in pancreatic cancer patients. Both are raised. However, no single marker alone is sufficiently sensitive or specific to be used as a screen. The CEA and CA 19-9 are the two markers used to monitor the effectiveness of treatment.

STAGING

The TNM system is the most commonly used staging tool. Staging is useful mainly for choosing treatment. The tumor status is defined by extension through the pancreatic capsule; nodal status is defined by the presence of regional pancreatic lymph-node involvement; and metastatic disease is defined by the presence of distal lymph node, peritoneal or visceral disease. Only stage I is considered resectable.

TREATMENT

Treatment varies according to staging. T1–2N0M0 is considered the only resectable disease, and surgery is considered the only potentially curative modality.[13] Curative surgery is feasible only in patients with cancer of the pancreatic head. Other patients will present with advanced disease for which resection is not an option. Even among the patients with a resectable tumor, 90% will die of tumor recurrence within 1–2 years. The median survival is 12–18 months after curative resection. The recurrence site is often local. Whipple resection is a pancreatoduodenectomy and is considered the standard surgical procedure for cancer of the head of the pancreas.[14]

Adjuvant radiotherapy can be used to prevent recurrence. Two small studies have been done showing only small gains including radiation post-surgery. These two trials were subject to criticism, and the incorporation of radiation into treatment with evidence from only two studies demonstrates the lack of treatment options for this cancer.

Adjuvant chemotherapy alone has not been systematically evaluated. In order for it to be evaluated an effective regimen would have to be found. No such regimen has been found to date for resectable pancreatic cancer. Frequently patients are offered chemotherapy, but refuse after discussion.

In unresectable disease palliative therapies are used. In the case of biliary obstruction a stent is placed endoscopically for percutaneous biliary drainage. This may not done in patients where no further therapy is planned because it can result in recurrent infections. Duodenal obstruction is relieved with bypass or laparscopic surgery.

Chemotherapy is generally very disappointing. 5-FU has a 28% response rate, and mitomycin also has a low level of activity against pancreatic cancer. A few trials have used intra-arterial chemotherapy. The results were again disappointing. Gemcitabine had only an 11% response rate, but there were substantial improvements in pain levels, and this in itself is valuable. It is not uncommon to use use gemcitabine as palliative care. Continuous infusion is also a possibility. When a continuous infusion schedule is used (via a belt pump), then gemcitabine or 5-FU is usually the agent of choice. The treatment is not for cure but for palliation of pain.

Hormonal therapies include tamoxifen and somatostatin. These seem to stop the secretion of cholecystokinin (CCK), which stimulates the growth of a human pancreatic adenocarcinoma cell line.[15] But no effect on disease progression or quality of life has been documented with either of these hormonal therapies.

Radiation has been used to control pain. Radiation with 5-FU has extended life by a few months. Intraoperative radiation has been used directly to the disease site while sparing normal tissue. Improved local control of the disease did not translate into improved survival. Iodine-125 seeds have not yielded better results. Biologic therapies such as monoclonal antibodies have been used to target tumor cells through antibody-dependent cell-mediated cytotoxicity (ADCC). Some reactivity has been found.

It is clear that the treatment of pancreatic cancer is difficult and generally unsuccessful.

Pain control is one of the primary treatment goals in pancreatic cancer. This pain is burning and severe. Anticonvulsants and tricyclic antidepressants are useful in treating this type of pain.[16] Steroids can be used to reduce edema associated with the cancer and lessen compression and pain. Pain may also be due to gastric or small bowel obstruction or bile duct dilatation, which leads to intense muscular spasm. This, in turn, leads to ischemia with cellular breakdown and the release of pain-producing substances. This type of pain is diffuse and poorly localised and is referred to dermatomes, implying that acupuncture techniques similar to those used in treating shingles (herpes zoster) would be useful. Oral narcotics are used. See the section on pain in Chapter 12 on concurrent issues.

Patients with intractable pain may require celiac axis block. Radiation is one form of celiac axis block. It is used to shrink the tumor and relieve compression on nerves. Its disadvantage is delayed relief, but it is effective when used with other therapies.[17] The most common form of intervention is surgical, which is, of course, permanent.

HEPATOCELLULAR CARCINOMA

Hepatocellular carcinoma (HCC) is one of the most common malignancies and causes an estimated 1 250 000 deaths every year worldwide. This cancer is high in incidence (20 per 100 000 per year) in China, South-East Asia, Western and Southern Africa, and in Chinese populations in Singapore, Taiwan, and Hong Kong. This is prob-

ably due to the higher incidence of hepatitis B virus (HBV) and hepatitis C virus (HCV) infection in those areas. Incidence is low (<5 cases per 100 000 per year) in the UK, US, Canada, Australia, Israel, Scandinavia, Latin America, India, and New Zealand.[18] Worldwide, HCC occurs three times more frequently in males than in females. Incidence increases with age. In high-incidence areas there is a shift towards increased incidence in younger age groups. One might assume that this is due to increased i.v. drug use in younger populations.

Risk factors for HCC are almost always associated with chronic underlying liver disease, principally HBV and HCV or cirrhosis from chronic alcoholism. Molecular studies have shown integrated HBV DNA in the livers of patients with chronic hepatitis and hepatocellular carcinoma.[19] Aflatoxin, a mycotoxin resulting from *Aspergillus* fungi, appears to be an important co-carcinogen in rural Africans.[20] In the West, 80–90% of cases are related to alcohol-induced cirrhosis. However, HCV infection caused by a contaminated blood supply and intravenous drug use with contaminated needles is becoming more common.

PATHOLOGY

Hepatocellular carcinoma occurs in a diffuse form and a nodular form.[21] Of all the histologic types of HCC, only the fibrolamellar variant is of importance in treatment and clinical behavior. This type is more frequent in females, occurs at an earlier age, is not associated with cirrhosis, and tends to be a solitary lesion, making it more amenable to surgical resection. Therefore, this type has a better prognosis than other types.

Invasion of the portal vein is found in about 14% of HCC specimens when the lesion is smaller than 2 cm, and in 71% of specimens when the lesion is larger than 5.1 cm. Thrombi may involve the hepatic vein, vena cava, and portal vein.[22]

CLINICAL FEATURES

The most common symptoms in HCC are abdominal pain, ascites, weight loss, weakness, anorexia, vomiting, and jaundice. About one-third of patients are asymptomatic. Metastatic disease can present as malignant ascites, skeletal pain from bone metastasis, dyspnea with lung involvement, and neurologic abnormalities due to brain metastases.[23]

Ascites can occur as a result of underlying chronic liver disease or may be due to portal vein occlusion due to obstruction. Other symptoms may include fever of unknown origin, intra-abdominal hemorrhage, upper gastrointestinal bleeding, bone pain, coma secondary to liver failure, hypercalcemia, and respiratory symptoms.

Hepatomegaly is common. Signs of cirrhosis include spider angiomas all over the body but especially on the abdomen, and gynecomastia. Abdominal bruits may be due to increased vascularity in the abdomen. Splenomegaly arises as a result of portal hypertension from underlying liver disease. Weight loss is common with rapidly growing tumors. Paraneoplastic syndromes can also be seen with HCC. Hypoglycemia, erythrocytosis, hypercalcemia, hypercholesterolemia, dysfibrinogenemia, carcinoid syndrome, sexual changes, and porphyria cutanea tarda can be present.

Laboratory changes are similar to those found in cirrhosis. Alkaline phosphatase, transaminases, and bilirubin levels can all be elevated, and if present predict short survival.[24] Alpha fetoprotein (AFP) and alpha-1-globulin are tumor markers usually associated with HCC.

DIAGNOSIS

Hepatocellular carcinoma is best diagnosed with the aid of CT scans. Ultrasonography cannot distinguish benign from cancerous tumors. Cysts in the liver are quite common. Ultrasound also cannot distinguish the portal and hepatic veins from a mass. The diffuse form of hepatic cancer can be indistinguishable from cirrhosis and chronic active hepatitis when using ultrasound. Magnetic resonance imaging (MRI) has not been proven to be more useful than CT. Laparoscopy provides a direct visualisation of the liver, peritoneal cavity, and local viscera, and also allows for percutaneous needle biopsy under direct vision.

Needle biopsy can be performed directed by ultrasound, CT, blindly, or with laparoscopy.

STAGING

Staging is done according to the TNM system. Stage I solitary tumors smaller than 2 cm without vascular invasion or lymph node spread have the best prognosis. Multiple tumors, vascular invasion, and lymph-node spread are considered adverse prognostic factors.

TREATMENT

Surgery is the only curative modality for HCC. Small encapsulated HCCs can be cured with resection in about 50% of cases. Stage I and II tumors are considered for surgery. However, if the hepatic reserve, the remaining portion of the liver, is non-functioning as in cirrhosis, even smaller tumors are not considered resectable. Intraoperative ultrasound can help detect satellite tumors. Death during or from the surgery increases with the extent of resection and with a decrease in the degree of function of the remaining liver tissue. Surgical mortality can range from 5% to 33%, and is often due to uncontrolled bleeding. There is no value in using chemotherapy after resection.

Cryosurgery involves the in-situ destruction of tumor by applying liquid nitrogen where temperatures reach less than −20°C. Although this would appear to be an ideal modality, especially for patients with cirrhosis, complications associated with the procedure and low survival rates have limited it to the research setting.

Chemotherapy is the only option for many patients. However, there is currently no effective regimen for HCC.[25] Doxorubicin, the single agent standard, has a response rate of only 20%. Combination therapy has increased toxicity with no improvement in survival. Interferon alfa-2a has been used without great benefit.[26] Ribavirin is a newer agent that is being used with better success.

Hepatic intra-arterial infusion (IAC) has been used somewhat successfully. Floxuridine, mitomycin, and interferon are delivered in high dose directly to the liver, with response rates as high as 50%. But the rates are not durable.[27] This technique is also subject to complications due to long-term percutaneous catheterisation of the hepatic artery. In China, IAC is used to deliver specially prepared herbal formulas directly to the liver. These formulas are combined with chemotherapy and work with the chemotherapy by opening the masses to better penetration by the cytotoxic agent.

Chemoembolisation is the administration of chemotherapy concomitant with percutaneous hepatic embolisation. The major blood supply to HCC is derived from the hepatic artery, while normal liver parenchyma is supplied primarily by the portal vein. Occlusion of the hepatic artery can cause relatively selective tumor ischemia. Gelatin sponge is the most widely used vaso-occlusive material. Starch, polyvinyl alcohol, collagen, and autologous blood clots have all also been used. The duration of blockade is predictable by the time it takes for each substance to degrade. Chemoembolisation for HCC produces partial responses in approximately 50% of patients.

Radiation therapy via external beam is used primarily in palliative therapy. Radiation hepatitis with subsequent fibrosis is one possible complication. A new technique uses radiation-labeled antibodies to ferritin. Ferritin is not only found in normal tissue but is also synthesised and secreted by HCC. Use of polyclonal antiferritin antibody has produced a remission rate in phase I and II trials. It has also downstaged larger tumors into resectable tumors. A radiolabeled antibody–chemotherapy regimen is used to target tumor cells via the ferritin connection with HCC.[28]

Liver transplantation has been used in patients with advanced bilobar HCC. However, the 3-year survival rate is less than 50%, and the long-term survival rate is 20%. The number of livers available is low and patients' status will determine their place on a waiting list. Patients with a history of alcoholism who do not have controlled alcoholism may not be placed on a waiting list at all. There is a whole 'industry' developing in the research of cloned liver tissue and/or fetal-cell-derived liver tissue for transplantation. Even baboon livers have been transplanted into humans. In the latter cases, antirejection drugs must then be used for the remainder of the patient's life.

GALL BLADDER CARCINOMA

This is now the fourth most common carcinoma of the gastrointestinal tract. Gall bladder cancer is an aggressive disease and the prognosis is dismal, with an overall 5-year survival rate of less than 5%, and a median survival of 6 months.

This cancer is mainly a disease of older people, with three times as many women as men affected. The incidence is higher in White women than Black women and 10 times higher in Mexican Americans, Native Americans, and Alaskan natives. There may be a connection between benign and malignant gall bladder disease. Cholelithiasis is present in almost 70% of patients. Other contributing factors may be chemical carcinogens, especially nitrosamines, and inflammatory processes like ulcerative colitis, which have a strong association with gall bladder cancer.

PATHOLOGY

Almost 85% of these cancers are adenocarcinomas. About 6% are squamous-cell carcinoma.

NATURAL HISTORY

Detection of gall bladder carcinoma is usually late and at an advanced stage when the prognosis is poor. Many of these cancers are discovered during removal of the gall bladder for chronic cholecystitis. It can be found as a polypoid projection into the lumen of the organ, with or without extension into the liver and other adjacent organs. Liver and regional lymph nodes are the most common sites of involvement. Spread to the liver is either direct or via the Luschka's ducts or various combinations of each process. The cystic and common bile ducts act as a route of metastatic spread to local lymph. The cystic node is invaded in almost 80% of cases. Invasion to colon, pancreas, and stomach is less common and is seen in only 20% of patients.

CLINICAL FEATURES

Patients with gall bladder carcinoma may be asymptomatic or they may present with abdominal pain, jaundice, weight loss, anorexia, or nausea and vomiting. There may be a right upper quadrant mass or complications like gastrointestinal hemorrhage. It is difficult sometimes to distinguish between benign disease and cancer. Serum bilirubin levels can be normal even in the presence of a gall bladder carcinoma. However, elevated alkaline phosphatase level with a normal serum bilirubin level is indicative of gall bladder carcinoma.

DIAGNOSIS

Ultrasound is very helpful in diagnosis of gall bladder cancer. It may show localised thickening or a mass. However, it can be difficult to differentiate from the wide spectrum of appearances associated with gallstones. In a series of 3000 patients who were treated for cholecystitis with gall bladder removal, 21 were found to have a malignancy, and of these 21 only two had been correctly diagnosed preoperatively.

Computerised tomography scanning is also helpful in diagnosis. Angiography can demonstrate irregularities and tumor vessels arising from the cystic artery. An upper gastrointestinal contrast study can show displacement of the stomach and duodenum when extensive disease is present.

STAGING

The TNM and the Nevin staging systems are commonly used. The Nevin & Moran system classifies tumors localised to the mucosa as stage I; stage II tumors penetrate the muscularis layer; stage III tumors involve all three layers; stage IV disease involves metastases to the cystic duct lymph nodes; and stage V disease involves invasion of metastases to liver or adjacent or distant organs.

TREATMENT

Treatment depends on the staging of the disease. Surgery is the primary modality for gall bladder carcinoma. Cholecystectomy may be the only required therapy in stage I and II disease. Patients with tumors confined in the wall of the gall bladder, which were resected, had a 5-year survival of 67%. Sometimes with more invasive disease the gall bladder is removed along with the regional lymph nodes. If the lesion invades the gall bladder serosa it is considered incurable. The 5-year survival rate in this case is 10–30%.

Radiation therapy is difficult to assess. However, it does seem to have a role in palliative and adjunctive therapy. Post-surgical radiation produces higher survival rates.

Chemotherapy

Fluorouracil has a 20% response rate and produces only transient responses. Ultimately, chemother-apy provides little benefit in either mid-stage or advanced gall bladder cancer.

CHINESE MEDICINE

PANCREATIC CANCER

The spleen function is commonly thought of as several upper and middle gastrointestinal functions in Western physiology. The character 'pi' is variably translated as spleen or pancreas. When we look at spleen function in traditional Chinese medicine, we see elements of water metabolism relating to small intestine and absorption, elements of food metabolism and assimilation relating to stomach (proteins), gall bladder (fats), pancreatic function (carbohydrates), and the jejunum end of the small intestine (water and nutrients), elements of blood manufacture relating to marrow (kidney), and the manufacture of blood from nutrition and oxygenation of tissue (lung and spleen), and the building of the body structure, especially muscle mass and some forms of connective tissue (fascia). The mucosal lining of the entire gastrointestinal tract and the immunity provided by the mucosal lining is also related to spleen function, through the ying, and possibly to the San Jiao (immunoglobulins), as well.

Therefore, when we talk about the Western disease of pancreatic cancer, we are probably discussing the functional orb of the spleen from the point of view of Chinese medicine. For example, there are a variety of ways in which long-term chronic spleen dysfunction can evolve into a cancerous process. According to the Pi Wei Lun, any chronic evolution of spleen deficiency can develop into an environment of stasis in the middle jiao. Simple spleen qi deficiency, if left untreated, can progress into spleen yin and/or yang deficiency. When this happens damp accumulations occur, which cause stasis and then heat. Heat burns fluids and causes yin deficiency on the one hand and phlegm and phlegm heat on the other. These conditions concurrently provide a foundation for blood stasis, which begins as blood dryness and progresses into blood deficiency. Blood deficiency often evolves into blood stasis, and, in the presence of phlegm heat will easily transform into blood heat. When blood heat and phlegm heat combine they can eventually become knotted with toxin. At this point, a malignancy begins to form. If the immune environment is low, due to malnutrition underlying and stemming from this condition, and also due to anemias from blood deficiency, then the malignancy can progress through a loss of surveillance.

It may be that a damp environment along with a damp pathogen is the cause of pancreatic cancer. No pathogens have been identified as causative for this cancer but alcoholism and resulting pancreatitis are certainly damp in nature. A high-sugar, high-fat diet has been identified as causative for pancreatic cancer. And so, as is common with spleen deficiency, dampness as an external and internal insult plays a major role in this cancer. It may be that we cannot know why similar internal environments evolve into pancreatic cancer and some do not. It would seem that some kind of pathogenic exposure is necessary for the transformation to a malignancy but this is unknown at this time. Is it genetic or some local familial exposure or habit? The diet and internal milieu for adult onset diabetes seems to be the same for pancreatic cancer. Diabetes is emblematic for dampness and almost all pancreatic cancer patients are diabetic at the time of diagnosis but this may be a result of the cancer rather than a cause of the cancer.

When the subject of liver cancer is discussed, the primary causes are either cirrhosis due to long-term alcoholism or chronic HBV or HCV infection. The liver/spleen environment is a complex one involving the shen and ko cycles of Five Phase theory. When the spleen is deficient, liver blood deficiency can evolve. This leads to liver qi stasis and eventually heat. This is one kind of constraint and is a Xiao Yao San pattern. When the spleen is deficient, it can also lead to dampness accumulating in the middle jiao. Dampness causes stasis, which then causes heat. Heat traverses the Ko cycle and injures the liver. This dampness is often an initial presentation in hepatitis. In other words, the hepatitis viral factors are damp pathogens, which injure the spleen as the primary hit and then the liver as a result of heat stasis traversing the Ko cycle. This is the nature of a transverse rebellion. And dampness is the primary nature in its initial form of the disease which conventional medicine calls hepatitis.

Therefore, although the end result is different, the environment is quite similar for both pancreatic and liver cancer. Spleen deficiency and dampness is the primary injury. In the case of pancreatic cancer, as far as we currently know, the main injury is spleen deficiency and dampness in the terms in which we usually think of spleen deficiency. In the case of HCC, the main injury is secondary to spleen injury and the pathogen is a damp viral pathogen that probably acts as a latent pathogenic factor (LPF), especially in a damp and yin deficient environment like cirrhosis from alcoholism or drug addiction. These environments draw the LPF deeper into the body. HBV and HCV must be damp pathogens that enter directly into the blood level both in the case of a contaminated blood transfusion or intravenous drug use with contaminated needles.

There are four types of pancreatic cancer:[29]

1. Interior damp heat stasis: carcinoma of the pancreatic head.
2. Blood and qi stasis: carcinoma of the body of the pancreas.
3. Yin deficiency with toxic heat: advanced stage with infection and injury by conventional treatment.
4. Deficient qi and deficient spleen qi and yang: advanced stage with anemia.

There are formulas commonly used to treat prior to and after surgery. In the case of a Whipple cytoreductive surgical procedure, it is important to remember that cure is not the goal and that prevention of spread during the procedure is most important. Therefore, treatment to prevent spread, decrease healing time, improve overall health, and address the constitution is the goal. The formulas used pre- and post-surgery have been given in other chapters and need only be modified to treat this presentation and the constitutional diagnosis for the individual patient. They can be used generally in any cancer with moderate modifications that treat the diagnostic pattern for that specific cancer and also take into account the constitution of the individual patient.

1. Interior damp–heat stasis

Symptoms: jaundice due to compression and/or obstruction of the common bile duct, dark urine, gray feces, possibly pruritis (common), bitter taste, anorexia, epigastric fullness, low fever or feeling of fever, probable palpable abdominal mass, no thirst, weight loss, hypochondrium pain that radiates around the middle and to the back. It is very common for a stent to be placed around the blockage of the bile duct. This blockage is what causes the stools to be gray like clay. The stent will relieve the jaundice and much of the pain but progression of the disease will cause a later obstruction.

Tongue: red, scarlet or purple with a greasy coat or no coat; it is common for there to be horizontal cracks in the stomach and spleen area on the tongue.

Pulse: normal, taut or slippery, rapid.

Treatment principle: clear damp heat, tonify spleen, reduce pain, antineoplasm.

Formula:[29]

yi ren (Coicis Semen; *Coix lacryma-jobi*)	30 g
bai mao teng (Solani lyrati Herba; *Solanum lyratum*)	30 g
yu jin (Curcumae Radix; *Curcuma longa* rhizome)	15 g
tu yin chen (Origani vulgaris Herba; *Origanum vulgare*)	15 g
mai ya (Hordei Fructus germinatus; *Hordeum vulgare*; barley sprouts; malt)	10 g
shen qu (Massa medicata fermentata; medicated leaven)	10 g
tai zi shen (Pseudostellariae Radix; *Pseudostellaria heterophylla*)	15 g
fu ling (Poria; *Poria cocos*)	15 g
zhu ling (Polyporus; *Polyporus – Grifola*)	15 g
gua lou ren (Trichosanthis Fructus; *Trichosanthes* seed)	20 g
bai zhu (Atractylodis macrocephalae Rhizoma; *Atractylodes macrocephala*)	15 g
ban zhi lian (Scutellariae barbatae Herba; *Scutellaria barbata*)	15 g
da huang (Rhei Radix et Rhizoma; *Rheum*)	6 g

gan cao (Glycyrrhizae Radix; *Glycyrrhiza*; licorice root)	6 g

There are several herbs in the formula that drain dampness. These are yi ren, tu yin chen, fu ling, zhu ling, and gua lou ren. Except for tu yin chen, these herbs are also antineoplastic. Da huang and ban zhi lian are also antineoplastic. Yu jin enters the liver and is a blood-cracking herb that breaks down masses and allows the antineoplastics to enter the tumor. It can also treat pain, a clinical feature of advanced pancreatic cancer, because of its blood-regulating qualities and because it enters the liver which regulates qi and moves blood to treat pain.

Tai zi shen, bai zhu, shen qu, mai ya, and gan cao all tonify the spleen qi or support the spleen to drain dampness. They also enable the spleen (pancreas) to fulfill its function of transforming and transporting. Cachexia is a major problem in pancreatic cancer. Increasing appetite and digestive fire can enable the pancreas/spleen, central to cachexia, to remain as functional as possible helping to lengthen life. Da huang can move stool, move blood, and clear heat. Fu ling and zhu ling, along with yi ren contribute various immunomodulatory functions and the two mushrooms are mildly analgesic. Tu yin chen also helps the gall bladder in secreting bile. When the gall bladder is obstructed the stools become gray. It regulates the qi and eliminates dampness; clinical studies show that it is useful in treating hepatitis, both infectious and non-infectious, and jaundice is a common presenting sign in this cancer. Bai mao teng also treats hepatitis, clears heat and toxins, promotes blood circulation, and reduces leukopenia.

2. Qi and blood stasis

Symptoms: epigastric fullness, pain radiating to the waist and back, worse when lying down/better when curled up, bitter taste, restlessness and insomnia, palpable mass possible, hepatomegaly, possible gastrointestinal hemorrhage, acid reflux.

Tongue: dark red with petechiae or red points.

Pulse: choppy or tight.

Treatment principle: invigorate the blood, regulate the qi, reduce pain, soften the hard, antineoplasm.

Formula:[29]

dan shen (Salviae miltiorrhizae Radix; *Salvia miltiorhiza* root)	20 g
chi shao (Paeoniae Radix rubra; *Paeonia lactiflora* root)	15 g
yan hu suo (Corydalis Rhizoma; *Corydalis yanhusuo*)	15 g
mo yao (Myrrha; *Commiphora myrrha*; myrrh)	15 g
zhe bei mu (Fritillariae thunbergii Bulbus; *Fritillaria thunbergii*)	10 g
chuan lian zi (Toosendan Fructus; *Melia toosendan*)	15 g
fu ling (Poria; *Poria cocos*)	15 g
bai zhu (Atractylodis macrocephalae Rhizoma; *Atractylodes macrocephala*)	10 g
gan cao (Glycyrrhizae Radix; *Glycyrrhiza*; licorice root)	6 g
mai dong (Ophiopogonis Radix; *Ophiopogon*)	15 g
ba yue zha (Akebiae Fructus; *Akebia*)	30 g
xian he cao (Agrimoniae Herba; *Agrimonia pilosa* var. *japonica*; agrimony)	20 g
tai zi shen (Pseudostellariae Radix; *Pseudostellaria heterophylla*)	15 g
bai qu cai (Chelidonii Herba; *Chelidonium*)	10 g
teng li (Actinidiae chinensis Radix; *Actinidia chinensis*)	15 g

The first four herbs in this formula are blood-moving and blood-cracking; they break up the tumor and treat pain. Zhe bei mu is a strong herb that clears heat and breaks up nodules. It is antineoplastic. Chuan lian zi clears and dries dampness, it regulates the qi and reduces pain. It is especially good for treating flank pain and it helps to resolve cholecystitis and hepatitis, both of which may exist if obstruction is present.

Tai zi shen, bai zhu, fu ling, and gan cao make up Si jun zi tang, the main spleen tonic formula. This formula goes beyond its classical uses here by helping the spleen to metabolise and assimilate the antineoplastics and the blood-cracking herbs in the formula. It also helps to maintain the spleen/pancreas function, lengthening life and quality of life. Mai dong is added to protect the yin in a warming formula. Tai zi shen supports this protection by being a neutral qi tonic herb that generates fluids while tonifying the spleen qi.

Xian he cao cools the blood to stop bleeding. It clears heat from the liver. It is antineoplastic and analgesic. Ba yue zha is also antineoplastic. Bai qu cai is an especially good herb for treating abdominal pain. The alkaloids in this herb have an anaesthetic effect on sensory nerve endings. It causes relaxation of the abdominal and gastrointestinal muscles relieving pain. Teng li is antineoplastic against this cancer.

3. Yin deficiency with heat toxin

Symptoms: dry mouth and tongue, restlessness, insomnia, emaciation, fatigue, anorexia, fever due to infection, epigastric distention and pain, constipation, frequent hematuria, ascites.

Tongue: red or crimson, no coat.

Pulse: fast, thready or faint.

Treatment principle: nourish the yin, clear heat, clear toxin, antineoplasm.

Formula:[29]

shi hu (Dendrobii Herba; *Dendrobium*)	15 g
zhi mu (Anemarrhenae Rhizoma; *Anemarrhena*)	15 g
bei sha shen (Glehniae Radix; *Glehnia*)	15 g
bai mao gen (Imperatae Rhizoma; *Imperata cylindrica* rhizome)	15 g
ou jie (Nelumbinis Nodus rhizomatis; *Nelumbo nucifera* rhizome node)	15 g
gua lou ren (Trichosanthis Semen; *Trichosanthes* seed)	10 g
ban zhi lian (Scutellariae barbatae Herba; *Scutellaria barbata*)	20 g
jin yin hua (Lonicerae Flos; *Lonicera* flowers)	10 g
bai hua she she cao (Hedyotis diffusae Herba; *Oldenlandia*)	30 g
ban bian lian (Lobeliae chinensis Herba; *Lobelia chinensis*)	20 g
tai zi shen (Pseudostellariae Radix; *Pseudostellaria heterophylla*)	15 g
jiao gu lan (Herba Gynostemmatis; *Gynostemma*)	15 g

bai zhu (Atractylodis macrocephalae   10 g
   Rhizoma; *Atractylodes macrocephala*)

da huang (Rhei Radix et Rhizoma;   8 g
   Rheum)

huo ma ren* (Cannabis Semen;   10 g
   Cannabis sativa [sterilised] seed)

Shi hu and sha shen are yin-nourishing herbs that help to alleviate dry mouth and throat. Zhi mu clears heat and generates fluids. Ou jie astringes and helps to stop bleeding. Together with bai mao gen, it cools the blood to stop bleeding, clears heat and promotes urination, and helps to resolve hepatitis. Gua lou ren, ban zhi lian, jin yin hua, bai hua she she cao, ban bian lian, and jiao gu lan are all antineoplastic by clearing heat and toxin. Ban bian lian also cools the blood and promotes urination.

Tai zi shen and bai zhu support the spleen but are neutral in temperature and therefore are not warming, which is important in a yin-deficient patient. Da huang moves the stool and cools the blood. Huo ma ren is mildly laxative. It also nourishes the yin and clears heat.

4. Deficient spleen and kidney yang

Symptoms: fatigue, dyspnea, anemias, sallow complexion (may or may not be jaundiced), spontaneous sweating, anorexia, cachexia, lower limb edema, ascites, abdominal masses, diarrhea, bitter taste or no sense of taste, serious weight loss.
Tongue: pale with a greasy coat.
Pulse: soft, weak, slow or rapid.
Treatment principle: nourish the blood, tonify the qi, strengthen the spleen, antineoplasm.

Formula:[29]

dang shen (Codonopsis Radix;   15 g
   Codonopsis pilosula root)

bai zhu (Atractylodis macrocephalae   15 g
   Rhizoma; *Atractylodes macrocephala*)

fu ling (Poria; *Poria cocos*)   15 g

gan cao (Glycyrrhizae Radix;   6 g
   Glycyrrhiza; licorice root)

bu gu zhi (Psoraleae Fructus;   15 g
   Psoralea)

ji xue teng (Spatholobi Caulis;   20 g
   Spatholobus suberectus)

huang qi (Astragali Radix;   20 g
   Astragalus membranaceus)

zhu ling (Polyporus; *Polyporus –*   20 g
   Grifola)

ze xie (Alismatis Rhizoma; *Alisma*)   10 g

nu zhen zi (Ligustri lucidi Fructus;   15 g
   Ligustrum lucidum fruit)

shu di (Rehmanniae Radix   15 g
   preparata; *Rehmannia*)

bai ren shen (Ginseng Radix; *Panax*   10 g
   ginseng; white ginseng)

bai mao teng (Solani lyrati Herba;   20 g
   Solanum lyratum)

The first four herbs are an unmodified version of Si jun zi tang, the main spleen qi tonic formula. Bu gu zhi is a yang tonic herb. Bu gu zhi especially helps resolve diarrhea due to spleen and kidney yang deficiency. It is very high in genistein and is antineoplastic without being cold or cooling, important in this yang-deficient condition.

Ji xue teng and huang qi are excellent herbs for supporting normal blood levels. Ji xue teng increases the red blood cells (RBCs) and huang qi increases the white blood cells (WBCs) and RBCs. Zhu ling also increases WBCs and natural killer (NK) cells to improve function and act antineoplastically. It is also mildly analgesic. These herbs all work to restore normal digestive function, prevent the loss of fluids from diarrhea, and can act to support the spleen and the kidneys to drain abnormal fluids like ascites in the abdomen and edema in the lower extremity. Nu zhen zi and dang shen are herbs that act synergistically to improve the complete blood count. Shu di nourishes the blood while bai ren shen tonifies the qi and yang. Bai mao teng acts as a classical antineoplastic herb, the only strong toxin-clearing herb of this kind in the formula.

Concerns

Pancreatic cancer affects a primary digestive organ, impacting the patient's ability to digest and assimilate. Anorexia is a major problem. Many patients with this cancer die partly from malnutrition. It is very difficult for them to eat and, therefore, to take herbal medicines or any medicines except intravenously. Many patients are fed intravenously with total parenteral nutrition (TPN). TPN can be an excellent remedy for cachexia and malnutrition, but it requires a larger fluid intake than is normal in order to protect the kidneys. As a result there may be edema and renal toxicity.

Finding ways to help a patient to continue to take food, fluids and herbal medicine via mouth is a contribution to quality of life. But finding ways to deliver herbal medicine can be problematic. One mechanism for delivering herbal medicine is via a congee or hsi fan.[30] Congee is the South-East Asian word for rice gruel; hsi fan is the Chinese word. To cook a congee use six parts of water to one part of rice. Usually white rice is used because it is very easy to digest. Other kinds of rice can be used based on what is comfortable for the patient. The cooking time for congee is between 8 and 10 hours. To the congee can be added various herbs. To drain dampness and tonify the spleen to improve nutrition and decrease fatigue and anorexia use:

1 cup rice.
6 cups water.
15 g of the following herbs:
  yi ren (Coicis Semen; *Coix lacryma-jobi*)
  ge gen (Puerariae Radix; *Pueraria*)
  fu ling (Poria; *Poria cocos*)
  dang shen (Codonopsis Radix; *Codonopsis pilosula* root)

These herbs are cooked with the congee for the full 8 hours. This long cook transforms the rice into a more yang food. Generally rice is thought to be neutral in temperature and quality; this means that the pH of rice is neither acid nor alkaline, and this is one reason why it is thought to be such a perfect food. The long cooking time makes the rice more warming and energetically nutritious. The herbs cook into the gruel and dissolve. The congee can be suited to taste by adding culinary herbs and other flavorings like salt, cinnamon, honey or maple syrup, thyme, cilantro (coriander), sage, and so on. To prepare 'to taste' means to prepare a food in such a way that an individual will eat that food. This is so important in a cancer patient who has an altered sense of taste and often no appetite at all. Preparing food that the patient can and will eat is an immense gift to them.

At the end of the cooking period vegetables or fruit can be added; meat or fish can also be added

near to the end of cooking, say 1 hour from the end, to ensure proper cooking. A breakfast congee is typically sweeter and is cooked with cinnamon, cardamom and warming culinary herbs. A lunch or dinner congee is cooked with more savory spices that are also warming but to which meats or fish can be added. This is an excellent way of helping patients to be able to eat and also to take their herbs to treat symptoms and improve quality of life. It is less about providing nutrition and more about providing comfort and palliative care through herbal medicines via food. Please see Chapter 13 on death and dying for more information about end-of-life issues.

Current research

An Ayurvedic formula used to treat diabetes mellitus has been tested by an Indian researcher at the National Cancer Institutes (NCI). It is now in phase-two clinical trials at the Mayo Clinic. This formula dramatically lowered blood sugar and substantially decreased glycosylated hemoglobin (another diabetes indicator). It did not affect the blood sugar of normal subjects. It also revitalised liver and kidney function. The formula reversed damage to pancreatic β-cells. It might be of value as a supplement to a herbal formula that is in the realm of Chinese medicine and is specific to the diagnosis for the patient.

The ingredients are:

Gymnema sylvestre: a vine common to India.
Momordica charantia (also used in Chinese medicine): the common name is balsam pear.
Tinospora cordifolia: a succulent shrub.
Trigonella foenum-graecum: fenugreek; xiao hui xiang.
Pterocarpus marsupium: the resin of a shade tree.
Azadirachta indica.
Ficus racemosa: a fig tree.
Aegle marmelos.
Szygium cumini.
Cinnamomum tamala.

LIVER CANCER

Liver cancer occurs in the presence of chronic and serious underlying disease. In patients without a history of alcoholism, the underlying disease is almost always viral, although there are occasions when parasitic infections like aflatoxins from

Aspergillus fungus are the culprit. This is more common in Africans living in Africa but aflatoxins can be found here in the USA in foods like peanut butter.

These viral infections are LPFs, and can exist asymptomatically for several years without anyone knowing the seriousness of the condition. It is very difficult to treat a visceral cancer with an underlying LPF. There are two prongs of intent; one is to clear the pathogen and the other is to clear (depurate) the toxin and move blood to treat the cancer. The pathogen is a constant irritation. HBV/HCV enters via the blood and injures the spleen function. It then finds its way to the liver according to conventional medicine. In Chinese medicine, the spleen injury leads to a damp accumulation that causes stasis. The stasis causes heat and this injures the liver via the Ko cycle. Also spleen injury can lead to blood deficiency. The liver blood when deficient can lead to liver qi stasis, liver yin deficiency, and liver blood stasis. In both cases liver stasis leads to liver blood stasis and blood stasis in the liver (cirrhosis) and heat.

Liver cancer is very difficult to treat and usually the diagnosis is very late. The best medicine is to prevent the cancer by treating the HBV/HCV. Therefore, if you have a patient at risk for HBV or HCV either through their behavioral history, that is, intravenous drug use, or through blood transfusion in the past before adequate screening for HCV (proper screening for HCV is a very recent public health implementation and began only in the early 1990s), then it is appropriate to refer them for screening. If they are found to be positive for HCV infection, it is extremely important to treat them even if asymptomatic. Treatment for HCV must happen concurrently, if at all possible, for patients with HCC. Palliative treatment is usual. Pancreatic and liver cancers are similar in this respect and their presentations are also similar, that is, when advanced disease is already present.

There are four diagnostic categories for HCC. They are very similar to those for pancreatic cancer and include the following:[31]

1. Qi and blood stasis: stage I and II.
2. Spleen deficiency with damp accumulation: stage II with or without ascites.
3. Damp heat in the liver gall bladder: stage III inflammatory type.
4. Liver/kidney yin deficiency: stage III–IV.

1. Qi and blood stasis

Symptoms: stabbing pain over the liver, anorexia, weakness, insomnia, restlessness, hepatomegaly, normal liver enzymes.
Tongue: dark with petechiae on the edges, thin coat.
Pulse: taut and thready.
Treatment principle: soothe the liver, regulate qi, invigorate blood, crack the blood, antineoplasm.

Formula:

hai zao (Sargassum; *Sargassum*)	15 g
yu jin (Curcumae Radix; *Curcuma longa* rhizome)	15 g
chai hu (Bupleuri Radix; *Bupleurum*)	10 g
chi shao (Paeoniae Radix rubra; *Paeonia lactiflora* root)	10 g
bai mao teng (Solani lyrati Herba; *Solanum lyratum*)	30 g
bai zhu (Atractylodis macrocephalae Rhizoma; *Atractylodes macrocephala*)	15 g
huang qin (Scutellariae Radix; *Scutellaria baicalensis*)	10 g
bai hua she she cao (Hedyotis diffusae Herba; *Oldenlandia*)	30 g
fu ling (Poria; *Poria cocos*)	15 g
zhi zi (Gardeniae Fructus; *Gardenia* fruit)	10 g

Hai zao is a phlegm-dissolving herb that is commonly used to treat goiter and thyroid tumors. It enters the spleen and liver channels and can help in the treatment of hepatomegaly. It is an anticoagulant similar to heparin and, as such, can act as a messenger herb to enable other herbs and cytotoxic agents into the liver. It is antifungal (aflatoxin, dampness) and can lower cholesterol (dampness) levels, which may be elevated in a patient where liver function is impaired. Yu jin is a blood-cracking herb that enters the liver channel and acts to break up the mass by reducing the fibrinogen outer capsule and by changing the viscosity of the blood. This also helps to prevent metastatic spread. Chi shao enters the spleen and liver, vitalises the blood, clears blood heat and liver fire. The liver is by nature an organ with a deep relationship with blood. Liver cancer is very much a blood-stasis type of cancer. Only the stroma of the liver is connective tissue (phlegm in nature), and there is very little of it. This cancer is almost completely pure blood stasis. Therefore, blood-cracking herbs are called for. Chi shao is antineoplastic against blood stasis tumors.

Chai hu relieves liver qi stagnation and lifts the yang. It relieves intercostal and hypochondrium pain and improves capillary permeability, which may be impaired in liver cancer if a lot of the organ is involved with tumor. Chai hu is a liver protectant and reduces elevated liver enzymes. Huang qin is a primary herb in clearing heat and drying dampness, especially damp heat in the liver. It lowers cholesterol and is especially useful in treating gall bladder disorders that may accompany this cancer. It is a broad-spectrum antibiotic and studies show that it can be used successfully to treat chronic hepatitis and cirrhosis of the liver.

Bai mao teng and bai hua she she cao are the two antineoplastics in the formula. Bai zhu and fu ling support the spleen function, which must always be supported in treating any cancer, a middle jiao cancer, and those organs related to transverse rebellion. Zhi zi drains damp heat, cools the blood to stop bleeding, is antineoplastic and useful in treating ascites. It is a liver protectant and is used to treat icteric hepatitis.

2. Spleen deficiency with damp accumulation

Symptoms: abdominal distention, diarrhea, hepatomegaly, slightly- to moderately raised liver enzymes, lower-extremity edema, ascites, anorexia, weight loss, hypochondrium pain.
Tongue: pale with white thick greasy coat.
Pulse: slippery or soft or soggy.
Treatment principle: tonify qi, strengthen the spleen, transform damp, antineoplasm.

Formula:[31]

dang shen (Codonopsis Radix; *Codonopsis pilosula* root)	15 g
bai zhu (Atractylodis macrocephalae Rhizoma; *Atractylodes macrocephala*)	15 g
fu ling (Poria; *Poria cocos*)	15 g
gan cao (Glycyrrhizae Radix; *Glycyrrhiza*; licorice root)	6 g
zhu ling (Polyporus; *Polyporus – Grifola*)	15 g
qian shi (Euryales Semen; *Euryale*)	15 g
che qian zi (Plantaginis Semen; *Plantago*)	15 g
da fu pi (Arecae Pericarpium; *Areca catechu*)	15 g
ze xie (Alismatis Rhizoma; *Alisma*)	15 g
yi ren (Coicis Semen; *Coix lacryma-jobi*)	15 g
ban zhi lian (Scutellariae barbatae Herba; *Scutellaria barbata*)	25 g
ban bian lian (Lobeliae chinensis Herba; *Lobelia chinensis*)	25 g
bai hua she she cao (Hedyotis diffusae Herba; *Oldenlandia*)	25 g

This formula begins with Si jun zi tang, the main spleen qi tonic formula, to address the main treatment principle in this presentation. Whenever dampness is a primary aspect in the presentation, then either spleen or kidneys need support to resolve the dampness. Zhu ling is added as a drain-damp herb that also helps to improve immune function by increasing WBCs and NK cells. Zhu ling is considered antineoplastic for this reason. It also promotes urination in order to provide a route for the dampness to leave and clears heat from the liver while working to resolve ascites, which is often present with liver cancer. Da fu pi is a qi-regulating herb that circulates fluids and promotes urination. It treats chronic hepatitis and edema. Ze xie drains dampness and promotes urination. It reduces edema and lowers cholesterol. Qian shi is an astringent herb that tonifies the spleen to stop diarrhea and dispels dampness without harming fluids. Yi ren functions similarly. And the last three herbs all act as antineoplastics.

3. Damp heat in the liver gall bladder

Symptoms: hypochondrium pain, fever, jaundice, restlessness, insomnia, cannot rest, bitter taste, dry mouth, nausea and vomiting, anorexia, dry stool, dark urine, oliguria, painful urinary dysfunction (PUD), hepatomegaly, ascites, abnormal liver enzymes, elevated bilirubin.

Tongue: red with yellow greasy coat.

Pulse: tight, wiry, slippery, fast.

Treatment principle: clear heat, drain damp, clear liver heat, clear gall bladder heat, antineoplasm.

Formula:[31]

da huang (Rhei Radix et Rhizoma; *Rheum*)	15 g
huang qin (Scutellariae Radix; *Scutellaria baicalensis*)	10 g
zhi zi (Gardeniae Fructus; *Gardenia* fruit)	10 g
shi hu (Dendrobii Herba; *Dendrobium*)	15 g
zhi mu (Anemarrhenae Rhizoma; *Anemarrhena*)	10 g
yu jin (Curcumae Radix; *Curcuma longa* rhizome)	15 g
jiao gu lan (Herba Gynostemmatis; *Gynostemma*)	20 g
yi ren (Coicis Semen; *Coix lacryma-jobi*)	20 g
bai mao teng (Solani lyrati Herba; *Solanum lyratum*)	25 g
hong da zao (Jujubae Fructus; *Ziziphus jujuba*; red jujube)	15 g
bai hua she she cao (Hedyotis diffusae Herba; *Oldenlandia*)	25 g
zhu ling (Polyporus; *Polyporus – Grifola*)	15 g
che qian zi (Plantaginis Semen; *Plantago*)	15 g
gua lou ren (Trichosanthis Semen; *Trichosanthes* seed)	30 g

This is a complicated diagnosis, which requires a complex approach. Da huang clears heat and moves stool. It cools and moves the blood when prepared correctly. It is antineoplastic. Huang qin and zhi zi clear heat and help to detoxify the liver. Huang qin is a liver-specific herb that also dries dampness. Yi ren, zhu ling, and che qian zi all drain dampness. They also open a pathway to drain dampness and clear heat via urination. Che qian zi can help to resolve PUD and blood in the urine. Yi ren and zhu ling also have some immunomodulating effects that give them antineoplastic properties. Shi hu and zhi mu nourish yin and benefit fluids. There are many symptoms of yin and fluid deficiency in this presentation. Shi

hu is especially good at moistening dry mouth. Zhi mu aids in this by clearing heat and generating fluids.

Yu jin cracks the blood to open the mass, treat pain, allow access of other antineoplastic herbs and possible cytotoxic agents. It helps to reduce the swelling in the liver. Bai mao teng in combination with hong da zao inhibits ascites. It is a clear-heat-and-toxin herb that also promotes urination. Gua lou ren moistens the stool to relieve dry stool and constipation. It is antineoplastic especially for liver cancer. Bai hua she she cao, bai mao teng, jiao gu lan, da huang, yi ren, and zhu ling are all also antineoplastics.

By clearing heat and nourishing yin many signs and symptoms in this diagnostic pattern are addressed. Pain is addressed through clearing heat, nourishing yin, cracking the blood, and detoxifying. By draining dampness the urinary dysfunction, hepatomegaly, and ascites are taken into account. All of these symptoms are produced by damp heat toxin. This is a strong formula and protecting the yin and the spleen is very important. No accommodations are made for spleen protection and so the formula will probably require some modification for most patients. As the dampness is drained and the heat cleared, the spleen should regain some normal function. This should manifest in some return of appetite. This corroborates the diagnosis. If the appetite does not return, the formula must be drastically modified to treat this complex presentation.

4. Yin deficiency of liver and kidney

Symptoms: dry mouth, restlessness, thirst, abdominal distention, low fever, night sweats, general body pain, emaciation, hepatomegaly, impaired liver function, hematuria.

Tongue: red with little coat.

Pulse: thready, tight, rapid, choppy.

Treatment principle: nourish yin, generate fluids, soothe the liver, nourish the blood, stop pain, antineoplasm.

Formula:[31]

mai dong (Ophiopogonis Radix; *Ophiopogon*)	15 g
tian dong (Asparagi Radix; *Asparagus*)	15 g

bei sha shen (Glehniae Radix; 10 g
    Glehnia)
shi hu (Dendrobii Herba; 15 g
    Dendrobium)
zhi mu (Anemarrhenae Rhizoma; 15 g
    Anemarrhena)
yu zhu (Polygonati odorati 10 g
    Rhizoma; Polygonatum
    odoratum)
jiao gu lan (Herba Gynostemmatis; 15 g
    Gynostemma)
mu dan pi (Moutan Cortex; Paeonia 1 g
    suffruticosa root cortex)
shan yao (Dioscoreae Rhizoma; 15 g
    Dioscorea opposita)
ze xie (Alismatis Rhizoma; Alisma) 15 g
shu di (Rehmanniae Radix 15 g
    preparata; Rehmannia)
zhi zi (Gardeniae Fructus; Gardenia 10 g
    fruit)
gui ban* (Testudinis Plastrum; 15 g
    Chinemys reevesii plastron)
bai mao teng (Solani lyrati Herba; 25 g
    Solanum lyratum)
tu yin chen (Origani vulgaris Herba; 15 g
    Origanum vulgare) or yin chen hao
    (Artemisia scoparia/A. capillaris)
gan cao (Glycyrrhizae Radix; 6 g
    Glycyrrhiza; licorice root)

The first five herbs all have to do with nourishing the yin to clear heat. Mu dan pi clears heat and cools the blood; it vitalises the blood and is especially good for blood stasis masses. It helps to treat pain by clearing heat and moving blood; it reduces liver fire rising symptoms. Shan yao nourishes the kidneys and astringes the essence while tonifying the spleen function to address abdominal distention and emaciation or cachexia. Cachexia is almost always due to spleen and kidney deficiency. Ze xie drains dampness via the urine and clears heat to address the urinary difficulty, and is used here because of its ability to move downward deficient kidney fire, which is common in a yin-deficiency presentation and in a heart/kidney cystitis. Shu di potentiates the yin-nourishing herbs and also works to root the kidney fire. Zhi zi clears heat, drains damp heat, cools the blood, inhibits ascitic carcinoma, and helps to resolve the urinary dysfunction as manifested in hematuria.

Gui ban nourishes the yin and brings down ascending yang. It nourishes the kidneys and cools the blood. It enters the liver and kidneys and is mildly analgesic. Jiao gu lan and bai mao teng are the main antineoplastics in the formula. Tu yin chen regulates the qi to lessen pain; it also drains dampness and is antiviral, especially in treating icteric hepatitis, and in this way helps to adjust liver enzyme levels. The general body pain is caused by several factors, liver qi stasis, blood stasis due to liver injury, and disharmony between the ying and wei. Tu yin chen releases the exterior by regulating the ying and wei thereby lessening pain. It treats jaundice.

TREATMENT FOR HEPATITIS C VIRUS

Diagnosis for hepatitis C is based on enzyme immunoassay that detects antibodies to HCV. AntiHCV antibody is not a protective antibody. The enzyme immunoassay has limitations since it is only moderately sensitive for diagnosis of acute hepatitis C (false negatives) and has a low specificity (50%) in healthy blood donors and some persons who are potentially infectious. Recombinant immunoblot assay (RIBA) is used for confirmation, and most RIBA-positive persons are potentially infectious. This is then confirmed by yet another advanced test using polymerase chain reaction (PCR)-based tests to detect HCV RNA. In patients who test positive in the first two screens but have no HCV RNA in the serum, it is assumed that they have recovered from past HCV infection. Testing for HCV in donated blood has helped reduce the risk for transfusion-associated hepatitis C from 10% in the early 1990s to 0.1% in the year 2000.

Viral forms of hepatitis B and non-A-non-B (HCV) are often treated with interferon-α or a new anti-retroviral regimen that includes Ribavirin. However, treatment generalisation is difficult: what is helpful for one patient may exert no noticeable influence on the next. The major forms of treatments include anti-inflammatory agents, antiviral agents, immunomodulators and bile resins. Treatment must curtail necrosis due to persistent inflammation, allaying the formation of lesions or granulomas, which may lead to life-threatening disease due to loss of parenchymal tissue or to cancer and then necessitate organ transplantation.

From the Chinese medical point of view, there are several treatment principles used:[32]

- boost immunity
- prevent necrosis by clearing heat and moving blood
- support regeneration of new liver tissue
- promote bile flow, waste elimination, and toxin clearing
- address any addictions, if necessary, e.g. alcoholism, recreational drug abuse
- improve diet, if necessary.

Botanicals

- Liver 52: Ayurvedic formula.
- *Cynara scolymus* fruit: globe artichoke.
- *Glycyrrhiza glabra*: deglycyrrhised licorice (DGL).
- *Silybum*: silymarin (milk thistle).
- *Eclipta prostrata*: han lian cao; Ecliptae Herba
- *Phyllanthus amarus*: zhen zhu cao; Phyllanthi amari Herba
- *Schisandra*: wu wei zi; Schisandrae Fructus

There are several herbs in Chinese medicine that are especially antiviral for HCV:[33]

- *Artemisia scoparia*, which is one substitute for *A. capillaris*, yin chen hao; Artemisiae scopariae Herba. *Artemisia scoparia* is more active against HCV
- *Solanum lyratum* is a nightshade, which has antiviral activity for HCV. The pin yin is bai mao teng (Solani lyrati Herba).
- *Coptis*: huang lian; Coptidis Rhizoma
- *Arnebia/Lithospermum*: zi cao; Arnebiae/Lithospermi Radix
- *Hypericum*: di er cao; Hyperici japonici Herba
- *Isatis/Baphicacanthus* root: ban lan gen; Isatidis/Baphicacanthis Radix
- *Polygonum cuspidatum*: hu zhang; Polygoni cuspidati Rhizoma
- *Senecio scandens*: qian li guang; Senecionis scandens Herba
- *Scutellaria baicalensis*: huang qin; Scutellariae Radix
- *Taraxacum mongolicus*: pu gong ying; Taraxaci Herba.

These herbs when used in a formula specific to the patient diagnosis and presentation will help to lower HCV levels when measured with PCR technique. It is important to institute a broad approach including diet and nutrition, exercise, sleep, and detoxification.

Hepatitis moves through several phases from acute to chronic to cirrhosis to cancer:

- acute is the equivalent of damp heat
- chronic is the beginning of spleen and liver qi and blood deficiency
- chronic moves into cirrhosis with ascites which is the equivalent of damp heat in the blood level
- damp heat in the blood level leads to turbid phlegm and phlegm heat with severe blood stasis; this is the environment in which a malignancy evolves.

Several studies have been conducted in China on the treatment of chronic HBV and HCV infections of the liver with Chinese herbal medicine. One study using the following formula[34] used over a period of 6 months showed that the level of liver cirrhosis lowered by one grade and the liver transaminase levels returned to normal. There were 63 patients in the study, all of whom had been treated with either interferon or lamivudine.

yin chen hao (Artemisiae scopariae Herba; *Artemisia scoparia/A. capillaris*)	250 g
bai shao (Paeoniae Radix alba; *Paeonia lactiflora* root)	125 g
huang qi (Astragali Radix; *Astragalus membranaceus*)	250 g
huang jing (Polygonati Rhizoma; *Polygonatum*)	125 g
shan zha (Crataegi Fructus; *Crataegus*)	100 g
gan cao (Glycyrrhizae Radix; *Glycyrrhiza* licorice root)	100 g
ban lan gen (Isatidis/Baphicacanthis Radix; *Isatis/Baphicacanthus* root)	125 g
dan shen (Salviae miltiorrhizae Radix; *Salvia miltiorhiza* root)	250 g
dang shen (Codonopsis Radix; *Codonopsis pilosula* root)	125 g
shu di (Rehmanniae Radix preparata; *Rehmannia*)	125 g

shen qu (Massa medicata fermentata; medicated leaven)	100 g
dang gui (Angelicae sinensis Radix; *Angelica sinensis*)	125 g
yu jin (Curcumae Radix; *Curcuma longa* rhizome)	125 g
ze xie (Alismatis Rhizoma; *Alisma*)	125 g
shan yao (Dioscoreae Rhizoma; *Dioscorea opposita*)	125 g
qin jiao (Gentianae macrophyllae Radix; *Gentiana macrophylla*)	100 g

Nutritional therapy

- Magnesium.
- Zinc picolinate.
- Vitamin A.
- Vitamin E.
- Vitamin C.
- Vitamin B$_{12}$.
- Folic acid.
- Liver extracts.

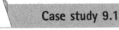

Case study 9.1

This was an 82-year-old female diagnosed with an infiltrating pancreatic ductal adenocarcinoma that was moderately differentiated. She had suffered a 30 lb weight loss in the 4 months prior to diagnosis. It was jaundice and hypochondrium pain that took her to her doctor. A chest, abdomen and pelvis CT scan was performed and metastatic disease was found in the left lower lobe of the lung and several paratracheal nodes were visualised with disease. The right lobe of the thyroid gland was also involved. The head and uncinate process of the pancreas were seen to be involved with masses. The common hepatic duct, the common bile duct, and the intrahepatic ducts were all dilated, and the gall bladder was enlarged. The left lobe of the liver showed a mass, with several masses in the dome of the liver, and both the left and right lobes. The infrarenal abdominal aorta was dilated. This was stage IV disease.

A non-cytoreductive surgery was performed to place a stent to reroute bile around the bile ducts. The large amount of local and metastatic disease precluded any approach besides palliation. Chemotherapy was offered but the patient refused, realising that her prognosis was very poor and chemotherapy would aid in palliation but perhaps at the expense of quality of life. This is not always true but it was the belief of the patient that her life would be made miserable by chemotherapy.

All of the liver transaminase levels were elevated above 200. The bilirubin was elevated to 5.8 and the RBC level was slightly low. Blood glucose levels were around 130 mg/dL. Triglycerides were high normal and total cholesterol had gradually fallen off to 135 mg/dL from over 200 mg/dL 4 months earlier. The CA 19-9 was elevated, as well as the CEA and alpha-fetoprotein (AFP).

The patient history included colon polyps and diverticulitis. The polyps demonstrated an underlying historical diagnosis of spleen deficiency with dampness pouring down. The diverticulitis was probably a reference to a liver/spleen disharmony with a transverse rebellion. She also had been living with a rectocele for several years, another manifestation of spleen deficiency and prolapse. She was hypertensive. She had delivered four children, all of whom were still alive.

General signs and symptoms

- Appetite: very low.
- Digestion: above navel normal except for excessive salivation.
- Below navel: bloating, distention, gas, cramping.
- Stool: very sluggish even with metamucil, cramping, hemorrhoids, three times daily, hard and dry to well-formed, clay-color prior to stent placement.
- Diabetes: no history although blood sugar was high.
- Sleep: hard to get to sleep; partly due to worry, but mostly due to pain.
- Energy level: slight improvement with pain relief, but still low at 4/10.

Case study continues

- Thirst: slight thirst but no desire to drink fluids, prefers drinks at room temperature.
- Temperature: tending to run cold, no fevers.
- Sweating: none.
- Pruritis: general itching without rash.
- Urination: frequent and difficult due to obstruction from rectocele.
- Pain: low-back, across abdomen and radiating to the flank and back, especially on right, partly from surgery; twisting and stabbing, worse at night and in morning after eating.
- Spirits: afraid and sad but wishes to live until 'not living', very positive and life-affirming, humorous.
- Tongue: scarlet with no coat, horizontal cracks across stomach/spleen area, gross vein distention (+4).
- Pulse: liver/kidney sho, left pulses very weak, very rapid (95), slippery.
- Hara: hard masses across pancreas reflex (Matsumoto); cold spleen and kidney reflex, clammy lung reflexes, concave stomach reflex, spider angiomas across abdomen, tight above and flaccid below, liver reflex very tight and tender, blood stasis reflex hard at deep level.

Medications

- Norvasc.
- Atenolol.
- Vitamin K.
- Calcium.
- Aspirin.

Diagnosis

1. Damp heat with toxin and qi and blood stasis.
2. Underlying qi and spleen qi deficiency.

Both of these presentations were present in this patient at the time of diagnosis. After being treated for one year with combined care, the diagnosis did change as stated later in this text.

Treatment plan

1. Palliative care, focusing on pain control and any other symptoms that arise.

Except for managing the side effects of pain-control medication, this is one rare occasion when treating strictly with Chinese herbal medicine is possible. It means that there is no need to interface with conventional care and this, in turn, allows the full force of herbal medicine to be used. Of course, the circumstances are dire and no two cases are the same, but the expectation is only for palliation with supportive care being given both by conventional and Chinese medicine.

Since this patient had never been treated before and was in stage IV pancreatic cancer, it was necessary and very important to approach treatment with caution and with a gentle formula to test the environment of the patient and their ability to metabolise and assimilate the formula. The following formula was given as a test:

dang gui (Angelicae sinensis Radix; *Angelica sinensis*)	6 g
chuan xiong (Chuanxiong Rhizoma; *Ligusticum wallichii* root)	6 g
xiao hui xiang (Foeniculi Fructus; *Foeniculum vulgare*; fennel seed)	10 g
pei lan (Eupatorii Herba; *Eupatorium fortunei*)	6 g
huang qi (Astragali Radix; *Astragalus membranaceus*)	12 g
ji nei jin (Gigeriae galli Endothelium corneum; *Gallus gallus domesticus* chicken gizzard lining)	10 g
mai ya (Hordei Fructus germinatus; *Hordeum vulgare*; barley sprouts; malt)	10 g
da fu pi (Arecae Pericarpium; *Areca catechu*)	6 g
bai xian pi (Dictamni Cortex; *Dictamnus*)	6 g
gan cao (Glycyrrhizae Radix; *Glycyrrhiza*; licorice root)	6 g

The dose was 4 grams three times daily.

Dang gui nourishes the blood, vitalises the blood to stop pain, moistens the intestines to treat constipation, is analgesic, lowers blood pressure, and is a liver protectant. Chuan xiong regulates the blood and helps to relieve flank pain. It is also antihypertensive. Xiao hui xiang regulates the qi and enters the liver and, therefore, treats abdominal pain. It improves appetite and increases peristalsis to move stool. Pei lan aromatically dries dampness and harmonises the middle jiao. It is a neutral herb that is mild and transforms dampness,

Case study continues

treats jaundice, and improves appetite. Huang qi is a major spleen and lung tonic herb that improves whole body function, increases WBCs to prevent infection, RBCs to treat anemia and improve energy, increases NK cell activity and surveillance against tumor cells. Although it is warming, it was felt that its presence was necessary to support the spleen and for its immunomodulatory benefits.

Ji nei jin and mai ya work together to prevent food stagnation in a seriously ill patient with a middle jiao cancer. They help to reduce distention, gas and bloating. Da fu pi regulates the qi, dispels dampness, and moves the stool. Bai xian pi is the only cooling herb in the formula and clears heat and drains dampness. It treats damp heat jaundice and can provide relief in the wind-generated pruritic itching condition that often accompanies pancreatic cancer.

This is a mild formula to address several of the main symptoms of this patient. Its intent is to stimulate digestion, resolve the damp heat portion of the diagnosis without being too cooling and injurious to the stomach/spleen axis, move stool, and reduce pain to enable the patient to sleep.

The patient was on this formula with minor variations for 4 months and did well; the pain was reduced and sleep improved with the addition of acetaminophen and diphenhydramine hydrochloride (Tylenol PM). The fact that she did well on this formula seemed to undermine the diagnosis of damp heat because the formula is quite warming. However, it worked well without side effects and so it was assumed that damp heat was some component along with spleen deficiency dampness. She began to eat again and had at least one meal per day that was eaten with gusto. The appetite improved partially because the stool began to move. Stasis at one end of the gastrointestinal tube will eventually shut down the other end. In this case, the anorexia was partly due to dampness in the middle jiao, spleen deficiency, and qi flushing upwards caused by constipation. Regulating the whole mechanism of digestion helped everything, including sleep. Sleep was improved because there was no longer a back-up in the digestion, which caused the qi to flush upward, a disturbing energetic mechanism; this allowed the patient to eat more regularly and this

nourishment regulated the blood sugars, allowing the patient to sleep more easily; the heart/spleen axis was nourished finally. All of these resolutions helped reduce the pain, as well, and sleep was, therefore, improved.

The next evolution of this cancer began 4 months later. Once again pain was the precipitating issue. Without cytotoxic therapy, the cancer continued to spread. The stent continued to provide a bypass for bile but the abdominal metastases began to cause more and more obstructive symptoms. The primary result was pain. This was a stabbing and dull pain that was better with warmth and pressure. Some of the masses had become necrotic and the tissue necrosis caused an inflammatory process that stimulated nerve receptors in the abdomen. The patient was put on oxycodone (Oxycontin) to manage the pain. This recreated constipation and sluggish stool and the whole cascade of upper, middle and lower digestive tract symptoms recurred.

The following formula was used to act more antineoplastically, treat the pain more directly, move stool, and treat fatigue. The dose was increased to 6 g four times daily:

dan shen (Salviae miltiorrhizae Radix; *Salvia miltiorhiza* root)	15 g
yan hu suo (Corydalis Rhizoma; *Corydalis yanhusuo*)	15 g
mo yao (Myrrha; *Commiphora myrrha*; myrrh)	15 g
mai ya (Hordei Fructus germinatus; *Hordeum vulgare*; barley sprouts; malt)	15 g
shen qu (Massa medicata fermentata; medicated leaven)	15 g
ji nei jin (Gigeriae galli Endothelium corneum; *Gallus gallus domesticus* chicken gizzard lining)	20 g
tai zi shen (Pseudostellariae Radix; *Pseudostellaria heterophylla*)	20 g
xi yang shen (Panacis quinquefolii Radix; *Panax quinquefolium*)	10 g
da huang (Rhei Radix et Rhizoma; *Rheum*)	15 g
fan xie ye (Sennae Folium; *Cassia*; senna leaf)	15 g

Case study continues

ba yue zha (Akebiae Fructus; *Akebia*) 25 g
chong lou (Paridis Rhizoma; *Paris*) 30 g
fu ling (Poria; *Poria cocos*) 20 g
huang qi (Astragali Radix; *Astragalus membranaceus*) 30 g
tu fu ling (Smilacis glabrae Rhizoma; *Smilax glabra*) 20 g
bai hua she she cao (Hedyotis diffusae Herba; *Oldenlandia*) 20 g
bai mao teng (Solani lyrati Herba; *Solanum lyratum*) 25 g
lai fu zi (Raphani Semen; *Raphanus sativus*) 15 g
ling zhi (Ganoderma; *Ganoderma*) 40 g
hong da zao (Jujubae Fructus; *Ziziphus jujuba*; red jujube) 10 g

Dan shen, yan hu suo, mo yao all crack the blood to treat pain and allow the antineoplastics and clear-heat herbs into the necrotic center of the masses. Mai ya, shen qu, ji nei jin, and lai fu zi work to prevent food stagnation and to stimulate the digestive enzymes to improve digestion, appetite, and absorption. Tai zi shen and xi yang shen tonify the qi and yin. Nourishing qi and fluids is important in a patient who is not eating well, who is constipated primarily because of pharmaceutical drugs, and who is in pain. Tonifying qi helps to move the qi and blood; and nourishing yin helps soothe and calm both physiologically and emotionally. Da huang and fan xie ye are stronger purgatives to move stool. Moving stool is very important in treating abdominal pain and maintaining upper digestion including appetite.

Chong lou and bai mao teng are the main antineoplastic herbs in the formula. They are very important in order to attack the cancer. They clear heat to reduce inflammation and help to detoxify the products of necrosis. Once the patient had been tested with the first formula, these two antineoplastics were added and had been present for about 2 months prior to the latest events. Tu fu ling was added because it clears damp heat toxins and is especially good in this kind of inflammatory process. And bai hua she she cao was added because it is especially antineoplastic for digestive tumors. Ba yue zha is also antineoplastic for this type of cancer. Ling zhi tonifies the qi and nourishes the fluids, removes toxins, and calms the spirit. It is a strong immunomodulating herb that increases WBCs to reduce risk of infection, increases RBCs to treat fatigue, decreases platelet aggregation to reduce metastatic spread, and is mildly analgesic. Fu ling and hong da zao support the spleen to metabolise these herbs and prevent dampness, which is already present. They are ameliorating herbs for the spleen in such a strong formula. Fu ling is also immune modulating.

The patient did well on variations of this formula for another 4 months. The tumors did not reduce but did not progress. The side effects of the Oxycontin were well managed. The patient was able to eat and to sleep. Pain was well controlled with the pharmaceutical drug and herb combination. The patient's weight remained stable for the duration of treatment. Her spirit was calm and centered. She was able to see everyone in her life that she wanted to and to have many immensely meaningful conversations. This gave her great comfort and joy. She was, in fact, often radiant.

At month 9 from diagnosis and initiation of treatment with Chinese herbal medicine the patient began to experience pain that was intractable. She was given a fentanyl patch to place over the area of greatest pain; her liver and gall bladder area. This patch delivered a transcutaneous steady dose of opioid analgesic to the area. After 1 month utilising this method, a hospice was called and arrangements were made to treat the patient at home with a PCA (personal computerised analgesia or personally controlled analgesia). This push-button system allowed the patient to have some control over her pain by releasing medication herself in measured doses. Eventually she became bedridden.

She was fed herbs via congee, which contained 100 g of granulated Li zhong tang added the last hour of cooking the congee. Crude herbs were added at the beginning of the cooking and consisted of yi ren (Coicis Semen; *Coix lacryma-jobi*), fu shen (Poriae Sclerotium pararadicis; *Poria cocos*), gui zhi (Cinnamomi Ramulus; *Cinnamomum cassia* twigs), and ding xiang (Caryophylli Flos;

Case study continues

Syzygium aromaticum). Although the original diagnosis was one of damp heat, the environment at this point in the cancer was one of spleen and kidney yang deficiency. With the gui zhi and ding xiang, the Li Zhong tang became a modification of Fu zi li zhong tang. This tasted good to the patient and helped with the pain. It provided some nourishment and was made into various styles of congee. Meat no longer interested her but sometimes fish was added. Miso (fermented soy) was the best substitution for protein and the saltier flavor tonified her kidney deficiency. Ren shen was double-boiler cooked for 5 hours at 40 g ren shen per cook. The juice from this process was added to the congee or given in a common tea to sip. This was immensely helpful in treating the fatigue, tonifying the whole body qi and calming the spirit. With the pain well controlled she was able to rest easily. During this time she lost another 15 lb for a total of 45 lb weight loss during her illness.

Eventually she stopped eating and drinking and remained only on the ren shen (Ginseng Radix; *Panax ginseng*) for the last week of her life. The patient passed calmly and quietly without struggle and without rattle 12 months after she was diagnosed with stage IV pancreatic cancer. Her family did not suffer by her bedside; they were also peaceful with her death.

References

1. American Cancer Society. Cancer Statistics – 2000. J Am Cancer Society 2000; 45:8–30.
2. Gloeckler LA. Cancer Statistics Review, 1973–1988 (NIH Publ 91-2789). Bethesda, Md: National Institutes of Health; 1988.
3. Krain L. The rising incidence of carcinoma of the pancreas: an epidemiological appraisal. Am J Gastroenterol 1970; 54:500.
4. Roebuck BD. Promotion by unsaturated fat of asazerine-induced pancreatic carcinogenesis in the rat. Cancer Res 1981; 41:3966.
5. Offerhaus GJA. Gastric, pancreatic and colorectal carcinogenesis following remote peptic ulcer surgery. Mod Pathol 1988; 1:352–356.
6. Pour P. The effect of N-nitrosobis-(2-oxopropyl)-almine after oral administration to hamsters. Cancer Lett 1977; 2:323.
7. Karmody A. The association between carcinoma of the pancreas and diabetes mellitus. Br J Surg 1969; 56:362.
8. Brooks J. Cancer of the pancreas. In: Brooks JR, ed. Surgery of the pancreas. Philadelphia: WB Saunders; 1983:263.
9. Legg MA. Pathology of the pancreas. In: Brooks JR, ed. Surgery of the pancreas. Philadelphia: WB Saunders; 1983:41–77.
10. Freeny PC. Endoscopic retrograde cholangiopancreatography (ERCP) and percutaneous transhepatic cholangiography (PTC) in the evaluation of suspected pancreatic carcinoma: diagnostic limitations and contemporary roles. Cancer 1981; 47:1666–1678.
11. Taylor KJW. Grey scale ultrasonography in the diagnosis of jaundice. Arch Surg 1977; 112:820–825.
12. Pasquali C. Evaluation of carbohydrate antigens 19-9 and CA-125 in patients with pancreatic cancer. Pancreas 1987; 2:34–37.
13. Romond EH. Adjuvant therapy of gastrointestinal cancer. Cancer Treat Res 1990; 33:273–295.
14. Whipple AO. Treatment of carcinoma of the ampulla of Vater. Ann Surg 1935; 102:763.
15. Theve NO. Adenocarcinoma of the pancreas – a hormone sensitive tumor? A preliminary report on Nolvadex treatment. Clin Oncol 1983; 9:193.
16. Leung JWC. Coeliac plexus block for pain in pancreatic cancer and chronic pancreatitis. Br J Surg 1983; 70:730–732.
17. Thompson GE. Abdominal pain and alcohol coeliac plexus block. Anaesthesia Analgesia 1977; 56:1–5.
18. International Union Against Cancer: Workshop on Biology of Human Cancer. Rep. 17: Hepatocellular carcinoma. Geneva; 1982.
19. Beasley RP. Prevention of perinatally transmitted hepatitis B virus infections with hepatitis B immune globulin and hepatitis B vaccine. Lancet 1983; 2:1099–1122.
20. Adamson RC. Carcinogenicity of aflatoxin B1 in rhesus monkeys: two additional cases of primary liver cancer. J Natl Cancer Inst 1976; 57:67–78.
21. Beazley R. Tumors of the pancreas, gallbladder, and extrahepatic ducts. ACS Textbook of Clin Onc 1994; 16:219–231.
22. Okuda K. Surgical management of hepatoma: the Japanese experience. In: Wnaebo JH, ed. Hepatic

and biliary surgery. New York: Marcel Dekker; 1987:219–238.

23. Okuda K. Prognosis of primary hepatocellular carcinoma. Hepatology 1997; 4:3–68.

24. Chin H. Hepatocellular carcinoma: statistical analysis of 78 consecutive patients (abstract). Proc Am Soc Clin Oncol 1994; 3:6.

25. Lewis BJ. Current status for chemotherapy for hepatoma. In: Ogawa M, ed. Chemotherapy of hepatic tumors. Princeton, NJ: Excerpta Medica; 1996:63–74.

26. Gastrointestinal Tumor Study Group. A prospective trial of recombinant human interferon alpha 2B in previously untreated patients with hepatocellular carcinoma. Cancer 1990; 66:135–139.

27. Yodono H. Arterial infusion chemotherapy for advanced hepatocellular carcinoma with EPF and EAP therapies. Cancer Chemther Pharmacol 1992; 31:S89–S92.

28. Order SE. Iodine 131 antiferritin, a newer treatment modality in hepatoma: an ROTG study. J Clin Oncol 1991; 3:1573–1582.

29. Sun, Gui Zhi. Kanh Ai Zhong Yao Fang Xuan (Treatment of cancer with Chinese herbal medicine); 1992:192–200.

30. Pitchford P. Healing with whole foods. Berkeley, CA: North Atlantic Books; 2002:477–479.

31. Zhang, Dai Zhao. Zhang Dai Zhao Zhi Ai Jing Yan Ji Yao (A collection of Zhang Dai Zhao's experiences in the treatment of cancer). Beijing: Chinese Medicine and Pharmaceutical Publishing House; 2001.

32. Ergil K. The treatment of viral hepatitis with TCM. Protocol Journal of Botanical Medicine 1995; Autumn:145–150.

33. Wang, Xiao Tao. Zhong Yao Pao Zhi Du Zeng Xiao Lun (Discussion of increasing the effectiveness of different preparations of Chinese materia medica). Zhong Guo Zhong Yao Za Zhi (Journal of Chinese Materia Medica) 1999; 24:146–148.

34. Yang LM. Clinical pathologic study on the effect of Qianggan capsule in treating patients with chronic hepatitis B with liver cirrhosis. Chinese Journal of Integrated Traditional and Western Medicine 2002; 8:85–99.

Chapter 10

Lymphomas

CHAPTER CONTENTS

General overview   253

Non–Hodgkin's lymphoma   254
    Indolent lymphomas   254
    Intermediate and high-grade non-Hodgkin's
        lymphomas   263

Hodgkin's disease   266

Violence was part of the very context of discovery of pesticides during World War I. The manufacture of explosives had a direct spin-off effect on the development of synthetic insecticides. The tear gas, chloropicrin, was found to be insecticidal in 1916 and thus changed from a wartime product to a peacetime one. DDT's discovery was the culmination of a research effort motivated purely by commercial concerns, but the compound's adoption was inextricably enmeshed in the politics of war. Pesticides were born as devastating weapons in man's war against his own kind. Organophosphates, of which parathion and malathion are the most widely used, are aimed at destroying the nervous system, whether the victim is an insect or a warm blooded animal.

from *Staying Alive* by Vandana Shiva, 1989

GENERAL OVERVIEW

Leukemias and lymphomas have a relationship to one another through hematopoiesis. Stem cells evolve either towards myeloid lines or towards lymphoid cell lines. The myeloid cell lines evolve, under normal circumstances, into reticulocytes, megakaryocytes, promyelocytes, or promonocytes. These cells then evolve into RBCs, platelets, neutrophils, monocytes, or eosinophils or basophils. In the myeloid lines these are the end cells of hematopoiesis. Lymphoid cell lines evolve only into prolymphocytes, which then become either B-cells or T-cells.

Lymphomas are divided into two types: Hodgkin's Disease or Non-Hodgkin's lymphoma (NHL). NHL is of two types, either B-cell NHL or T-cell NHL. Both of these types involve malignancies within the major lymph node groups.

In staging lymphomas, the Ann Arbor–Cotswolds staging system is used for both Hodgkin's disease and NHL.

- Stage I: involvement of a single lymph node region or involvement of a single extralymphatic site (stage IE).
- Stage II: involvement of more than two node regions on the same side of the diaphragm, which may include localised extralymphatic involvement of the same side of the diaphragm (stage IIE).
- Stage III: involvement of lymph node regions on both sides of the diaphragm, which may include involvement of the spleen (stage IIIS) or localised extranodal disease (stage IIIE).
- Stage IV: diffuse extralymphatic disease, such as liver, bone, marrow, lung, skin, even breast.

Modifiers of these stages are included:

- A: no symptoms
- B: fever, night sweats, weight loss
- C: extranodal sites
- X: bulky disease.

NON-HODGKIN'S LYMPHOMA

Non-Hodgkin's lymphoma includes a group of lymphoproliferative disorders with a wide variation in growth rate, progression and response to therapy. Approximately 70000 new cases are diagnosed each year in the United States. Types vary with age and sex. The death rate is 13 times higher than Hodgkin's disease. Currently NHL is considered an epidemic disease because of a rise in incidence of almost 200% since 1970.[1] The incidence of NHL is five times higher in farmers than in the general population. This rate does not include farm workers, who are generally not screened.

Of NHLs, 80% are of B-cell origin. The T-cell lymphomas tend to be aggressive. Follicular lymphomas are tumors of germinal centers of lymph nodes and are more indolent and of B-cell origin. Low-grade NHL is indolent and does not respond well to chemotherapy. The intermediate and high-grade types are more aggressive, but do respond well to chemotherapy and radiation.

INDOLENT LYMPHOMAS

Indolent non-Hodgkin's lymphomas are a heterogeneous group of lymphoproliferative disorders usually associated with relatively long survival. They are almost all of B-cell origin and include follicular small cleaved, follicular small and large-cell, small lymphocytic, immunosecretory (Waldenstrom's), marginal zone, and some cases of mantle-cell lymphoma (MCL). Indolent lymphomas can also be classified as low-grade lymphomas. There can be variable histology within the same patient, causing confusion. These mixed types are referred to as either composite lymphoma or as discordant lymphoma depending on the types.

Biology

Lymphocytes arise in the bone marrow from a hematopoietic stem cell. Their differentiation can be divided into two stages: early, antigen-independent, and late, antigen-dependent. Just as T-cells undergo early differentiation in the thymus, early B-cell differentiation occurs in the bone marrow.

Several steps occur in the rearrangement of Ig (immunoglobulin) through chromosomal activity ending in a pre-B-cell. If this rearrangement on the first chromosome is unsuccessful, the second allele can rearrange beyond the normal stage and proceed to pathogenesis. Because of a given relationship with Ig, the expression of surface immunoglobulin (sIg) is the hallmark of a mature B-cell. As the pre-B-cells express sIgM, they gradually change from large, rapidly dividing cells (small non-cleaved cells) to small resting cells. These are called naive or virgin mature B-cells. They leave the bone marrow and circulate briefly and then move to the perifollicular lymphoid tissue or the splenic marginal zone. Most mature B-cells entering a germinal center, like the spleen, will undergo apoptosis or programmed cell death. For B-cells to continue into postfollicle stages, they need a dual signal, one from antigen engagement with sIg receptor, and the second mediated by T-cell help.[2]

One model for lymphomagenesis posits that clonal B-cells carrying a specific translocation (t[14;18]) are subject to the same regulatory mechanisms as normal cells, but on antigen exposure these cells behave differently, failing to differentiate further and undergo apoptosis. The outcome is follicular lymphoma, a disease initiated by a chromosomal translocation and then promoted by an antigen-driven process.

Follicular lymphomas are the most common B-cell neoplasm in the West. They constitute 45% of all NHLs and 80% of all indolent lymphomas.[3] In follicular lymphomas the median survival is 8–10 years. These are exclusively adult and occur equally among males and females. Approximately 80–90% of patients present with advanced-stage disease (stage III or IV) with generalised adenopathy and a high incidence of bone marrow involvement.

Chinese medicine

The pathogenesis of lymphomas in Chinese medicine is not necessarily different for each type, although there are several patterns. What follows is not specific but is a general pathogenic theory for low-grade, intermediate grade, and high-grade types and Hodgkin's disease. The pathogeneses of lymphomas and leukemias according to Chinese medicine share a commonality. In conventional terms these two non-solid cancers can transform back and forth to one another; treatment for one can result in the transformation of one kind of cancer into the other. The blood and lymph progenitor cells are intimately related. In Chinese medicine, the relationship is similar. However, another shared characteristic is perhaps of greater significance. The shared common pathogen in both is most likely a latent pathogenic factor (LPF). Conventional medicine does not have an overall concept that expresses the idea of a latent pathogen as stated by Zhang Zhong Jing in the Shang Han Za Bing Lun, the first text in which this concept was presented.[4] However, latent viral infection exemplifies the concept of a latent pathogenic factor as it has become to be known in later wen bing theory.

The idea of latent pathogens may be related to many cancers. The concept has become intimately entwined with warm disease theory.[5] However, in modern times it may be necessary to expand the theory of LPFs to include chemical contamination. This is especially true in the developed world where almost all of life's creatures now have measurable levels of chemical contamination. It is not known how these contaminants can combine to create disease in humans.

One example is DDT,[6] which has been outlawed for use for over 40 years now. DDT is a xenoestrogenic organochlorine pesticide. Xenoestrogens look like normal endogenous estrogen to the human body. Normal body estrogen breaks down every 24 hours. The xenoestrogenic exposure from DDT breaks down after 44 years. So the effect of this exposure is long term and cumulative, not unlike a latent pathogenic factor. DDT also encourages the body to form new estrogen receptors with the end result of a long-lasting, increasing, and cumulative exposure to estrogen over the years. Chemical exposures act in much the same way as LPFs; they smolder in deeper levels of the body remaining ostensibly asymptomatic but eventually manifesting as a serious and chronic illness.

Even though the use of DDT was made illegal many years ago, it persists in the soil and water of the lands where it has been applied. It persists and accumulates downwind and downwater from the site of application and does not biodegrade for many years. The body of the outside environment is no different from the body of the internal animal environment. The carcinogenic effect of the increased exposure to estrogen-like substances through many fat-soluble organochlorine pesticides and herbicides is a modern example of a latent pathogenic factor. One toxic chemical that has been linked to non-Hodgkin's lymphoma is 2,4-D, an agricultural herbicide.[7] This may explain the higher incidence of NHL in farmers. The incidence of NHL in farmers is measured only in landowners who farm their land and not in the migrant farmworker populations. The actual rate of incidence of NHL in people who work on lands that are farmed according to modern agricultural monoculture techniques that require heavy inputs of pesticides, herbicides, nitrogen fertilisers, water, etc., is unknown.

Terms that are used to describe stuck latent pathogens:

- Fu: a latent, dormant, deep-lying pathogen that is barely perceptible; this term is also used to describe abdominal masses and lymph nodes
- Fu qi: refers to a latent pathogen that can symptomatically emerge later, long after the exposure to the pathogen
- Fu qi wen bing: refers to interior latent diseases caused by a pathogen that obstructs the qi mechanism; the pathogen sits until a later season when it emerges or until another evil causes it to emerge to the surface symptomatically.

These latent pathogens are typically heat, damp heat, or cold pathogens.[8] When we look at heat as an exterior pathogen usually we will see a fever caused by the wei qi battling with the pathogen, a sore throat when the taiyang layer or lung is attacked by heat in the superficial level, chills due to obstruction, and a rapid and floating pulse with a tongue that is normal but may have a red tip. When a heat pathogen is trapped interiorly, we see a low-grade fever with low-grade heat signs. The tongue may be red with no coat and a thick sticky dry yellow coat. There may be thirst due to heat lingering and scorching the fluids. This looks like yin deficiency but isn't. It also looks like category B symptoms.

LPF etiology

1. A pathogen can enter the body, manifest a few brief signs and/or move to the interior where it may lay dormant or it may emerge due to proper treatment or the body's own process. The ongoing exposure to chemical pathogens is impossible to differentiate symptomatically. Currently, an ongoing attempt is being made to not only understand how these chemicals may affect us but also how to get them out of the human body, how to disperse the pathogen.[9]
2. A wind invasion with an acute pathogen enters the body and is not expelled and sinks to the ying or deeper level. Again there is usually no way to differentiate pre- and post-exposure to chemical pathogens, which may have similarities to a wind pathogen. For example, many chemical exposures elicit a red, raised rash, which is a typical manifestation of wind heat. But most often the exposure goes unnoticed

and is insidious, eliciting a response only when acute toxicity from gross heavy exposure occurs. And so, little is known about how they may or may not affect us, and the exposures are so persistent, most of us never know we have ever been exposed until we are tested.[9]

Classical predispositions[10]

1. A weak constitution, which may be at the jing level (traditionally) or from acquired constitutional injuries (likely) allows penetration by an exterior pathogen in an individual.
2. Poor self-care leads to a weak constitution or a moment of indisposition; it is probable that typical promoting factors for cancer also are promoting factors for LPFs in the modern sense; for example, promoting factors for cancer include a diet that promotes diabetes and cardiovascular diseases, and these diseases imply a damp environment with phlegm stasis and middle jiao injury. LPFs are potentiated by a damp environment; fat soluble chemical exposures accumulate in fat tissues and the more fat cells you have (and a damp environment), the more exposure you suffer as those fat cells store chemicals that have a very long half-life.
3. Overwork may lead to not resting when sick (but working through the illness) and this then limits the body's ability to heal itself; overwork also implies a lifestyle in which regular detoxification does not occur and this can allow for toxic accumulation over and beyond what would be considered typical. Sleep is included in this category. Sleep is essential to detoxification and the release of growth hormone for the rebuilding of normal tissue and function. Poor or little sleep leads to yin deficiency, among other things, and yin deficiency potentiates LPFs by drawing the pathogen deeper into the body. Resting allows for detoxification and depuration.
4. Increased or overuse or improper use of herbs, supplements, pharmaceutical drugs may, in fact, be a form of a LPF. For example, antibiotics typically cause damage to the middle jiao, which leads to damp (candidiasis) and requires further treatment to drain dampness. Damp is a potentiating agent for LPFs. Another

example is the use of steroids, which dampen the effect of the adrenals and drive the wei qi back to the source. This continual dampening effect stifles immune function and leaves one more open to external exposures of any kind. These are just two examples. Steroids lead to yin deficiency, and yin deficiency also potentiates LPFs. There is a slightly longer list of pharmaceutical drugs that contribute to breast cancer in Chapter 4.

Of course, predispositions may not play an initial role when we have no choice regarding environmental exposures. However, as these exposures accumulate, it may occur that a threshold is met in which their bioaccumulative role in injury becomes a trigger for a malignant event. It is difficult to know if these exposures have a greater impact in people with the traditional predispositions. But it appears likely that this is true.

Traditionally, early-stage pathogens enter the exterior and are dispersed through the exterior. If the wrong herbs or other treatment are used or drugs that cool the interior are used, then these interventions drag the pathogen inward. The treatment may have cleared the exterior symptoms but the pathogen remains. Antibiotics have side effects, which include gastrointestinal dysfunction – symptoms which we see as the result of a damp phlegm accumulation due to spleen injury. We say that antibiotics are cold, bitter, internally cooling and toxic. They affect the lung, spleen, stomach, bladder, and kidney. The cold nature of antibiotics causes contraction and this does not allow the pathogen to be released to the exterior. The qi and yang of the spleen and kidneys is impaired. The patient appears to recover because the heat is cleared but the cold nature of the drugs causes the pathogen to smolder internally, thus injuring the yin. LPFs often look like deficiency heat. Although the yin is scorched, the yin is not the key to treatment, the root is heat and scorched yin is the branch. When a pathogen becomes latent, heat is the end result and, therefore, the treatment principle is primarily to vent the heat outwards in some way. We could say that releasing the heat is a form of detoxification or depuration. Depuration refers to the release of a toxic chemical from its binding place

in the body tissue and the discharge of it. Chelation therapy is a form of depuration for heavy metals.

In classical theory, the pathogen is there and can emerge when the resistance is low and/or another pathogen enters to exacerbate the deeper level injury. Chronic fatigue syndrome is a symptom of a LPF in which the course of the disease moves back and forth from improvement to worsening, all for no apparent conventional medical reason. This traditional analysis of LPFs is possibly what happens when our bodies become repositories for chemical exposures that are cumulatively toxic.

Predisposing factors[10]

1. A yin-deficient constitution leads to empty heat, which attracts inwardly unresolved pathogens; children are naturally yin-deficient and this may explain why toxic exposures result in acute disease so quickly. For example, acute childhood and adult leukemias commonly present like a flu. The onset is acute but then moves into a more chronic presentation of toxicity. In adults, the onset of NHL is commonly asymptomatic with nodal swelling or long-term fatigue with nodal swelling.
2. Spleen deficiency leads to a propensity of damp accumulations; dampness can attract or transform external pathogens to wind dampness, which can lead to damp heat in the interior. It is difficult in the developed world among people who chronically overeat to find individuals who are not spleen deficient. This modern problem then becomes a predisposing factor for profound LPF exposures that become cumulative in a way never seen before. If left untreated spleen deficiency leads to cardiovascular diseases and diabetes. But when the damp phlegm foods that have been eaten are contaminated with organochlorine agricultural additives, then the result can be cancer.
3. Qi stasis also generates heat and stasis and a vicious cycle, which often includes the middle jiao and spleen/liver axis.
4. Diet (alcohol, spicy foods, sweets, refined foods, and so on) can lead to phlegm heat.

Latent pathogenic factors are interior and, therefore, have no exterior signs or symptoms.

Their direction is interior and they move to the exterior as they resolve. When modern chemical exposures are thought of as analogs for the classical concept of an LPF it becomes very difficult to understand how to approach the concept clinically. Frequently, practitioners of conventional medicine will not even commit to the idea that chemical exposures, like organochlorine pesticides and herbicides, cause cancer. There is not much to go on. But classical Chinese medical theory says that the interior refers to the qi, ying or blood levels. At the qi level we are looking at symptoms or signs that reside in the lung, stomach, gall bladder, urinary bladder or intestines. At the ying or blood level we are looking at signs and symptoms that reside in the kidney, heart or liver. The level at which eventual symptoms or signs arise may give a hint as to which level is injured and, therefore, which level to treat.

Spleen, lungs, kidneys, San Jiao

Put another way, the complex transformative cycle of lymphomas can begin at the yuan qi, where a possible template for a predisposition may occur either at the genetic level or at the acquired constitutional level. This cycle proceeds to the ying and wei level, particularly of the kidneys, lung and spleen and their corresponding functional units. The wei qi has its origins in the source qi of the kidney, the ying originates in the spleen function as it relates to the acquired qi, and in the lung where it mixes to form zheng qi. All three of these functional organ units have to do with the transformation and movement of normal yin fluids and with the normal immune response at various levels. In the early qi-deficient end of this disease cycle the presentation is one in which injury to the functional activities of these organs, especially the spleen and lung, is pronounced. Fatigue, lowered appetite, mild damp accumulations, deficiency cold symptoms, and gastrointestinal deficiency syndromes with exterior pernicious influences (EPIs) are common.

If we were to observe early-stage HIV infection without antiretroviral therapy, we would see a very similar progression. An acute onset that looks like a flu-like illness appears to resolve. Then spleen-deficient symptoms like chronic loose stools and fatigue appear. This is followed by persistent generalised low-grade lymphadenopathy with a long series of acute infections and then chronic infections like candidiasis. Is it possible that LPFs that are chemical in nature act to some degree like chronic viral infections?

There are several functional units involved in water metabolism and, therefore, lymph in Chinese medicine. Much has been said about the lung, spleen and kidney axis but not as much has been said about the San Jiao. In modern times, the lymphatic system has typically been translated, at least anatomically, as the San Jiao. However, the San Jiao is one of those units of functional activity in Chinese medicine that has no simple analog in conventional medicine.

The yuan qi of the kidneys is the source of warming energy for the San Jiao, which is within the fire phase. This heat allows the San Jiao to control qi transformation, the products of which, according to the Ling Shu (Chapter 36),[11] go to warm and nourish the muscles and flesh, and to make the skin firm and taut. In the Jin Gui Yao Lue (Essentials from the Golden Cabinet), it says: 'The crevices in the surface tissues on the exterior of the body and the organs are the place where the San Jiao gathers the True Qi, the area suffused with qi and blood.'[12] The transformation and then the transportation of qi, blood and fluids by the zang fu require the qi transformation and movement, the function of the San Jiao. The San Jiao is located, at least in terms of palpable anatomy, just below the surface in what we call the surface interstitial spaces and the lymph nodes. The nodes around the joints, in the axilla, the cervical chain and all of the nodes of the Jade Screen around the neck are all quite superficial and palpable. The San Jiao is thought of as a Shaoyang unit, it is in-between. It is also ubiquitous.

According to Stephen Birch, in *Hara Diagnosis: Reflections on the Sea*, the San Jiao may be the very complex system of fascia that wraps every muscle fiber and organ in the body.[13] It is the mesenterium, the lymph system, and the means by which intercommunication occurs throughout the body. Certainly lymph progenitors in the marrow are part of an intimate feedback loop that runs immunity. This intimate loop also runs the formation of all of the blood progenitors.

The Zhu Bing Yuan Hou Lun[14] first suggested mechanisms between the San Jiao and phlegm. It says 'phlegm and thin mucus disease is a result of weak yang qi failing to maintain open pathways for qi, so that the body fluids are unable to transit smoothly' and 'the qi of yin and yang cannot circulate smoothly so that the upper Jiao blockage produces heat and, therefore, phlegm'. The Ji Sheng Fang (Formulas to Aid the Living) contains this passage: 'If the San Jiao is blocked, channel flow will be obstructed causing water and fluids to stop and gather without proper circulation, collecting to form phlegm and leading to diseases innumerable'.[15]

All of the mechanisms for health that involve the lungs, spleen, kidneys, and San Jiao can lead to phlegm when injured. These same functional units have a relationship to ying (spleen and lung) and wei (lung and kidney), as well, and, therefore, to immune function. Normal lymph fluids may have a propensity, by their very nature, for phlegm and phlegm accumulations. They have a proximity to the substance of phlegm, they interact with all fluids of the body, they have a relationship to and, in fact, may be the San Jiao, which is directly related to all fluid metabolism in the body through many interactive relationships.

Given the above as the environment in which lymphoma can occur, the following may be a good representation of the natural history of the disease. A deep level of spleen deficiency caused by promotional factors and by chronic exposure to various substances, as yet to be fully identified, leads to deficient blood symptoms, to qi and blood stasis, to clumping and yang deficiencies. When these deficiencies and static conditions are left untreated, the deficient qi aspect of the process can become overactive, almost like kidney yang deficiency that fails to ground the yang and manifests signs of what looks like yin deficiency but is, in fact, yang floating to the surface because of yang deficiency. This is an Er Xian Tang-like presentation. The yang floats to the surface and appears hyperactive. This hyper qi aspect is actually due to toxicity. It leads to allergies and to autoimmune disease. This happens when the qi moves primarily internally rather than externally and is emblematic of a latent pathogenic factor.

This internal movement of qi is combined with what appears to be a wei qi excess, but is actually a manifestation of an interruption in the internal/external cycle of wei qi, which normally moves inwardly for 12 cycles per day and outwardly for 12 cycles per day. It is also emblematic of an LPF. It is an example of the immune system being on alert because of hyperexcitability caused by toxicity; underlying this is adrenal exhaustion. When this apparent wei qi excess and qi deficiency are symptomatic over a long period of time, the entire process, one which was originally due to spleen deficiency and blood deficiency in combination with a latent pathogen, can switch entirely inward. As a result, the wei qi resides only in the interior at its source, the kidneys (the adrenals?); and the fire within water (Mingmen/adrenals) begins to smolder. This may be the place where, and time when, the marrow level genetic injury takes place.

Qi and blood deficiency with dampness then transforms to phlegm, phlegm heat, and blood heat. This transformation occurs due to the grinding stasis of the deficiency syndrome combined with dampness – a form of clumping. Phlegm arises out of this dampness, blood heat, and stasis. Phlegm with qi deficiency with smoldering wei qi cannot transform or correct itself and again transforms to heat. The phlegm dries and becomes stickier, which prevents the blood from moving smoothly. This contributes to blood heat. The weak spleen allows more dampness and phlegm to accumulate and then to dry in the smoldering heat environment. This vicious cycle turns upon itself if not detected and treated.

In the final transformation, the hot sticky phlegm complex has again nowhere to go. The spleen-deficient root combined with the inward movement of the unresolved LPF becomes so severe that it becomes disassociated with the San Jiao, which is the mother of earth in the Five Phase cycle. It is not only the mother but also is very closely related in terms of ying, wei qi, and fluid transformation. This causes a heart/kidney incoordination within the Five Phase cycle and this, in turn, allows the phlegm heat complex to move into the lymph, the San Jiao. The kidney is no longer nourished and the heart is uncontrolled (the water/fire axis). Kidney deficiency usually manifests as yin and yang deficiency. Yin is more predominant. The yin deficiency acts as a magnet for the LPF. Heat and phlegm gets stuck in the blood mechanism, the marrow. This pumps the adrenals and gives rise to heat and depletion cycles. The pernicious cycle feeds back upon itself over and over again and is very difficult to turn around.

When these transformations get stuck in the blood mechanism and move to the marrow entirely, then leukemias result. When they get stuck in the lymphatic system, the San Jiao, lymphomas result. The transformative cycle back and forth is very close. Perhaps this is why the mechanism for and treatment of leukemias and lymphomas can result in either disease and also why they may transform into one another as they progress.

Pathological heat in the blood with stasis and toxins knotted inside can evolve to later stages slowly or quickly. But usually in non-indolent lymphomas the evolution can occur over a period of weeks or months. Once the transformation has taken place at this level, the evolution of the disease occurs much more quickly than in solid tumors. The pathological heat toxins can enter:

- as an external pathogen or disease from the wei to ying to blood levels
- in an environment of chronic blood and yin deficiency with especially lung yin deficiency
- in an environment of chronic blood deficiency with specifically lung yin deficiency.

The lungs irrigate the body and the downward and upward motion of breathing acts like a pump and affects the lymphatic system, circulation and drainage. Lymphadenopathy with local edema in a patient with lung yin deficiency indicates that fluids are not moving well. Patients who present in this way, and with nodal swelling above the diaphragm only, will often have a history of chronic upper respiratory tract infections and allergies, asthma, and skin diseases.

Non-Hodgkin's lymphoma is a cancer that occurs in later stage HIV/AIDS. The use of steroidal treatments for skin disorders, to treat allergic sinusitis and asthma (all of which are common ailments in HIV infection) contribute to the mechanism of NHL in AIDS patients. These drugs put a damper on all reactions blocking the wei qi. This drives it inward and creates an atrophication of the humoral and cellular immune systems, which are already being replaced by HIV as part of the disease process. The adrenals are the pump for corticosteroids, and if we can accept that

the adrenals are an analog for Mingmen, then there is a dampening of the kidney function that creates a pathway for heart/kidney incoordination, which also creates stasis and heat at this deep level. Heat is rising from the inside out. This is pathological heat that smolders and not the warming affect of the kidney yang. Since the wei qi and the San Jiao evolve out of the moving qi between the kidneys, and the kidneys are stressed in chronic illness (HIV infection), these other functions are disrupted. The stress of chronic spleen/kidney deficiency is compounded by the use of steroidal drugs. The kidney/heart axis is continually injured, the yin and yang are damaged, the spleen is not supported and fluid metabolism is damaged all along the way. In HIV-related NHL, the long-term use of several drug therapies contributes to a lymphoma environment by acting as an additional LPF alongside HIV, by causing spleen deficiency and dampness, and by creating yin deficiency, the last two of which potentiate the LPFs. Unfortunately the number of LPFs in HIV infection can be a long list including HIV, herpes simplex virus (HSV), cytomegalovirus (CMV), hepatitis B virus (HBV), and human papillomavirus (HPV). The knot of all of these LPFs is potentiated by the use of steroids.

The above information gives a foundation for all the lymphomas.

Natural history of follicular lymphomas

Lymphomas usually grow in a nodular pattern. The nodules are of a uniform size and can result in the total effacement of normal nodal structure. The nodules are homogeneous clumps of neoplastic cells. Scattered within the follicles within the nodules is a dense meshwork of dendritic reticulum cells. The cells evolve through different stages with distinct cytologic features: small cleaved, large cleaved, large non-cleaved. This last cell type is more proliferative.

Subtyping of these follicular lymphomas is difficult, but they generally form a continuum from small cleaved to mixed to large-cell predominance. The types are divided based on the proportion of large cells in the nodules. Follicular small-cleaved lymphoma should have no more than five large non-cleaved cells visible per high power field.

All subtypes of follicular lymphomas demonstrate gene rearrangements. There may also be a T–B-cell interaction as well. The loss of genetic material is another common secondary abnormality. These deletions are non-random and the thought is that the areas where these deletions occur may be related to areas where as yet unidentified tumor-suppressor genes are carried. The overexpression of *Bcl-2* plays a critical role in blocking apoptosis and seems to be a major breakpoint region in these lymphomas.[16]

Clinical features, diagnosis, staging

The presence or absence of B symptoms is important for diagnosis and staging. They include fever, drenching night sweats, and significant weight loss of more than 10% of total body weight within 6 months. There may be symptoms of obstructive disease, especially in the neck and the retroperitoneum. Splenomegaly is more common in chronic lymphocytic leukemia (CLL) and small lymphocytic lymphomas (SLL) than in follicular lymphomas, and may be the only sign of disease. Mediastinal lymph node involvement may lead to superior vena cava syndrome. There may be symptoms of anemia, or thrombocytopenia. Gastrointestinal involvement may produce nonspecific symptoms including abdominal pain, change in bowel habits, and gastrointestinal bleeding.[17] All lymph nodes should be palpated and an abdominal exam should be performed as well.

Excisional lymph node biopsy is crucial to diagnosis. Fine needle aspiration (FNA) is considered inadequate since it does not preserve the nodal architecture and changes in nodal structure are a sign of disease. Bilateral bone marrow biopsies are necessary and when positive will show paratrabecular infiltration with small-cleaved cells. Assessing marrow and central nervous system (CNS) involvement is important in diagnosis and staging.

Common blood work (CBC with a Chem 23) may show anemia or thrombocytopenia. These abnormalities are relative to direct bone marrow involvement, splenomegaly, or may be autoimmune in nature. The latter is more commonly seen in CLL/SLL. Patients with anemia should have a direct Coombs' test. This test is used to diagnose

acquired autoimmune hemolytic anemias. Also lactate dehydrogenase (LDH) and beta2-microglobulin levels may be elevated and are important in prognosis.

Imaging should include a chest X-ray and a chest CT scan if the X-ray is suspicious. Abdominal and pelvic CT are essential. The Ann Arbor Staging sytem is as follows:

- Stage I: a single lymph-node region or extra-lymphatic site.
- Stage II: two or more lymph-node regions on the same side of the diaphragm or localised extralymphatic site with one or more lymph-node regions on the same side of the diaphragm.
- Stage III: lymph-node regions on both sides of the diaphragm and possible localised involvement of an extralymphatic site or the spleen.
- Stage IV: disseminated involvement of one or more extralymphatic organs or tissues.
- A or B: denotes absence (A) or presence (B) of: unexplained weight loss >10% body weight, unexplained fever >38°C, or night sweats.

Prognosis

Histology is a major predictor in distinguishing clinical course but there is no clear difference in long-term survival between subtypes. Patients with the follicular mixed lymphomas have a more prolonged initial remission than those with follicular small cleaved. High LDH and beta2-microglobulin levels[18] correlate with a poor prognosis.[19] Also *Ki-67* expression and an increased S-phase fraction are indicators for a poorer prognosis.

The extent of the tumor burden, host factors, and response to therapy are all prognostic indicators. The size of nodal disease, bone marrow involvement, and the number of extranodal sites are indicators as well. Early-stage disease is obviously associated with a more favorable outcome. Two or more sites of extranodal involvement correlates with a poorer prognosis.[20]

Other types of low-grade lymphomas

Small lymphocytic lymphoma is immunotypically identical to chronic lymphocytic leukemia. This type also includes low-grade B-cell lymphoma of mucosa-associated tissue (MALT), monocytoid B-cell lymphoma (spleen lymphoma), and extranodal SLL. The MALT lymphomas include those of the gastrointestinal tract, lungs, salivary glands, thyroid, thymus, breast, orbit, and conjunctiva. There seems to be a causal relationship between *Helicobacter pylori* and MALT lymphoma. In some studies where patients with MALT lymphoma were treated with antibiotic therapy for *H. pylori* a remission was maintained. Immunoproliferative small intestinal disease (IPSID), seems to share a relationship with gastric MALT and may be secondary to bacterial infections in the gastrointestinal tract.

Mantle-cell lymphoma is a more recently recognised entity (1970s) and is named because the neoplastic cells arise from the mantle zone of secondary follicles and give rise to a diffuse pattern of nodal involvement. Mantle-cell lymphoma constitutes 10% of all NHL. Patients are usually males older than 55 who present with advanced disease and generalised lymphadenopathy, bone marrow involvement, with liver and spleen frequently involved. The clinical course varies with some patients having very aggressive disease while other cases behave more like indolent lymphomas. There seems to be a relationship between Mantle-cell lymphoma and plasma-cell leukemia.[21]

Treatment

Most patients with advanced-stage low-grade NHL will respond to chemotherapy. However, most patients will relapse and most will die of this disease. The hallmark of advanced stage disease is its continuous recurring nature and incurability.[22] New therapies are difficult to assess because of the heterogeneity of the low-grade lymphoma. Also, the disease has a long natural history requiring long-term follow-up of patients. Biological markers are not identified as yet, although PCR for *bcl-2* may be such a marker. The frequency of having to restage can affect the comparability of relapse-free survival and the use of multiple therapies in an individual patient makes analysis of each regimen difficult. In limited-stage follicular lymphoma about 15–20% of patients have this history and about half of these patients may be curable. These patients are treated with radiation.

The long-term failure-free survival after radiotherapy is 40%. Patients treated with total-lymphoid irradiation (TLI), appeared to be more likely to remain relapse-free than those treated with involved-field or extended-field radiation.[23]

In combined therapy, stage I–II disease is commonly treated with 10 cycles of COP-Bleo (cyclophosphamide, vincristine, prednisone, bleomycin) or with CHOP-Bleo (COP-Bleo plus doxorubicin) with radiation to involved sites sandwiched after the third cycle. CHOP followed by rituximab (Rituxan) is also used. The 5-year survival rate with this combined regimen is 77%.

Advanced-stage follicular lymphoma – stages III and IV – is more difficult to assess because patients vary widely and the response rate also varies according to the status of the patient. Because low-grade lymphomas are sensitive to radiation, radiation has been incorporated in primary therapy for some advanced-stage disease. The CHOP-Bleo regimen including radiation therapy has produced 5-year disease-free survival rates of 52% in patients with stage III disease.[24]

However, the role of radiation in stage IV patients is less clear. There seems to be a clear advantage in combined therapy for patients with advanced nodular lymphomas. Sequential three-combination chemotherapy including CHOD-B (cyclophosphamide, doxorubicin, vincristine, dexamethasone, bleomycin)/ESHAP/NOPP (mitoxantrone, vincristine, procarbazine, prednisone) for a total of 12 cycles produced a 4-year survival of 94%. These statistics are inconclusive when compared to the survival rate of those left untreated. The complexity of staging and typing these lymphomas contributes to the confusion in analysing outcomes, especially for late-stage disease.[24] CHOP-R is the most common treatment regimen in use now.

The combined immunosuppressive effects of steroids and certain chemotherapeutic regimens in advanced stage CLL, especially, are of concern, because these combinations can result in serious infections including listeriosis, CMV, and pneumocystis pneumonia (PCP). Because of this certain antibiotics are commonly added to certain regimens.

Because low-grade lymphomas have a long indolent course and since no therapy has clearly impacted the continuous recurring nature of the disease, many clinicians feel that withholding therapy in relatively asymptomatic patients until symptoms warrant treatment may be an appropriate approach.[25] A study by the NCI looked at patients who were treated with intensive therapy at the time of diagnosis versus those who were in a watch-and-wait group. It was found that the complete response rate (CR) to therapy of those in the watch-and-wait group was lowered at the time they were finally treated compared to the CR in the group treated immediately. In other words, bulky disease with secondary genetic abnormalities may have contributed to resistance to treatment. One of the preliminary conclusions of this study has been to favor early treatment in terms of quality-of-life issues, because those treated early actually enjoyed more time in remission than those who were not treated early.[26]

Interferon (IFN) is of interest in treating chemotherapy-resistant patients and in maintenance therapy after chemotherapy. It is used as an induction agent for treatment at presentation and in relapse. It is sometimes used with chemotherapy as part of an induction therapy. Generally, IFN has been found to help prolong remission when used in combination with chemotherapy but does not affect long-term survival.[27]

Rituxan, or rituximab, is used more commonly today but the results are mixed as to whether it is a good choice for maintenance in patients with low-grade lymphomas.

There is currently no satisfactory treatment for mantle-cell lymphoma.

High-dose chemotherapy with autologous bone marrow transplantation (ABMT) has been reserved for young patients who have failed previous systemic therapy. A common scenario is high-dose cyclophosphamide with fractionated total body irradiation (TBI) and autologous bone marrow rescue. This lowered recurrence rates but did not change long-term survival.[28]

Chinese medicine

The combined treatment of all lymphomas is included at the end of the section. Although this treatment is differentiated in terms of interfacing with conventional medical treatment, it is not differentiated in terms of pattern differentiation.

INTERMEDIATE AND HIGH-GRADE NON-HODGKIN'S LYMPHOMAS

The NHLs are a collection of lymphoid malignancies of diverse pathology and natural history. This is exemplified by the many systems of classification that have been used over the years. The NCI initiated a new system in the 1970s called the Working Formulation.[29] It is a useful source of information for assessment of prognosis and is used as a tool for treatment planning. However, it has some limitations. Nearly 10% of all lymphomas elude precise classification, especially those presenting primarily in extranodal tissues where there is no lymph node architecture. Also within the many histologic categories of low, intermediate and high-grade lymphomas there is a wide spectrum of biologic behavior. Histopathologic classification alone is often inadequate. There are clinically unique subtypes of NHL that are immunophenotypically, cytogenetically, and oncogenically different to any classified within this system. There are other newer systems used but the Working Formulation remains the main system for classification of NHL. It is included under the staging section of this chapter.[17]

Epidemiology and etiology

The incidence of NHL has risen dramatically since the 1940s. This rise is considered to be an unexplained epidemic. The incidence in 1947 was 6.9 per 100 000 and was 17.4 per 100 000 in 1984. The rise appears to be in intermediate-grade lymphomas among the elderly, but also is seen across age and gender status. The incidence in males has risen slightly as well. This rise is addressed in the past section on pathology in Chinese medicine. Since 1970, the rates for NHL have risen by almost 200%.[30]

Intermediate- and high-grade tumors comprise nearly 55% of NHLs with a proportionately higher number of high-grade tumors in children and young adults. Burkitt's lymphoma and T-cell acute lymphoblastic lymphoma (T-ALL) comprise 90% of childhood NHLs.

There is no single defect that causes a lymphoma. The etiology is considered to be a multi-step process in which the malignant phenotype develops gradually. Please see the Chinese medicine analysis of pathogenesis. Hereditary and environmental factors contribute to the process. Three factors appear common:

- certain patients may be predisposed because of a specific immune defect
- the occurrence of a specific infection that is difficult to eradicate and that may alter normal lymphoid tissues can contribute to development of lymphoma
- single specific mutation or a number of mutations or chromosome translocations can alter suppressor genes or oncogenes.[31]

Any or all of these factors may be at work. Again, please note the Chinese medicine section on pathogenesis. Amongst farmers the rates for NHL are six times higher than in the non-farming population and a relationship has been found between 2-4D, an agricultural pesticide, and NHL.

Many specific lymphomas are the result of immune factors. For example, Duncan's syndrome is an X-linked lymphoproliferative syndrome in which males are unable to mount an appropriate immunological response to an Epstein–Barr virus (EBV) infection and develop a fatal lymphoproliferative syndrome. This exact immune defect is unknown. Post-transplant lymphoproliferative syndrome is very similar. Immunosuppression following organ transplanation can cause an EBV infection-related polyclonal lymphoproliferative disease that can develop into NHL. And the primary CNS lymphomas associated with HIV infection may develop in a similar way following EBV infection. Burkitt's lymphoma is an African endemic NHL. The assumption is that it arises in areas in Africa where there is a high incidence of malaria and that malaria may cause a defect in the immune system in children living in these areas. This defect results in their inability to resolve EBV infections successfully. The lymphoma develops when a chromosome translocation brings the *c-myc* oncogene on a certain chromosome[32] into the proximity of an immunoglobulin gene on another chromosome, thus overexpressing the *c-myc* oncogene causing cellular proliferation and Burkitt's lymphoma. In this case, solving a public health problem (malarial mosquito infestations) may help eradicate a cancer. This evolution is a classic example of how a LPF works to cause a serious disease.

EBV, human T-cell lymphotrophic virus (HTLV)-1 and HIV are three infectious agents that interact to cause lymphomas. *Helicobacter pylori* is another related to gastric lymphomas, as discussed above. However, reversing immunosuppression and treating these infections does not, after a certain point, stop the disease progression. A non-reversible phenotype for malignancy may be present as a step in the process. This last step may relate to the mutation of a suppressor gene or a chromosomal translocation causing the abnormal expression of an oncogene.[30]

Clinical features and diagnosis

The manifestations of intermediate- and high-grade NHLs are diverse, depending on the site of involvement. These tumors have a more rapid growth rate than indolent types of lymphoma. They may infiltrate tissue and obstruct organs. Burkitt's lymphoma in children commonly presents as a head and neck mass. T-ALL frequently presents with a mediastinal mass in younger patients. A clinically distinct primary mediastinal B-cell diffuse large-cell lymphoma presents in young women. Patients with Hashimoto's thyroiditis are predisposed to primary thyroid lymphomas, and patients with Sjögren's syndrome are predisposed to salivary and lacrimal gland primary NHL. Patients with celiac disease are predisposed to enteropathy-associated T-cell NHL.[33]

Non-Hodgkin's lymphoma can present with systemic B symptoms, including fever, Pel–Ebstein relapsing pattern, drenching night sweats, 10% weight loss, generalised pruritis. Also paraneoplastic syndromes may develop with lymphomas. Non-parathyroid-hormone-induced hypercalcemia can occur, and subacute motor neuropathy and polymyositis may be present.[34]

Pathologic exam of the lymph node is necessary whenever possible. Again, FNA is variable in terms of accuracy. It may be necessary to establish clonality to confirm malignancy. This is done with montypic immunohistochemical staining for kappa or lambda light chain. In some cases gene studies must be done on T-cell receptor rearrangements or on the B-cell immunoglobulin gene.[35]

Staging and treatment

Staging in these lymphomas is an area of intense study. NHL was staged anatomically (above and below the diaphragm), but NHL does not spread anatomically to contiguous nodal regions and cannot be staged solely by anatomic methods.

For intermediate-grade NHL several staging systems are in use. These include the Ann Arbor system, the International Index and the MD Anderson Tumor Score System. They are used primarily as prognostic models and, therefore, as a means to determine treatment. Box 10.1 shows the Working Formulation for Staging NHLs.

The treatment of Hodgkin's disease and NHL has formed the modern paradigm of all cancer chemotherapy. The concepts were first established for infectious diseases and then applied to oncol-

---

> **Box 10.1   Working formulation for staging NHLs**
>
> **Low grade**
>
> - Small lymphocytic (CLL)
> - Follicular, predominantly small-cleaved cell
> - Follicular mixed, small-cleaved and large-cell
>
> **Intermediate grade**
>
> - Follicular, predominantly large-cell
> - Diffuse small-cleaved cell
> - Diffuse mixed small- and large-cell epithelioid component
> - Diffuse large-cell cleaved, non-cleaved
>
> **High grade**
>
> - Large-cell, immunoblastic plasmacytoid
> - Clear-cell, polymorphous, epithelioid
> - Small non-cleaved cell
> - Burkitt's lymphoma
> - Follicular areas
>
> **Miscellaneous**
>
> - Composite
> - Mycosis fungoides/Sezary syndrome
> - Histiocytic
> - Unclassifiable

---

ogy. These include the concepts of tumor resistance and combination chemotherapy including non-cross-resistant chemotherapeutic regimens. The principle treatment for NHL is combination chemotherapy and radiation therapy. Surgery is used only for diagnosis. The basis for chemotherapy has been CHOP. Second- and third-generation non-cross-resistant regimens have been developed for especially high-grade NHL.

Patients are stratified in most advanced disease studies for age, marrow development, histology, bulky disease sites, and LDH levels.[36] Newer combination therapies include m-BACOD (methotrexate, bleomycin, doxorubicin, cyclophosphamide, vincristine, and dexamethasone), and ProMACE-CytaBOM (prednisone, methotrexate, doxorubicin, cyclophosphamide, etoposide, cytarabine, bleomycin, vincristine). However, CHOP remains the standard of therapy. Rituxan is used either in combination or as a maintenance drug after remission has been achieved.

Older patients tend to fare poorly and there is some question as to whether the biology of tumors in the elderly is different to that in younger age groups. However, some elderly patients who present with no complicating disease are treated for NHL with lower doses of chemotherapy in order to avoid increased toxicity. Dose intensity seems to alter outcome in these tumors in the sense that less is bad but more is not necessarily better.[37,38]

Confirming the presence of early relapse can be difficult. CT can pick up residual mass in 40% of patients. But there is no other diagnostic tool available. There is no accepted standard of therapy for refractory disease. Allogenic BMT is limited to patients under the age of 60. Salvage therapies include MIME (mesna, ifosfamide, methotrexate, and etoposide), DHAP (dexamethasone, high-dose cytarabine, and cisplatin), and ESHAP (etoposide, methylprednisolone,high-dose cytarabine, and cisplatin). Some new approaches include continuous infusion chemotherapy and some biologic agents. Allogeneic BMT has been explored with poor results.

High-grade tumors include lymphoblastic NHL, Burkitt's NHL, and non-Burkitt's NHL. They double in size more quickly than any other tumor and they are rapidly fatal. Tumor lysis syndrome can be seen even prior to therapy. Rapid destruction of malignant cells can result in the release of cellular breakdown products and intracellular ions causing potentially fatal metabolic derangements. Oddly, in these high-grade tumors, the disease-free state rates average from 35% to 60%, depending on the prognosis for a given patient.

HODGKIN'S DISEASE

Hodgkin's disease accounts for 1% of all cancers, with approximately 7000–8000 cases diagnosed each year in the United States. The distribution is about 85% in males with a bimodal distribution by age in the 15–35 age range and then again in the over-50 age range. It almost always arises in the lymph nodes and is a disorder of the lymphoid system that is now highly treatable. The tumors are largely composed of normal cells with a higher proportion of Reed–Sternberg cells, which is the differentiating characteristic defining Hodgkin's disease as opposed to NHL. There seems to be a higher risk for Hodgkin's in higher social classes and more educated individuals. Why this is true has never been explained.[39]

Subtypes of Hodgkin's disease are:

- nodular sclerosing, which occurs mostly in females and in ages between 13 and 34[40]
- lymphocyte-dominant, which occurs more between the ages of 40 and 50 years[41]
- mixed cellularity, which occurs mostly in males between the ages of 30 and 40[42]
- lymphocyte-depleted, which occurs mostly in elderly males.[42]

The symptoms of Hodgkin's disease include painless lymphadenopathy, especially in the neck, supraclavicular, and axillary nodes. Systemic symptoms may include category B symptoms, which are fever, night sweats, fatigue, and weight loss of more than 10% of total body weight in less than 6 months. Pain can be neurogenic, alcohol-induced, or bone pain.

Diagnosis is via lymph node biopsy, chest X-ray to rule out pleural effusions, abdominal X-ray to rule out hepatic/splenic enlargement or masses, palpating for bony tenderness especially of the sternum, and computerised tomography (CT) scan of the chest and abdomen. A complete blood count (CBC) and a chemistry panel are done. Lymph node and/or bone marrow biopsy is performed. In differential diagnosis, one must rule out AIDS, or other systemic autoimmune disease. The final diagnosis is given by the hematologist.

Surgery is performed only for diagnosis or symptom control, for example splenectomy. Radiation is used alone as primary treatment in many cases of Ia or IIa disease. Chemotherapy is used for stages IIIb and IV. Chemotherapy plus radiation is used for stages IIb and IIIa. The MOPP chemotherapeutic regimen (mechlorethamine, Oncovin [vincristine], procarbazine, and prednisone) is commonly used for Hodgkin's disease and NHL. Its toxicities include marrow suppression, nausea, neuropathy, infertility, and leukemia.

Another regimen is ABVD (Adriamycin [doxorubicin], bleomycin, vinblastine, dacarbazine). This regimen causes less leukemia and infertility and may be more effective than MOPP. A common intervention is the combination of ABVD and MOPP for 12 alternating cycles.[43,44]

In Hodgkin's disease the stage is the most important factor in terms of prognosis.[45] The histopathology is only slightly related to prognosis. Category B symptoms indicate a poorer prognosis. Stage I and II patients include 60% of all patients at diagnosis. And of these stage I–II patients, 75% should be cured. Most relapses occur in the first 3–4 years after treatment. Relapses are rare after 48 months. And of the stage IIIa and IVa patients 80% survive past the 10-year mark. Those who fail to respond to treatment usually go on to bone marrow transplantation (BMT).

There are sequelae after treatment for Hodgkin's disease. These include hypothyroidism in 10–20% of patients. Sterility is nearly universal with the MOPP regimen, especially in females. Radiation pneumonitis and pericarditis occur frequently. And aseptic necrosis of the femoral heads can lead to severe complications with aging. There are also secondary neoplasms as a result of treatment, which include myelodysplasia in 2–10% of patients, acute myelogenous leukemia (AML) 3–10 years post-treatment, and NHL. Epithelial tumors and sarcomas occur in up to 20% of patients treated for Hodgkin's disease.[32]

The presence of the Reed–Sternberg cell is what identifies Hodgkin's disease. This distinctive cell was first described by Sternberg in 1898, and more clearly by Reed in 1902, thus the name. The origin of this cell still remains a point of dissension. The CD40 antigen is strongly represented on the surface of Reed–Sternberg cells and helps in distinguishing between nodular sclerosing Hodgkin's disease and other lymphoid malignancies; it remains the only marker of clinical use.[46]

Histologic classification is based on the ratio of Reed–Sternberg cells to other normal background cells in tissue samples. The Rye modified classification system divides Hodgkin's disease into four histologic types:

- lymphocyte-predominant
- nodular sclerosis
- mixed cellularity
- lymphocyte-depleted.

Lymphocyte-predominant disease is further subtyped nodular and diffuse. Nodular lymphocyte-predominant Hodgkin's disease is now regarded as B-cell lymphoma and is the only subtype for which the cell of origin is known. Nodular sclerosis Hodgkin's disease may be difficult to differentiate from large-cell lymphoma. This type is divided into grade 1 and grade 2 because there are differences in the overall survival and disease-free rates between the two grades. More recent studies do correlate a difference in grade and prognosis, but the classification remains intact. A third type of Hodgkin's disease, mixed cellularity, has much more variation in cell type, has rare Reed–Sternberg cells, and can be easily confused with other types of lymphomas, especially peripheral T-cell lymphoma.[46]

Epidemiology

Hodgkin's disease is uncommon and accounts for only 7500 cases annually in the USA. The nodular sclerosing type occurs predominantly in females and the other types predominantly in males. It appears to be a disease of more developed countries. Those in the First World countries present at an earlier age.

Strangely, investigators have found that possible risk factors may include small family size, single-family dwellings, and high parental education. The factors may be explained by the delayed-infection hypothesis, which applies more readily to young patients than to the elderly. Epstein–Barr virus has been implicated because cases of Hodgkin's disease have occurred following bouts of infectious mononucleosis, and the EBV genome is found in many cells in involved lymph nodes. HIV1 has also been associated with Hodgkin's disease.[47,48]

Staging

Box 10.2 describes the Ann Arbor staging for Hodgkin's disease.

Patient evaluation includes common blood analysis, the level of beta-2-microglobulin, erythrocyte sedimentation rate (ESR), X-ray evidence, and other possible procedures depending on the presentation. CT evaluation of the liver and spleen

---

Box 10.2 Ann Arbor staging for Hodgkin's disease

Stage I

Involvement of a single lymph-node region (I) or a single extralymphatic organ or site (Ie).

Stage II

Involvement of two or more lymph-node regions on the same side of the diaphragm (II) or localised involvement of an extralymphatic organ or site (IIe).

Stage III

Involvement of lymph-node regions on both sides of the diaphragm (III) or localised involvement of an extralymphatic organ or site (IIIe), spleen (IIIs), or both (IIIse).

Stage IV

Diffuse or disseminated involvement of one or more extralymphatic organs, with or without associated lymph-node involvement; the organ(s) involved should be identified by a symbol: (P) pulmonary, (O) osseous, or (H) hepatic. In addition, (A) indicates an asymptomatic patient; (B) indicates the presence of fever, night sweats, or weight loss >10% of body weight.

and abdomen, and bilateral bone marrow biopsy should be performed routinely. Lymphangiography may be a valuable tool and can help to detect early nodal disease missed by CT scan. X-ray films can also be used to determine the response to treatment.

About 30–50% of patients will have microscopic abdominal involvement that has not been detected by CT or lymphangiography. Therefore, a staging laparotomy may be used. B symptoms are usually indicative of abdominal disease.[49] Male gender, age greater than 40, B symptoms, and mixed cellularity disease are predictive risk factors for abdominal disease. Also a high number of positive upper torso nodal sites may be indicative of abdominal disease. Patients with stage I disease above the cricoid cartilage, patients with lymphocyte-predominant stage I disease, and women with nodular sclerosis stage IA disease are the only patients that can be confidently predicted to have no abdominal disease.

Treatment

In patients with early laparotomy-staged supradiaphragmatic disease and no mass or only a small mediastinal mass, radiation therapy may be the only treatment.[50] Even in early stage, however, there is a high rate of disease relapse in a disseminated pattern. Because of this, prophylactic abdominal radiation in these same patients has been used. Extended field radiation has been used with 10-year survival rates of up to 83% for stages I and II. Low-dose radiation to the lungs and liver has been added.[45]

Some adverse prognostic features have been identified that are predictive for relapse. These include the presence of a mediastinal mass greater than 7.5 cm, hilar lymphadenopathy, B symptoms, advanced age, extension of disease into the pulmonary parenchyma, mixed cellularity histology, stage II disease, and increased number of nodal sites. These adverse signs have encouraged the use of combined therapy.[45]

The optimal therapy for stage I and II Hodgkin's disease remains controversial. However, the focus has become one in which less intense or less toxic treatment can give equivalent results with decreased long- and short-term complications. The challenge continues to be the identification of prognostic risk factors that will allow a regimen to be specifically designed for an individual patient. MOPP followed by mantel irradiation or extended field radiation is commonly used.[51]

It is unusual for Hodgkin's disease to present initially with infradiaphragmatic disease. These patients are treated with an inverted Y radiotherapy that reaches the splenic pedicle. MOPP is also used, especially in those patients with stage IIA and IIB disease. Most patients with this presentation and with stage I and II disease are treated with combined therapy. The outcomes when chemotherapy was added changed from a 50% disease-free survival rate to a 92% disease-free survival rate.[52]

Stage III disease treatment is controversial and is dependent on the extent of disease. Combined therapy is the norm. The number of nodes involved, their location, and the size of the tumors all affect the prognosis and the treatment. When combined therapy is used the extent of abdominal involvement does not change the survival outcomes. Patients with stage III3B disease are generally treated more intensively. MOPP continues to be the first line of chemotherapy for these stages of Hodgkin's disease.[53]

Treatment of stage IV disease depends on the presence of B symptoms, previous doses of vincristine administered, extent of extranodal involvement, mechlorethamine doses, bone marrow involvement, anemia, elevated ESR, and advanced age. The difference in CR between patients with one extranodal site compared with those with two or more extranodal sites is 75% versus 25%. Overall survival is greatly influenced by this factor alone. Those who can tolerate a higher dose of mechlorethamine also have a higher survival rate.[54]

MOPP and ABVD (doxorubicin, bleomycin, vinblastine, and dacarbizine) are the standards for chemotherapy. These two are combined to produce better overall survival rates with better complete response rates and better disease-free survival rates.

Salvage therapy depends primarily on the initial therapy. If radiotherapy was given for early stage Hodgkin's disease then any of the above regimens will be 80–90% successful. Therefore, patients who had once achieved a complete remission are again likely to achieve a complete remission. If recurrence happens in less than the first year after remission, a second regimen may produce varied results depending on prognosis.[55]

Complications caused by treatment predispose patients for secondary malignancies. Alkylating agents are associated with hematologic malignancies whereas radiation therapy has been associated with an increased incidence of solid tumors. The most common malignancies to occur after chemotherapy for Hodgkin's disease are acute non-lymphocytic leukemia, myelodysplastic syndrome, NHL, and solid tumors. The cumulative risk for acute non-lymphocytic leukemia is 10–15%. The risk factors for this occurrence are prolonged exposure to alkylating agents and advanced age. Diffuse NHL is the next most common secondary malignancy with a cumulative 10-year risk of 4–5%. This incidence is also increased in untreated patients. The risk for solid tumors appears to be related to radiation therapy. The cumulative risk is 9% at 10 years.

Endocrine abnormalities limited mainly to the thyroid and gonads are another complication of treatment for Hodgkin's disease. Thyroid hyperplasia, hypothyroidism, and thyroid malignancy are possibilities.[56] Fertility, especially in men, can be decreased; radiotherapy scatter may effect testicular function. But alkylating agents are the most problematic regarding male fertility. Cyclophosphamide, mechlorethamine, chlorambucil, and procarbazine are most commonly associated with male infertility. MOPP causes prolonged testicular dysfunction in 80% of patients, with only 10% showing partial recovery in 1–7 years. ABVD impairs spermatogenesis in 54% of men, but recovery usually occurs in 2 years. More recently, young males with this diagnosis have the option of saving their sperm prior to treatment so as to allow for option of having children later.

Women are also affected by chemotherapy. Menopausal symptoms can develop even several years after treatment. Ovarian ablation can cause anovulatory or irregular cycles. Alkylating agents are the main inducer. As many as 80% will have some ovarian dysfunction and 20–30% will have permanent amenorrhea. Young women also have the option of saving their eggs prior to treatment.[32]

Cardiovascular complications are caused by chemotherapy and radiation injury. Pericarditis is common in irradiation and occurs 5–9 months after completion of radiotherapy. Many patients will remain asymptomatic, but others will present with cardiomegaly, friction rub, effusion, tamponade, fever, electrocardiogram (ECG) changes, and pleuritic pain. Steroidal and non-steroidal agents are used to treat these symptoms; digoxin and diuretics may also be used. Pericardial effusions develop in 25–30% of patients, and usually occur within 2 years of therapy, but can arise even later.[57,58] Myocardial damage can also be experienced after radiation, especially of the right ventricle, because of its location, exposing it to a greater dose. Valvular abnormalities can develop, causing aortic and mitral regurgitation. Accelerated atherosclerosis has resulted in myocardial infarction (MI) in some patients who were otherwise healthy.

Doxorubicin (Adriamycin) can cause chronic and acute side effects. Carditis and arrhythmias can occur, and the mortality rate from doxorubicin-induced cardiomyopathy is 50%. Patients are closely monitored during treatment for toxicity through endocardial biopsy. Advanced age and uncontrolled hypertension with previous radiotherapy all contribute to an increased risk of cardiomyopathy in patients treated with doxorubicin. Mitomycin and cyclophosphamide may act synergistically with doxorubicin to produce heart damage.[59]

Pulmonary complications primarily arise from radiotherapy. Acute radiation pneumonitis is the most common side effect. Patients with mediastinal disease and those who receive total body irradiation for BMT are most prone to this side effect. The presentation includes shortness of breath, cough, fever, pain, and wheezing. Pleural effusions may be present. Some patients may not require treatment but others may need treatment with corticosteroids. Rapid discontinuation of steroidal treatment after MOPP may precipitate acute radiation pneumonitis. There may be synergy with certain drugs; bleomycin, cyclophosphamide, and methotrexate. Radiation recall is a phenomenon characterised by signs and symptoms of chronic restrictive fibrosis occurring after completion of therapy and doxorubicin, bleomycin, and dactinomycin have all been implicated.[60]

Chemotherapeutic drugs associated with pulmonary toxicity include bleomycin and carmustine (BiCNU). Bleomycin toxicity most commonly presents as interstitial pneumonitis. Pulmonary fibrosis has been associated with carmustine and procarbazine.

Patients with Hodgkin's disease may also experience musculoskeletal complications. Avascular necrosis of the bone is a condition connected to Hodgkin's and made worse by radiotherapy to the bone. Children may grow assymmetrically due to premature closure of the epiphyseal plates. Soft tissue irradiation may cause fibrosis, edema, venous thrombosis, and nerve entrapment. And those treated with mantle or cervical radiotherapy may have an increased risk for dental caries.[61]

Chinese medicine

Treatment

The modern treatment of this large category of lymphatic cancers is according to the presentation and the pattern differentiation. The presentation includes the type, the anatomical location of involvement, and the stage. To a large extent the early stage lymphomas include the treatment principle of smoothing qi and moving blood stasis, regulating the qi, transforming phlegm, softening hardness, dispersing nodules, and acting antineoplastically. The late-stage presentations carry the treatment principles of clearing heat and toxin, releasing the LPF, and sometimes nourishing yin, if necessary. This is especially true in the non-indolent lymphomas. But in later stage indolent lymphomas a more aggressive approach may be considered because of the projected lifespan of the patient and the relative nature of the disease, which is not aggressive even in late stage. As always, these aspects of treatment are combined with potentiating the chemotherapeutic regimen and radiation along with managing the side effects of these treatments. When in remission, the patient is treated according to the Chinese medicine parameters.

1. Early stage with tumor above the cricoid process including the parotid gland, e.g. Burkitt's lymphoma[62]

fang feng (Ledebouriellae Radix; *Ledebouriella* root)	10 g
zhi zi (Gardeniae Fructus; *Gardenia* fruit)	10 g
lian qiao (Forsythiae fructus; *Forsythia*)	15 g
da huang (Rhei Radix et Rhizoma; *Rheum*)	10 g
chi shao (Paeoniae Radix rubra; *Paeonia lactiflora* root)	10 g
dang gui (Angelicae sinensis Radix; *Angelica sinensis*)	10 g
jin yin hua (Lonicerae Flos; *Lonicera* flowers)	30 g
di gu pi (Lycii Cortex; *Lycium*)	10 g
long yi (Serpentis Periostracum; *Elaphe/Zaocys*; snake slough)	3 g
jie geng (Platycodi Radix; *Platycodon grandiflorus* root)	15 g

In this early-stage presentation, the involved node or nodes may be surgically resected and then followed by radiation and/or chemotherapy. Fang feng relieves the surface and dispels wind. It dissipates wind damp bi syndrome, and treats this level of lymphoma. It has an antibacterial and antiviral effect. Zhi zi clears heat, drains damp heat, cools the blood, and is antineoplastic and antibiotic. All of these actions are especially beneficial in treating lymphoma since it combines elements of LPF exposure related to wind, damp heat, and heat in the blood level. Lian qiao clears heat and resolves toxic heat. It also disperses swellings and pus and is antibacterial and antiviral. It is especially beneficial in clearing wei and qi stage heat which may be appropriate to this early stage and contained lymphoma.

Wine-prepared (jiu jun) da huang vitalises and cracks stagnant blood. It clears blood heat and fire toxins. This herb is antineoplastic and antibiotic and antiviral. Chi shao moves the blood while clearing heat and cooling the blood. It is antineoplastic and reduces swellings. Dang gui acts in consort with chi shao by nourishing the blood and mildly moving the blood. Jin yin hua clears heat and toxic heat. It resolves abscesses and is antibacterial and antiviral. These antibacterial and antiviral herbs are important because these latent infections may be implicated in this neck lymphoma (Burkitt's). Di gu pi clears heat and cools the blood. It is especially beneficial for treating the nasopharyngeal cavity and related lymph nodes.

Long yi is the sloughed dry skin of three different types of snakes (*Elaphe carinata, E. taeniura,* and *Zaocys dhumnades*). According to *Essential Prescriptions Worth a Thousand Gold Ducats*, 'To treat malignant boils lingering for 10 years, a slough is burnt and mixed with lard for external application to the lesion, and another slough is burnt and taken with wine'. Jie geng acts as a messenger herb that directs the formula to the head and neck.

2. Stage I and II abdominal lymphoma[63]

mu li (Ostreae Concha; *Ostrea* shell)	30 g
xia ku cao (Prunellae Spica; *Prunella vulgaris*)	15 g
hai zao (Sargassum; *Sargassum*)	15 g
kun bu (Eckloniae Thallus; *Ecklonia kurome*; kelp thallus)	15 g
xuan shen (Scrophulariae Radix; *Scrophularia*)	15 g
tian hua fen (Trichosanthis Radix; *Trichosanthes* root)	15 g
zhe bei mu (Fritillariae thunbergii Bulbus; *Fritillaria thunbergii*)	10 g
nan sha shen (Adenophorae Radix; *Adenophora*)	30 g
ba yue zha (Akebiae Fructus; *Akebia*)	10 g
dan shen (Salviae miltiorrhizae Radix; *Salvia miltiorhiza* root)	15 g
shan yao (Dioscoreae Rhizoma; *Disoscorea opposita*)	15 g
wang jiang nan (Cassiae Semen; *Cassia occidentalis*)	30 g

Mu li, hai zao, kun bu are all soften-hard-mass herbs that reduce phlegm tumors and act as antineoplastics. Tian hua fen also clears and dissolves heated phlegm and is antineoplastic. These herbs work together with xia ku cao, xuan shen (a blood-regulating-blood-heat-clearing herb) and zhe bei mu to clear toxin and heat from phlegm tumors. Ba yue zha and dan shen help to crack the blood to provide access to the tumor tissue. They are also antineoplastic. Sha shen protects the yin while draining and transforming dampness and phlegm. Wang jiang nan is the seed of the *Cassia* plant. The high dose indicates that this herb is antineoplastic and is included in anticancer preparations in traditional Chinese medicine.

3. Stage II to III with qi and blood deficiency[64]

dang gui (Angelicae sinensis Radix; *Angelica sinensis*)	15 g
chi shao (Paeoniae Radix rubra; *Paeonia lactiflora* root)	15 g
bai shao (Paeoniae Radix alba; *Paeonia lactiflora* root)	15 g
huang qi (Astragali Radix; *Astragalus membranaceus*)	30 g
xia ku cao (Prunellae Spica; *Prunella vulgaris*)	15 g
hai zao (Sargassum; *Sargassum*)	15 g
mu li (Ostreae Concha; *Ostrea* shell)	15 g
chuan bei mu (Fritillariae cirrhosae Bulbus; *Fritillaria cirrhosa*)	10 g
pu gong ying (Taraxaci Herba; *Taraxacum mongolicum*)	15 g
sheng di huang (Rehmanniae Radix; *Rehmannia*)	15 g
xuan shen (Scrophulariae Radix; *Scrophularia*)	15 g
tu bie chong (Eupolyphaga; *Eupolyphaga sinensis*)	10 g
nan sha shen (Adenophorae Radix; *Adenophora*)	30 g
fu ling (Poria; *Poria cocos*)	15 g
chen pi huang (Citri reticulatae Pericarpium; *Citrus reticulata* pericarp)	10 g
tian nan xing (Arisaematis Rhizoma preparatum; *Arisaema erubescens* rhizome)	10 g
bai jie zi (Sinapis Semen; *Sinapis*)	10 g
zhi ban xia (Pinelliae Rhizoma preparatum; *Pinellia ternata* rhizome)	6 g

This formula has many herbs that clear heat and toxin and are antineoplastic. These are combined with herbs that transform phlegm and soften hardness. This last group acts like blood-cracking herbs in that they open the nodes to allow the antineoplastic herbs into the center of the active tumor sites. Similarly, they allow any chemotherapeutic regimen into the nodal sites. There are also herbs that clear heat from the blood level. Overall this formula acts to eliminate blood level LPFs by using these blood-heat-clearing herbs as messenger herbs to target the site of the LPF and then clear toxin. Nan sha shen nourishes and protects the yin. Fu ling transforms dampness but also protects the spleen. Ban xia acts in a similar way, and chen pi protects the middle jiao.

4. Early stage[65]

zhi ban xia (Pinelliae Rhizoma preparatum; *Pinellia ternata* rhizome)	10 g
fu ling (Poria; *Poria cocos*)	10 g
chen pi (Citri reticulatae Pericarpium; *Citrus reticulata* pericarp)	10 g
xia ku cao (Prunellae Spica; *Prunella vulgaris*)	15 g
kun bu (Eckloniae Thallus; *Ecklonia kurome*; kelp thallus)	10 g
huang yao zi (Dioscoreae bulbiferae Rhizoma; *Dioscorea bulbifera*)	10 g
mu li (Ostreae Concha; *Ostrea* shell)	15 g
xuan shen (Scrophulariae Radix; *Scrophularia*)	10 g
chuan bei mu (Fritillariae cirrhosae Bulbus; *Fritillaria cirrhosa*)	10 g
chai hu (Bupleuri Radix; *Bupleurum*)	10 g
hai zao (Sargassum; *Sargassum*)	10 g
mao zhua cao (Ranunculi ternati Radix; *Ranunculus ternatus* root)	30 g

Many of these various formulas demonstrate similar selections to arrive at the same goal: to soften hardness, transform and detoxify phlegm, clear heat and toxin, and harmonise the blood level. The tuber, mao zhao cao, is a bitter and cold herb that enters the liver and spleen. It is a clear-heat-and-toxin herb that also cracks the blood and promotes water metabolism, making it useful in treating ascites. It is antineoplastic against lymphoma and is used here as the main antineoplastic herb.

5. Late stage[65]

qing hao (Artemisiae annuae Herba; *Artemisia annua*)	10 g
di gu pi (Lycii Cortex; *Lycium*)	10 g
sheng di huang (Rehmanniae Radix; *Rehmannia*)	15 g

xuan shen (Scrophulariae Radix; *Scrophularia vulgaris*)	10 g
xia ku cao (Prunellae Spica; *Prunella*)	15 g
dan shen (Salviae miltiorrhizae Radix; *Salvia miltiorhiza* root)	30 g
mu li (Ostreae Concha; *Ostrea* shell)	10 g
bai shao (Paeoniae Radix alba; *Paeonia lactiflora* root)	10 g
dang shen (Codonopsis Radix; *Codonopsis pilosula* root)	15 g
huang qi (Astragali Radix; *Astragalus membranaceus*)	15 g
jin yin hua (Lonicerae Flos; *Lonicera* flowers)	15 g
huang yao zi (Dioscoreae bulbiferae Rhizoma; *Dioscorea bulbifera*)	10 g

The main antineoplastic herb in this formula is dan shen, which is at the highest dose. The surrounding herbs clear heat and toxin from the qi and blood level, and also tonify qi and nourish blood. The assumption is that the patient with later stage disease has longer-term qi and blood injury. The formulas usually take this into account and act antineoplastically in a more indirect way that is less injurious to the qi and blood and the middle jiao.

All of these formulas demonstrate various practitioners' approaches to treating lymphomas via stage.

6. Gastric lymphoma[66]

add: hu tao ruo (Juglandis Semen; *Juglans* seed)	15 g

When the addition of a herb is suggested it is assumed that it will be added to the formula written based on the pattern identification, along with the conventional treatment and the symptom picture.

Unripe walnuts are steeped in wine for 1 month. The wine is condensed to 60% when prepared and this is then called Qing long yi jiu. Walnut twigs are also used in decoction with other herbs.[67]

7. Thymus gland involvement

add: dan shen (Salviae miltiorrhizae Radix; *Salvia miltiorhiza* root)	15 g

Dan shen has been studied extensively in cancer treatment as a radiosensitising and chemotherapy herb. It has also been studied as an herb for direct treatment against several cancers, including lymphoma where the thymus gland is involved. This herb is included in a paper presented on thymus gland lymphoma.[68]

8. Parotid gland involvement

add: hai zao (Sargassum; *Sargassum*)	15 g
ju ruo (Amorphophalli Rhizoma; *Amorphophallus rivieri*; konjac)	10 g
ma lan jin (Wedeliae Herba; *Wedelia chinensis*)	10 g

Hai zao clears heat and transforms phlegm. It is especially beneficial in treating thyroid and neck tumors, not just because it is a seaweed and contains iodine. It reduces lymph tumors and phlegm nodules of all kinds. Ju ruo is the rhizome of *Amorphophallus*, a herb that transforms phlegm and moves blood. It has been found to be antineoplastic against leukemic cell lines, particularly the *A. sinensis* variety. Ma lan jin clears toxin, transforms phlegm and disperses swellings. It has been found to be antineoplastic and is included in the *Reference for the Essentials of Properties of Medicinal Herbs*.

9. Late stage large–cell with heat and pain, i.e. B symptoms and metastatic disease[69]

niu bang zi (Arctii Fructus; *Arctium lappa*)	15 g
tian hua fen (Trichosanthis Radix; *Trichosanthes* root)	15 g
chai hu (Bupleuri Radix; *Bupleurum*)	10 g
tu bei mu (Rhizoma Bolbostemmae; *Bolbostemma paniculatum*)	15 g
shan dou gen (Sophorae tonkinensis Radix; *Sophora tonkinensis*)	30 g
tu fu ling (Smilacis glabrae Rhizoma; *Smilax glabra*)	30 g
lu feng fang (Vespae Nidus; *Vespa*; wasp/hornet nest)	30 g
ban lan gen (Isatidis/Baphicacanthis Radix; *Isatis/Baphicacanthus* root)	30 g
xuan shen (Scrophulariae Radix; *Scrophularia*)	30 g
xian feng cao (Bidentis pilosae Herba; *Bidens pilosa*)	30 g
di jin cao (Herba Euphorbiae humifusae; *Euphorbia humifusa*)	30 g
lian qiao (Forsythiae fructus; *Forsythia*)	30 g

This formula is a case in point that nourishing yin in B-symptoms is not the correct approach with toxic heat and a smoldering LPF as the causative factor. Niu bang zi reduces swellings and neutralises toxins. It is antineoplastic and is commonly used to bring on the expression of rashes. The outward expression of smoldering diseases carries with it the same treatment principle as LPF treatment. Therefore, some of the same herbs are used. Tian hua fen clears and dissolves hot phlegm. It clears toxins and generates fluids while doing so. It is antineoplastic for phlegm tumors. Chai hu is used here because it is an excellent herb to treat Shaoyang stage heat, and in many ways LPFs and stuck pathogens have a similarity to Shaoyang stage disease. Herbs that move pathogens either out or downward help to unlock LPFs. Chai hu is one of these herbs. Tu bei mu is a phlegm-transforming herb that is 'good for scattering carbuncles, removing pus, dispelling wind and damp pathogenic factors and resolving phlegm.' (*Mirror of a Hundred Herbs*).

Shan dou gen removes toxic heat and disperses swellings. It is a clear-heat-and-toxin herb that has been found to be antineoplastic for many cancers. Tu fu ling is also a clear-heat-and-toxin herb that is antineoplastic. It is especially good for damp heat toxins. Lu feng fang is antineoplastic against several cancers including phlegm tumors. It is also analgesic. Ban lan gen and xuan shen work together to clear heat from the blood and the qi level. They are both antineoplastic against lymphoma and leukemia. Xian feng cao (or gui zhen cao; Bidentis bipinnatae Herba; *Bidens bipinnata*) clears heat and toxins and vitalises the blood. As reported in *Treatment Based on the Differentiation of Symptoms and Signs*, it has been found to have bacteriophagic anticancer activity against lymphoma. Di jin cao has been found to have anticancer activity against lymphomas and lymphosarcoma. It is a phlegm-transforming herb that also kills some parasites and removes toxin. Lian qiao clears heat and resolves toxic heat. It reduces swellings and drains pus. It is antibacterial and antiviral. It is beneficial for treating phlegm nodules, inflamed lymph nodes and abscesses. It also enhances immune function by increasing antibody formation.

10. Deficient qi, wei qi, qi and blood with heart and kidney disharmony[70]

huang qi (Astragali Radix; Astragalus membranaceus)	30 g
dang gui (Angelicae sinensis Radix; Angelica sinensis)	15 g
huang qin (Scutellariae Radix; Scutellaria baicalensis)	10 g
zi cao (Arnebiae/Lithospermi Radix; Arnebia/Lithospermum root)	15 g
xuan shen (Scrophulariae Radix; Scrophularia)	15 g
sheng di huang (Rehmanniae Radix; Rehmannia)	15 g
mu li (Ostreae Concha; Ostrea shell)	20 g
long gu (Fossilia Ossis Mastodi; fossilised bone)	15 g
long yan rou (Longan Arillus; Dimocarpus longan aril)	10 g
jin yin hua (Lonicerae Flos; Lonicera flowers)	15 g
shan yao (Dioscoreae Rhizoma; Dioscorea opposita)	15 g
yi ren (Coicis Semen; Coix lacryma-jobi)	15 g
mu xiang (Aucklandiae Radix; Saussurea)	5 g
ji nei jin (Gigeriae galli Endothelium corneum; Gallus gallus domesticus chicken gizzard lining)	15 g
tian dong (Asparagi Radix; Asparagus)	15 g
mai dong (Ophiopogonis Radix; Ophiopogon)	15 g
tian hua fen (Trichosanthis Radix; Trichosanthes root)	15 g
wu wei zi (Schisandrae Fructus; Schisandra)	5 g
shan zhu yu (Corni Fructus; Cornus officinalis fruit)	10 g
bai shao (Paeoniae Radix alba; Paeonia lactiflora root)	15 g
gui ban* (Testudinis Plastrum; Chinemys reevesii plastron)	20 g

This formula nourishes the heart and kidneys to strengthen the heart/kidney axis. It also strengthens the spleen to enrich the blood and tonify the qi. The only antineoplastics in the formula are specifically in the realm of moving blood and clearing blood heat and in the realm of softening hard mass to reduce tumor. The remaining herbs nourish the blood and yin. The lead herb, huang qi, is in the highest dose and strongly tonifies the qi to move qi. Moving qi is a form of treatment for phlegm, which is transformed by moving qi. Zi cao clears heat and cools and vitalises the blood, clears toxic heat, and is antineoplastic against lymphoma and leukemia. Although there are yin-nourishing herbs in the formula, this formula describes medicinally the very picture of the analysis of lymphoma pathogenesis via LPF. It is a more advanced-stage presentation, as well, in terms of the mechanics of this formula. As a result, it is used in its entirety in presentations where more injury has occurred and a less antineoplastic formula may be necessary to avoid further damage.

11. Hodgkin's disease[70]

dang gui (Angelicae sinensis Radix; Angelica sinensis)	10 g
chuan xiong (Chuanxiong Rhizoma; Ligusticum wallichii root)	10 g
chi shao (Paeoniae Radix rubra; Paeonia lactiflora root)	10 g
sheng di huang (Rehmanniae Radix; Rehmannia)	10 g
xuan shen (Scrophulariae Radix; Scrophularia)	15 g
shan ci gu* (Cremastrae/Pleiones Pseudobulbus; Cremastra/Pleione pseudobulbs)	15 g
huang yao zi (Dioscoreae bulbiferae Rhizoma; Dioscorea bulbifera)	15 g
hai zao (Sargassum; Sargassum)	15 g
kun bu (Eckloniae Thallus; Ecklonia kurome; kelp thallus)	15 g
xia ku cao (Prunellae Spica; Prunella vulgaris)	15 g
mu li (Ostreae Concha; Ostrea shell)	30 g
chong lou (Paridis Rhizoma; Paris)	30 g

The first five herbs of this formula direct the qi of the formula to the blood level. The remaining herbs direct the qi of the formula to the phlegm and are antineoplastic. They also potentiate radiation and chemotherapy by cracking the blood and phlegm and improving circulation to nodal sites.

12. Formula for combined chemotherapy and radiotherapy[70]

huang qi (Astragali Radix; Astragalus membranaceus)	30–60 g
dang shen (Codonopsis Radix; Codonopsis pilosula root)	15–30 g
bai zhu (Atractylodis macrocephalae Rhizoma; Atractylodes macrocephala)	15 g
fu ling (Poria; Poria cocos)	10 g
chen pi (Citri reticulatae Pericarpium; Citrus reticulata pericarp)	10 g
ji xue teng (Spatholobi Caulis; Spatholobus suberectus)	15 g
dang gui (Angelicae sinensis Radix; Angelica sinensis)	10 g
gou qi zi (Lycii Fructus; Lycium chinensis fruit)	10 g
bei sha shen (Glehniae Radix; Glehnia)	10 g
nu zhen zi (Ligustri lucidi Fructus; Ligustrum lucidum fruit)	10 g
tu si zi (Cuscutae Semen; Cuscuta seed)	10 g
yin yang huo (Epimedii Herba; Epimedium grandiflorum)	10 g

Si jun zi tang is embedded in this formula and helps to support and protect the middle jiao which, in turn, supports the blood. The blood-regulating and blood-nourishing herbs potentiate the yin-nourishing herbs to support normal blood levels, which are injured during chemotherapy. The yin-nourishing and blood-regulating herbs also potentiate radiation and help to protect normal tissue from injury by toxic heat (radiation). The two yang tonic herbs support the source.

13. During MOPP or CHOP chemotherapy[71]

tian dong (Asparagi Radix; Asparagus)	30 g
bai hua she she cao (Hedyotis diffusae Herba; Oldenlandia)	40 g
fu ling (Poria; Poria cocos)	15 g
bai zhu (Atractylodis macrocephalae Rhizoma; Atractylodes macrocephala)	15 g
yu jin (Curcumae Radix; Curcuma longa rhizome)	15 g
shan yao (Dioscoreae Rhizoma; Dioscorea opposita)	15 g
gan cao (Glycyrrhizae Radix; Glycyrrhiza; licorice root)	5 g
huang qi (Astragali Radix; Astragalus membranaceus)	15 g
dang shen (Codonopsis Radix; Codonopsis pilosula root)	15 g
tai zi shen (Pseudostellariae Radix; Pseudostellaria heterophylla)	15 g
jin yin hua (Lonicerae Flos; Lonicera flowers)	10 g
xian he cao (Agrimoniae Herba; Agrimonia pilosa var. japonica; agrimony)	15 g
nu zhen zi (Ligustri lucidi Fructus; Ligustrum lucidum fruit)	15 g
zhu ling (Polyporus; Polyporus – Grifola)	15 g

This formula is specifically designed to protect heart muscle and renal function that is injured by either of these regimens. It maintains normal blood levels injured by cytotoxic myelosuppression. It maintains normal digestive function and it clears heat and prevents bleeding, especially from cystitis. Several of the herbs are also antineoplastic.

14. During radiation[72]

dan shen (Salviae miltiorrhizae Radix; Salvia miltiorhiza root)	15 g
mu dan pi (Moutan Cortex; Paeonia suffruticosa root cortex)	10 g
mai dong (Ophiopogonis Radix; Ophiopogon)	10 g
tian dong (Asparagi Radix; Asparagus)	15 g
bai mao gen (Imperatae Rhizoma; Imperata cylindrica rhizome)	15 g
zhu ling (Polyporus; Polyporus – Grifola)	15 g
fu ling (Poria; Poria cocos)	15 g

huang qi (Astragali Radix; *Astragalus membranaceus*)	15 g
bai hua she she cao (Hedyotis diffusae Herba; *Oldenlandia*)	25 g
bai zhu (Atractylodis macrocephalae Rhizoma; *Atractylodes macrocephala*)	15 g
chuan xiong (Chuanxiong Rhizoma; *Ligusticum wallichii* root)	10 g
yu jin (Curcumae Radix; *Curcuma longa* rhizome)	10 g
tai zi shen (Pseudostellariae Radix; *Pseudostellaria heterophylla*)	15 g
huang jing (Polygonati Rhizoma; *Polygonatum*)	10 g

This formula increases circulation and, thereby, potentiates radiation treatment by increasing oxygenation of tumor tissue. It clears blood heat to prevent blood stasis and resulting scarring. It nourishes yin, tonifies qi, and is antineoplastic. Zhu ling is a primary herb in potentiating radiation treatment. Combined radiation and chemotherapy is often used in intermediate- to high-grade lymphomas and in Hodgkin's disease. The side effects are severe when whole-body radiation is used. These side effects can persist for life. This formula is extremely valuable in potentiation of radiation therapy and in protection of normal cells and structures.

15. Prevention of recurrence[64]

ren shen (Ginseng Radix; *Panax ginseng*)	60 g
dang gui (Angelicae sinensis Radix; *Angelica sinensis*)	60 g
chen pi (Citri reticulatae Pericarpium; *Citrus reticulata pericarp*)	20 g
shu di (Rehmanniae Radix preparata; *Rehmannia*)	20 g
mu dan pi (Moutan Cortex; *Paeonia suffruticosa* root cortex)	30 g
hong da zao (Jujubae Fructus; *Ziziphus jujuba*; red jujube)	30 g
bai zhu (Atractylodis macrocephalae Rhizoma; *Atractylodes macrocephala*)	60 g
fu ling (Poria; *Poria cocos*)	60 g
xiang fu (Cyperi Rhizoma; *Cyperus rotundus* rhizome)	20 g

yuan zhi (Polygalae Radix; *Polygala*)	30 g
tian nan xing (Arisaematis Rhizoma preparatum; *Arisaema erubescens* rhizome)	30 g
chuan bei mu (Fritillariae cirrhosae Bulbus; *Fritillaria cirrhosa*)	30 g
bai zi ren (Biotae Semen; *Biota*)	30 g
long gu (Fossilia Ossis Mastodi; fossilised bone)	20 g

Recurrence is often the name of the game in lymphoma treatment. Prevention of recurrence, especially in low-grade lymphomas, can be the primary treatment in terms of time. This formula moves qi to transform phlegm, cracks the blood, clears LPFs and detoxifies. It should be modified to specifically fit the presentation of the patient being treated.

Radiation side effects The therapeutic principles for the treatment of side effects of radiation are the following:

- clear heat and dissolve toxins
- generate fluids and moisten dryness
- regulate blood and prevent blood stasis
- tonify qi and blood with neutral or cooler herbs
- invigorate the spleen and harmonise the stomach
- nourish and tonify the liver and kidneys.

The therapeutic principles for the treatment of the side effects of chemotherapy are the following:

- tonify and cultivate qi and blood
- invigorate the spleen and harmonise the stomach
- nourish the liver and kidneys
- clear heat and resolve toxicity.

The therapeutic principles in preventing recurrence include:

- tonify qi to maintain the source and zheng qi and prevent phlegm
- nourish the blood and clear blood heat to prevent the establishment of a LPF
- transform phlegm
- move the qi
- harmonise the heart and kidney axis.

Case study 10.1

This was a 56-year-old woman who referred herself to her primary care physician for inguinal lymphadenopathy. She had noticed two swollen lymph nodes, one in each groin, for several months. They were gradually enlarging, and more recently two more nodes were enlarging nearby in the same two areas. They did not change in size except for enlarging. They were non-tender. She had no fevers or night sweats, a normal CBC and a normal chest X-ray. There was no sign of local infection, no vaginal discharge or rectal bleeding or trauma or ingrown toenail, which might explain a swollen inguinal lymph node. There was no history of melanoma.

The nodes that were swollen were approximately 3 cm, smooth, mobile, and not consistent with a hernia. The newer swellings were 1.5–2 cm. A FNA was performed at the first visit. The aspirate confirmed malignancy and an excisional biopsy was performed. The biopsy showed a follicular B-cell low-grade non-Hodgkin's lymphoma. Further workup showed that the CNS was not involved but the bone marrow was involved. There was lymphadenopathy in the chest, abdomen, pelvis, inguinal area, mediastinum and retroperitoneum. The grade was 1, the stage was IV. She had no B symptoms, her LDH was in the normal range, and all of her blood work was normal. She had a Pap smear, which was found to normal.

With stage IV disease, she opted for immediate treatment. She did not seek a second opinion.

Presenting signs and symptoms

- Appetite: normal.
- Digestion
  - above the navel: no symptoms but a history of morning sickness (one child now age 17)
  - below the navel: mild gas on occasion.
- Stools: 'dependable'.
- Sleep: good, 8 hours nightly.
- Energy: 'slightly dragging since last summer'.
- Pain: none.

- Temperature: some flushing once per day in the early morning upon waking, otherwise runs neither hot or cold.
- Sweats: normal; no night sweats or other sweats; does not sweat easily.
- Thirst: yes; drinks a lot due to thirst.
- Fevers: none; some chills after flushing.
- Rashes: none.
- Cycle: post-menopausal for 4 years; still symptomatic but mildly so; pregnancies: three, two miscarriages, not known why, one son age 17.
- Exercise: walking, hiking, gardening, although less recently due to flagging energy.
- History: frequent cystitis due to teaching schedule, low hydration and inability to leave classroom, every 3 months; lots of coffee and tea; frequent antibiotic therapy for the last 5–8 years.
- Hospitalisations: once for birth of son.
- Tongue: very pale, thin white coat, no vein distention.
- Pulse: liver/kidney sho; left pulses very low; generally slow pulse.

Diagnosis

1. Deficient qi, wei qi, and blood with heart and kidney disharmony and possible LPF.

Treatment plan

For this low-grade presentation the patient was offered several options:

1. Watch and wait.
2. Rituxan alone.
3. Chlorambucil in pill form.
4. CVP with Rituxan (cytoxan, vincristine, prednisone with Rituxan).
5. CHOP with Rituxan.
6. FND with Rituxan (Fludarabine, mitoxantrone [Novantrone], dexamethasone)
7. A clinical trial of CHOP with Rituxan versus CHOP with Bexxar.

Case study continues

8. Bexxar with Zevalin, a radiolabeled antibody.
9. Stem cell tranplantation.
10. RICE, DHAP.

With stage IV disease this patient had a 50–60% chance of survival at 10 years. Recent studies show that earlier treatment provides better outcomes than waiting for disease progression or symptomatic progression. However, it still remains controversial and watch-and-wait remains an option. Because of this, the patient finally did seek another opinion but the number of options presented did not necessarily help the decision-making process. She opted for the most common regimen with the longest statistical record, CHOP-R (or CHOP with Rituxan). This regimen was given every 3 weeks for six infusions.

This patient was given a formula that combines elements from the Formula 10 with Formula 13 for CHOP chemotherapy, and a small part of Qing hao bai du yin and Qing hao bie jia tang. Following is the formula used during chemotherapy:

huang qi (Astragali Radix; *Astragalus membranaceus*)	30 g
dang gui (Angelicae sinensis Radix; *Angelica sinensis*)	15 g
dang shen (Codonopsis Radix; *Codonopsis pilosula* root)	15 g
nu zhen zi (Ligustri lucidi Fructus; *Ligustrum lucidum* fruit)	15 g
huang qin (Scutellariae Radix; *Scutellaria baicalensis*)	10 g
zi cao (Arnebiae/Lithospermi Radix; *Arnebia/Lithospermum* root)	15 g
xuan shen (Scrophulariae Radix; *Scrophularia*)	15 g
mu li (Ostreae Concha; *Ostrea* shell)	20 g
long yan rou (Longan Arillus; *Dimocarpus longan* aril)	10 g
yi ren (Coicis Semen; *Coix lacryma-jobi*)	15 g
ji nei jin (Gigeriae galli Endothelium corneum; *Gallus gallus domesticus* chicken gizzard lining)	15 g
qing hao (Artemisiae annuae Herba; *Artemisia* annua)	20 g
di jin cao (Herba Euphorbiae humifusae; *Euphorbia humifusa*)	30 g
shan dou gen (Sophorae tonkinensis Radix; *Sophora tonkinensis*)	20 g

This formula treats the diagnosis according to Chinese medicine by working as soon as possible to clear latent pathogens that may be lodged at the ying and blood level. Qing hao is a primary herb to lift the pathogen to the qi level. In many ways it is during the early treatment time, no matter the stage, that the best opportunity is available to clear pathogens. It is complicated to have several treatment principles engaged and the chemotherapeutic regimen adds to this complexity. However, qing hao is used in LPF treatment theory as an envoy herb. With this in mind, it is appropriate to use it within the context of both paradigms to deliver the chemotherapy to the scene of the crime while working to clear the unidentified latent pathogen. Huang qi strongly tonifies the qi and supports the spleen to transform phlegm, a given in lymphoma. Tonifying qi also helps to move qi and transform phlegm. Zi cao clears toxic heat and is antineoplastic against lymphoma. Di jin cao is also antineoplastic against lymphoma.

The formula also nourishes the heart/kidney axis. The diagnosis was derived partly from the pulse and partly from the presentation. The toxicities of the chemotherapeutic regimen also drive the use of the formula to strengthen the heart and kidneys. Shan dou gen removes toxic heat and disperses swellings. It is a clear-heat-and-toxin herb that is also antineoplastic. The remaining herbs work mainly to maintain normal blood levels, normal digestive function, and protect the heart and kidneys from toxicity.

In fact, the patient did not require colony-stimulating factors of any kind during her treatment. She stopped her antiemetics after two rounds of chemotherapy and never resumed them. She dramatically changed her diet to one that included far more vegetables, no coffee or tea, except for green tea; she increased her fluid intake, and she left the classroom to use the

Case study continues

bathroom when needed. She switched to only organic foods, stopped sweets and eating after 7 pm at night, and went to bed by 10 pm rather than midnight or 1 am. It was her habit to arise at 6 am for school and this meant in a typical day that she would get only 6 to 7 hours of sleep. This chronic sleep deprivation may have contributed to her diagnosis.

This patient has remained in remission for 12 years now. She has followed the dietary and lifestyle path and maintained her general health in the ways that evolved during treatment. Studies were done in the year after she ended chemotherapeutic treatment to determine if there were any latent pathogens or chemical exposures that could be attributed to her diagnosis. She was found to have higher levels of PCB and atrazine along with moderate levels of other organochlorine pesticides like DDE. She was treated with various nature cure methods along with Chinese herbal medicine to depurate these toxins (see Chapter 14). After 1.5 years of this kind of intermittent treatment, she was rescreened and findings showed that her levels of these latent toxins gradually reduced to just above the lowest limit of harmful toxins. The herbal formula used during that time is a combination of the final two formulas in the prevention chapter modified to meet other needs of the patient at that time.

After depuration, the formula used generally to prevent recurrence was usually a form of the following combination:

ren shen (Ginseng Radix; *Panax ginseng*)	20 g
dang gui (Angelicae sinensis Radix; *Angelica sinensis*)	15 g
huang qin (Scutellariae Radix; *Scutellaria baicalensis*)	15 g
zi cao (Arnebiae/Lithospermi Radix; *Arnebia/Lithospermum* root)	20 g
xuan shen (Scrophulariae Radix; *Scrophularia*)	15 g
sheng di huang (Rehmanniae Radix; *Rehmannia*)	20 g
mu li (Ostreae Concha; *Ostrea* shell)	30 g
long gu (Fossilia Ossis Mastodi; fossilised bone)	15 g

long yan rou (Longan Arillus; *Dimocarpus longan* aril)	20 g
jin yin hua (Lonicerae Flos; *Lonicera* flowers)	20 g
shan yao (Dioscoreae Rhizoma; *Dioscorea opposita*)	15 g
yi ren (Coicis Semen; *Coix lacryma-jobi*)	30 g
mu xiang (Aucklandiae Radix; *Saussurea*)	15 g
ji nei jin (Gigeriae galli Endothelium corneum; *Gallus gallus domesticus* chicken gizzard lining)	20 g
tian dong (Asparagi Radix; *Asparagus*)	15 g
mai dong (Ophiopogonis Radix; *Ophiopogon*)	15 g
tian hua fen (Trichosanthis Radix; *Trichosanthes* root)	25 g
wu wei zi (Schisandrae Fructus; *Schisandra*)	15 g
shan zhu yu (Corni Fructus; *Cornus officinalis* fruit)	15 g
gui ban* (Testudinis Plastrum; *Chinemys reevesii* plastron)	20 g

This is Formula 10 to strengthen the heart/kidney axis. It also strengthens the spleen function to transform phlegm and to re-establish and maintain normal digestive function after cytotoxic treatment. Maintaining spleen function is important in every cancer, but especially in lymphomas because of the mechanism of the pathogenesis of this cancer, which often begins with spleen injury and is further injured by conventional treatment. Other herbs in the formula nourish yin and blood. Once the LPF has been cleared then nourishing yin is an important element of treatment and one can assume that any heat symptoms at this point are probably due to deficiency and not to a latent pathogen residing in the interior.

Using herbs at this point that strengthen immune function is appropriate whereas it may not have been appropriate before the latent pathogen had been cleared, except in the case of maintaining normal WBCs during chemotherapy. The antineoplastics are left in to treat the memory

Case study continues

of the disease, which is deeply embedded in indolent lymphomas. This formula, or a formula similar to it, was used for several years after conventional treatment. A period of 1 month was taken off the formula once every 6 months. The formula was also adjusted every 6 months to avoid

habituation. At 5 years, the patient stopped the formula. She was monitored every 6 months via CT scan. No scan ever showed any cancer activity. She is now 12 years out from original treatment without any signs of recurrence.

References

1. Hartge P. Quantification of the impact of known risk factors on the trends in non-Hodgkin's lymphoma incidence. Cancer Res 1992; 52(Suppl):5566–5569S.
2. Sheibani K. Variability in interpretation of immuno-histologic findings in lymphoproliferative disorders by hematopathologist: a comprehensive statistical analysis of interobserver performance. Cancer 1998; 62:657–664.
3. Simon R. The non-Hodgkin's lymphoma pathological classification project. Long-term follow-up of 1152 patients with non-Hodgkin's lymphomas. Ann Intern Med 1998; 109:939–945.
4. Zhang Zhong Jing. Shang Han Za Bing Lun. 210 ACE. People's Health Publishing; 1987.
5. Zhejiang TCM College, eds. Wen Bing tiao bian Bai Hua Jie (Vernacular explanation of the systematic differentiation of warm diseases). People's Health Publishing; 1979.
6. Wolfe SM. Standards for carcinogens: science affronted by politics, in origins of human cancer. Cold Springs Harbor: Cold Springs Harbor Laboratory; 1977:1735–1748.
7. Schwetz BA. The Effect of 2,4-D and esters of 2,4-D on rat embryonal, fetal, and neonatal growth and development. Food Cosmetics Toxicology 1971; 9:801–817.
8. Ye Tian Shi. Wen Re Lun (Discussion of warmth and heat). 1766 ACE.
9. Wu Ju Tong. Wen Bing Tiao bian (Systematic differentaition of warm diseases). 1798 ACE.
10. Ma Shou Cun. Interpretations from lectures on Shang Han and Wen Bing Theory. 1990–1992.
11. Hebei Medical Institute. Ling Shu Jing Giao Shi (Comparative explanation of the Ling Shu). People's Health Publishing; 1982.
12. Zhu Dan Xi. Jin Gui Gou Xuan (Scythe of mysteries of the golden cabinet). Xuan Dynasty.
13. Matsumoto K, Birch S. Hara diagnosis: reflections on the sea. Brookline, Ma: Paradigm Publications; 1988: Chapters 7,8,9.
14. Chao Yuan Fang. Zhu Bing Yuan Hou Lun (Generalized treatise on the etiology and symptomotology of disease). 610 ACE.
15. Yan Yong He. Ji Sheng Fang (Formulas to aid the living). 1253 ACE.
16. Horning ST. The natural history of initially untreated low-grade non-Hodgkin's lymphomas. N Engl J Med 1994; 311:1471–1475.
17. Harris N. A revised European American classification of lymphoid neoplasms: a proposal from the International Lymphoma Study Group. Blood 1994; 84:1361–1392.
18. Litam P. Prognostic value of serum B2 microglobulin in low-grade lymphoma. Ann Intern Med 1991; 114:755–810.
19. McLaughlin P. Stage III follicular lymphoma. Durable remissions with a combined chemotherapy–radiotherapy regimen. J Clin Oncol 1997; 6:867.
20. Leonard RCF. The identification of discrete prognostic groups in low-grade non-Hodgkin's lymphoma. Ann Oncol 1991; 2:655–662.
21. Fisher RI. A clinical analysis of two indolent lymphoma entities. Mantle-cell lymphoma and marginal zone lymphoma (including mucosa-associated lymphoid tissue and moncytoid subcategories). A SWOG study. Blood 1995; 85:1075–1082.
22. Bookman M. Lymphocytic lymphoma of inermediate differentiation: Morphology, immunophenotype, and prognostic factors. J Natl Cancer Inst 1998; 82:742–748.
23. Horning ST. Low-grade lymphoma, 1993: state of the art. Ann Oncol 1994; 5(Suppl 2):523–527.
24. Klasa RJ. BP-VACOP and extensive lymph node irradiation for advanced stage low-grade lymphoma (Abstract 1117). Proc Am Soc Clin Oncol 1992; 11:328.
25. Portlock C. No initial therapy for stage III and IV NHL of favorable histologic types. Ann Intern Med 1995; 90:10–13.
26. Robertson LE. Induction of apoptotic cell death in CLL by 2-chlorodeoxyadenosine and 9-beta-D-Arabinosyl-2-fluoradenine. Blood 1995; 81:143.
27. Hagenbeek A. Interferon-alfa-2a versus control as maintenance therapy for low-grade NHL: results from a prospective randomized clinical trial on

behalf of the EORTC Lymphoma Cooperative group. Proc Am Soc Clin Oncol 1995; 14:386.

28. Schouten HC. Autologous bone marrow transplantation for low-grade NHL: The European Bone Marrow Transplant Group experience. Ann Oncol 1994; 5(Suppl 2):S147–149.
29. Simon R. The Non-Hodgkin's Lymphoma Pathological Classification Project. Long-term follow-up of 1152 patients with NHL. Ann Intern Med 1998; 109:939–945.
30. Wotherspoon AC. Regression of primary low-grade B-cell gastric lymphoma of mucosal-associated lymphoid tissue type after eradication of *Helicobacter pylori*. Lancet 1993; 342:575–577.
31. Sander CA. p53 mutation is associated with progression in follicular lymphomas. Blood 1993; 82:1994–2004.
32. Bookman MA. Concomitant illness in patients treated for Hodgkin's disease. Cancer Treat Rev 1986; 13:77.
33. Coleman NC. Treatment of lymphoblastic lymphoma in adults. J Clin Oncol 1986; 4:1628–1637.
34. Seymour JF. Calcitriol production in hypercalcemic and normocalcemic patients with non-Hodgkin's lymphoma. Ann Intern Med 1994; 121:633–640.
35. Cossman J. Gene rearrangements in the diagnosis of lymphoma/leukemia guidelines for use based on a multi-institutional study. Hematopathology 1991; 95:347–354.
36. Shipp MA. Prognostic factors in aggressive non-Hodgkin's lymphoma: who has high-risk disease? Blood 1994; 83:1165–1173.
37. Shipp MA. A predictive model for aggressive NHL: The International non-Hodgkin's Lymphoma Prognostic Factors Project. N Engl J Med 1993; 329:987.
38. Grogan L. Comparable prognostic factors and survival in elderly patients with aggressive non-Hodgkin's lymphoma treated with standard-dose Adriamycin-based regimens. Ann Oncol 1994; 5(Suppl 2):S47–51.
39. Banks PM. The pathology of Hodgkin's disease. Semin Oncol 1990; 17:683.
40. Ferry J. Hodgkin's disease, nodular sclerosis type. Implications of histologic subclassification. Cancer 1993; 71:457–463.
41. Hagemeister FB. Controversies in management of Hodgkin's disease. In: Freireich EJ, Kantarjian H, eds. Therapy of hemtaopoietic neoplasia. New York: Marcel Dekker; 1991:249.
42. Hellman S. Hodgkin's disease. In: De Vita, ed. Cancer: principles and practice of oncology. Philadelphia: JB Lippincott; 1999:1696.
43. Hagemeister FB. Two cycles of MOPP and radiotherapy: effective treatment for stage IIIA and IIIB Hodgkin's disease. Ann Oncol 1990; 2:25.
44. Canellos GP. Chemotherapy of advanced Hodgkin's disease with MOPP, ABVD, or MOPP alternating with ABVD. N Engl J Med 1992; 327:1478–1484.
45. Tubiana M. Toward comprehensive management tailored to prognostic factors of patients with clinical stages I and II in Hodgkin's disease. The EORTC lymphoma group controlled clinical trial: 1964–1987. Blood 1989; 73:47–56.
46. Banks PM. The pathology of Hodgkin's disease. Semin Oncol 1990; 17:683.
47. Evans AS. A population-based case-control study of EBV and other viral antibodies among persons with Hodgkin's disease and their siblings. Int J Cancer 1984; 34:149.
48. Ree HJ. Human immunodeficiency virus-associated Hodgkin's disease: clinicopathologic studies of 24 cases and preponderance of mixed cellularity type characterized by the occurrence of fibrohistiocytoid stromal cells. Cancer 1991; 67:1614.
49. Glatstein E. The value of laparotomy and splenectomy in staging of Hodgkin's disease. Cancer 1969; 24:709.
50. Hagemeister FB. Controversies in management of Hodgkin's disease. In: Freireich EJ, ed. Therapy of hematopoietic neoplasia. New York: Marcel Dekker; 1991:249.
51. Leslie NT. Stage IA and IIB supradiaphragmatic Hodgkin's disease: long-term survival and relapse frequency. Cancer 1985; 55:2072–2078.
52. Longo DL. Radiation therapy versus combination chemotherapy in the treatment of early stage Hodgkin's disease: seven-year results of a prospective randomized trial. J Clin Oncol 1991; 9:906–917.
53. Mauch P. Stage III Hodgkin's disease: improved survival with combined modality as compared with radiotherapy alone. J Clin Oncol 1985; 3:1166.
54. Yahalom J. Impact of adjuvant radiation on the patterns and rate of relapse in advanced-stage Hodgkin's disease treated with alternating chemotherapy combinations. J Clin Oncol 1991; 9:2193.
55. Philip T. High dose chemotherapy and autologous bone marrow transplantation in refractory Hodgkin's disease. Br J Cancer 1986; 53:737.
56. Tamura K. Thyroid abnormalities associated with treatment of lymphoma. Cancer 1981; 47:2704.
57. Byhardt R. Dose and treatment factors in radiation-related pericardial effusion associated with the mantle-technique for Hodgkin's disease. Cancer 1975; 35:795.

58. Burns RJ. Detection of radiation cardiomyopathy by gated radionuclide angiography. Am J Med 1983; 74:297.

59. Minow RA. Adriamycin (NSC-123127) cardiomyopathy: an overview with determination of risk factors. Cancer Chemother Rep 1975; 6:195.

60. Hellman S. The place of radiotherapy in the treatment of Hodgkin's disease. Am J Med 1978; 60:152.

61. Engel IA. Osteonecrosis in patients with malignant lymphoma. A review of 25 cases. Cancer 1981; 48:1245.

62. Cao Shi Long. Zhong Liu Xin Li Lun Yu Xin Ji Shu (New theories and treatments for tumors). Shanghai Medical University Press; 1997.

63. Cao Guang Wen. Xian Dai Zhong Liu Sheng Wu Zhi Liao Xue (Current biological treatment of tumors). People's Military Medical Publishing Press; 1995.

64. Sun Yan. Zhong Xi Yi Jie He Fang Zhi Zhong Liu (Combination of Chinese and Western medicine in the prevention and treatment of tumors). Beijing Medical University and Peking Union Medical University Joint Press; 1995.

65. Zhang Dai Zhao. Zhang Dai Zhao Zhi Ai Jing Yan Ji Yao (Collection of Zhang Dai Zhao's experiences in the treatment of cancer). China Medicine and Pharmaceutical Publishing House; 2001.

66. Zhang Tian Ze. Zhong Liu Xue (Oncology). Tianjian Science and Technology Publishing House; 1996.

67. Chang Mingyi. Anticancer preparation. Traditional Chinese Medicine 1980; 2:176–177.

68. Chang Mingyi. New Traditional Chinese Medicine 1983; 11:77.

69. Tang Zhai Qiu. Xian Dai Zhong Liu Xue (Current oncology). Shanghai Medical University Press; 1993.

70. Zhang Dai Zhao. E Xing Zhong Liu Fang Hua Zhong Xi Zhi Liao (Chinese materia medica in the treatment of malignant tumors with chemotherapy and radiation). People's Medical Publishing House; 2000.

71. Yang Shi Yong. Sheng Wu Fan Yong Tiao Jie Ji Yu Zhong Liu Mian Yi Zhi Liao (Regulation of biological formulas and the treatment of tumor immunity). Xian Science and Technology Publishing House; 1989.

72. Li Pei Wen. Ai Zheng De Zhong Xi Yi Zui Xin Dui Ce (New cancer strategies in Chinese and Western medicine). China TCM Publishing House; 1995.

Chapter 11

Leukemia

CHAPTER CONTENTS

Introduction   283

Epidemiology   284

Etiology   284
 Genetic factors   284
 Viral factors   284
 Immunologic factors   284
 Chinese medicine   285
 Etiology of specific leukemias   286

Acute lymphocytic leukemia   287
 Etiology   287
 Clinical features of ALL   287
 Classification of ALL   287
 Prognosis   288
 Treatment of ALL   288

Acute myelogenous leukemia   288
 Clinical features of AML   288
 Diagnosis and classification of
   AML   288
 Prognosis   288
 Treatment of AML   289

Chronic lymphocytic leukemia and similar
 disorders   289
 Etiology of CLL   289
 Diagnosis of CLL   289
 Treatment of CLL   289

Chronic myelogenous leukemia   290
 Allogeneic bone marrow
   transplantation   290

Stem cell transplants   291
Autologous transplantation   292

Chinese medicine   293
 Patterns   293
 Complications   296
 Treating children   297

> Do all you can
> with what you have
> in the time you have
> in the place you are.
>
> Nkosi Johnson, age 11, at the 2000
> International AIDS Conference in
> Durban, South Africa. Nkosi was born
> HIV-positive and died at the age of 12 years.

INTRODUCTION

Leukemias are neoplasias in which there are two major defects: unregulated proliferation and incomplete maturation of hematopoietic or lymphopoietic progenitors. Leukemia originates in the marrow. Leukemic cell lines may infiltrate lymph nodes, liver, spleen, and other tissues. The main clinical manifestation is a decrease of red blood cells, granulocytes, and platelets as a result of suppression of normal hematopoiesis by malignancy.

In the chronic or well-differentiated leukemias, unregulated proliferation, accumulation of leukemic cells, and elevated white blood cell (WBC) count dominate. The differentiation and maturation of the leukemic cells may be largely preserved. In acute leukemias, unregulated proliferation also occurs, but maturation of the leukemic progenitors is profoundly impaired. Therefore, therapy for the chronic leukemias is directed towards suppressing the excessive proliferation to reduce the accumulation of leukemic cells and to allow for improvement in effective hematopoiesis. In acute leukemias, very strong treatment, like bone marrow transplantation, is used to obliterate the leukemic clone.[1]

EPIDEMIOLOGY

Incidence varies with the type of leukemia. The rate of incidence also varies depending on age, sex, race, and geographic location. In general, acute lymphocytic leukemia (ALL) is a disease of childhood; chronic lymphocytic leukemia (CLL) is a disease of the aged; acute myelogenous leukemia (AML) occurs with similar frequency at all ages; and chronic myelogenous (or myeloid) leukemia (CML) occurs most frequently in middle life. Gender differences are negligible, except in CLL where male dominance is significant.[2]

ETIOLOGY

Environmental and genetic factors are causal in leukemia. Ionising radiation is documented as a casative factor in leukemia by the Atomic Bomb Casualty Commision in Hiroshima and Nagasaki. Leukemias have been observed after therapeutic irradiation for Hodgkin's disease. Low-level irradiation very likely plays a role in leukemia.[3]

Chemicals and drugs like benzene, arsenic, chloramphenicol, and phenylbutazone cause bone marrow aplasia, which leads to leukemia. Alkylating agents, especially melphalan, can cause AML in patients treated for solid tumors with this agent. The MOPP (mechlorethamine, Oncovin [vincristine], procarbazine, prednisone) regimen is also a causative factor in leukemia.[4]

Environmental factors can predispose to leukemia. Examples include maternal irradiation, in utero irradiation, early childhood viral diseases, and maternal history of fetal wasting.[5] Wide geographic and seasonal differences have been reported for different types of leukemia. These differences are not explainable in conventional medicine but may be explainable in Chinese medicine. Refer to the section on Chinese medicine below.

GENETIC FACTORS

Leukemias occur frequently in those with Down's syndrome, Fanconi syndrome, and Klinefelter's syndrome. This suggests a genetic predisposition to leukemia. Studies in Japan and New Zealand suggest a time–space clustering in childhood leukemia but not in adult leukemia. There is a 40-fold increase in frequency of leukemia in infant identical twins, as compared with siblings, which points to a genetic influence. At the same time, the risk of leukemia in the second of identical twins falls after infancy, suggesting an interaction of developmental or environmental factors with the hereditary predisposition to leukemia.[6,7]

VIRAL FACTORS

Overwhelming evidence implicates RNA viruses in the etiology of animal leukemia. This same etiologic agent may play a role in human leukemia. Evidence is accumulating to link RNA viruses to leukemogenicity in human cells. The viruses are called retroviruses and carry the gene for the enzyme reverse transcriptase.[8]

IMMUNOLOGIC FACTORS

Immune deficiency may favor the development of leukemia. Immune capabilities in a host individual may contribute to the development and progression of tumors of any kind. Intriguing relationships between immune alterations in relatives of leukemic patients have been reported.

There appear to be multiple host and environmental factors in the etiology of leukemia. Animal studies indicate that irradiation and chemically-induced leukemia may be mediated through the interaction of a latent RNA virus, or may require other accompanying host insults. Those exposed to irradiation from the atomic bomb explosions in Hiroshima and Nagasaki developed leukemias characteristic of the subpopulations. For example, ALL occurred predominantly in children, and the myelogenous types occurred in their typical age distribution. CLL, which is extremely rare in the Japanese population, did not occur at all.[9]

CHINESE MEDICINE

The pathologies that occur at the blood and lymph level are very complex. See Chapter 10 on lymphomas and the etiology of lymphomas and leukemias in the context of latent pathogenic factors (LPFs). Several factors come together to cause leukemias and preleukemias. Leukemia is the resulting complication of the following factors:[10]

- an internal latent pathogenic factor
- a physiological imbalance
- an external inducement.

Latent pathogenic factors

A latent virus, sometimes called a fetal toxin, is a heritable factor. For example, leukemia may exist in many normal animals and, as such, be heritable through many generations. It has a latent force for causing disease, much like a latent pathogen. Only when an external inducement is present does the disease manifest. Infantile leukemias, for example, seem to be more relative to Epstein–Barr virus (EBV).

Acute leukemia often presents like epidemic disease, especially viral disease, such as measles or chicken pox. However, measles and chicken pox, once fully erupted, resolve, giving immunity for life. But the 'virus' of leukemia is hidden and latent, and if it cannot erupt causes a physiological maladjustment, acting much like an LPF in the classical sense of the term. This maladjustment then leads to symptomatic changes.

Physiological imbalances

There are five major features of the physiological maladjustment. These include a deep, hidden latent virus (in the classical sense), deficiency in kidney jing and yin (as part of the heritable feature), hyperactivity disorder, which is a kind of yang excess described in the lymphoma section

that can look like yin-deficient heat, blood deterioration, and disharmony of the embryological channels, the Ren, Chong and Du channels..

If we look at these features one by one we see the following:

1. A deep, hidden virus is rooted in the bone marrow. In the infant the WBCs suffer injury and deformity from poison. Poison can be considered in the classical sense or the modern sense (for example, arsenic or a heavy metal or chemical exposure).
2. This deep hidden virus ferments or smolders, consuming jing and damaging the DNA, which decreases the yin.
3. The WBCs in the marrow are proliferating but making abnormal cells. This hyperactivity, if sudden and frequent, can affect the blood, causing hemorrhage, mouth sores, bleeding gums.
4. The bleeding combined with kidney jing and yin deficiency leads to blood dryness and deficiency. The yang excess leads to a shortened cell cycle and increased metabolism. The yang excess leads to hyperplasia in the WBC count but deficiency in the RBC count and this causes anemia of various kinds.
5. The Du channel relates to and refers to the yang of the whole body. The Ren relates to and refers to to yin of the whole body. The Chong assists the Ren and connects the 12 collaterals in adjusting growth and flow of blood. All major troublesome diseases are associated with the Eight Extraordinary Channels since these are embryologically the main channels and the primary deep channels. Blood diseases especially relate to the Ren and Chong.

External triggers

There are many possible external triggers that can act as the induction for leukemia. The six climatic factors are all inducements and can include environmental pollution like ionising radiation and chemical exposures. Topographical disturbances like earthquakes and sunflares, and UV exposures due to loss of the ozone layer are examples of some modern exposures.

Unsuitable foods and drugs, unclean food, too much food, too much meat, chemicals coming via the food chain, impure water, pharmaceutical drugs are examples of external triggers entering the oral route. Overwork, loss of proper life routine leads to exhaustion of qi and yin. Trauma from a fall or accident can cause qi and blood stasis, which acts as an induction. Unresolved emotions can also cause a deep injury, which then acts as an external trigger. For example, the sudden loss of a loved one can act as a trigger. Other diseases can induce leukemia. Common examples are Hodgkin's disease or other lymphomas, tuberculosis, and festering diseases like the poxes.

There are two trends of pathological change: one is inward and the other is outward.[11]

1. When a virus comes out to the surface this is called venting. It erupts into papules, macules, or other rashes, demonstrating that a healthy vital force is present and can 'oust' the virus to the surface.
2. When the virus goes to the interior it becomes a hidden latent virus, which can end up lodged in the bone marrow. In children this is a kind of 'latent metaplasia of poxes and measles'. The skin reaction is mostly insignificant.
3. If chemotherapy or some other cytotoxic therapy is given, immunity is suppressed or checked and so the pox and skin venting through papules is difficult to accomplish. In the adult, the latent virus and the inability to cause eruption or venting outward leads to an undulatory state with the blood being 'injured and corrupted'. In chronic leukemia, the long-term deep-rootedness of this condition leads to liver, spleen and lymph swelling.
4. Therefore, the latent virus is the remote lurking internal cause. Physiological maladjustment is the intermediate development of the disease. The external cause of induction is the recent igniting fuse of the disease. And the trends of pathological changes become the demarcation line of the leukemia and the non- or preleukemia. An example of a preleukemia would be myelodysplastic syndrome, or MDS.[10]

According to Chinese medicine, chemotherapy in the treatment of leukemia is used differently than in any other form of cancer. Chemotherapy, or suppressive and cytotoxic therapy, ignores the viral factors underlying leukemia and destroys the

'innocent', that is, the normal qi. It ignores the host (the patient) and encourages the negative pattern already set deeply into place. It sacrifices immunity for temporary alleviation of the disease results without actually treating the cause, the latent pathogenic factor (which we are calling, and may in fact be, a virus-like pathogen). In doing so, it causes four fatal injuries post-chemotherapy: fever, hemorrhage, anemia, and recurrence.

ETIOLOGY OF SPECIFIC LEUKEMIAS

Leukemias account for 2–3% of all malignancies in the general population. However, certain kinds of leukemia account for 30–35% of childhood malignancies.

- Factors in acute leukemia:[12]
  - differentiation of progenitor stem cells is blocked
  - this results is an accumulation of various immature cells (blasts)
  - there is an abrupt onset that looks like an acute flu-like disease
  - then there is very rapid progression
  - there is almost always short survival
  - the acute leukemias include acute myelogenous leukemia (AML) and acute lymphoblastic leukemia (ALL).
- Factors in chronic leukemia:[13]
  - unregulated proliferation of more mature cells
  - gradual onset without an acute episode
  - a prolonged course that is often years rather than months
  - longer survival
  - the chronic leukemias include chronic myelogenous leukemia (CML), and chronic lymphocytic leukemia (CLL).

The general symptoms of leukemias include:

- fatigue
- malaise
- weight loss
- recurrent infections
- unexplained bleeding
- progressive anemia
- pain
- lymphadenopathy
- gingival hypertrophy
- splenomegaly.

ACUTE LYMPHOCYTIC LEUKEMIA

The clonal proliferation of lymphoid precursors with arrested maturation gives rise to B- or T-cell leukemias and sometimes mixed types of B- and T-cell leukemia. ALL was one of the first malignancies to respond to chemotherapy and it is the first malignancy to have been cured in children. Most cases are found in children and, therefore, most of the studies done on ALL have been in children. More studies are now being done on adult populations, which comprise one-third of this type of leukemia. The median age at diagnosis is 12 and ALL accounts for 25% of all childhood cancers. The peak in incidence is at age 3–5 and then slowly declines until age 50, when it begins to rise again until the age of 65. In all ages the incidence is higher in males than in females and higher in white than in black populations.[14]

ETIOLOGY

Genetic factors seem to play a role. Down's syndrome is a risk factor and a history of a twin or sibling with ALL is a risk factor. Socioeconomic issues are implicated, and parents whose occupations expose them to agents like benzene and pesticides have increased risk for producing offspring who are diagnosed with ALL. Mothers older than 35 years produce children with increased risk, only partially explained by the increased risk of having a Down's syndrome child. Exposure to radiation is a definite risk, especially in utero. Electromagnetic fields are linked to ALL but the evidence is currently inconclusive.

CLINICAL FEATURES OF ALL

There is impairment of normal hematopoiesis and infiltration of non-hematopoietic tissues by leukemic cells. Presenting symptoms are attributable to anemia, neutropenia, and thrombocytopenia. There is fatigue, weakness, fever, weight loss, and abnormal bleeding. The onset is usually abrupt. There may be severe pain resulting from overgrowth of leukemic cells in the bone marrow, which affects especially the sternum and some large joints. Lymphadenopathy will be present in 80% of patients with painless and movable nodes. Hepatosplenomegaly is representative of a large

tumor burden and correlates with a poor prognosis. There may be lung and heart involvement and 5% of children will present with CNS involvement. The testicles are a 'sanctuary site', where disease may persist after systemic treatment. They are frequently the site of recurrence.[12]

The WBC count is often elevated and accompanied by low neutrophil counts. Thrombocytopenia is present in more than 90% of patients at presentation. Normocytic, normochromic anemia and reticulocytopenia are universal. Hypereosinophil syndrome is sometimes present and can lead to death from cardiorespiratory failure. High lactate dehydrogenase (LDH) levels are common and reflect a large tumor burden. A diagnosis of ALL is confirmed when bone marrow aspirates contain 30% lymphoblasts.[15]

CLASSIFICATION OF ALL

Acute lymphocytic leukemia is actually a heterogeneous group of disorders that comprise several subgroups that are somewhat distinct from one another. A morphologic grouping from the French–American–British (FAB) Cooperative Working Group identifies three groupings. L1 is most common in children; L2 is most common in adults; and L3 is the least common.

Immunophenotypic classification is based on the expression of certain antigens on the surface of leukemic cells. Markers that are used include CD 19, CD 2, and CD 4, which are also found in some other forms of leukemia. These markers are used clinically but are not necessarily diagnostic.[16]

Early pre-B-cell ALL is a common form of ALL in children and adults. It carries a poor prognosis when CD 10 is not expressed. Pre-B-cell ALL accounts for 20% of ALL and almost all patients express CD 10. This group includes more African-American patients. This type correlates with a worse prognosis than early pre-B-cell ALL. Transitional pre-B-cell ALL is a newer group that accounts for only 1% of cases.[17]

Mature B-cell ALL represents a leukemic phase of Burkitt's lymphoma. There is frequent CNS involvement. This type often corresponds with the L3 morphological classification. Only 5% of patients have this type.[18]

T-cell ALL comprises 20% of ALL patients. It is associated especially with male gender, very high

WBC counts, CNS involvement, and mediastinal involvement. The prognosis for this type with no expression of CD 10 is poor.

PROGNOSIS

- Age: infants and children over age 10 have a worse prognosis.[19] Adults have a worse prognosis than children, especially if over age 60.[20]
- WBC count: the higher the count, the worse the prognosis.
- Cytogenetic characteristics: ploidy is very significant; hyperdiploid seems to infer hypersensitivity to chemotherapy and thus a better outcome.[21]
- Chromosomal abnormalities: translocation is less in children than in adults of certain chromosomes. The Ph chromosome is significant.[22]
- Immunophenotype: T-cell ALL and mature B-cell ALL have poor outcomes.
- Other: CD 34 expression is correlated with a more favorable outcome.

TREATMENT OF ALL

In adults, 75% will achieve a complete remission, but still there is only a 20–40% cure rate overall. Therapy includes induction, consolidation, maintenance, and CNS prophylaxis.

Induction usually includes vincristine and corticosteroids or a combination of two to three anthracyclines. Consolidation is used frequently in childhood ALL. High-dose methotrexate with cytarabine or asparaginase is used.[23] Maintenance consists of mercaptopurine and methotrexate and is continued for 2 years. CNS prophylaxis has reduced the incidence of relapse to less than 10%. Cranial radiation and intrathecal (IT) chemotherapy (methotrexate) are used. Allogeneic bone marrow transplantation (BMT) is an alternative therapy sometimes used in the first remission.

Induction is used to kill as many blasts as possible and includes vincristine, prednisone, and asparaginase. CNS prophylaxis kills cells in the CNS to prevent relapse. Consolidation and maintenance is low-dose treatment to maintain remission. It includes methotrexate and 6-mercaptopurine, typically for 3 years.

ACUTE MYELOGENOUS LEUKEMIA

This type of leukemia is marked by infiltration of bone marrow by abnormal hematopoietic progenitors. These cells are unable to differentiate in a normal manner into myeloid, erythroid, and/or megakaryocytic cell lines. They infiltrate vital organs. They also lead to thrombocytopenia, anemia, and granulocytopenia. Patients rarely survive past 6–12 months. This is a rare malignancy and is fatal 80% of the time.

CLINICAL FEATURES OF AML

Weakness, bleeding and infections usually cause patients to present for diagnosis. Vague upper respiratory tract infections are common in presentation. Disseminated intravascular coagulopathy (DIC) is a hallmark. Gum hypertrophy, leukemia cutis (a skin condition) and bone pain may be present. Abdominal pain secondary to hepatosplenomegaly or adenopathy is also common.

DIAGNOSIS AND CLASSIFICATION OF AML

The French–American–British Working Group has set criteria for this diagnosis.[24] AML is confirmed by morphological and cytochemical staining techniques – 30% of nucleated cells in the bone marrow or peripheral blood are blasts. Cytogenetic information has proven more useful clinically than the FAB group system. There are several chromosomal abnormalities characteristic of AML but these do not necessarily affect prognosis.

PROGNOSIS

The prognosis is changing continually based on new information regarding AML.[25] The cure rates are very low, however, and death often occurs during chemotherapy. Death occurs in relation to resistance to chemotherapy, age, performance status, prior chemotherapy or radiation for another malignancy, antecedent blood disorders, and pretreatment karyotype. There is a 60–70% chance of remission with a 15–25% survival rate of 5 years or more. Most relapses occur in the first 3 years. Remission rates are inversely related to age. The median survival is 12–24 months.

TREATMENT OF AML

Of all AML patients 25% do survive. Chemotherapy in the form of cytarabine followed by daunorubicin in the 'three plus seven' regimen is part of the standard of care. This regimen comprises 3 days anthracycline in i.v. bolus followed by 7 days of continuous daunorubicin i.v. infusion.[26] Generally post-remission therapy is used. BMT is sometimes used as post-remission therapy. This is done during the first remission after treatment. Allogeneic BMT is used in patients who have relapsed or with refractory AML.

Treatment is similar to treatment for ALL and is in three phases. Combinations of an anthracycline and cytosine are used.[27] Induction therapy is done in the hospital due to severe side effects which include severe marrow depression, nausea, vomiting, stomatitis, and risk of infection. Remission is achieved in 65% of patients (higher in children). CNS therapy is done only if there is evidence of cells in the CNS. Post-remission maintenance is done with chemotherapy, allogeneic or autologous BMT.[28,29]

CHRONIC LYMPHOCYTIC LEUKEMIA AND SIMILAR DISORDERS

Chronic lymphocytic leukemia is the most common adult leukemia in the West and accounts for 30% of leukemias.[30] CLL always involves the bone marrow and peripheral blood. It can also be found in lymph nodes, liver and spleen. Bone marrow failure can occur as a late event. There is great heterogeneity between subgroups. Cytogenetic and molecular analysis mainly provides information on disease development and prognosis. Nucleoside analogs and BMT have improved survival rates.

Chronic lymphocytic leukemia is a progressive accumulation of mature lymphocytes in the blood, nodes, spleen and marrow. There is a clonal expansion of abnormal B lymphocytes with low proliferation. The B-cells are functionally ineffective. The early symptoms may be non-existent. Later, lymphadenopathy, fatigue, weight loss, night sweats, hepatosplenomegaly, anorexia, and infections may present. An autoimmune

hemolytic anemia may be present. Risks include exposure to fertilisers, pesticides, nitrate, and working in the rubber and asbestos occupations. Hair-coloring agents have also been found to be a causative factor.[31]

There is no known cure for CLL. Supportive care is offered and sometimes oral alkylating agents like fludarabine, chlorambucil, or cyclophosphamide are given. A splenectomy may be necessary to reduce pain. CLL is the only leukemia that is staged. Staging is 0–4. CLL can transform to AML. Marrow failure is a risk, as is skin cancer and renal involvement.

ETIOLOGY OF CLL

B-cell CLL is the only leukemia that has not been associated with radiation exposure, chemicals, or drugs. Relatives of patients with CLL have an increased risk that is between two- and seven-fold. There are common cytogenetic abnormalities, especially trisomy 12, which is detected by using fluorescent in situ hybridisation (FISH).

DIAGNOSIS OF CLL

Diagnosis is done via several criteria including abnormal lymphocyte levels, atypical cells in large quantities, bone marrow involvement, and B phenotype. It is staged according to the Rai system for CLL, which stages from 0 to 4, or the Binet system which stages A, B, C. These systems both stage according to the tumor burden via lymphadenopathy, hepatomegaly, splenomegaly, and bone marrow failure via anemia and thrombocytopenia.[32] Interestingly, there is a conventional medical term called 'smoldering CLL', which has been proposed for patients who belong in a subgroup of early-stage CLL.[33]

TREATMENT OF CLL

Chlorambucil is a nitrogen mustard derivative commonly used to treat CLL. There is some question as to whether treating patients with early-stage disease with chlorambucil actually shortens lifespan when compared to observation alone. Cyclophosphamide is as effective as chlorambucil.[34] Cyclophosphamide, vincristine, doxorubicin and prednisone (COP) and the nucleoside analogs fludarabine, cladribine, and pentostatin are also used. Alpha interferon and recombinant IL-2 are used to activate natural killer (NK) cells.[35] Allogeneic BMT and autologous BMT are being used. Sometimes splenectomy is performed, or splenic irradiation as an alternative to surgery.

There are many subcategories of CLL that include Richter's syndrome, prolymphocytic leukemia, T-cell chronic lymphocytic leukemia, large granular lymphocyte proliferation, and hairy cell leukemia.

CHRONIC MYELOGENOUS LEUKEMIA

Chronic myelogenous leukemia accounts for 15% of all leukemia cases. It usually occurs in adults between the ages of 50 and 60 years. The hallmark of this type of leukemia is the translocation of chromosomes between 9 and 22, known as Philadelphia syndrome.[36] Overproduction of mature WBCs and immature blasts produce vague symptoms and malaise. CML is not staged but is categorised as:

- stable, with mild splenomegaly and few blasts
- accelerated, with moderate splenomegaly, erratic WBCs and increased blasts
- blast crisis, with marked splenomegaly, variable WBCs, and >25% blasts.

In patients with Philadelphia syndrome, 60–70% will progress to blast phase. The average overall survival is 42–45 months. CML is not curable by standard chemotherapy. If chemotherapy is used it is used in the form of hydroxycarbamide (Hydrea) or busulfan (Myleran). Alpha-interferon is also used with good results.[37] Staging is important and predictive of response and survival with interferon treatment. Patients who are over 60 have a worse prognosis. Allogeneic BMT is the only chance for long-term survival. Allopurinol is used to limit uric acid buildup from the death of leukemic cells.

ALLOGENEIC BONE MARROW TRANSPLANTATION

Allogeneic marrow transplantation is used to reconstitute hematopoiesis in several situations, including in patients who have received myeloab-

lative therapy for a malignancy, in patients with bone marrow failure for various reasons, to reconstitute the immune system in patients with severe immunodeficiency, and to normalise metabolism in patients with certain inherited metabolic deficiency disorders.[38]

Allogeneic marrow transplantation is very intense and very toxic. Therefore, it is generally reserved for patients under the age of 55 whose graft is being donated by a related donor who has been matched for human leukocyte antigen (HLA). In younger patients, it is sometimes possible to use partially matched and unrelated donors. Improvements in supportive care have allowed this procedure to be used in greater numbers of patients. In 1998, approximately 4000 BMTs were reported to the International Bone Marrow Transplant Registry.

Mobilisation

Eradication of the malignancy and successful engraftment of allogeneic marrow requires the use of a preparative regimen of very high doses of chemotherapy with or without radiation. New regimens are being developed but the two most commonly used in leukemia are:

- cyclophosphamide plus total body irradiation (TBI)
- busulfan plus cyclophosphamide.

Due to the high incidence of pneumonitis in TBI, fractionated TBI with lung shielding in combination with cyclophosphamide via i.v. drip for 2 days provides antileukemic activity and toxicity. When busulfan is used it is administered orally every 6 hours for 16 doses, followed by four doses of cyclophosphamide.[39]

Successful engraftment of allogeneic bone marrow requires myeloablation and immunosuppression. The combination of busulfan, which is myeloablative but not immunosuppressive, with cyclophosphamide, which is immunosuppressive but not myeloablative, with TBI, which is both, has become the standard preparative regimen.

Marrow harvesting and processing

Marrow is harvested from the posterior iliac crests of the donor under general anaesthesia. It is usually performed on an outpatient basis. About

150 aspirations are performed during the procedure, and about 10–15 ml of bone marrow are removed. This amount should contain 1–4×10^8 nucleated cells per kilogram. There is very low risk of complications to the donor, but pain is common after the procedure.[40]

If there is no blood group (ABO) incompatibility between the patient and the donor, then the marrow is filtered through bone particles and infused i.v. Day 0 is designated as the day of marrow infusion. If there is incompatibility, the red cells, plasma, or both may need to be removed from the donor marrow to prevent hemolytic reaction during infusion. Hemolytic reactions can lead to prolonged red cell aplasia caused by circulating red cell antibodies. Infusion of the new marrow from the donor saves the patient and allows them to begin again with clean marrow.

STEM CELL TRANSPLANTS

Allogeneic stem cell transplantation is used as an alternative to BMT. The donor receives granulocyte colony stimulating factor (filgrastim [Neupogen]) injections subcutaneously for mobilisation, and stem cells are collected by apheresis in a manner similar to collecting platelets. No general anaesthesia is necessary and the cost is lower. Stem cell transplants are being used increasingly, because of these factors and because the incidence of graft-versus-host disease (GVHD) is not greater, nor are the outcomes reduced. Stem cell transplantation is gradually replacing BMT.[41]

Another technique involves transplanting allogeneic cord blood stem cells. This technique greatly reduces the risk of GVHD because the immaturity of the cord cells means they have not yet 'self-identified', making them somewhat universal. The outcomes have been equal to BMT. A national registry is now available for parents who wish to donate cord blood postpartum. It is a matter of educating the public about this life-saving possible donation. There is absolutely no reason, either medical or philosophical or religious, not to donate the cord blood.

Complications

Nausea, vomiting, stomatitis, alopecia, erythema, rash, and diarrhea occur in most graft recipients. Phenytoin is routinely given to prevent seizures from high-dose busulfan. More serious complications occur in some patients and include idiopathic interstitial pneumonitis, hemorrhagic cystitis, pericarditis, hepatic veno-occlusive disease (VOD), and sometimes pulmonary hemorrhage. These life-threatening complications can occur in 20% of patients; the mortality rate is 5%.[42,43]

Screening to determine risk factors is done prior to transplantation. VOD liver toxicity syndrome is characterised by fluid retention, weight gain, hepatomegaly with pain, ascites, hyperbilirubinemia. This condition may result in liver failure. The occlusion of the central veins of the liver can lead to centrilobar necrosis. Risk factors for this complication include a history of hepatitis of any kind, elevated transaminase levels at the time of transplantation, the use of methotrexate to prevent GVHD, high-dose chemotherapy, and mismatched or unrelated donor marrow grafts.

Because of myelosuppression, fatal bleeding and infection can occur.[44] Transfusions and standard antibiotic therapy are used. Growth factors are also used to shorten the period of aplasia. If methotrexate is used as GVHD prophylaxis then the effectiveness of growth factors in enhancing engraftment is limited.

Graft failure occurs in about 5% of patients and is usually due to rejection, infection (usually viral), drugs, and insufficient stem cells. An increased risk of rejection is present when the T-cells are depleted, there is HLA incompatibility, or the nucleated marrow cell dose is too low. Failure in these cases can be as high as 15%.

Infection from profound neutropenia can occur early after transplantation. The risk for infection can last as long as 1 year after transplantation. Restrictions on possible exposures to pathogens are imposed during this period. Some specific infections are especially opportunistic. The most common include:[45,46]

- bacterial: *Streptococcus pneumoniae*
- fungal: *Candida, Aspergillus*
- viral: herpes simplex virus (HSV), adenovirus, cytomegalovirus (CMV), herpes zoster
- Others: toxoplasma, pneumocystis.

Fluconazole (Diflucan) is given prophylactically to reduce risk for candidiasis. Inhalation amphotericin-B is given for aspergillosis pneumonitis. Trimethoprim-sulfamethoxazole is given twice weekly for a year to prevent pneumocystis pneumonia (PCP) and pneumococcal infections. Pentamidine is given in patients allergic to sulfas. Immunoglobulin is sometimes also given i.v.

Viral infections are challenging in immuno-compromised patients. Aciclovir reduces the reactivation of HSV. Ganciclovir (Cytovene) is given to decrease CMV reactivation until day 100. EBV-related lymphoproliferative disease (LPD) occurs in a small number of patients with leukemia during transplantation. This risk is increased when anti-CD 3 monoclonal antibody is used to prevent GVHD. Peripheral blood donor lympho-cytes are now infused as treatment for what used to be a fatal complication.

Organ dysfunctions can also evolve after transplantation and, therefore, patients are evaluated on an annual basis for hypothyroidism, gonadal failure, pulmonary fibrosis, obstructive lung disease, cataracts, and leukoencephalopathy.[47]

Second malignancies occur in 4–10% of long-term survivors after allogeneic transplantation.

Graft–versus–host disease

Graft-versus-host disease is a reaction of the donor's immune system against the marrow recipient's tissue. It is mediated by T-cells, NK cells, and inflammatory cytokines. Patients with HLA-matched related donors have the best chance of avoiding GVHD.[48]

Patients are monitored for acute GVHD through until day 100. Clinical manifestations include skin rash, fever, nausea, vomiting, diarrhea, and hyperbilirubinemia. A clinical grading system for these symptoms has been devised. Risk factors include older age, a pregnant donor, less intense immunosuppression, and genetic disparity between the donor and recipient. The grading system includes stages through 4 and grades through IV.[49]

To prevent GVHD a combination of ciclosporin and methotrexate is used. When this two-drug combination is used only 20–30% of patients exhibit acute symptoms. This regimen is administered 1–2 days prior to marrow infusion. Ciclosporin is given at full dose for at least 180 days after transplantation and then is tapered, possibly up until 1 year after transplantation.[50]

Chronic GVHD occurs in 20–50% of long-term survivors. Risk factors include older age, prior acute GVHD, and prior HSV infection. Risk begins at about month three after transplantation. Common manifestations are sicca syndrome, lichen planus-like rash, sclerodermatous skin reactions, esophageal and intestinal fibrosis, obstructive lung disease, and elevated alkaline phosphatase levels. There is a resemblance to autoimmune disease.[51]

Chronic GVHD that is limited has a good prognosis; 60–70% long-term survival. Extensive chronic GVHD with multiple organ involvement has a poorer long-term outcome; 20–30% survival. High-dose prednisone is the first line of therapy for low-risk GVHD. This therapy continues for up to 9 months before tapering. High-risk patients are treated with prednisone and ciclosporin together.

AUTOLOGOUS TRANSPLANTATION

High-dose chemotherapy (HDCT) with autologous stem cell transplantation is effective against leukemia. It is now used more than allogeneic transplants. Standard-dose combination chemotherapy is given before autologous transplantation, in order to reduce the tumor burden. This is a form of induction therapy to reduce the volume of disease as much as possible. Patients then undergo stem cell collection, cryopreservation, and storage of either bone marrow or peripheral-blood stem cells. Bone marrow is collected from the posterior iliac crests as in allogeneic collection. The marrow must not contain any malignant cells. These stored cells are viable for more than 5 years, and some higher risk patients have their stem cells collected in the case they need them for treatment in the future. Peripheral blood cells are collected by apheresis via the subclavian vein. Leukapheresis is repeated by using continuous flow cell separation. To collect an adequate amount for transplantation, 8–12 daily leukaphereses are needed. Progenitor cells are mobilised to a higher level during the recovery phase following cytoreduction and treatment with GM-CSF or G-CSF.[52]

The dose of HDCT and/or radiation is limited by that regimen's toxic effects.[53] The transplantation procedure is considered to be a rescue from

HDCT and severe myelosuppression. The neo-plasm must exhibit a response so that one or some-times more courses eradicate the malignant cells. Dose intensity varies according to the aggressive-ness of the disease. A benefit-to-risk ratio is app-lied on an individual basis.

Marrow cells or peripheral blood progenitor (PBP) cells are infused intravenously after the preparative regimens. The stem cells home to the marrow and restore hematopoiesis. Usually recovery occurs within 3–4 weeks with PBP cells. G-CSF, GM-CSF or other cytokines are used to accelerate marrow recovery. After full recovery of the bone marrow the neoplasm is then restaged.[42,54]

Autologous transplantation is less likely to produce major side effects than allogeneic transplantation because the issue of rejection is eliminated. GVHD does not occur in autologous transplantation. The main cause of treatment failure is recurrence. A major concern is that the marrow or the PBP cells may be contaminated by malignant cells at the time of collection. Many techniques are under evaluation for detecting occult malignant cells. Ex vivo treatment with antitumor monoclonal antibodies, antibody-toxin conjugates, or chemotherapy is done to ensure non-malignant marrow. Also hematopoietic cells are selected that carry the CD 34 marker, ensuring non-toxicity and a more rapid recovery. Also the Thy-1 antigen is being evaluated as a more specific marker.[55]

Potential complications

Infections from granulocytopenia and systemic reactions from the conditioning or induction regimen are the most common complications. Fatal complications occur in 10% of patients. The immune reconstitution in patients undergoing autologous transplantation is more complete than in allogeneic transplant patients.

High-dose chemotherapy induces pancy-topenia, which lasts about 2–4 weeks until the stem cells restore hematopoiesis. G-CSF and GM-CSF are used to accelerate recovery of the blood system. Thrombopoietin is used to stimulate recovery of platelets.

Organ toxicity from the preparative regimens can be severe and affects primarily the lungs, heart, liver and nervous system. VOD is present in autologous transplantation in about 5% of patients, depending on their past history and age. Cardiac toxicity is also common, especially with high-dose cyclophosphamide regimens and when com-bined with carmustine or other alkylating agents. Hypothyroid can occur as a delayed reac-tion. Cystitis is not uncommon and mesna is com-monly used as prophylaxis against hemorrhagic cystitis. Post-transplant immunodeficiency recov-ers more quickly in autologous transplantation.[56]

Autologous transplantation is used to treat acute myelogenous leukemia, acute lymphoblastic leukemia, chronic myelogenous leukemia, chronic lymphocytic leukemia, lymphomas, Hodgkin's disease, multiple myeloma, and some other solid tumors.

CHINESE MEDICINE

Entrance of a pathogenic process into the blood level is a profound occurrence and generally implies a very poor prognosis. There are many transformations that take place in order to reach the blood level and it is very difficult to reverse these and cure a patient. In childhood leukemias the transformative process can happen very quickly because of the lack of maturity and con-solidation in several organ systems in children.

The etiology for leukemia remains quite con-stant in Chinese medicine. Therefore, the staging and grade of the leukemia become the main factors for determining treatment. Leukemias are considered in a general sense to be manifestations of pathogenic heat in the ying and blood level. This is described in Chapter 10 (lymphoma) and the earlier section of this chapter. Pathogenic heat can evolve into first deficient qi and blood stasis and then progress into liver and kidney yin defi-ciency with pathogenic heat caused by an LPF.

PATTERNS

1. Pathogenic heat at the ying and blood level[57]

Early stage or acute phase:

Symptoms: may have a high fever or sweating, dry mouth, headache, irritability and restless-ness, fatigue, abnormal bleeding, ecchymosis, weight loss, possible abdominal pain, abdominal masses like hepatosplenomegaly, hematuria, constipation.

Tongue: red with yellow thick coat.

Pulse: fast and full.

Treatment principle: clear toxin from the ying level, clear heat from the blood level, tonify qi, antineoplasm.

Formula: Xi jiao tang he hua ban tang

mu dan pi (Moutan Cortex; *Paeonia suffruticosa* root cortex)	15 g
shu di (Rehmanniae Radix preparata; *Rehmannia*)	40 g
shui niu jiao (Bubali Cornu; *Bubalus* horn)	30 g
jin yin hua (Lonicerae Flos; *Lonicera* flowers)	15 g
zi hua di ding (Violae Herba; *Viola yedoensis*)	18 g
xuan shen (Scrophulariae Radix; *Scrophularia*)	15 g
gui ban* (Testudinis Plastrum; *Chinemys reevesii* plastron)	18 g
qing dai (Indigo naturalis; *Indigofera tinctoria*)	18 g
chi shao (Paeoniae Radix rubra; *Paeonia lactiflora* root)	20 g
xian he cao (Agrimoniae Herba; *Agrimonia pilosa* var. *japonica*; agrimony)	25 g
hong hua (Carthami Flos; *Carthamnus tinctorius* flowers)	15 g
tai zi shen (Pseudostellariae Radix; *Pseudostellaria* heterophylla)	20 g

2. Qi deficiency with blood stasis[58]

Symptoms: frequent low-grade fever, fatigue, dyspnea, vague bone pain, hypochondrium pain, hepatosplenomegaly, lymphadenopathy, possible yellow stool, petechiae, hematuria, melena.

Tongue: dark with ecchymosis.

Pulse: weak, tight, choppy.

Treatment principle: tonify qi, invigorate blood, crack blood, antineoplasm.

Formula: special formula

ren shen (Ginseng Radix; *Panax ginseng*)	10 g
xi yang shen (Panacis quinquefolii Radix; *Panax quinquefolium*)	10 g
dan shen (Salviae miltiorrhizae Radix; *Salvia miltiorhiza* root)	25 g
chi shao (Paeoniae Radix rubra; *Paeonia lactiflora* root)	15 g
dang gui (Angelicae sinensis Radix; *Angelica sinensis*)	15 g
chuan xiong (Chuanxiong Rhizoma; *Ligusticum wallichii* root)	10 g
tao ren (Persicae Semen; *Prunus* seed)	10 g
ji xue teng (Angelicae sinensis Radix; *Spatholobus suberectus*)	20 g
huang qi (Astragali Radix; *Astragalus membranaceus*)	15 g
fu ling (Poria; *Poria cocos*)	15 g
bai zhu (Atractylodis macrocephalae Rhizoma; *Atractylodes macrocephala*)	10 g
gan cao (Glycyrrhizae Radix; *Glycyrrhiza*; licorice root)	5 g
xian he cao (Agrimoniae Herba; *Agrimonia pilosa* var. *japonica*; agrimony)	20 g
tai zi shen (Pseudostellariae Radix; *Pseudostellaria heterophylla*)	15 g

3. Liver and kidney yin deficiency[59]

Symptoms: low or moderate fever, spontaneous sweating, night sweats, dizziness, dry throat, five center heat, palpitations, dyspnea, weak knees and low back, irritability and restlessness, insomnia.

Tongue: deep red or purple or scarlet with no coat.

Pulse: fast and thready.

Treatment principle: nourish the blood, clear blood heat, clear LPF or toxin, nourish yin, antineoplasm.

Formula: special formula

mai dong (Ophiopogonis Radix; *Ophiopogon*)	15 g
bei sha shen (Glehniae Radix; *Glehnia*)	15 g
zhi mu (Anemarrhenae Rhizoma; *Anemarrhena*)	15 g

shu di (Rehmanniae Radix   15 g
    preparata; *Rehmannia*)

tai zi shen (Pseudostellariae Radix;   15 g
    Pseudostellaria heterophylla)

xuan shen (Scrophulariae Radix;   10 g
    Scrophularia)

gou qi zi (Lycii Fructus; *Lycium*   15 g
    chinensis fruit)

gui ban* (Testudinis Plastrum;   15 g
    Chinemys reevesii plastron)

fu ling (Poria; *Poria cocos*)   15 g

bai zhu (Atractylodis macrocephalae   10 g
    Rhizoma; *Atractylodes macrocephala*)

gan cao (Glycyrrhizae Radix;   5 g
    Glycyrrhiza; licorice root)

qing hao (Artemisiae annuae Herba;   15 g
    Artemisia annua)

jin yin hua (Lonicerae Flos; *Lonicera*   10 g
    flowers)

xi yang shen (Panacis quinquefolii   10 g
    Radix; *Panax quinquefolium*)

shi hu (Dendrobii Herba;   15 g
    Dendrobium)

jiao gu lan (Herba Gynostemmatis;   15 g
    Gynostemma)

4. Deficient qi and blood[57]

Symptoms: late stage presentation with pallor, dizziness, tinnitus, palpitations, dyspnea, generalised edema, anasarca, night sweats, spontaneous sweating, hemorrhagic tendency, anorexia, weight loss.

Tongue: pale with no coat.

Pulse: weak and minute.

Treatment principles: replenish qi and nourish blood, antineoplasm.

Formula: special formula

ren shen (Ginseng Radix; *Panax*   10 g
    ginseng)

huang qi (Astragali Radix; *Astragalus*   25 g
    membranaceus)

bai zhu (Atractylodis macrocephalae   15 g
    Rhizoma; *Atractylodes macrocephala*)

fu ling (Poria; *Poria cocos*)   15 g

wu wei zi (Schisandrae Fructus;   10 g
    Schisandra)

dang shen (Codonopsis Radix;   15 g
    Codonopsis pilosula root)

dang gui (Angelicae sinensis Radix;   10 g
    Angelica sinensis)

he shou wu (Polygoni multiflori   15 g
    Radix preparata; *Polygonum*
    multiflorum root)

yin yang huo (Epimedii Herba;   15 g
    Epimedium grandiflorum)

yu zhu (Polygonati odorati   15 g
    Rhizoma; *Polygonatum odoratum*)

nu zhen zi (Ligustri lucidi Fructus;   15 g
    Ligustrum lucidum fruit)

suan zao ren (Ziziphi spinosae   10 g
    Semen; *Ziziphus spinosa* seed)

san qi (Notoginseng Radix; *Panax*   2 g
    notoginseng)

bai hua she she cao (Hedyotis   25 g
    diffusae Herba; *Oldenlandia*)

The above formulas are the constitutional formulas that provide a guide for treatment of the underlying cancer presentation. These formulas are modified to address individual signs and symptoms. They are also modified to address the staging, the aggressiveness of the leukemia, the age and performance status of the patient, and the issues, usually organ-related, that are dominant. Alongside all of these factors is the conventional treatment and its side effects, which must also be taken into account.

Induction therapy is HDCT and, therefore, can induce severe symptoms. Because of severe myelosuppression and immunosuppression it is extremely important that any supplements or herbal formulas be delivered in as close to sterile form as possible. It may be necessary to prepare the herbal formula in sealed individual-dose packs, which are then irradiated. This means that the herbal preparation only contacts the surroundings when the pack is opened and is placed in water for taking orally, or when the sealed plastic container with the decocted formula is opened. It may happen that the conventional providers will disallow their patients any preparations outside of conventional medicine. This would be especially true in BMT.

During BMT, the intent of induction therapy is to destroy the marrow and, therefore, immunity.

This means that utilising fu zheng therapies may be contraindicated. Herbs that nourish the blood and improve immunity, like huang qi and others, would actually work against the intention of the conventional therapy. Stimulating the bone marrow to produce progenitor cells is contraindicated until reinfusion with the donor bone marrow. And then, unless the herbals used are close to sterile, it remains contraindicated until the immune system of the patient reconstitutes itself and can fight against any impurities in their food or medicines. This strict adherence to no contamination begins approximately 4–6 weeks prior to the transplant. As the immune system goes down in HDCT with the preparatory conditioning regimen, its ability to stop any biological contaminants becomes less and less. If there are fungal spores, for example, in the decoctions or the prepared herbal materials, these can linger asymptomatically in the body and then become severely symptomatic and even life-threatening during the transplant. This is a serious issue requiring skill and knowledge of all of the issues surrounding induction therapy and/or transplantation.

COMPLICATIONS

Many complications can arise as a result of leukemia and treatment for leukemia. Following are formulas that that can be used to treat conditions and complications that may arise in treating leukemia.

1. Leukocytopenia and thrombocytopenia[60]

huang qi (Astragali Radix; Astragalus membranaceus)	25 g
ji xue teng (Spatholobi Caulis; Spatholobus suberectus)	20 g
jiao gu lan (Herba Gynostemmatis; Gynostemma)	15 g
bai zhu (Atractylodis macrocephalae Rhizoma; Atractylodes macrocephala)	15 g
gou qi zi (Lycii Fructus; Lycium chinensis fruit)	15 g
ren shen (Ginseng Radix; Panax ginseng)	10 g

he shou wu (Polygoni multiflori Radix preparata; Polygonum multiflorum root)	15 g
dang shen (Codonopsis Radix; Codonopsis pilosula root)	15 g
shi wei (Pyrrosiae Folium; Pyrrosia leaves)	15 g
nu zhen zi (Ligustri lucidi Fructus; Ligustrum lucidum fruit)	15 g
fu ling (Poria; Poria cocos)	15 g
tu si zi (Cuscutae Semen; Cuscuta seed)	15 g
shu di (Rehmanniae Radix preparata; Rehmannia)	15 g
bu gu zhi (Psoraleae Fructus; Psoralea)	10 g

2. Diffuse intra-arterial coagulopathy (DIC)[61]

shu di (Rehmanniae Radix preparata; Rehmannia)	20 g
dang gui (Angelicae sinensis Radix; Angelica sinensis)	15 g
tao ren (Persicae Semen; Prunus seed)	15 g
hong hua (Carthami Flos; Carthamnus tinctorius flowers)	15 g
ba yue zha (Akebiae Fructus; Akebia)	15 g
da huang (Rhei Radix et Rhizoma; Rheum)	15 g
qian cao gen (Rubiae Radix; Rubia cordifolia root)	15 g
san qi (Notoginseng Radix; Panax notoginseng)	2 g
dan shen (Salviae miltiorrhizae Radix; Salvia miltiorhiza root)	15 g
gan cao (Glycyrrhizae Radix; Glycyrrhiza; licorice root)	5 g

3. Hemorrhage or abnormal bleeding of any kind due to blood heat and yin deficiency[62]

shui niu jiao (Bubali Cornu; Bubalus horn)	10 g
mai dong (Ophiopogonis Radix; Ophiopogon)	15 g
shu di (Rehmanniae Radix preparata; Rehmannia)	15 g

chi shao (Paeoniae Radix rubra;   15 g
Paeonia lactiflora root)

mu dan pi (Moutan Cortex; *Paeonia*   10 g
suffruticosa root cortex)

dan shen (Salviae miltiorrhizae   15 g
Radix; *Salvia miltiorhiza* root)

ou jie (Nelumbinis Nodus   30 g
rhizomatis; *Nelumbo nucifera*
rhizome nodes)

xuan shen (Scrophulariae Radix;   15 g
Scrophularia)

shi hu (Dendrobii Herba;   15 g
Dendrobium)

4. Hemorrhagic cystitis[63]

Urinary bleeding is a toxic side effect of Ifos-famide, which is sometimes used to treat leukemia. Mesna is given to prevent this bleeding. Urinary bleeding is also a symptom of the disease, which can be due to thrombocytopenia and blood heat.

bai mao gen (Imperatae Rhizoma;   15 g
Imperata cylindrica rhizome)

chi xiao dou (Phaseoli Semen;   10 g
Phaseolus calcaratus)

da ji gen (Cirsii japonici Herba sive   10 g
Radix; *Cirsium japonizum* root)

sheng di huang (Rehmanniae Radix;   10 g
Rehmannia)

che qian zi (Plantaginis Semen;   10 g
Plantago)

lu cao (Herba Humuli scandentis;   10 g
Humulus scandens)

ji cai (Herba Capsellae; *Capsella*)   10 g

ou jie (Nelumbinis Nodus   10 g
rhizomatis; *Nelumbo nucifera*
rhizome nodes)

xiao ji (Cirsii Herba; *Ciraium*)   10 g

mu tong (Akebiae Caulis; *Akebia*   10 g
stem)

5. Toxic myocarditis/pericarditis[64]

Several of the regimens in leukemia treatment are cardiotoxic. There are several ways to protect heart muscle including supplementation with CoQ10, folic acid, and L-carnitine. The following formula is for the acute presentation and for prophylaxis during chemotherapy.

ren shen (Ginseng Radix; *Panax*   10 g
ginseng)

san qi (Notoginseng Radix; *Panax*   10 g
notoginseng)

tai zi shen (Pseudostellariae Radix;   15 g
Pseudostellaria heterophylla)

dan shen (Salviae miltiorrhizae   10 g
Radix; *Salvia miltiorhiza* root)

wu wei zi (Schisandrae Fructus;   10 g
Schisandra)

shan zhu yu (Corni Fructus; *Cornus*   10 g
officinalis fruit)

huang jing (Polygonati Rhizoma;   10 g
Polygonatum)

fu ling (Poria; *Poria cocos*)   15 g

zhu ling (Polyporus; *Polyporus –*   10 g
Grifola)

huang qi (Astragali Radix;   15 g
Astragalus membranaceus)

6. CNS leukemia[65]

tian ma (Gastrodiae Rhizoma;   15 g
Gastrodia elata)

gou teng (Uncariae Ramulus cum   15 g
Uncis; *Uncaria*)

fo shou (Citri sarcodactylis Fructus;   10 g
Citrus sarcodactylis)

long chi (Fossilia Dentis Mastodi/   30 g
Draconis Dens; fossilised teeth)

huang lian (Coptidis Rhizoma; *Coptis*)   10 g

TREATING CHILDREN

Two-thirds of all leukemias are diagnosed in children. Children's organs are delicate and the qi is still immature. The lung qi is barely consolidated at birth. The spleen qi only begins to reach consolidation around age eight. Children are considered to be pure yang. Young children are generally thought of as either young yin or young yang.[66] The first category refers to a child with delicate skin, deficient qi and blood, immature zang fu, weak muscles and vessels, and with deficient yin and yang. The second category refers to a child who is thriving and exuberant. It is important to know where on the continuum a child lies prior to the onset of leukemia. Leukemia can be diagnosed in either child but the constitution of the child will determine to some extent the way in which the cancer will be treated. In weaker children great care must be taken to protect digestive function and to protect the essence and yin and yang. In stronger children it may be possible to treat more vigorously.

In children with young yin and young yang there tend to be more diseases of the lung and spleen since these are the last organ units to consolidate. These children are more easily injured by cold. Most current chemotherapy is very cold in nature. Digestive problems will arise more easily in children in general and even more easily in children who are weaker constitutionally. Guard these children by prophylaxis against these injuries. Understand that they need especially detailed care in choosing the correct herbs.

Younger children have diseases that are often characterised by rapid transformation. Excess syndromes can rapidly change into deficiency syndromes or combinations of excess and deficiency together. For example, a cold in these children may transform into pneumonia almost immediately.

Visceral disease in children can be detected on the skin. Inspection of the skin is important as well as inspection of the urine and stool. Veins will be visible and small patches of roughness or scales or rash will be evident. These are indicators of underlying disease and inflammation. The superficial venules of the index finger are also used. In pulse taking, only one position is felt at cunkou.

Feeling for floating, deep, slow or fast gives an indication of whether the syndrome is exterior or interior, cold or hot. The rest of the body should be observed and palpated. Palpate the abdomen, the nodes, the head and neck and chest. Palpate for lumps, for heat and cold, and tenderness. Inspect for changes in coloration, red, raised rashes or scaly areas. All of these are very important and full of diagnostic meaning in young children.

The treatment of pediatric cancers, including leukemia, is a specialty area. The dosage is different for children depending on their weight and the status of their gastrointestinal function and ability to metabolise herbal medicine. Very young children may not be able to take herbs. Granules, syrups and tablets put into food, injections and suppositories are all used for children rather than decoction. If decoction is given then it can be mixed with sugar or into hot milk or cereal. Dosing is more frequent in children and in smaller amounts.

For children of 3 years of age who weigh approximately 40 lb, the dosage of herbs in any given formula is usually at least half that of the written dosage for adults. The dosing of the formula varies depending upon the disease being treated, but is commonly six times daily rather than three times daily in half the common dose. In children who are extremely weak, the dosage of a single herb in a formula may be changed based on the nature of the herb and the child's ability to metabolise that herb. The formula will be much smaller in terms of the number of the herbs and also the dose of each herb in the formula.[66]

References

1. Sawyers CL. Leukemia and the disruption of normal hematopoiesis. Cell 1991; 64:337–350.
2. Brincker H. Population-based age-and sex-specific incidence rates in the four main types of leukemia. Scand J Haematol 1982; 29:241–249.
3. Stewart A. Radiation dose effects in relation to obstetric X-rays and childhood cancers. Lancet 1970; 1:1185–1188.
4. Buckley HD. Occupational exposures of parents of children with acute nonlyphocytic leukemia: a report from the Children's Cancer Study Group. Cancer Res 1989; 49:4030–4037.
5. Kaye SA. Maternal reproductive history and birth characteristics in childhood acute lymphoblastic leukemia. Cancer 1991; 68:1351–1355.
6. De Oliveira MSP. Lymphoblastic leukemia in Siamese twins: evidence for identity. Lancet 1986; 2:969–970.
7. Robinson LI. Down syndrome and acute leukemia in children: a 10-year retrospective study from

the Children's Cancer Study Group. J Pediatr 1984; 105:235–244.

8. Alexander FE. Viruses, clusters, and clustering of childhood leukemia. A new perspective. Eur J Cancer 1993; 29A:1424–1443.

9. Greaves MF. An infectious etiology for common acute lymphoblastic leukemia in childhood? Leukemia 1993; 7:349–360.

10. Li Yan. Zhong Liu Lin Zheng Bei Yao (Essentials of clinical pattern identification of tumors), 2nd edn. Beijing: People's Medical Publishing House; 1999.

11. Wu Ju Tong. Wen Bing Tiao Bian Bai Hua Jie (Vernacular explanation of the systematic differentiation of warm diseases). Zhengjian Traditional Chinese Medicine College, eds. People's Health Publishing; 1979. Original from 1798 ACE.

12. Poplack DG. Clinical manifestations of acute lymphoblastic leukemia. In: Hoffman R, et al, eds. Hematology: basic principles and practice. New York: Churchill Livingstone; 1991:776–784.

13. Montserrat E. Presenting features and prognosis in of chronic lymphocytic leukemia in younger adults. Blood 1991; 78:1545.

14. Robinson LL. Epidemiology of childhood leukemia. ASCO Educational Book; 1994:120–123.

15. Lukens JN. Acute lymphocytic leukemia. In Lee GR, et al, eds. Wintrobe's clinical hematology, 9th edn. Philadelphia: Lea and Febiger, 1993:1892–1919.

16. Pui CH. Serum CD4, CD8, and interleukin-2 receptor levels in childhood acute myeloid leukemia. Leukemia 1991; 5:249–254.

17. Crist WM. Immunologic markers in childhood acute lymphocytic leukemia. Semin Oncol 1995; 12:105–121.

18. Magrath IT. Bone marrow involvement in Burkitt's lymphoma and its relationship to acute B-cell leukemia. Leukemia Res 1979; 4:33–59.

19. Ribeiro RC. Prognostic factors in childhood acute lymphoblastic leukemia. Hematol Pathol 1993; 7:121–142.

20. Cortes J. Leukemia in the elderly. Cancer Bull 1995; 7:171–175.

21. Smith M. Towards a more uniform approach to risk classification and treatment assignment for children with acute lymphoblastic leukemia (ALL). ASCO Educational Book; 1994:124–130

22. Ribeiro RC. Clinical and biologic hallmarks of the Philadelphia chromosome in childhood acute lymphoblastic leukemia. Blood 1987; 70:948–953.

23. Kasparu H. Intensified induction therapy for ALL in adults: a multicenter trial. Onkologie 1991; 14(Suppl 1):80.

24. Bennet JM. Proposed revised criteria for the classification of acute myeloid leukemia. Ann Intern Med 1985; 103:620–625.

25. Estey EH. Prediction of survival during induction therapy in patients with newly diagnosed acute myeloblastic leukemia. Leukemia 1989; 3:257–263.

26. Mayer RJ. Intensive post-remission chemotherapy in adults with acute myeloid leukemia. N Engl J Med 1994; 331:896–903.

27. Bishop JF. High-dose cytosine arabinoside (ara-C) in induction prolongs remission in acute myeloid leukemia (AML): updated results of a randomised phase III trial. Blood 1994; 84:232a.

28. Horousseau JL. Double intensive consolidation chemotherapy in adult acute myeloid leukemia. J Clin Oncol 1991; 9:1432–1437.

29. Gamberi B. Acute myeloid leukemia from diagnosis to bone marrow transplantation: Experience from a single center. Bone Marrow Transplant 1994; 14:69–72.

30. Call TG. Incidence of chronic lymphocytic leukemia in Olmstead county, Minnesota, 1935 through 1989, with emphasis on changes in initial stage at diagnosis. Mayo Clin Proc 1994; 69:323–328.

31. Zahm SH. Use of hair coloring products and the risk of lymphoma, multiple myeloma, and chronic lymphocytic leukemia. Am J Public Health 1992; 82:990.

32. Cheson BD. Guidelines for clinical protocols for chronic lymphocytic leukemia. Am J Hematol 1988; 29:152.

33. Rai KR. Clinical staging of chronic lymphocytic leukemia. Blood 1975; 46:219.

34. Begleiter A. Mechanism of resistance to chlorambucil in chronic lymphocytic leukemia. Leuk Res 1991; 15:109.

35. French Cooperative Group in Chronic Lymphocytic Leukemia. A randomized clinical trial of chlorambucil versus COP in stage B chronic lymphocytic leukemia. Blood 1990; 75:1422.

36. Kantarjian HM. Chronic myelogenous leukemia: a concise update. Blood 1995; 82:691–703.

37. Kantarjian HM. Prolonged survival following achievement of a cytogenetic response with alpha interferon therapy in chronic myelogenous leukemia. Am Intern Med 1995; 6:347–349.

38. Bortin MM. Increasing utilization of bone marrow transplantation. Ann Intern Med 1992; 116:505.

39. Clift RA. Allogeneic marrow transplantation in patients with acute myeloid leukemia in first remission: a randomized trial of two irradiation regimens. Blood 1990; 76:1867.

40. Petz LD. Bone marrow transplantation. In: Petz LD, ed. Clinical practice of transfusion medicine, 2nd edn. New York: Churchill Livingstone; 1989:485.

41. Kessinger A. Utilization of peripheral blood stem cells in autotransplantation. Hematol Oncol Clin North Am 1993; 7:535–545.
42. Kennedy MJ. Phase I trail of interferon gamma to potentiate cyclosporine-induced graft-versus-host disease in women undergoing autologous bone marrow transplantation for breast cancer. J Clin Oncol 1994; 12:249–257.
43. Gilmore MJML, Hamon HG. Failure of purged autologous bone marrow transplantation in high-risk acute lymphoblastic leukemia in first complete remission. Bone Marrow Transplant 1991; 8:19–26.
44. Rowley SD. Efficacy of ex-vivo purging for autologous bone marrow transplantation in the treatment of acute nonlymphoblastic leukemia. Blood 1989; 74:501–506.
45. Noga SJ. Using elutriation to engineer bone marrow allografts. Prog Clin Biol Res 1990; 333:345–362.
46. Champlin RE. Early complications of bone marrow transplantation. Semin Hematol 1984; 21:101–108.
47. Nemunaitis J. Use of recombinant human granulocyte-macrophage colony-stimulating factor in graft failure after bone marrow transplantation. Blood 1990; 76:245–253.
48. Braverman AC. Cyclophosphamide cardiotoxicity in bone marrow transplantation: a prospective evaluation of new dosing regimens. J Clin Oncol 1991; 9:1215–1223.
49. Vogelsang GB. Acute graft-versus-host disease: clinical characteristics in the cyclosporine era. Medicine 1988; 67:163.
50. Przepiorka D. Evaluation of anti-CD5 ricin A chain immunoconjugate for prevention of graft-versus-host disease after HLA-identical marrow transplantation. Ther Immunol 1994; 1:77.
51. Martin PJ. A retrospective analysis of therapy for acute graft-versus-host diasease: initial treatment. Blood 1990; 76:1464.
52. Meagher RC. Techniques of harvesting and cryopreservation of stem cells. Hematol Oncol Clin North Am 1993; 7:501–533.
53. Champlin R. Preparative regimens for autologous bone marrow transplantation. Blood 1993; 81:1709–1719.
54. Peters WP. Comparative effects of GM-CSF and G-CSF on priming peripheral blood progenitor cells for use with autologous bone marrow after high-dose chemotherapy. Blood 1993; 81:277– 280.
55. Civin CI. Identification and positive selection of human progenitor/stem cells for bone marrow transplantation. Prog Clin Biol Res 1992; 377:461–473.
56. McDonald GB. Veno-occlusive disease of the liver and multi-organ failure after bone marrow transplantation: a cohort study of 355 patients. Ann Intern Med 1993; 118:255–267.
57. Tang Zhaiqiu. Xian Dai Zhong Liu Xue (Current oncology). Shanghai: Shanghai Medical University Press; 1993.
58. Zhang Dai Zhao. Zhang Dai Zhao ZhiAi Jing Yan Ji Yao (Collection of Zhang Dai Zhao's experiences in the treatment of cancer). Beijing: China Medicine and Pharmaceutical Publishing House; 2001.
59. Yang Shi Yong. Sheng Wu Fan Ying Tiao Jie Ji Yu Zhong Liu Mian Yi Zhi Liao (Regulation of biological reactions and the treatment of tumor immunity). Xian: Xian Science and Technology Publishing House; 1989.
60. Lang Wei Jun. Kang Ai Zhong Yao Yi Qian Fang (One thousand anti-cancer prescriptions). Beijing: Traditional Chinese Medicine and Materia Medica Science and Technology Publishing House; 1992.
61. Zhou Ju Ying. Fu Zheng Qu Yu Fa Zhi Liao Zhong Liu Hua Liao Suo Zhi Ji Xing Gan Zang Sun Hai (Supplementing vital qi and dispelling stasis method in the treatment of liver damage caused by chemotherapy). Shanxi J of TCM 1993; 9:18.
62. Li Pei Wen. Zhong Yi Za Zhi (J TCM) 1993; 34:693.
63. Tumor Research Group of Chinese Materia Medica Institute, Chinese Academy of Traditional Chinese Medicine. Ke Ji Zi Liao Hui Bian (Collection of scientific papers) 1972:140.
64. Wang xiao Ming. Bian Zheng Zhi Liao Zhong Liu Hua Liao Ji Qi Du Fu Fan Ying 108 Li (Treatment based on pattern identification for 108 cases of toxic side effects caused by chemotherapy for tumors). Liaoning J TCM 1994; 21:117–118.
65. Li Pei Wen. Zhong Xi Yi Lin Chuang Zhong Liu Xue (Clinical oncology in Chinese and Western medicine). Beijing: China TCM Publishing House; 1996.
66. Cao Ji Ming. Essentials of traditional Chinese pediatrics. Beijing: Foreign Language Press; 1990.

Chapter 12

Concurrent Issues

CHAPTER CONTENTS

Introduction   302

General anemias   302
  Conventional medicine   302
  Chinese medicine   303

Neutropenia and neutropenic fevers   304
  Conventional medicine   304
  Chinese medicine   305

Bone marrow suppression and
  thrombocytopenia   307
  Conventional medicine   307
  Chinese medicine   308

Nausea and vomiting   309
  Conventional medicine   309
  Chinese medicine   310

Stomatitis/mucositis   312
  Conventional medicine   312
  Chinese medicine   312

Other issues caused by chemotherapy   313
  Toxic hepatitis   313
  Toxic myocarditis   313
  Toxic nephritis   314
  Hemorrhagic cystitis   314
  Pancreatitis   314
  Skin rashes   314

Peripheral neuropathy   314

Anxiety and depression   317
  Anxiety   317
  Depression   319

Cancer pain syndromes   322
  Chinese medicine   323

Pleural effusion   324
  Chinese medicine   324
  External treatment   326

Ascites   327
  Chinese medicine   327

A plant is the manifestation of the beingness of Earth, the ensouling life of the planet which you may call the Earth Logos. Plants serve a function for this being. They also serve the function of providing an environment for higher forms of life to enter and be comfortable within this physical dimension. We are far more ancient than the physical Earth itself and we draw freely upon the powers of cosmic creativity. Before a planet can come into existence, we exist; we bring the planet into existence.

From *The Findhorn Garden,*
by the Findhorn Community.

INTRODUCTION

The progression of cancer carries with it certain disease processes that are inherent in each case depending on the type of cancer involved, the degree of disease, the individual involved, and the treatment utilised. These injuries and conditions, no matter what the cause, require treatment in order to maintain normal function. Maintaining normal function enables a patient to better survive the cancer and to live with a higher quality of life. Therefore, this aspect of treatment can be as important as cytotoxic intervention.

Cytotoxic treatment mainly kills cancer cells. In the process, it also damages other healthy cells. Cytotoxic treatment does not change the overall environment in which the cancer evolved in terms of moving that environment away from one that promotes cancer. Although some hormonal therapies have a more positive systemic effect, generally cytotoxic therapies cause damage. The continual repair of the damage caused by conventional treatments helps to create an ecology within the body that is more healthy and better able to survive the cancer. This repair and the repair of general body health makes a profound contribution to survival.

GENERAL ANEMIAS

CONVENTIONAL MEDICINE[1]

The blood is an organ with its own anatomy, physiology, and developmental natural history. Every second 2 million red cells, 2 million platelets, and 700 000 granulocytes are produced. Red cells have an approximately 120-day lifespan and travel 175 miles during that lifespan. The function of blood is to provide oxygen to the tissues, prevent invasion by micro-organisms, and to promote hemostasis. Fetal hematopoiesis is somewhat different than that of the adult body.

The physical examination of blood as an organ includes the determination of the status of the hemoglobin, the hematocrit, the white blood cell count, the red blood cell count, the differential count, platelet count, and the blood cell morphology from a smear.

The bone marrow has well-defined architecture that is specifically designed for specific cell–cell interactions and the delivery of mature blood cells to the circulation. The delivery of these mature blood cells to the circulation requires the ability of these cells to traverse the endothelial lining of the bone marrow sinuses. Within the marrow the cells undergo organisation into distinct pools. For example, myeloid and erythroid precursors can be divided into proliferating and non-proliferating pools. The complexity of cell lines within the marrow is astonishing. A red cell will reach maturation in 7 days. Marrow transit time can be shortened when there is a demand, and reticulocytes can be released prematurely into the bloodstream.

Mature red cells lack the capacity to synthesise proteins and, therefore, cannot replace enzymes and structural proteins as they age. The reticuloendothelial system removes these cells and they are catabolised, releasing iron for reutilisation. Bilirubin is also released in the form of heme, which is converted and transported to the liver for conjugation and excretion.

Myelopoiesis and megakaryocytopoiesis are other functions of the marrow controlling the generation of myelocytes, neutrophils, monocytes, granulocytes, and megakaryocytes, which act as precursors for platelets. Hematopoietic progenitor cells within the marrow are capable of differentiating to maintain the pool of circulating blood cells, but are incapable of replenishing themselves. Another population of marrow cells capable of differentiation and self-renewal maintains the pool of progenitor cells. These are called stem cells. These cells have no identifiable features and their identification is based purely on their function.

The mechanisms that control the proliferation and differentiation of hematopoietic cells are not fully understood.

Erythropoietin is a glycoprotein produced in the kidney and possibly also in the liver. Production of this hormone is regulated by levels of oxygen supply and demand in tissues. Hypoxia stimulates erythropoetin production. The oxygen sensor is located in the kidney.

Anemia is biomedically defined quantitatively as a reduction in the circulating red cell mass below what is considered normal for individuals of the same sex and body mass. Three measurements are used to quantify red blood cell (RBC) counts: the red cell count, the blood hemoglobin concentration, and the volume of packed red cells known as the hematocrit. Electronic particle counters assay the blood for these levels. All of these counts are influenced by the plasma volume. Patients given intravenous fluids will have lowered levels because of the increased serum plasma levels that dilute the counts.

Anemia develops when the demand for red cells exceeds the capacity of the marrow to produce them. Acquired anemia is always a consequence of another disorder, therefore transfusion alone is not curative. The symptoms and signs associated with anemia depend on the cause, its extent, and rapidity of onset, and the presence of other disorders affecting the patient's health. In pernicious anemia, which has an insidious onset, the reduction in red cell mass may be tolerated for a period of time with few symptoms.

Types of anemia include microcytic, macrocytic, normocytic, pernicious, megaloblastic, hemolytic, aplastic, infection deficiency anemia, anemia associated with systemic disease, anemia associated with infiltrative disease of the bone marrow, pure red cell anemia (PRCA), iron deficiency anemia, sideroblastic anemia, and many more.

CHINESE MEDICINE

In Chinese medicine, the term blood includes the substance and also the force of movement of blood in the body. Therefore, a level of activity is implied that is involved particularly with the sensitivity of the sense organs and with a deep level in the body relative to the progression of febrile diseases. Diseases at the blood level are considered very serious and are treated differently than diseases at the qi level. This is important since most cancers are considered to be blood level diseases.

The blood is manufactured mainly in the middle jiao, using the qi derived from prana in the lungs and food digested by the spleen, the gu qi. This combination is called zheng qi when it is completed by the addition of ying and wei qi. The blood is also generated at the kidney essence level by the marrow. So blood can be found to be deficient at two different levels – spleen and kidney.

The relationship between blood and jin ye is extremely close. Both are fluids, both travel together in the vessels, both function as moistening nourishers, both are yin, and they both have the same source: the essence of foods and fluids.

Ying qi comes out of the middle burner and secretes jin ye fluids like a life-giving fog. From above it pours into the confluences of the tissues, then seeps into the delicate collaterals where, if the jin and ye are harmonious and through the qi transformative process of the lungs and heart, they become red blood. If this blood remains harmonious, it will first fill the delicate collaterals, and then pour into the collaterals proper – the luo mai. When these are full, the blood will pour into the major channels – the jing mai – of the body, both yin and yang, ensuring the abundance of protective nourishing qi and blood, flowing through the body with the rhythmic impetus of the lung's breath.
Ling Shu; Chapter 81

Jin ye is produced in the middle jiao, transported through the San Jiao, and acted upon by the lungs and heart so that a portion of the fluids becomes blood. Anatomically, the lungs surround the heart and are the equivalent of the qi surrounding the vessels through which the blood flows. Part of the jin ye goes to the lungs and moves with the qi outside the vessels, and part goes to the heart and moves into the vessels mixing with and becoming part of the blood. This happens within the body wherever there is this structure of surrounding the blood.

In pathological situations, blood and jin ye influence each other. For example, when there is excessive blood loss the jin and ye fluids outside the vessels can permeate into the vessels to make up for fluid loss. If there is a huge amount of fluid, the resulting depletion outside the vessels can lead to fluid deficiency. Blood stasis in the channels, as another example, also leads to obstruction of the moistening effect of the jin ye on the surface, resulting in dry, rough, thick skin. The opposite can also occur; when the fluids have been damaged severely this can cause an exodus of fluids from the blood leaving the vessels empty. This condition is called jin withered and blood parched – jin ku xue zao. This can lead to severe shen disturbance, as the heart is not nourished. Extreme diaphoresis can cause this condition.

Qi and blood also have a strong relationship. Qi is the commander of blood. Blood is the mother of qi. They are said to magnetise one another. In many cases the diseases of blood parallel those of qi. Stagnant qi can lead to stagnant blood. Blood nourishes qi and deficient blood can predispose a person to deficient qi. Deficient blood can result from loss of blood, malnutrition, deficient spleen, deficient kidneys, and congealed blood. Deficient blood can also result from systemic disease where stasis of some kind causes the blood to move unsmoothly. This causes a mild heat, which dries the blood. Blood dryness leads to blood deficiency. All of the above can transform into blood heat and blood heat causes more blood dryness, then blood heat, and then blood stasis. When carried to an extreme, masses can evolve.

Possible diagnostic patterns for anemia:

- liver constraint with underlying blood deficiency due to transverse rebellion
- liver blood deficiency
- internal injury due to consumption (xu lao)
- middle jiao deficiency with sunken yang
- straight qi and blood deficiency due to source qi deficiency
- spleen qi deficiency leading to heart blood deficiency
- kidney essence injury.

Treatment principles:

- to raise the RBC counts and tonify the qi and blood
- to raise the white blood cell (WBC) counts and invigorate the yang
- to raise the platelet levels and nourish the yin and essence.

NEUTROPENIA AND NEUTROPENIC FEVERS

CONVENTIONAL MEDICINE

Neutropenia is a major predisposing factor for infection in cancer patients. Risk for infection begins to increase when neutrophil counts drop below 1000/mm^3 and is greatest when counts are at or below 100/mm^3. Twenty percent of fevers in a neutropenic patient are caused by bacterial infection. Intensive chemotherapeutic regimens used to achieve maximal antitumor activity can produce severe and prolonged neutropenia in many patients.

It is not always possible to document an infection in a febrile neutropenic cancer patient. In high-risk patients prophylactic antibiotics are used. The micro-organisms commonly causing infection are: Staphylococcus aureus, enterococci, and different streptococci. Most staphylococcal infections are cutaneous, and most enterococcal infections are gastrointestinal. Escherichia coli, Klebsiella, and Pseudomonas are frequently found. Heavy antibiotic use in neutropenic patients has led to the emergence of other, often resistant, Gram-negative organisms. P. aeruginosa is one of these.

Febrile neutropenic patients are often hard to evaluate. The fevers may be intermittent and low-grade and there may be no other manifestation of serious infection. This may be due to an impaired inflammatory response. Therefore, all sites for culturing are used including blood, urine, and stools. Infections can develop rapidly and progress as rapidly and cause death. The response rate to antibiotics in the first 24 hours is very high, but falls off rapidly if antibiotics are administered in the following 24 hours after the initiation of a fever.

Some of the combinations of antibiotics are very strong, synergistic in effect and have broad-spectrum applicability. Some are combined with vancomycin to include activity against Gram-positive infections. Cephalosporins are being used less since they are only moderately active against Gram-positive organisms, and they seem to have a relationship with the emergence of drug-resistant Gram-negative organisms and the development of super-infections.

The duration for antibiotic treatment in a febrile neutropenic patient is debatable. Some recommend continuation until the resolution of the neutropenia. This increases the possibility for the development of super-infections caused by resistant bacteria or fungi. It may also increase drug toxicity. Others say to treat for a minimum of 7–9 days and until the patient has no evidence of infection and is clinically stable and without fever for 5 days.

Up to 20% of infections in neutropenic patients fail to respond to antibiotic therapy. Sometimes in these cases hematopoietic growth factors are used. Granulocyte-macrophage colony stimulating factor (GM-CSF), can be used (sargramostim [Leukine]), or granulocyte colony stimulating factor (G-CSF; filgrastim [Neupogen]). Some medical oncologists use Neupogen as a matter of course to act prophylactically in those patients whose chemotherapeutic regimen is predicted to cause lowered WBC counts.

The prevention of infection in myelosuppressed patients is a main concern. Two strategies are used: propylactic antibiotics and colony-stimulating factors, and the prevention of infection through strict handwashing precautions, well-cooked, and sometimes even irradiated food, and, rarely, isolation techniques or protected environments (most commonly in leukemia patients or others who are undergoing high-dose chemotherapy).

CHINESE MEDICINE

There are many causes of fever according to Chinese medical theory. Infection may be one cause. Neutropenic fevers without evidence of infection may be caused by qi deficiency. In fact, intermittent and low-grade fevers are the hallmark of qi-deficient fevers. The fever should resolve quickly with the use of qi tonic herbs and acupuncture techniques. The ability to recognise these kinds of fevers, as differentiated from those caused by external pernicious influences, is a skill of great importance in cancer treatment. Even in fevers caused by an exterior pernicious influence (EPI) during cancer treatment, the ability to read the pattern in the context of the constitutional presentation of the patient determines what treatment will be used to clear the pathogen and the fever. Please refer back to Chapter 1 and the rules of treatment.

The tongue and pulse, the onset and predisposing factors relative to recent exposures, and the symptom transformations should be clues. Since the gastrointestinal tract is usually moderately-to-severely impacted by chemotherapy, it is important to be able to limit or eliminate the use of prophylactic antibiotics or antibiotic treatment for non-infectious fevers in a cancer patient. Antibiotics kill off normal flora in the gut and use up spleen qi in order to rehabilitate normal function, which is already injured by many chemotherapeutic agents (see *Nausea and vomiting* section in this chapter).

Besides infection due to external exposures other causes of fever may be:

- stagnation caused by tumor tissue metabolites, which cause qi and phlegm stasis leading to heat
- necrosis and ulceration of tumor tissue due to a loss of blood supply in the center of the lesion, which leads to blood stasis and blood heat
- an inflammatory process caused by leukocytes infiltrating the tumor leading to organ level heat stasis
- bacterial infection of the tumor itself, which clinically depends on the stage of the infection
- an allergic response to antitumor drugs, which results in wind heat, or blood heat, or heat at the qi level
- loss of jin ye due to chronic disease or to drug therapies, which leads to yin deficient heat.

When fever is due to infection the WBC counts will be elevated unless they are so low in number an elevation is impossible to read. In these cases, the patient can be treated based on the analysis of the infection according to Chinese medical parameters. In the neutropenic patient, however, the WBC counts will have already been low for some time. This makes analysis more difficult. It also brings up another issue, which must be discussed here. The issue of contamination of herbs is a particularly difficult one when treating neutropenic patients. Conventional oncologists say that Chinese herbs have contained cultures of *Aspergillus* (fungal growth) and other bacterial or viral factors in crude form. Chinese practitioners say that decocting the herbs will kill any bacterial or fungal contamination in crude herbs. It is a dilemma. The answer is to use granulated herbs; Western patients often do not know well enough the proper means by which to decoct herbs. If they are unwell, it becomes even more difficult for them. Provide your patients with the cleanest and easiest product to use. Develop relationships with other providers; this allows for more and better communication, and will give you the opportunity to explain what you are doing and the quality of the medicine you are using. Always write a letter of introduction to the providers for every patient you ever see.

Suggestions currently under evaluation regarding the issue of herbal contamination are to irradiate granulated herbs in single-dose packets. This achieves a level of purity and almost sterility that is beyond the levels commonly accepted in conventional settings in the United States for the food that is served to cancer patients at high risk. Another suggestion is to have the formulas compounded and extracted into sterile solution, almost as though they were going to be used intravenously. The cost would be fairly great and it is not clear what effect this handling of the herbs would have on the synergism of a given formula. Since herbs in any form are considered 'food' and are metabolised in the same way as food when taken orally, then can we apply similar standards to our medicines? This is one current approach and one that has been negotiated successfully with many institutions.

In order to differentiate a non-infectious fever from an infectious fever it is possible to look at the many symptoms accompanying fever due to infection. These include the following symptoms and therapeutics for each:

- A lack of sweat when it would be appropriate in order to release the pathogen: use ma huang (Ephedrae Herba; *Ephedra*) or hot bath with ginger tea to induce sweat. Make sure that adequate fluids are taken.
- Continuous sweating that will lead to dehydration: use ge gen (Puerariae Radix; *Pueraria*), lian qiao (Forsythiae fructus; *Forsythia*), huang qi (Astragali Radix; *Astragalus membranaceus*), xi yang shen (Panacis quinquefolii Radix; *Panax quinquefolium*), mai ya (Hordei Fructus germinatus; *Hordenm vulgare*; barley sprouts; malt) to consolidate the exterior and close the pores while releasing the pathogen. Many patients are already subclinically dehydrated. Therefore, recognising and treating this pattern is very important.
- Constipation: huo ma ren* (Cannabis Semen; *Cannabis sativa* [sterilised] seed), da huang (Rhei Radix et Rhizoma; *Rheum*), to move and moisten the stool.

- Thirst: bei sha shen (Glehniae Radix; *Glehnia*), shi hu (Dendrobii Herba; *Dendrobium*) to nourish the fluids of the stomach and lung.
- Restlessness: Gan mai da zao tang to benefit the spleen in order to nourish the heart blood.
- Bleeding gums: sheng di huang (Rehmanniae Radix; *Rehmannia*; unprepared root) and mu dan pi (Moutan Cortex; *Paeonia suffruticosa* root cortex) to clear heat from the blood level.
- Anorexia due to cold in the stomach/spleen: Si jun zi tang with zhi ban xia (Pinelliae Rhizoma preparatum; *Pinellia ternata*).

The above symptoms when combined with a fever can indicate an infectious cause. The herbs suggested are to be combined with the formula of choice for the pattern diagnosed, except in the case of the first, second, and last presentations, where the herbs listed can be used as a formula in and of itself.

When fevers are clearly not due to infection they are most often caused by the cancer itself in some way, or by deficiency. In these cases the fever will consistently be low-grade with spikes in the afternoon, or with malar flush. There will be a dry mouth and throat but often an inability to drink, or only the capacity to wet the mouth and throat by sipping small amounts only. The tongue coat is commonly a mirror or smooth coat, there will be five center heat, constipation, and dark urine. It is important to note that cancer pain is often increased by fever.

Presentations not caused by infection is caused by a combination of yin deficiency, blood heat and toxin, or by qi deficiency, so the treatment principles are to lower the fever, clear blood heat, and nourish the yin or tonify the qi. The particular herbs chosen are specific to the site or mechanism of the heat. In the case of a qi-deficient fever, qi tonic herbs are added to the general formula being used during treatment. Useful herbs are shown in Box 12.1.

Using a whole formula to tonify the qi is also appropriate. The most common is Si jun zi tang, which is generally added to many formulas for use during chemotherapy. To specifically raise the WBC count then invigorate the yang. Kidney yang tonic herbs or general tonic herbs that raise the WBC count are shown in Box 12.2.

Box 12.1   Herbs to treat infection

Herbs that nourish the yin

- mai dong (Ophiopogonis Radix; *Ophiopogon*): especially good for stomach and lungs
- tian dong (Asparagi Radix; *Asparagus*): general yin nourishing
- zhi mu (Anemarrhenae Rhizoma; *Anemarrhena*): especially good to generate fluids while clearing heat
- gui ban* (Testudinis Plastrum; *Chinemys reevesii* plastron): especially good for the kidneys
- tai zi shen (Pseudostellariae Radix; *Pseudostellaria heterophylla*): especially good to generate fluids while tonifying the qi without warming

Herbs that clear blood heat

- mu dan pi (Moutan Cortex; *Paeonia suffruticosa* root cortex)
- sheng di huang (Rehmanniae Radix; *Rehmannia* unprepared root)
- xuan shen (Scrophulariae Radix; *Scrophularia*)

Herbs that clear toxic heat

- bai hua she she cao (Hedyotis diffusae Herba; *Oldenlandia*)
- jin yin hua (Lonicerae Flos; *Lonicera* flowers)
- tu fu ling (Smilacis glabrae Rhizoma; *Smilax glabra*)
- ge gen (Puerariae Radix; *Pueraria*)

Herbs that tonify the qi

- huang qi (Astragali Radix; *Astragalus membranaceus*)
- dang shen (Codonopsis Radix; *Codonopsis pilosula* root)
- tai zi shen (Pseudostellariae Radix; *Pseudostellaria* heterophylla)

Box 12.2   Kidney yang tonic herbs or general tonic herbs that raise the WBC count

- huang qi (Astragali Radix; *Astragalus membranaceus*)
- bu gu zhi (Psoraleae Fructus; *Psoralea*)
- yin yang huo (Epimedii Herba; *Epimedium grandiflorum*)
- dong chong xia cao (Cordyceps; *Cordyceps*)
- lu rong (Cervi Cornu pantotrichum; *Cervus nippon*; deer velvet)

BONE MARROW SUPPRESSION AND THROMBOCYTOPENIA

CONVENTIONAL MEDICINE[2]

Myelosuppression during and after chemotherapy is one of the contributing factors in the incidence of infection. Anemias can be barriers to the early resolution of cancer, and sometimes in myelodysplastic syndromes anemias caused by treatment can lead to refractory anemias and new malignancies. It is not uncommon for patients to be released from cytotoxic therapy and into monitoring alone without an analysis of their current status with regard to common blood levels. If this is true in the case of your patient, make sure that at least a complete blood count (CBC) with differential is done. It sometimes happens that patients are still anemic 6 months or even longer after conventional treatment.

Hematopoietic growth factors are being used to accelerate recovery from chemotherapy-induced anemias. There are toxicities related to hematopoietic growth factors. GM-CSF can be accompanied by flushing, tachycardia, dyspnea, hypoxemia, and nausea. It can induce fever and chills, which are difficult to distinguish from infection. Lethargy, myalgia, bone pain, and anorexia are common complaints. A capillary-leak syndrome may develop as characterised by edema, effusions, and inflammation. GM-CSF may exacerbate thrombocytopenia and reactivate autoimmune disorders that were underlying the cancer in certain patients. The most frequent G-CSF toxicity is bone pain. Fever, rash and arthralgia are

Appropriate choices made from these lists would be added to another formula based on the presentation of the patient and the pattern they manifest.

sometimes present, and mild splenomegaly may occur. Thrombocytopenia is sometimes reported.

These growth factors, colony stimulating factors, erythropoietin, thrombopoietin, and retinoids are commonly used as biologic therapies to treat the side effects of chemotherapy as they relate to myelosuppression. They are sometimes self-injected by patients within the context of their chemotherapeutic cycle dosing in order to prevent myelosuppression.

Thrombocytopenia is evidenced by bruising easily, gum bleeding, and, if severe, by hemorrhagic disorders such as hematemesis, hemoptysis, melena, and hematuria, which are all signs of an inability of the blood to clot. Neutropenia is evidenced by a proneness to infection. A RBC insufficiency, indicated by low hemoglobin and a low hematocrit, is primarily evidenced by fatigue.

CHINESE MEDICINE

The injuries caused by cytotoxic treatment, and especially many chemotherapeutic regimens affect the qi, blood, yin, and yang. The RBC counts can be raised by tonifying the qi, which will in turn nourish the blood. The platelet levels can be raised by nourishing the yin and essence. The WBC counts can be raised by invigorating the yang.

For general bone marrow suppression use:[3]

ren shen (Ginseng Radix; *Panax ginseng*)	10 g
lu jiao (Cervi Cornu; *Cervus* deer antler)	12 g
yin yang huo (Epimedii Herba; *Epimedium grandiflorum*)	15 g
shan zhu yu (Corni Fructus; *Cornus officinalis* fruit)	10 g
e jiao (Asini Corii Colla; *Equus asinus*; donkey-hide gelatin)	12 g
huang qi (Astragali Radix; *Astragalus membranaceus*)	20 g
ling zhi (Ganoderma; *Ganoderma*)	12 g
yun zhi (Coriolus; *Coriolus versicolor*)	12 g
bai mu er (Tremella; *Tremella*)	12 g
fu ling (Poria; *Poria cocos*)	15 g

If estrogen, progesterone, or androgen hormonal levels are of concern in specific cancers (breast, adrenal, prostate, ovarian, cervical), then do not use ren shen, lu jiao jiao, or e jiao. These animal products are hormonally active and can contribute to exposures in certain patients that may not be beneficial.

For thrombocytopenia:[4]

shu di (Rehmanniae Radix preparata; *Rehmannia*; prepared root)	15 g
shan zhu yu (Corni Fructus; *Cornus officinalis* fruit)	20 g
shan yao (Dioscoreae Rhizoma; *Dioscorea opposita*)	15 g
ze xie (Alismatis Rhizoma; *Alisma*)	10 g
mu dan pi (Moutan Cortex; *Paeonia suffruticosa* root cortex)	6 g
fu ling (Poria; *Poria cocos*)	12 g
ren shen (Ginseng Radix; *Panax ginseng*)	12 g
bai mu er (Tremella; *Tremella*)	15 g
ji xue teng (Spatholobi Caulis; *Spatholobus suberectus*)	15 g
liu zhi (Salicis babylonicae Ramulus; *Salix babylonica* branches)	10 g
zhi mu (Anemarrhenae Rhizoma; *Anemarrhena*)	10 g
chi shao (Paeoniae Radix rubra; *Paeonia lactiflora* root)	8 g
pu gong ying (Taraxaci Herba; *Taraxacum mongolicum*)	10 g
xiao ji (Cirsii Herba; *Cirsium*)	10 g

For a general formula during chemotherapy to maintain normal blood levels:[5]

huang qi (Astragali Radix; *Astragalus membranaceus*)	20 g
dang shen (Codonopsis Radix; *Codonopsis pilosula* root)	15 g
bai zhu (Atractylodis macrocephalae Rhizoma; *Atractylodes macrocephala*)	12 g
fu ling (Poria; *Poria cocos*)	12 g
gan cao (Glycyrrhizae Radix; *Glycyrrhiza*; licorice root)	5 g
shu di (Rehmanniae Radix preparata; *Rehmannia*; prepared root)	15 g
gou qi zi (Lycii Fructus; *Lycium chinensis* fruit)	12 g
he shou wu (Polygoni multiflori Radix preparata; *Polygonum multiflorum* root)	12 g

huang jing (Polygonati Rhizoma;   10 g
    Polygonatum)

nu zhen zi (Ligustri lucidi Fructus;   15 g
    Ligustrum lucidum fruit)

bei sha shen (Glehniae Radix; *Glehnia*)   10 g

mai dong (Ophiopogonis Radix;   10 g
    Ophiopogon)

ji xue teng (Spatholobi Caulis;   25 g
    Spatholobus suberectus)

qian shi (Euryales Semen; *Euryale*)   12 g

shan yao (Dioscoreae Rhizoma;   12 g
    Dioscorea opposita)

NAUSEA AND VOMITING

CONVENTIONAL MEDICINE[6]

Some types of chemotherapy can cause nausea; there are three types of nausea and vomiting. The first occurs within the first 24 hours after chemotherapy infusion and is called acute emesis. It occurs, for example, in about one-third of patients on cisplatin even when treatment is given with pharmaceutical antiemetics. The second type is called delayed emesis and occurs 24 hours or more following chemotherapy administration. The mechanism for this type is not well known. Risk factors include female gender, cisplatin in high dose, and prior acute emesis. This type can be quite severe and require hospitalisation. The third type is anticipatory emesis, which begins prior to chemotherapy administration and affects nearly 25% of patients who have undergone several rounds of chemotherapy, especially with poorly controlled emesis reactions. It is considered to be a part of a conditioned response.

The chemoreceptor trigger zone (CTZ) is the end neurologic structure for many pathways that receive stimuli from the vestibular areas, the cerebral cortex, and from the gut through vagal and splanchnic nerves. The CTZ is in an area characterised by the absence of an effective blood–brain barrier. It is thought that this center is directly stimulated by chemotherapeutic agents. Neuroreceptors in the gastrointestinal tract are also stimulated. Serotonin has been identified as the principal mediator of chemotherapy-induced emesis. Factors that affect emesis and its control are divided into those inherent to the patient and those inherent to the chemotherapy regimen. These are the factors used to determine which antiemetic program to use.

The patient-related factors are:

- prior exposure to chemotherapy
- age: older patients are more prone to nausea
- gender: females are more prone to nausea
- history of alcohol abuse
- history of motion sickness.

The chemotherapy-related factors are:

- emetic potential and pattern of the agent
- dose, route, and schedule of the chemotherapy
- the combination used.

Antiemetic drugs are usually used in combination. Phenothiazines (used less now due to inferior effect), substituted benzamides (metoclopramide), serotonin-receptor antagonists (ondansetron), corticosteroids (dexamethasone), antihistamines (diphenhydramine), benzodiazepines (lorazepam), and cannabinoids (nabilone) are all used. They are commonly given in combination together or singly in varying schedules just before chemotherapy is administered and then afterwards as indicated.

Some commonly used antiemetics are listed in Box 12.3. Many of these antiemetics have side effects. These include headache, constipation, fatigue, and diarrhea. Of these, constipation is the most prevalent and most difficult.

Box 12.3   Some antiemetic drugs (brand name in parentheses)

Lorazepam (Ativan)
Tetrohydrocannabinol (THC)
Prochlorperazine (Compazine)
Chlorpromazine (Thorazine)
Dexamethasone (Decadron)
Trimethobenzamide (Tigan)
Diazepam (Valium)
Dronabinol (Marinol)
Ondansentron (Zofran)
Metoclopramide (Reglan)

CHINESE MEDICINE:[7]

Many epigastric and abdominal symptoms arise from middle jiao injury caused by chemotherapeutic regimens. Some regimens are more problematic than others, especially those that are based in platinol-derived substances like cisplatin and carboplatin. Chemotherapeutic agents have varying mechanisms of action. Some are alkylating agents, others are antibiotics, others are antimetabolites, and so on. What they have in common from the point of view of Chinese medicine is that they are designed to treat toxins and toxic heat or fire-related pathogenic processes in the body. Because of this they are generally, but not always, very cold in nature.

A main site of injury, therefore, is the middle jiao. Injury to the stomach/spleen function by cold undermines the qi and the transformative and transportative process. This causes qi deficiency and dampness accumulation leading to a stomach/spleen disharmony, which causes the stomach qi to flush upward as it loses its normal qi flow. Spleen deficiency can result in transverse rebellion especially if the patient enters treatment with a pre-existing spleen deficiency. Damp accumulation in the middle jiao can also lead to lower abdominal symptoms since the spleen is symptomatic below the navel and the stomach is symptomatic above the navel. Lower abdominal pain and distention can result from spleen deficiency as well as loose stools or even diarrhea. Anorexia or reduced appetite and loss of taste may also be present. Fatigue is a common manifestation of this pattern and is caused by dampness and later by blood deficiency.

When this pattern persists over time the damp cold accumulation will cause stasis. Stasis will cause heat and the pattern can transform into one where there are signs and symptoms of stomach heat or yin deficiency with dry mouth, constipation, and insomnia. There may be concurrent spleen qi or yang deficiency with constipation and diarrhea alternating, lower abdominal cramping and pain, and thirst but an inability to drink. It is important to evaluate the pattern of injury based on the phase(s) of chemotherapy in order to understand if this presentation is more complex than a damp accumulation. Often in later stage rounds of chemotherapy, the injury to the digestive tract becomes more complex with elements of heat and yang deficiency. It is also possible that patients who enter chemotherapy do so with digestive tract injuries already in place. This means it is not always a simple matter to diagnose nausea and vomiting during treatment.

When treating the combinations of symptoms that are present, take into account the side effects of all of the medications the patient is taking. These can include supplement therapies, as well. Try to understand the presentation in the light of all oral medications. Often what we are doing clinically is treating the side effects of drug interventions, supplementation, and our herbal formula in a seriously ill patient. It is a complex interaction that requires levels of knowledge and skill that can only be obtained through experience.

Using the original formula for treatment during chemotherapy, adjust it in the following ways to address gastrointestinal symptoms. The dose for each herb will vary depending on the diagnosis and the strength of the symptoms and strength of the pattern.

To reduce nausea and vomiting add combinations of the following herbs according to pattern differentiation.[8,9]

- wu zhu yu (Evodiae Fructus; *Evodia*): warms the middle jiao
- huang lian (Coptidis Rhizoma; *Coptis*): resolves damp heat
- zhi ban xia (Pinelliae Rhizoma preparatum; *Pinellia ternata* rhizome): transforms phlegm
- zhu li (Bambusae Succus; *Bambusa* dried sap): transforms phlegm or damp heat
- shi di (Kaki Calyx; *Diospyros kaki* calyx): transforms phlegm
- ding xiang (Caryophylli Flos; *Syzygium aromaticum*; clore): warms the middle jiao,

and decrease:

- ji xue teng (Spatholobi Caulis; *Spatholobus suberectus*)
- he shou wu (Polygoni multiflori Radix preparata; *Polygonum multiflorum* root).

These herbs are blood-nourishing and cloying in nature and can contribute to nausea and vomiting.

To decrease abdominal distention add combinations of the following herbs:

- mu xiang (Aucklandiae Radix; *Saussurea*)
- fo shou (Citri sarcodactylis Fructus; *Citrus sarcodactylis*)
- chen pi (Citri reticulatae Pericarpium; *Citrus reticulata* pericarp)
- shen qu (Massa medicata fermentata; medicated leaven).

To decrease abdominal pain add combinations of the following herbs according to pattern:

- yan hu suo (Corydalis Rhizoma; *Corydalis yanhusuo*)
- bai qu cai (Chelidonii Herba; *Chelidonium*)
- wu yao (Linderae Radix; *Lindera*).

To improve appetite add a combination of the following herbs:

- ji nei jin (Gigeriae galli Endothelium corneum; *Gallus gallus domesticus* chicken gizzard lining)
- mai ya (Hordei Fructus germinatus; *Hordeum vulgare*; barley sprouts; malt)
- su ya (Setariae Fructus germinatus; *Setaria italica*; millet sprouts)
- shan zha (Crataegi Fructus; *Crataegus*)
- shen qu (Massa medicata fermentata; medicated leaven)
- qian shi (Euryales Semen; *Euryale*)
- lian zi (Nelumbinis Semen; *Nelumbo nucifera* seed),

and decrease:

- shu di (Rehmanniae Radix preparata; *Rehmannia*; prepared root)
- ji xue teng (Spatholobi Caulis; *Spatholobus suberectus*)
- he shou wu (Polygoni multiflori Radix preparata; *Polygonum multiflorum* root).

These blood-nourishing herbs are cloying in nature and are difficult to digest contributing to poor appetite.

To alleviate dry mouth add combinations of the following herbs:[10]

- shi hu (Dendrobii Herba; *Dendrobium*)
- zhi mu (Anemarrhenae Rhizoma; *Anemarrhena*)
- yu zhu (Polygonati odorati Rhizoma; *Polygonatum odoratum*)
- ou jie (Nelumbinis Nodus rhizomatis; *Nelumbo nucifera* rhizome nodes)
- xuan shen (Scrophulariae Radix; *Scrophularia*)

- bai mao gen (Imperatae Rhizoma; *Imperata cylindrica* rhizome)
- sheng di huang (Rehmanniae Radix; *Rehmannia*; unprepared root)
- tian dong (Asparagi Radix; *Asparagus*)
- tai zi shen (Pseudostellariae Radix; *Pseudostellaria heterophylla*)
- zhu li (Bambusae Succus; *Bambusa* dried sap),

and decrease:

- huang qi (Astragali Radix; *Astragalus membranaceus*)
- dang shen (Codonopsis Radix; *Codonopsis pilosula* root)
- shi di (Kaki Calyx; *Diospyros kaki* calyx)
- he shou wu (Polygoni multiflori Radix preparata; *Polygonum multiflorum* root)
- qian shi (Euryales Semen; *Euryale*)
- shan yao (Dioscoreae Rhizoma; *Dioscorea opposita*).

These herbs are warming in nature and will contribute to dry mouth. Dry mouth is a troublesome symptom and an important one to treat. Dry mouth is one step towards mouth sores of various kinds and proper treatment can prevent mouth sores and pain and possible weight loss during cytotoxic treatment.

To alleviate constipation add combinations of the following herbs according to the strength of the laxative needed:

- huo ma ren* (Cannabis Semen; *Cannabis sativa* [sterilised] seed)
- gua lou ren (Trichosanthis Semen; *Trichosanthes* seed)
- da huang (Rhei Radix et Rhizoma; *Rheum*)
- rou cong rong (Cistanches Herba; *Cistanche*)
- fan xie ye (Sennae Folium; *Cassia*; senna leaf),

and decrease:

- he shou wu (Polygoni multiflori Radix preparata; *Polygonum multiflorum* root)
- shi di (Kaki Calyx; *Diospyros kaki* calyx)
- dang shen (Codonopsis Radix; *Codonopsis pilosula* root)
- qian shi (Euryales Semen; *Euryale*)
- shan yao (Dioscoreae Rhizoma; *Dioscorea opposita*).

These herbs are generally warming and can exacerbate a dry constipation.

To manage diarrhea add combinations of the following according to the pattern differentiation:

- huang lian (Coptidis Rhizoma; *Coptis*)
- qin pi (Fraxini Cortex; *Fraxinus*)
- hou po (Magnoliae officinalis Cortex; *Magnolia officinalis* cortex)
- bu gu zhi (Psoraleae Fructus; *Psoralea*),

and decrease:

- mai dong (Ophiopogonis Radix; *Ophiopogon*)
- bei sha shen (Glehniae Radix; *Glehnia*)
- ji xue teng (Spatholobi Caulis; *Spatholobus suberectus*).

These herbs are yin-nourishing or cloying and can exacerbate diarrhea. Diarrhea is an important symptom and condition to treat since many cancer patients tend to be borderline dehydrated. Diarrhea becomes another way in which bodily fluids are lost. It is important to treat even intermittent diarrhea, and to make sure that the patient remains hydrated.

STOMATITIS/MUCOSITIS

CONVENTIONAL MEDICINE

Stomatitis is an inflammation of the oral mucosa and can present differently depending on the type. There may be a very bright and shiny erythema, itching and dryness, burning pain, ulceration, accompanying thrush, fever, and lymphadenopathy. These inflammations can be due to infections like candidiasis (thrush) or herpes simplex virus (HSV), trauma from irradiation therapy, dryness caused by chemotherapeutic agents or radiotherapy, irritants, toxic agents like chemotherapy that strip the mucosal lining, or autoimmune conditions that are part of underlying disease, such as hairy leukoplakia.

Recurrent aphthous stomatitis or canker sores may be due to deficiencies in iron, vitamin B$_{12}$, and folic acid. These deficiencies are common in cancer patients and adding these in supplement form to the diet is valuable for many reasons, including the possible prevention of cankers in the mouth.

Oral erythema multiforme is an acutely painful stomatitis characterised by hemorrhagic lesions of the lips and the mucosa and may be accompanied by systemic symptoms. These lesions make it difficult to swallow even fluids and are, therefore, important to diagnose and treat since dehydration can become an issue.

Oral herpetic lesions are also common during chemotherapy. These are acute, painful vesicular eruptions of the oral mucosa caused by an activation of HSVI. The cold nature of chemotherapeutic agents will often activate a latent HSV infection that was never before symptomatic. Also, patients who are neutropenic may have a mild to moderately lowered immunity and be more susceptible to this ubiquitous virus.

Glutamine in supplement form is an excellent addition during chemotherapy. Several studies have shown that glutamine is very useful in preventing oral inflammations of any kind. Some other studies have shown a possible risk for interference with some chemotherapeutic regimens.

CHINESE MEDICINE

Oral lesions are differentiated according to appearance. The main chemotherapy formula is based on the presentation and is constructed according to pattern differentiation. Herbs may be added to this formula that are pharmaceutically specific for a known pathogen if one is present. There are several possible patterns and it is important not to assume that stomach heat is the one and only pattern associated with mouth sores. Incorrect treatment can actually grossly exacerbate stomatitis and add insult to injury in a patient who is already suffering.

Pattern differentiations[10]

1. Stomach cold

The lesions are pale, painful, recurrent, and either raised or flat. The tongue body is pale. The whole body feels either normal in temperature or cold. The pulse may be full because this is an excess condition, even though the tongue is pale. The key is the pale tongue and the use of chemotherapy in the early rounds of treatment. As time progresses this pattern may transform into the second pattern.

Treatment principles: to warm the central axis and move qi.

Formula: Fu zi li zhong tang.

2. Spleen/stomach stasis due to the cold nature of chemotherapy that transforms and flares upward to steam and scorch the oral cavity.

This presentation looks like gingivitis, cankers, or perhaps oral HSV. The flesh breaks down. When a cold excess is present for a period of time, the stasis will eventually cause heat. This heat will lead to heat excess, or more probably, deficiency heat. The pulse is wiry forceful and fat. The tongue is red.

Treatment principles: to clear heat in the stomach and nourish the yin.

Formula: Liang ge san or Huang lian jie du pian.

3. Empty fire flaring

Here there are sparse and scattered ulcerations. The pain is worse at night, and there is five-center heat. The heart is involved in this presentation and so insomnia may be present. This is a more systemic condition, which includes kidney deficiency. The pulse is thin and fast. The tongue is red, dry and cracked.

Treatment principles: to clear heat in the stomach and nourish the yin of the stomach, lung and kidneys.

Formula: Zhi bai di huang tang or Qing re bu qi tang.

4. Middle jiao deficiency

This presentation includes repeated episodes of mouth sores that heal slowly or not at all. The lesions are light-colored. The appetite is low and there are spleen-qi-deficient symptoms. The pulse is weak or soft or moderate. The tongue is pale. There may be signs in the mouth of candidiasis.

Treatment principles: to tonify the middle jiao and lift the qi, and transform damp if present.

Formula: Bu zhong yi qi tang jia wei.

External treatments are available for this painful syndrome. A wash made from decocting gan cao (Glycyrrhizae Radix; *Glycyrrhiza*) and huang lian (Coptidis Rhizoma; *Coptis*) is made in a ratio of 2 parts licorice and 1 part *Coptis*. This is used as a swish-and-swallow gargle to cool the lesions and treat pain. Xi gua shuang, or watermelon powder, can be spritzed on the lesions or even to treat the mouth and throat made dry by radiation therapy. Gargling green tea with jin yin hua (Lonicerae Flos; *Lonicera* flowers) steeped in it is also very helpful. Gargling with a decoction of xuan shen (Scrophulariae Radix; *Scrophularia*) is also helpful. In many patients where this syndrome can be expected, the addition of glutamine to the supplement list can help prevent mouth sores.

OTHER ISSUES CAUSED BY CHEMOTHERAPY[11]

TOXIC HEPATITIS

bai mao teng (Solani lyrati Herba; *Solanum lyratum*)	10 g
yin chen hao (Artemisiae scopariae Herba; *Artemisia scopiaria/ A. capillaris*)	15 g
tai zi shen (Pseudostellariae Radix; *Pseudostellaria heterophylla*)	12 g
yu jin (Curcumae Radix; *Curcuma longa* rhizome)	10 g
dan shen (Salviae miltiorrhizae Radix; *Salvia miltiorhiza* root)	10 g
fu ling (Poria; *Poria cocos*)	12 g
zhu ling (Polyporus; *Polyporus – Grifola*)	10 g

TOXIC MYOCARDITIS

ren shen (Ginseng Radix; *Panax ginseng*)	8 g
san qi (Notoginseng Radix; *Panax notoginseng*)	12 g
tai zi shen (Pseudostellariae Radix; *Pseudostellaria heterophylla*)	15 g
dan shen (Salviae miltiorrhizae Radix; *Salvia miltiorhiza* root)	10 g
wu wei zi (Schisandrae Fructus; *Schisandra*)	8 g
shan zhu yu (Corni Fructus; *Cornus officinalis* fruit)	8 g
huang jing (Polygonati Rhizoma; *Polygonatum*)	10 g
fu ling (Poria; *Poria cocos*)	12 g
zhu ling (Polyporus; *Polyporus – Grifola*)	10 g
huang qi (Astragali Radix; *Astragalus membranaceus*)	15 g

TOXIC NEPHRITIS

yi ren (Coicis Semen; *Coix lacryma-jobi*)	12 g
yi zhi ren (Alpiniae oxyphyllae Fructus; *Alpina oxyphylla* fruit)	10 g
che qian zi (Plantaginis Semen; *Plantago*)	10 g
bai mao gen (Imperatae Rhizoma; *Imperata cylindrica* rhizome)	10 g
bi xie (Dioscoreae hypoglaucae Rhizoma; *Dioscorea hypoglauca*)	10 g
dan shen (Salviae miltiorrhizae Radix; *Salvia miltiorhiza* root)	10 g
ren shen (Ginseng Radix; *Panax ginseng*)	8 g
fu ling (Poria; *Poria cocos*)	15 g
zhu ling (Polyporus; *Polyporus – Grifola*)	15 g
guang jin qian cao (Desmodii styracifolii Herba; *Desmodium styracifolium*)	12 g
lu cao (Herba Humuli scandentis; *Humulus scandens*)	8 g

HEMORRHAGIC CYSTITIS

bai mao gen (Imperatae Rhizoma; *Imperata cylindrica* rhizome)	12 g
chi xiao dou (Phaseoli Semen; *Phaseolus calcaratus*)	10 g
da ji gen (Cirsii japonici Herba sive Radix; *Cirsium japonicum* root)	10 g
sheng di huang (Rehmanniae Radix; *Rehmannia*)	10 g
che qian zi (Plantaginis Semen; *Plantago*)	10 g
lu cao (Herba Humuli scandentis; *Humulus scandens*)	8 g
ji cai (Herba Capsellae; *Capsella*)	8 g
ou jie (Nelumbinis Nodus rhizomatis; *Nelumbo nucifera* rhizome nodes)	10 g
xiao ji (Cirsii Herba; *Cirsium*)	8 g
mu tong (Akebiae Caulis; *Akebia* stem)	8 g

add for heavy bleeding:

pu huang (Typhae Pollen; *Typha* pollen)	8 g

PANCREATITIS

lu cao (Herba Humuli scandentis; *Humulus scandens*)	8 g
yu jin (Curcumae Radix; *Curcuma longa* rhizome)	10 g
shu yang quan (Solani lyrati Herba; *Solanum lyratum*)	10 g
huang qin (Scutellariae Radix; *Scutellaria baicalensis*)	8 g
ren shen (Ginseng Radix; *Panax ginseng*)	8 g
bai hua she she cao (Hedyotis diffusae Herba; *Oldenlandia*)	12 g

SKIN RASHES

Add to the working formula in amounts appropriate to the working formula and the presentation:

sheng di huang (Rehmanniae Radix; *Rehmannia*)
shan zhu yu (Corni Fructus; *Cornus officinalis* fruit)
mu dan pi (Moutan Cortex; *Paeonia suffruticosa* root cortex)
rou cong rong (Cistanches Herba; *Cistanche*)

for an external wash use:

ku shen (Sophorae flavescentis Radix; *Sophora flavescens*)
huang bai (Phellodendri Cortex; *Phellodendron* cortex)
bai xian pi (Dictamni Cortex; *Dictamnus*)

All should be in equal portions and decocted in 10 times the amount of water.

PERIPHERAL NEUROPATHY

Peripheral neuropathy is a condition commonly seen in those patients whose cancers have been treated with paclitaxel (Taxol). Some other agents also cause peripheral neuropathy. In cancer patients, peripheral neuropathy is an iatrogenic injury. The symptoms can persist long after treatment has ended. In some cases the initial reaction is so severe that cessation of treatment with the drug is necessary, and hospitalisation may be required followed by a period of rehabilitation.

Ambulation may be difficult because of abnormal sensation, weakness, and pain in the feet and lower extremity. The ability to treat this side effect is highly valued by patients. There is little that conventional medicine has to offer. Patients will present with numbness and tingling of hands of feet, abnormal and overly sensitive reactions to touch, heat, cold and other external stimuli. There can be pain and difficulty walking that can range from mildly disturbing to extremely disturbing leading to an inability to walk. Hands can also be painful; grasping and movement in general can be painful. The hands may blanch or turn red in cold or hot temperatures. The discomfort in the hands can range from mild numbness and tingling to severe numbness and an inability to grasp. All of the above symptoms can persist for even 3 years post-treatment. Some symptoms in some patients appear to be permanent.

In Chinese medicine peripheral neuropathy is classified as a form of 'wilting impediment syndrome' or wei suo or wei bi. It implies a vast array of disorders of the nerves and soft tissue. The manifestations are myriad and it is difficult to diagnose and treat accurately. Nerves were not described in Chinese medical literature until exposure to Western medicine, so wilting impediment syndrome was mainly associated with the effect of various etiologies on the channels. It was first described in the Neijing.

The main symptoms of wei suo are atrophy and weakness, primarily of the limbs and especially the lower limbs. The Su Wen states that the main pathological mechanism is heat, which scorches the lungs. This scorches the essence, and since the lungs control the vessels, leads to a failure in the distribution of essence to the whole body, especially the peripheral body. This was usually in reference to polio. There are several types of wei suo including vessels atrophy and tendon atro-phy, which leads to contractures, muscle atrophy, which leads to emaciation, and bone atrophy, which leads to extreme emaciation.

Zhang Jing Yue, from the 16th century, stated that kidney yin is the root of the body and the kidney yang was an expression of the one sun in the body. Therefore, he concluded that both were very important. He used Zuo gui wan and You gui wan together to nourish source qi exhaustion. His thought was that wei suo was a form of source qi exhaustion manifesting as a result of severe kidney essence injury. He said that the kidney essence was failing to irrigate the whole body and that the blood, in part as a form of yuan qi derived directly from the essence, was failing to nourish the body. Since the muscles were failing to be nourished, the treatment principle was to nourish the essence and blood.

His treatment principle for every type of wei suo was to treat the stomach/spleen axis. He said this was necessary because the lung fluid came from stomach/spleen, the liver blood was also produced by the stomach/spleen, and the kidney essence was replenished by nutrients from the post-natal essence. He suggested that the herbs used be not too greasy because they would reduce the stomach/spleen function. He also said that the herbs be not too bitter or dry because they would injure the wei qi. He felt that exterior wind-releasing herbs were contraindicated because they are drying. Only in patients with excessive damp could exterior releasing wind herbs be used because they would dry damp.

Paclitaxel, a main example of an agent with this side effect, generally does not cause the same kinds of symptoms as other agents. There are few gastrointestinal symptoms and few symptoms of bone marrow suppression. The primary symptoms for most patients are muscle and joint pain, numbness and tingling in the extremities, depression and other mood changes. Although paclitaxel appears to cause a combination of wei syndrome and bi syndrome, it is usually treated primarily as a form of wei syndrome.

The following are simplified traditional classifications of this syndrome, and may correspond to the peripheral neuropathy induced by paclitaxel.[12]

1. Heat damages the lung and body fluids

This has a sudden onset, possible fever, dry skin, dry stools, dark, yellow and scanty urine. The tongue is red with a thin dry yellow coat. The pulse is rapid and thin. This is the classical presentation for poliomyelitis, an acute infectious disease. It may also be a clinical manifestation for the following conventional medical diagnoses: multiple sclerosis, poliomyelitis, myasthenia gravis, and progressive acute myelogenous leukemia (AML). A heat toxin, which has traditionally been an infectious warm febrile disease, but here may be chemical in origin, combines with dampness, which is environmental and affects the spleen/stomach axis and the liver/kidney axis. This affects the qi and blood. The lung qi is damaged and fails to distribute fluids to the whole body. As a result, the fluids are damaged and fail to nourish the extremities; this results in wei syndrome.

- Treatment principles: clear lung heat, moisten dryness, and nourish the lung and stomach.
- Formula: Qing zao jiu fei tang: to correct heat damaging the fluids, plus Sha shen mai dong tang: to correct fluid deficiency in the lung.

2. Damp heat macerates the flesh

This pattern has traditionally implied that there is an environmentally related problem and/or an improper diet. In either case the end result is injury to the stomach/spleen, which in turn creates damp heat and injury to the tendons and vessels caused by poor qi and blood circulation. There is commonly nerve damage. There may be slight swelling and a loss of sensation in the skin. Damp heat especially attacks the lower body. The tongue has a yellow and greasy coat. The pulse is slippery or soft.

Treatment principles: drain damp heat.
Formula: Si miao wan.

3. Stomach/spleen deficiency

If the stomach/spleen axis is weak or weakened by chronic debilitating disease or other injuries, it fails to produce enough qi and blood to nourish the tendons, muscles, and vessels, which leads to wei syndrome. Spleen/stomach deficiency may also exacerbate a pre-existing wei syndrome. This is one way of looking at stomach/spleen deficiency in this context.

Another approach is to view the Yangming, the stomach, spleen, and large intestine, as the sea of food and water. If the Yangming is weak, then the tendons are weak. If the Yangming has been weakened by damp heat, then it fails to produce enough qi and blood to nourish the tendons. This type of wei syndrome accompanies muscle atrophy and weakness, loose stools, and poor appetite.

Treatment principles: tonify the central qi and nourish the blood.
Formula: Shen ling bai zhu tang.

4. Liver and kidney yin deficiency

This pattern is found when there is chronic and debilitating disease or during the climacteric. It implies liver blood deficiency with kidney essence deficiency. The liver nourishes the tendons; the kidneys nourish the bone. There may be signs of perimenopause or menopause, dizziness, sore and weak low back and knees. The onset is usually gradual with increasing weakness or pain.

Treatment principles: tonify liver and kidney, nourish the yin, and clear heat.
Formula: Jian bu hu qian wan.

Portions of the above formulas can be added to the main formula being used during chemotherapy. Generally all of the above patterns, whether they are wei or bi in nature, are grossly identified by determining if the causative factor is internal or external in origin, yin or yang in nature, excess or deficient, and are characterised by wind, cold, damp, or heat symptoms. The complexity of wei suo and the identification of the specific disorder creates a variety of treatment principles. It is further complicated by the fact that each patient may report differences in their subjective symptoms. This may create a mixture of treatment principles that ends in a very individualised treatment.

In iatrogenic disease it is always difficult to define internal and external injury. Careful observation and questioning is very necessary in order to treat accurately and successfully. In the context of modern drug reactions, treatment becomes somewhat experimental. What is known is that prevention of onset of peripheral neuropathy is much easier to do than trying to resolve peripheral neuropathy that has already occurred. One combination of herbs seems to ameliorate this difficult side effect:

- gu sui bu (Drynariae Rhizoma; *Drynaria*)
- chuan xiong (Chuanxiong Rhizoma; *Ligusticum wallichii*)
- dan shen (Salviae miltiorrhizae Radix; *Salvia miltiorhiza*).

Acupuncture is traditionally used in the treatment of all wei and bi syndromes. Points carrying the strongest yang qi are chosen on the channels affected, and especially on the Yangming and Shaoyang channels. Additional points are added in relation to the diagnosis.

ANXIETY AND DEPRESSION

(Ma Shoucun, lecture notes, 1988.)

ANXIETY

Conventional medicine

Anxiety is a common condition accompanying the diagnosis of cancer. Patients bring themselves and their coping mechanisms and history to the treatment realm of any life-threatening illness. Treatment of the whole being is immensely important and valuable in the treatment of cancer. Maintaining a well spirit will enable patients to do better physically to survive the cancer. At the same time, receiving a potentially life-threatening diagnosis necessarily places one in different and possibly unfamiliar territory, territory that is fraught with painful anxiety, grief, and fear.

Anxiety states usually include panic disorder, generalised anxiety disorder, obsessive-compulsive disorder, and post-traumatic stress disorder. Anxiety is described as 'running at a high idle with the sympathetic nervous system inappropriately on alert'. This sympathetic response leads to an increased alertness for both mind and body. Mania has many of the same signs and symptoms, but is associated with a sense of wellbeing or euphoria.

Anxiety is a normal state when an individual is avoiding danger or is in the midst of a high-stress situation, and having a diagnosis of cancer is certainly a high-stress situation. However, patients' responses to diagnosis vary. This variation may be the result of underlying pathology prior to diagnosis, or the pathology may come about as a result of persistent anxiety. For example, it is not uncommon for a cancer patient to develop insomnia, exhaustion, panic attacks, increased heart and respiration rates, palpitations, and increased pain as a result of anxiety.

Conventional medicine treats anxiety with anxiolytics, many of which have their own set of complicating side effects. Many patients do not wish to add more drugs to their increasing arsenal of pharmaceuticals to treat the cancer and the side effects of other drugs. Therefore, being able to treat anxiety as part of one herbal formula is a great advantage, and helping a patient cope during this trial is immensely valuable.

Chinese medicine

Treating the spirit is part of the deeper tradition of Chinese medicine. The heart is thought of as the 'great void'; the only dwelling place for the spirits (spirits can only rest and dwell in a void). The art of the heart in Chinese philosophy is the way to obtain and conserve this void, which allows the various organ shen to be present and to impart spiritual essences and power to the blood. Therefore, the art of the heart becomes part of overall health. The heart, as a void, has the possibility of receiving spiritual influences in the form of shen. When a patient is diagnosed with a life-threatening illness like cancer, the need for a spiritual concentration of shen is immense. Those patients who can remain in control of their deeper destiny, even when they have lost control of their outer destiny, seem to do far better than those who cannot. The functions of the mind and heart are intricately interwoven and must be aligned so that internal and external life events may be accurately perceived.

Shen and jing have a deep relationship because the heart/kidney axis is the central axis of spiritual stability and power. This axis is contained and continues through all of the other yin and yang relationships of the zang fu. By restoring the communication between yin and yang, shen and jing, inner and outer, what is actually touched is the depth of all separations in that person's being. Helping to re-establish this relationship helps patients to know themselves better, and may provide a more profound opportunity for a peaceful passing or a deeper living, whether they survive physically or not.

When the shen is disturbed there is a scattering of qi. Anxiety is one manifestation of shen disturbance. It is caused by the irregular movement of qi, which then agitates the heart shen. Anxiety is traditionally linked to the heart and kidneys but can often be mixed with the emotional energies of other organ systems as well. Some people are more prone to anxiety than others. Anxiety manifests differently in different people depending upon which zang organs are involved and what type of agitation is occurring, that is, is it excess, deficient, or stasis.

Etiology

1. Excesses disturb and agitate the heart shen, causing it to be more irregularly active and intense.
   - Fire: results from heart fire combined with either liver or stomach fire. Suppressed emotions, smoking, alcohol, hot/greasy foods, lack of exercise and a hectic lifestyle are causative factors.
   - Phlegm fire: results from spleen deficiency and stasis giving rise to phlegm, which combines with heart fire.
2. Deficiencies all combine to create and intensify anxiety. Lack of sleep or rest, overwork, stress, illness, and malnutrition do not allow the shen to be adequately anchored by blood, yin, qi or essence.
   - Deficient heart qi: combines with deficient kidney and/or spleen qi.
   - Deficient heart blood.
   - Deficient heart yin: combines with kidney yin deficiency.
3. Stasis gives rise to irregularity of movement, which disturbs the free circulation of qi and shen. This can result in the accumulation of phlegm.
   - Heart qi stasis: combines with liver qi stasis, liver yang rising, or heart phlegm.

Clinical presentations

1. Anxiety and the heart.
   - Emotions: agitation, panic, hysteria.
   - Physical: insomnia, palpitations, hypertension, cardiac pain, pallor, cold extremities.
2. Anxiety and the kidneys: heart anxiety rooted in kidney fear.
   - Emotions: apprehension, fear, easily startled.
   - Physical: trembling, urinary frequency, loose stools.

3. Anxiety and the liver: combination of fear, anger, anxiety stemming from kidney, liver, and heart.
   - Emotions: fear, anger, anxiety, gall bladder – uncertainty, indecision, hypersensitivity.
   - Physical: headaches, stiffness, tremors, muscle and joint pain, insomnia.
4. Anxiety and the spleen: anxiety that interferes with the ability to think clearly.
   - Emotions: worry, anticipation of problems (real or imaginary), insecurity, fear.
   - Physical: digestive complaints, insomnia, fatigue, nausea.
5. Anxiety and the lungs: fear of loss, imagined or real, that manifests as grieving before an event that actually warrants it
   - Emotions: fear of loss.
   - Physical: asthma, difficulty breathing.

Patterns

1. Heart fire.
   Emotions: agitation, feelings of desparation, restlessness, quick movements, impulsive, can not concentrate.
   Physical: nervous talking, palpitations, red face, whole body heat.
   Tongue: red or dark red with dry yellow coat.
   Pulse: full and rapid.
   Treatment principles: clear heat, calm the spirit, nourish yin.
   Formula: Tian wang bu xin tang (heart/kidney disconnect), or Huang lian e jiao tang (fire from yin deficiency after illness).
2. Heart qi stasis.
   Emotions: anxiety, depression, irritability.
   Physical: sensation of epigastric and chest fullness (men), palpitations, chest constriction.
   Tongue: normal or slightly purple/dark.
   Pulse: wiry and/or full.
   Treatment principles: regulate the liver qi, calm the spirit.
   Formula: Xiao yao san, can add Suan zao ren tang.
3. Deficient heart qi.
   Emotions: exaggerated emotional response, anxiety.
   Physical: palpitations, conditions worse with fatigue, cold hands and feet.
   Tongue: pale.

Pulse: empty.

Treatment principles: tonify the source qi, tonify the qi and blood, calm the spirit.

Formula: Yang xin tang, or Bai zi yang xin tang, or Ding zhi wan.

4. Deficient heart blood.

Emotions: anxiety, poor memory, easily startled, sadness, confused, depressed, inability to concentrate.

Physical: palpitations, insomnia, fatigue, dizziness, pale face.

Tongue: pale and dry.

Pulse: thin, possibly choppy.

Treatment principles: nourish the blood, calm the spirit.

Formula: Tian wang bu xin tang or Suan zao ren tang

Herbal anxiolytics

Ashwagandha (*Withania somnifera*)
Kava (*Piper methysticum*)
Lemon grass (*Cymbopogon citratus*)
Panax ginseng: for anxiety due to stress
Ginkgo biloba extract
St John's wort (*Hypericum perforatum*): not to be taken concurrently with monoamine oxidase inhibitors
Siberian ginseng (*Eleutherococcus senticosus*)

DEPRESSION

Depression is a confusing term because both in conventional and Chinese medicine it is both a symptom and a diagnosis. When depression is used as a diagnostic category in Chinese medical terms it refers to two possible patterns: plum pit qi and organ agitation. When depression is used as a symptomatic expression of a certain psychoemotional state it can be part of an overall presentation in plum pit qi, organ agitation, and constraint disorder. All of these disorders have in common depression as a symptom, but their underlying etiology is not the same.

The ancient texts called the condition/symptom of depression 'knotted qi'. They said that the syndrome of depression was caused by the symptom of depression. Depression was said to be caused by a person thinking and worrying, which led to the spirit becoming trapped. The qi

was thought to follow the trapped spirit and this is how 'knotted qi' came about. According to the definition of this syndrome in the classic texts, it would be necessary for the individual's organ qi to be weak in order for knotted qi to happen. Therefore the scenario for depression would have the following etiology:

- depression is caused by excessive melancholy, pensiveness, and organ qi weakness
- the heart stores the spirit and controls thinking
- this syndrome can develop in any of the five organs and not just in the heart
- depending upon which organ has weakness, the condition will develop in that organ.

Therefore, if the spleen is weaker, then the qi will knot in that organ, and so on. The normal condition of the body is moderated and circulating throughout. As soon as a person begins to become depressed or sad this disrupts the regular movement of qi and blood. The organ that is weak acts like a magnet for this disruption of qi and blood flow. And the condition will develop in that organ. All organs have some relationship to the heart. The heart rules the blood and if the blood becomes weak, then this can affect the spirit since the heart stores the spirit. We often misunderstand this syndrome of depression as liver qi stagnation.

Depression has many indications:

- some patients tend towards melancholy
- some tend towards anger
- some tend towards fear
- some tend towards apprehension and doubt
- some tend towards insomnia.

To correctly diagnose depression, the individual symptoms of the patient must be made clear.

Depression symptoms and organ correlations are shown in Box 12.4.

A clear understanding of these emotional expressions can help us better understand patients' underlying patterns, and this can help us better treat them not only for emotional disorders but for all kinds of disorders.

Etiology and pathological mechanism for plum pit qi

Depression and anger injure the liver and excessive thinking injures the spleen. Liver qi stasis

Box 12.4 Depression symptoms and organ correlations

Tendency to cry	heart qi deficiency
Tendency to anger	liver qi stasis
Tendency to fear	kidney qi deficiency
Tendency to men	liver qi stasis or phlegm
Tendency to be quiet	yang qi deficiency
Tendency to apprehension	phlegm
Tendency to insomnia	phlegm, heart blood deficiency, liver fire blazing
Tendency to melancholy	heart qi deficiency, kidney yang deficiency

caused by depression and anger transforms into fire. Spleen stasis generates dampness. Together dampness and fire combine to form phlegm. The phlegm qi lodges or settles in the throat and leads to a sensation of something caught there that won't go away by swallowing or coughing. This is called plum pit qi. Plum pit qi is an excess and a deficient condition.

Treatment principles: dispel the phlegm, move the qi (which implies a descending direction), disperse the qi (which implies spreading the qi in all directions).
Formula: Ban xia hou pou tang

Etiology and pathological mechanism of organ agitation

Long-term depression (symptom) leads to reduced appetite, which leads to the qi and blood losing their source of nourishment. This loss of nourishment causes either spleen qi deficiency or kidney qi deficiency. Organ agitation has come to be understood as primarily a women's complaint and part of gynecology. This is because organ agitation refers to the heart being hurried and agitated, especially during the premenses. When this happens the shen is disturbed. The heart is the ruler of blood. When a woman is depressed and agitated during the premenses then certain symptoms express this agitation. For example, moodiness, crying and a craving for sweets are all

symptoms of the heart being pressed. Organ agitation is a syndrome of deficiency and is not an excess condition.

Treatment principles: tonify the qi, nourish the blood, calm the spirit.
Formula: Gan mai da zao tang.

There are three basic considerations to take into account regarding the diagnosis of depression:

- is the pattern one of excess or deficiency?
- what is the underlying constitution of the patient?
- are there accompanying problems?

Excess presentations of depression are much less prevalent and usually the liver and heart are involved. There is qi stasis, a floating and surging pulse, or wiry and forceful pulse. Anger and irritability are primary expressions involving more recent content.

Deficient presentations are far more prevalent. The content of the depression is not recent but often ancient and forgotten. There is underlying organ deficiency, a deep and fine pulse or a wiry but forceless pulse. The patient is quiet and melancholy. This type of melancholy or depression is more common in cancer patients. Whether or not this is to be the end of one's life, this time is frequently used to look back and resolve the past. It is a deeply meaningful time and can be used in many ways. Sometimes a patient appears depressed but is actually contemplative. It is very important to support the process of the patient, whatever that may be.

The constitution can reflect tendencies towards the knotting of qi. Yang deficiency more easily leads to knotted qi and the organ agitation type of depression. A phlegm-damp constitution more easily leads to the development of phlegm and plum pit qi depression.

Accompanying deficiency conditions can evolve into excess conditions like phlegm, dampness and blood stasis.

Provide comfort to these patients. Refer when necessary. Advise the patient to refrain from eating too many cold or uncooked foods, because these foods can exacerbate the problem of qi stasis by depleting the middle jiao function. Often needles and moxa combined are applied to back shu points in one treatment. Avoid dispersing points like P6, LV3, and CV17. In deficiency depression these points only scatter the qi, making the condition worse. If the patient cries on the treatment table, it may not be a sign of discharge but rather a sign that they have been improperly treated and are losing heart qi as a result.

Emotional constraint

Constraint has a very broad meaning and includes any form of stagnation. When speaking of emotional constraint the reference is to the stagnation of emotions where there is a blockage or lack of flow on the emotional level. Historically, constraint has been thought to affect all of the organs. The Neijing talks about constraint and how it can effect the lung, heart, liver, and so on.

There are six different types of constraint described by the Yuan Dynasty. These include:

- qi constraint
- damp constraint
- heat constraint
- lung constraint
- blood constraint
- food constraint.

Emotional constraint can cause any one of these constraint syndromes, depending on which organ or level of disease attracts injury.

Emotional constraint is often accompanied by a change in perception regarding pain. Therefore, it is important when differentiating pain syndromes to understand if a psychological or emotional problem is the cause of the pain or disease or if it is the result of the pain or disease. This problem in differentiation is especially important in cancer treatment. Later stages of cancer can cause pain due to obstruction. This same pain can be exacerbated by emotional constraint and anxiety. Often there are two levels of treatment in pain management in cancer patients. One is the physical cause of the pain, the other is the emotional constraint contributing to the pain.

If a person is in chronic pain, they will often develop constraint. In conventional medicine, this would be a form of depression and some types of pain are treated with antidepressants. The question becomes whether a patient has pain because of a psychological predisposition or whether being in pain for long periods of time causes psychological problems. This is often difficult to discover but it makes a difference in the way that the patient is treated.

If a patient has a psychological problem as the underlying cause of pain, or another disease, then it is important to get to the root of the problem in order to treat the pain. Paying attention to this, especially when looking at treatment failures by looking at why a patient did not improve when the case should have been easy to treat, may demonstrate that we did not treat the appropriate level of the emotions.

If a patient has pain and this causes a depressive emotional state, the condition should be easier to treat than one caused by an emotional problem as the root cause. The differentiation between a physical cause for pain and a psychological cause for pain can be discerned with the following clues:

- many patients with constraint will often interpret relaxation as a more intense throbbing and discomfort than a release and relief
- many patients with constraint will interpret all sensations as uncomfortable and negative
- if you are convinced that your needling technique, for example, is correct and the patient becomes more uncomfortable during treatment, this is a sign of constraint
- if you treat a patient for pain and you feel your treatment is correct but there is no improvement, this may be a sign of constraint as the problem rather than a physical injury

Emotional constraint is primarily a pathology of the liver and gall bladder and is related to a lack of the free-flowing and spreading function of the liver. Constraint is the accurate diagnosis for the symptom of depression when accompanied by liver qi stagnation. With liver constraint you will often see heart problems as a result of shen cycle flow injury and spleen problems as a result of ko cycle flow injury.

When the spleen is adversely affected by the liver then the transformation and transportation function is affected. This result in the formation of dampness and phlegm. This is a qi problem. When the heart is affected by the liver this is a mother/child relationship. The heart loses its nourishment and this leads to a blood level problem.

In early-stage constraint there is a qi level problem that results in phlegm and dampness. As this constraint evolves it can develop into heat depending on the person's constitution. As this problem progresses, more damage to the qi will be seen, which then produces a blood level problem. In severe cases, constraint can lead to a form of consumption due to blood exhaustion. Consumption is a group of disorders marked by some chronic process that has consumed qi and blood. This process can result from many things including overwork, chronic blood stasis, which prevents the generation of new blood, and so on. This condition is usually marked by fatigue combined with other fairly severe symptoms. Emotional constraint can lead not only to mental illness but also to chronic and serious illness. In a cancer patient it is very important to treat this condition, which is often called depression.

There are two types of emotional constraint; excess and deficient. It is common to see aspects of both together. When looking at a patient with constraint it is important to find not only the cause but also what is the environment for the problem. For example, the constitutional make-up, a chronic deficiency, a particular life event like giving birth or being diagnosed with cancer, all work together with the pattern for emotional constraint to manifest in a particular way.

Excess constraint

Etiology: chronic frustration, intense anger, both of which lead to stagnation of emotions and qi.
Main indications: the patient is constantly wound up, there is chronic irritability, there is hypochondrium tightness when emotions occur, there is distention and pain in the chest and flanks that is not fixed in location.
Tongue: thin body and greasy coat.
Pulse: wiry and forceful.
Treatment principle: focus on smoothing the liver qi.
Formula: Shu gan wan.

With this type of constraint, treating liver qi stasis as an excess condition is correct. Using moving and dispersing points in acupuncture treatment is appropriate.

Deficiency constraint

In this presentation the patient is disoriented or confused. They are upset as opposed to angry. The patient feels melancholy and sadness; they are withdrawn, crying and sighing.

Tongue: pale body with a thin coating.
Pulse: thin and possibly wiry but forceless.
Treatment principle: tonify the spleen to nourish liver blood.
Formula: this is a true Xiao yao san presentation.

CANCER PAIN SYNDROMES[13]

The World Health Organization (WHO) states that 25% of all cancer patients die with unrelieved pain. Pain is a sensory and a physical symptom. Parallel neural pathways transmit stimuli from the periphery, through the spinal cord, to multiple areas in the brain. Pain signals, or nociceptive inputs, are localised and interpreted, and the affective component assigned at the cerebral cortical level. Modulation of nociceptive input by opioid and non-opioid mechanisms occurs in the periphery, at the dorsal horn of the spinal cord, in the brainstem, and possibly in higher centers.

In conventional medicine, pain is classified and this classification forms the basis for therapeutic choices. Nociceptive pain relates broadly to that with ongoing tissue damage. Neuropathic pain is caused by nervous system dysfunction in the absence of ongoing tissue damage.

Damage to the nervous system may result in pain in an area of reduced sensation. This pain is usually described as burning or lancinating. Patients often complain of bizarre symptoms like painful numbness, itching pain, or crawling sensations. Most commonly, psychological factors affect the reporting of pain but not the pain itself. Chronic unrelieved pain has psychological consequences but is not a psychiatric disease.

Cancer pain varies by tumor type and is related to patterns of tumor growth and metastasis. Pain can also be related directly to antineoplastic therapy and is sometimes unrelated to the neoplasm.

There are subgroupings of patients with cancer pain. These include:

- patients with acute cancer-related pain, which includes that associated with the cancer and that associated with treatment for the cancer
- patients with chronic cancer-related pain, which includes that associated with cancer progression and with cancer therapy
- patients with pre-existing chronic pain and cancer-related pain
- patients with a history of drug addiction with cancer-related pain who include those actively involved in illicit drug use, or in a methadone treatment program, or with a past history of drug abuse
- patients who are in the process of dying with cancer-related pain.

All of the above factors are taken into account when determining how to manage pain in a cancer patient. The steps used to make this decision include:

- determine if primary antineoplastic therapy is needed for pain palliation
- tailor the pharmacological analgesia to the individual
- consider concurrent non-pharmacological methods
- monitor for response and modify if necessary.

The WHO has a three-step analgesic ladder, which progresses from non-opioid analgesics to opioid analgesics and adjuvants for progressively severe pain. There is a ceiling to the effects of non-opioid drugs, and exceeding these maximum dose ranges can result in organ toxicity especially of the liver, kidneys and gastrointestinal tract.

There are many opiate-derived analgesics, including many morphine agonists, meperidine, methadone, oxycodone, fentanyl, nalbuphine, pentazocine, and codeine. Adjuvant drugs used for pain include steroids, such as prednisolone, dexamethasone, and progestin, antidepressants such as amitriptyline and imipramine, anxiolytics such as hydroxyzine and diazepam, phenothiazines such as haloperidol and chlorpromazine, and anticonvulsants such as carbamazepine and phenytoin. Amphetamines are also used.

Transcutaneous electrical nerve stimulation (TENS) is also used, as a neuroablative procedure. On occasion a nerve will be surgically severed to reduce pain in a terminally ill patient.

CHINESE MEDICINE

The treatment of pain with herbal medicine is complex. There are many causes and many interventions. Some pain may be due to inflammatory processes from the cancer itself; some is due to compression of nerves and other structures by the tumor tissue; some may be due to tumor metabolites stimulating nerve tissue abnormally. It is important to treat the underlying condition causing the pain.

The treatment principles to alleviate pain will include objectives that:

- activate circulation
- regulate and invigorate blood
- regulate and move the qi
- dredge the channels that are blocked
- eliminate heat
- detoxify static fire toxin
- nourish yin
- clear blood heat
- calm and tranquilise
- invigorate the spleen
- benefit the spleen and kidney yang
- clear dampness and heat and reduce swelling.

Herbal analgesics are added to the main formula in order to address the chief area of diagnostic concern. For example, if the pain is primarily due to blood stasis and blood heat, then herbs are added that clear blood heat and move blood. If the pain is due to edematous swelling, as in ascites, then herbs are added that move blood and drain damp. If the pain is mainly in the upper jiao due to obstruction or atelectasis, then the diagnosis for the presenting symptoms is addressed by adding herbs that treat that specific chest presentation including herbs that will adjust the qi of the lung.

Herbs commonly used to treat pain include:

- xi yang shen (Panacis quinquefolii Radix; *Panax quinquefolium*)
- long dan cao (Gentianae Radix; *Gentiana*)
- wei ling xian (Clematidis Radix; *Clematis chinensis*)
- chi shao (Paeoniae Radix rubra; *Paeonia lactiflora* root)
- yu jin (Curcumae Radix; *Curcuma longa* rhizome)

- yan hu suo (Corydalis Rhizoma; *Corydalis yanhusuo*)
- bai zhi (Angelicae dahuricae Radix; *Angelica dahurica*)
- chuan xiong (Chuanxiong Rhizoma; *Ligusticum wallichii* root)
- mu xiang (Aucklandiae Radix; *Saussurea*)
- ru xiang (Olibanum; *Boswellia sacra*; frankincense; gum olibanum)
- mo yao (Myrrha; *Commiphora myrrha*; myrrh)

Almost all blood-cracking herbs are analgesic, and many herbs that enter the liver and move qi and blood are analgesic.

Patients with later stage cancer are often unable to take food or fluids, including herbal medicine. Acupuncture, moxibustion and other techniques are valuable substitutes.

When using acupuncture to treat pain there are some contraindications:

- When bone pain is present in the vertebral column it is important to understand if a protective muscle spasm is actually stabilising the vertebral column. Needling this juncture may destabilise the vertebra, causing damage to the spinal column.
- Avoid needling areas of lymphedema because there is increased risk of infection, not from the needle but via the hole made by the needle.
- Coagulopathies indicated by a high normalised ratio or low platelets may result in atypical bruising.
- Electroacupuncture is contraindicated in patients with a pacemaker.
- Do not needle into areas where there is malignant infiltration.

A segmental approach to pain treatment is used and Yangming channel points are selected just as in treating a Bi syndrome. Front and back points can be used during one treatment. The same points are selected as would be in other circumstances. In treating shingles, segmental paraspinal points are selected along with LI4 and LV3.

The greater the tumor burden, the shorter the length of pain relief. If the metastatic spread is successfully treated and the tumor burden is lessened, then the length of acupuncture pain relief will revert back to its original length of time.

Acupuncture also works well for other non-pain related conditions. These include:

- dyspnea
- anxiety
- nausea and vomiting
- dysphagia
- radiation rectitis
- lower limb deep vein thrombosis (DVT)
- stroke and during brain tumor rehabilitation
- flushing
- abdominal pain
- decubitus ulcers
- constipation from pain medications.

PLEURAL EFFUSION

Pleural effusion is a complication commonly seen in lung cancer and in cancers that metastasise to the lungs. The term refers to fluid accumulation in the thoracic cavity. A pleural effusion makes a curative resection more difficult. It can lead to reduced cardiac and pulmonary function as the fluid accumulates and applies pressure to the organs. Atelectasis occurs when the fluid pressure against the lung actually makes it collapse. The collapse can involve a large or a small area of the lung lobe. Repeated infection also can evolve from a pleural effusion, and pneumonia is a common cause of death in patients with a pleural effusion.

Fluid accumulation due to a primary or metastatic tumor in the lung is difficult to treat with conventional medicine. Draining of the fluid is done by thoracentesis during which a hollow needle or tube is placed through the chest wall and the fluid is drained manually. Needle thoracentesis is used when less fluid is present. A temporary indwelling tube can be placed. The fluid drained contains blood and tumor cells along with WBCs and serum plasma. The thoracentesis must be repeated as the fluid continues to accumulate. Diuretic drugs can be given to reduce the fluid buildup but the mechanical means of draining is the primary method in intermediate to large effusions. Until the cancer itself is reduced the need will persist to intervene and drain the pleural effusion.

CHINESE MEDICINE[14]

Pleural effusion is called 'suspended fluids', or xuan yin, in Chinese medicine. The distribution and excretion of water and jin ye depends primarily on the San Jiao function. It is the external fu organ and governs qi transformation for the entire body. It manages the routes for transportation and movement of water, food and jin ye. In cancer, tumors can affect qi transformation in the San Jiao and impair its diffusing function. This also can affect the yang, which leads to yang deficiency. Then water and jin ye do not move well, resulting in the collection of retained fluids. The mechanism for fluid retention was first put forward in the Sheng Ji Zong Lu (The General Collection for Holy Relief).

The lungs control water regulation in the upper jiao, the spleen in the middle, and the kidneys in the lower jiao. If the functions of the San Jiao are impaired, the lungs cannot regulate the water passages properly and the spleen then becomes injured, losing some of its transportation function. The kidneys fail to steam and transform water, which results in retained fluids, or xuan yin. Tumors that affect the lungs, spleen and kidneys can all lead to pleural effusion.

The spleen plays a vital role in transporting fluids and if the yang of the spleen is deficient then the essence cannot be transported upward to nourish the lungs and this, in turn, results in water and food not transformed properly. Phlegm will form and dry the lungs. The spleen will not be able to help the kidneys in governing water and pathogenic water and cold will damage the kidney yang. Water and fluids will then accumulate in the middle jiao and flood. The flooding can penetrate between the skin and the membranes, form in the hypochondrium and then lead to a pleural effusion. Therefore, pleural effusion is generally caused by lung qi deficiency and yang deficiency of the spleen and kidneys, which impairs the qi transformation function so that water and jin ye accumulate. Middle jiao yang and qi deficiency is the basic internal pathology. If water is yin then it must be moved by yang. If yang is deficient, the qi cannot transform jin ye. Yin accumulates and cold fluids collect internally.

Patterns for pleural effusion

Heat or cold attacking the chest and lungs

Symptoms: pleural effusion with alternating fever and chills, general low-grade fever, no sweating, or fever with aversion to cold, fever does not resolve the condition, cough with no phlegm, rapid breathing, stabbing pain in the chest made worse with inhalation and with rotating trunk, dry throat.
Tongue: red with yellow or thin coat.
Pulse: wiry and rapid.

This is a combination presentation that requires harmonising the Sahoyang, clearing heat, transforming phlegm and opening the chest.
Formula: Chai zhi ban xia tang jia jian

chai hu (Bupleuri Radix; *Bupleurum*)	10 g
huang qin (Scutellariae Radix; *Scutellaria baicalensis*)	10 g
gua lou shi (Trichosanthis Fructus; *Trichosanthes* fruit)	15 g
zhi ban xia (Pinelliae Rhizoma preparatum; *Pinellia ternata* rhizome)	10 g
zhi ke (Aurantii Fructus; *Citrus aurantium*)	10 g
jie geng (Platycodi Radix; *Platycodon grandiflorus* root)	10 g
chi shao (Paeoniae Radix rubra; *Paeonia lactiflora* root)	10 g

Retained fluids collecting in the chest

Symptoms: pain on coughing, expectorating, difficult inhalation, dyspnea, wheezing, rales, can lie only on the side of the effusion.
Tongue: pale with thin white or greasy white coat.
Pulse: deep and wiry, or wiry and slippery.
Formula: Shi zao tang.

gan sui (Kansui Radix; *Euphorbia kansui*)	10 g
jing da ji (Euphorbiae pekinensis Radix; *Euphorbia pekinensis*)	10 g
yuan hua (Genkwa Flos; *Daphne genkwa*)	10 g
da zao (Jujubae Fructus; *Ziziphus jujuba*; jujube)	30 g

Special herbs that drain fluids from the chest and lungs include:

ting li zi (Lepidii Semen; *Lepidium* seed)
sang bai pi (Mori Cortex; *Morus alba*)
jiao mu (Zanthoxyli Semen; *Zanthoxylum*)
fu ling (Poria; *Poria cocos*)

sheng jiang pi (Zingiberis Rhizomatis Cortex; *Zingiber officinale*; fresh peel)

tong cao (Tetrapanacis Medulla; *Tetrapanax papyriferus*)

lu lu tong (Liquidambaris Fructus; *Liquidambar formosana*)

dong gua pi (Benincasae Exocarpium; *Benincasa hispida* exocarp)

Disharmony of qi in the network vessels

Symptoms: pleural effusion with pain in the chest and hypochondrium, mun (chest oppression), burning and stabbing pain, inhibited inhalation.
Tongue: dark red with thin or no coat.
Pulse: wiry.
Formula: Xiang fu xuan fu hua tang jia jian.

xuan fu hua (Inulae Flos; *Inula* flowers [wrapped])	10 g
su zi (Perillae Fructus; *Perilla frutescens*)	10 g
ku xing ren (Armeniacae Semen amarum; *Prunus armeniaca*)	10 g
zhi ban xia (Pinelliae Rhizoma preparatum; *Pinellia ternata* rhizome)	10 g
yi ren (Coicis Semen; *Coix lacryma-jobi*)	30 g
fu ling (Poria; *Poria cocos*)	15 g
xiang fu (Cyperi Rhizoma; *Cyperus rotundus* rhizome)	10 g
chen pi (Citri reticulatae Pericarpium; *Citrus reticulata* pericarp)	10 g

The above formula regulates the qi, transforms phlegm, and harmonises the network vessels.

Internal heat due to yin deficiency

Symptoms: pleural effusion and intermittent choking cough, expectoration of sticky phlegm, dry mouth and throat, tidal fevers, red cheeks, irritability, five center heat, night sweating, mun, emaciation.
Tongue: red with no coat.
Pulse: small and rapid.
Formula: Sha shen mai dong tang he Xie bai jia jian.

bei sha shen (Glehniae Radix; *Glehnia*)	10 g
mai dong (Ophiopogonis Radix; *Ophiopogon*)	15 g
yu zhu (Polygonati odorati Rhizoma; *Polygonatum odoratum*)	15 g
tian hua fen (Trichosanthis Radix; *Trichosanthes* root)	15 g
sang bai pi (Mori Cortex; *Morus alba*)	15 g
di gu pi (Lycii Cortex; *Lycium*)	15 g
gan cao (Glycyrrhizae Radix; *Glycyrrhiza*; licorice root)	6 g

The above formula nourishes yin and clears heat. The Xie bai tang portion bears fire downward and is used for a choking cough, dypsnea, and heat steaming to the skin and flesh.

EXTERNAL TREATMENT[15]

Herbs that transform blood stasis, disperse masses, aromatically open the orifices, and expel water and retained fluids are used in combination to relieve pressure on the blood vessels and lymphatics. This allows for greater movement within the vessels and helps the resorption of jin ye in the thoracic cavity. The lungs are relieved and pain is lessened.
Powder very finely:

da huang (Rhei Radix et Rhizoma; *Rheum*)	6 g
jing da ji (Euphorbiae pekinensis Radix; *Euphorbia pekinensis*)	6 g
bing pian (Borneolum; *Dryobalanops aromatica*; borneol)	10 g
san qi (Notoginseng Radix; *Panax notoginseng*)	6 g
shan ci gu* (Cremastrae/Pleiones Pseudobulbus; *Cremastra/Pleione* pseudobulb)	10 g
e zhu (Curcumae Rhizoma; *Curcuma zedoaria*; zedoary)	6 g

Infuse these ingredients in castor oil of high quality and purity (not rancid) at very low heat for 1 hour. Cool and refrigerate. For each application warm the infusion or a small portion. Warm the area above the location of the effusion and open the pores of the skin by warming with a hot washcloth. This opens the pores of the skin. Apply a thick slather over the warmed area. Quickly spread Saran wrap or some such non-porous product to act as a barrier so that the castor oil will not flow outward. Then cover the entire area with a warm towel and then apply a hot water bottle for 2 hours. Do this procedure twice daily. Combine this technique with the oral decoction according to the pattern diagnosis.

ASCITES

Ascites is an accumulation of fluid in the abdominal cavity. The most common disorders that cause ascites are chronic liver disease, tumors, and congestive heart failure. Physical signs include bulging of the flanks and shifting percussion dullness of the abdomen when the patient shifts to one side. Laying one's hand on the abdomen and pressing downward and to one side will elicit a visible wave motion.

Diagnostic paracentesis is usually performed by drawing 50 ml of fluid and analysing the fluid for protein content, amylase, cell count and differential, bacterial and fungal cultures, and cytologic examination. On the basis of protein concentration, ascitic fluids are divided into exudates or transudates. Inflammatory reactions from tumors are usually exudative in nature. Bloody ascitic fluid suggests a neoplasm. Ascites frequently happens in chronic liver disease and is the result of complex processes.

Metastatic disease in the abdomen from any tumor, including lymphoma and leukemia, can cause exudative ascites. Transudative ascites is a risk when veno-occlusive disease (VOD) is present. VOD often accompanies leukemia and treatment for leukemia. Infiltrative processes of the liver caused by tumors can cause ascites. Increased abdominal pressure may affect venous return causing DVT and damage to the heart, lung and kidney functions. Susceptibility to infection is increased and can lead to bacterial peritonitis, lung infection, and other infections. Because of these issues, ascites is a difficult but important condition to treat. Lack of treatment or failure in treatment for ascites can lead to death.

Ascites is a kind of abdominal effusion. However, unlike a pleural effusion, paracentesis is not considered good treatment because it can lead to hypovolemia, hypokalemia, hyponatremia, and renal failure. Ascites fluid contains between 10 and 30 g protein in each liter of fluid. Draining this fluid through centesis can deplete the serum albumin, promoting the reaccumulation of fluid. If ascites causes severe respiratory difficulty, then paracentesis might be performed.

About 5–10% of patients with ascites also develop pleural effusions, especially in the right hemithorax. Salt restriction and diuretics are the best approach to treatment. Too rapid diuresis can lead to severe electrolyte imbalance.

CHINESE MEDICINE

Ascites comes under the category of diseases called gu zhang, or drum distention. Liver, spleen and kidney functions are all impaired by the metastatic spread of tumors in the abdomen or by primary abdominal tumors. This results in qi and blood stasis and water accumulation in the abdomen.

Liver qi stasis leads to general li stasis, which inhibits the movement of blood. The blood vessels and network vessels of the blood and liver are intermingled. This creates a situation in which a vicious cycle of stasis can feed upon itself. It also causes a transverse rebellion injuring the spleen, which then fails to transform and transport fluids. Fluids accumulate and fight with blood stasis. Fluid and blood stasis block the middle jiao and gradually this affects the kidneys leading to gu zhang.

The patterns for ascites are excess and deficiency. When the liver, spleen and kidneys are all impaired this means that any deficiency will be severe in patients manifesting with this pattern. At the same time, stasis of blood and fluid in the abdomen with no transforming power for water and dampness means that excesses will be severe for patients manifesting an excess pattern. Ascites patterns are characterised by root deficiency and manifestation excess. Treatment requires a differentiation of this complex in terms of percentage of deficiency and percentage of excess.

Patterns

Excess type

Symptoms: abdominal distention, rolling fluid accumulation, possibly hard lumps in the abdomen, anorexia, pale complexion, frequent but scant urination, loose stools or constipation.

Tongue: pale body with white greasy or yellow greasy coat.

Pulse: soggy and moderate or deep and wiry.

Formula: Si jun zi tang he Wu ling san jia jian.

additions:

yi ren (Coicis Semen; *Coix lacryma-jobi*)	30 g
e zhu (Curcumae Rhizoma; *Curcuma zedoaria*; zedoary)	15 g
long kui (Solani nigri Herba; *Solanum nigrum*)	15 g
ban zhi lian (Scutellariae barbatae Herba; *Scutellaria barbata*)	20 g

Deficiency type

Symptoms: abdominal distention and distending pain, worse in the evening, jaundice, anorexia, fatigue, hardly moving, cold limbs with lower extremity edema, very little urination, thin and loose stools.

Tongue: pale or purple, swollen, white greasy coat.

Pulse: deep and thready, forceless.

Formula: Ji sheng qi wan jia jian.

Additions:

chen pi (Citri reticulatae Pericarpium; *Citrus reticulata* pericarp)	10 g
huai niu xi (Achyranthis bidentatae Radix; *Achyranthes bidentata*)	10 g
shen qu (Massa medicata fermentata; medicated leaven)	30 g
long kui (Solani nigri Herba; *Solanum nigrum*)	20 g
bai hua she she cao (Hedyotis diffusae Herba; *Oldenlandia*)	30 g

Deficient liver and kidney yin

Symptoms: distention and fullness with an enlarged abdomen, cachexia, anorexia, fatigue, irritability, dry mouth, little urination, constipation.

Tongue: dry red or crimson.

Pulse: deep and wiry or thready and rapid.

Formula: Liu wei di huang wan jia jian.

Additions:

fu ling (Poria; *Poria cocos*)	15 g
zhu ling (Polyporus; *Polyporus – Grifola*)	15 g
chen pi (Citri reticulatae Pericarpium; *Citrus reticulata* pericarp)	10 g
lai fu zi (Raphani Semen; *Raphanus sativus*)	15 g
long kui (Solani nigri Herba; *Solanum nigrum*)	20 g
bai ying (Solani lyrati Herba; *Solanum lyratum*)	15 g

External application:

huang qi (Astragali Radix; *Astragalus membranaceus*)	60 g
qian niu zi (Pharbitidis Semen; *Pharbitis*)	20 g
gan cao (Glycyrrhizae Radix; *Glycyrrhiza*; licorice root)	15 g
zhu ling (Polyporus; *Polyporus – Grifola*)	20 g
e zhu (Curcumae Rhizoma; *Curcuma zedoaria*; zedoary)	30 g
tao ren (Persicae Semen; *Prunus* seed)	15 g
yi ren (Coicis Semen; *Coix lacryma-jobi*)	60 g

Double decoct the above ingredients. Add starch or some similar medium and make a paste of the liquid. Spread the paste on the disinfected abdomen about 1–2 mm thick. If the liver area is grossly tense, do not apply over this area. Cover with Saran wrap or some equivalent to keep the paste moist and also immobile. Change the dressing and the application once per day. You may leave in place all day and night.

References

1. Treseler K. Clinical laboratory and diagnostic tests. Norwalk, CT: Appleton and Lange; 1995.

2. Groopman JE. Hemopoietic growth factors. N Engl J Med 1989; 321:1449–1469.

3. Han Rui. Zhong liu hua xue yu fang ji yao wu zhi liao (Chemical drugs and preparations in the prevention and treatment of tumors). Beijing: Beijing Medical University and Peking Union Medical University Joint Press; 1992.

4. Liao Junxian. Study of the pathology of ultrastructural changes in bone marrow induced by formulae for supplementing the kidneys and invigorating the blood. Shi Yong Zhong Xi Yi Jie He Za Zhi 1991; 4:731.

5. Lang Weijun. Kang Ai Zhong Yao Yi Qian Fang (One thousand anti-cancer prescriptions). Beijing: Traditional Chinese Medicine and Materia Medica Science and Technology Publishing House; 1992.

6. Mitchell EP. Gastrointestinal toxicity of chemotherapeutic agents. Semin Oncol 1992; 19:566–579.

7. Wang Yusheng. Zhong Yao Yao Li Yu Ying Yong (Pharmacology and applications of Chinese materia medica, 2nd edn). Beijing: People's Medical Publishing House; 1998.

8. Yang Zongming. Zhong Yao Ji En Xi Tong Yu Fang Fang Hua Liao E xing Ou Tu Fan Ying 50 Li (Combination of Chinese materia medica and ondansetron in the treatment of 50 cases of severe nausea and vomiting caused by chemotherapy and radiotherapy). Zhong Guo Zhong Yi Xi Jie He Za Zhi 2000; 20:58.

9. Wang Xiaoming. Bian Zheng Zhi Liao Zhong Liu Hua Liao Ji Qi Du Fu Fan Ying (Treatment based on pattern identification for 108 cases of toxic side effects caused by chemotherapy for tumors). Liao ning Zhong Yi Za Zhi 1994; 21:117–119.

10. Liu Li. Qi Ji Tang Han Fu Zhi Liao Hua Liao Bing Ren Kou Qiang Kui Yang Lin Chuang Guan Cha (Clinical observation of a formula in the treatment of patients with mouth ulcers caused by chemotherapy). Shan Xi Hu Li Za Zhi 1999; 2:2.

11. Wang Yongyan. Xian Dai Zhong Yi Nei Ke Xue (Modern traditional Chinese medicine internal medicine). Beijing: People's Medical Publishing House; 1999.

12. Sun Peilin. The treatment of pain with Chinese herbs and acupuncture. Edinburgh: Churchill Livingstone; 2002.

13. Enck R. The medical care of terminally ill patients. Baltimore: Johns Hopkins University Press; 1994.

14. Li Peiwen. Zhi Tong Xiao Shui Fang De Zhi Tong Yuan Li (Principle of alleviating pain in formulae for alleviating pain and dispersing water). J TCM 1991:11.

15. Li Peiwen. Zhong Yao Xiao Shui Gai Zhi Liao Ai Xing Fu Shui 120 Li Lin Chuang Ji Shi Yan Yan Ji U (Clinical and experimental study of Xiao Shui Gao in the treatment of 120 cases of ascites as a complication of cancer). Zhong Yi Za Zhi 2000; 41:358–359.

Chapter 13

Death and Dying

CHAPTER CONTENTS

Introduction   331

How we die – the Western approach   331

General symptoms of dying patients   333
   Nausea and vomiting   333
   Anorexia and cachexia   333
   Dehydration   333
   Constipation   334
   CNS symptoms   334
   Depression   334
   Dyspnea   334
   Urinary incontinence   334
   Pressure sores   335

The time of death   335

The process of dying   336
   The outer dissolution   337
   The inner dissolution   337

The pulses   337

Conclusions   338

> Poles apart, I'm the color of dying,
> You're the color of being born.
> Unless we breathe in each other,
> There can be no garden.
>
> Kahlil Gibran

INTRODUCTION

The emergence of the hospice movement in the 1980s – to a large extent in response to the HIV/AIDS epidemic, plus the rising rates of the incidence of cancer, and the rising rates of chronic disease in an aging population – clearly focused for the public the medical community's deficiencies in dealing with end-of-life issues for terminal patients. It has been primarily a patient-based community impetus that has driven physicians to become more knowledgeable and humane in caring for dying patients. As a result, a great deal of research has been and is being conducted in this area of medicine. The most recent pressure on the medical community regarding terminal patients is that of euthanasia and other medical ethics problems, for which answers are not currently available.

HOW WE DIE – THE WESTERN APPROACH

There are many ways in which an individual can die physiologically.[1] Depending on the cause of death, a varying cascade of events occurs. For example, in trauma or septic shock, a predictable series of events occurs that very much resembles hypovolemic or cardiogenic shock. If this shock does not respond to treatment, then the vital organs fail one after the other. The occurrence of septic shock is not restricted to subjects of trauma. It can also be seen in advanced diabetes, cancer, pancreatitis, cirrhosis, and in extensive burns. In an environment where the patient's defense mechanisms have become seriously impaired, septic shock kills between 40 and 60% of patients. Septic shock is the leading cause of death in intensive care units in the United States.[2]

Several things happen in septic shock that can lead to death.[3] Once the lung has lost some of its ability to oxygenate the blood and the circulation is impaired by a generally depressed myocardium then pooling begins to happen in the vessels of the gut. At this point several organs begin to demonstrate the effects of decreased nourishment. The liver loses its ability to make some of the compounds the body needs and to destroy some of those it does not. Liver failure compounds a simultaneous depression of the immune system. At the same time, the decreased blood flow to the kidneys prevents proper filtering and results in an inadequate urinary output and gradually worsening uremia, causing toxicity in the blood.

The cells lining the stomach and intestine begin to die with resulting ulcerations and bleeding. Shock, kidney failure, and gastrointestinal bleeding are often the final events in people who die from the syndrome of post-traumatic multiple organ failure. Multiple organ failure is the endpoint of sepsis. All of the characteristics of this syndrome seem to be caused by the effects of toxins on various organs. Mortality is related to the number of organs affected. If three are involved, mortality is close to 100%. The entire process usually takes 2–3 weeks.[3]

The lethal events follow a predictable pattern. First there is fever, rapid pulse, and respiratory distress. An endotracheal tube is usually inserted, but is commonly of no benefit. If the patient is not already sedated, the level of consciousness will begin to fluctuate. Scans and studies are performed to find the source of the infection, often in vain. Antibiotics are started, changed and stopped, with the hope that some treatable germ

will finally be identified. In only about 50% of patients with multiple organ failure will study of the blood yield microbes that can be grown in a laboratory culture.[3]

Variations in the elements of the blood begin to appear, including the clotting mechanism. Spontaneous bleeding may occur. Liver failure may produce jaundice and the kidneys begin to fail. The patient and the family often begin to wonder if the relief given justifies the discomfort and invasiveness of treatment. At this point, often a process of depersonalisation may set in, where hospital staff and doctors and sometimes family begin to separate from the patient. The patient becomes less of a person and more of a medical problem to be solved.

Finally, the patient, if lucky, will enter a state of minimal responsiveness or coma. The treatment team separates more from the patient and focuses on the family and providing comfort to the family. At the end, there is a sense of relief from caregivers and family.[3]

In cancer patients, specifically, death takes a general route, depending on the type of cancer. Nutritional depletion results in cachexia, which is characterised by muscle wasting, weakness, poor appetite, and alterations in metabolism.[4] Changes in taste perception not caused by chemotherapy are common.[5] Abnormalities in the utilisation of carbohydrates, fats, and proteins also occur. The cause is not yet understood. The malignant cells release a substance called cachectin, which decreases appetite by direct action on the brain's feeding center. Tumors of all sorts release various hormone-like substances, which produce generalised effects on nutrition, immunity, and other vital functions, that until recently were attributed to the parasitic effects of the tumor's growth.[6]

Usually, when the body goes into a fasting state fat stores are utilised. However, in cancer this process is not effective and so protein is taken up from the muscle mass. The decreased protein levels contribute to the dysfunction of organs and enzyme systems and significantly affect immunity. This depressed immunocompetence, when magnified by chemotherapy and radiation, increases susceptibility to infection.

Pneumonia and abscesses, and urinary and other infections are frequently the immediate causes of death of cancer patients, and sepsis is their common terminal event. The profound weakness of severe cachexia does not permit effective coughing, expectoration and respiration, increasing the chances of pneumonia and aspiration of emesis. The final hours are sometimes accompanied by deep, gurgling respirations, called the death rattle, especially in patients who remain hydrated.[7]

In the end, the decreased volume of circulating blood and extracellular fluid leads to a gradual decrease in blood pressure. This either leads to shock or to liver and kidney failure. In elderly cancer patients, these depletions can lead to stroke, myocardial infarction, or heart failure.

GENERAL SYMPTOMS OF DYING PATIENTS

NAUSEA AND VOMITING

Nausea and vomiting occur even in patients who are not undergoing chemotherapy. The mechanism for this is not yet clear. Nausea and vomiting are reported more often in patients with stomach or breast cancer as the primary, in women in general, and in patients who are younger than 65 years.[8] These symptoms seem to begin to appear in the last 6 weeks of life. Common causes of nausea and vomiting are fluid and electrolyte imbalances like hypercalcemia, volume depletion, water intoxication caused by inappropriate antidiuretic hormone (ADH) secretion, and adrenocortical insufficiency. Gastrointestinal causes include candidiasis, abnormal taste sensations left from chemotherapy, candidiasis infection in the esophagus, stomach stasis, obstruction of the small intestine, and constipation. Herpes simplex and other forms of stomatitis, and esophageal infections all have been implicated. Liver metastasis also interferes with normal gastrointestinal function. Peritonitis also causes these symptoms as well as CNS involvement. Infections and septicemia, renal failure with uremia, and tumor toxins all interfere with normal digestion. Many opioid drugs have side effects of nausea and vomiting. Identifying the cause is primary to treatment. See the section on nausea and vomiting in Chapter 12 on concurrent issues for detail in terms of Chinese medicine.[2]

ANOREXIA AND CACHEXIA

Anorexia and cachexia are part of a syndrome with causes that are multiple and frequently overlapping. The symptom of anorexia inevitably leads to weight loss and cachexia. This can become a self-perpetuating vicious cycle. This cycle can exist even in patients who have a favorable prognosis, and significantly contributes to shorter survival. There seem to be three main causative factors; the systemic effects of the cancer, local effects of the cancer, and treatment-related complications. It is a remote effect of a paraneoplastic syndrome in that a tumor-associated substance is the causative factor(s). This syndrome includes weight loss, weakness, asthenia, anemia, and protein, lipid, and carbohydrate metabolism abnormalities. Tumor necrosis factor (TNF) is one substance contributing to cachexia caused by cancer.[9]

The local effects of cancer are generally mechanical or obstructive. Patients with head and neck cancer may have dysphagia, early satiety, obstruction and malabsorption.[10] Treatment problems such as radiation therapy injuries cause injury to local tissue and cause difficulties with nutrition. Surgical procedures can lead to chronic nutritional problems, especially when they are performed on the bowel. Corticosteroids are commonly used to overcome these local and systemic problems. Megestrol acetate is also used as an oral progestogenic agent and also as an appetite stimulant. Transparenteral nutrition (TPN) is often provided to ensure adequate nutrition.

DEHYDRATION

Hydration is a complex issue in dying patients. There is some controversy over whether or not to hydrate patients in the process of dying.[11] Dehydration and electrolyte imbalance may cause confusion and restlessness. Dying patients are generally more comfortable if they receive hydration. There is no evidence that fluids alone prolong life. Parenteral hydration is currently the minimum standard of care, and many believe that discontinuing this treatment breaks the bond with the patient.

On the other hand, parenteral hydration may prolong the dying process. Most hospice workers (not MDs) support this view.[12] Fewer urinary accidents prevent the bed-wetting that causes decubitus ulcers. Fewer pulmonary secretions mean less coughing, choking, congestion and no death rattle.[13] There is less GI secretion with fewer bouts of vomiting. Edema and ascites are minimised. Diminished fluids and raised serum electrolyte levels may serve as a natural anesthetic and lessen the patient's level of consciousness. It is natural and more comfortable to die dehydrated. Perhaps patients should be encouraged to consider these issues when composing a living will.[14,15]

CONSTIPATION

Constipation is almost always caused by narcotic bowel syndrome.[16] Opioid analgesics affect gastrointestinal (GI) function through sigma receptors for muscle tone located throughout the GI tract. These drugs reduce GI motility while at the same time causing an increase in muscle tone in the gastric atrium and the first part of the duodenum. Gastric emptying is therefore significantly delayed, contributing to nausea and vomiting. Sphincter tone is enhanced intestinal peristalsis is decreased, and so stool moves very slowly through the GI tract and becomes desiccated. Autotoxicity may result. This picture is called narcotic bowel syndrome. It is caused by opioid analgesics, anticholinergics, and antidiarrheal agents. It is characterised by chronic abdominal pain, nausea and vomiting, abdominal distention, constipation, and at least one episode of pseudo-obstruction. Gastric, biliary and pancreatic secretions are also reduced.[17] The pain and discomfort of this kind of constipation caused by narcotic bowel syndrome are no longer treated with castor oil packs due to lack of nursing time. Managed care has ruled out the time and hands-on nature of modern nursing care.

CNS SYMPTOMS

Delirium (acute confusional states) has been called 'everyone's psychosis'. The reported incidence for this delirium in dying cancer patients ranges from 53 to 85%. Delirium manifests as disorders of perception, thinking, memory, and the disruption of a normal sleep–wake cycle. These symptoms commonly develop acutely. There is a wide range of causes, all of which can lead to diffuse cerebral dysfunction.[18] Some of these include metastases to the CNS, metabolic encephalopathy not caused by metastases, encephalopathy related to organ failure, electrolyte imbalance, infections, vascular disorders, side effects of therapy including opioid analgesia, and paraneoplastic syndromes. So delirium becomes superimposed on a broader process that must first be identified.[19] Acupuncture based on a traditional pattern diagnosis is very helpful in calming patients.

DEPRESSION

Reactive depression is the most frequent psychological problem diagnosed in patients with cancer. The clinical symptoms are anorexia, weight loss, and fatigue. Sadness, anxiety, feelings of hopelessness and worthlessness are all common. Those patients who are at higher risk are those with poor pain control, a more deteriorated physical condition, advanced stages of disease, and a history of depression prior to the diagnosis of cancer. Management is similar to the general population.[20,21] Please see Chapter 12 on concurrent issues.

DYSPNEA

Dyspnea is one of the 10 major symptoms of a dying patient.[22] Dyspnea can occur by differing mechanisms in patients with pulmonary metastases. A pleural effusion, bleeding into a metastases, or a pneumothorax caused by ulceration are all possibilities. Other causes include radiotherapy or chemotherapy (bleomycin) leading to lung injury, generalised debility, pulmonary embolism, aspiration pneumonia, chronic obstructive pulmonary disease (COPD) or congestive heart failure (CHF) as underlying or secondary conditions in elderly patients, massive ascites compromising pulmonary function, anxiety, and lung infection due to compromised immunity.[23] Even if the patient is unable to take herbs orally, the use of acupuncture can be very helpful to redirect lung qi.

URINARY INCONTINENCE

The involuntary loss of urine is another of the 10 majors symptoms of dying.[24] Although there are many often interacting factors causing incontinence, in a terminal patient the value of pursuing an evaluation of this symptom remains questionable. In modern medicine, this problem is managed usually with a catheter, absorbent pads, or intermittent catheterisation. These protective mechanisms are valuable in that they protect a patient from developing decubitus ulcers.

PRESSURE SORES

Decubitus ulcers can be a serious problem. Pressure, shearing forces, friction, and moisture are the causes of pressure sores. When the external pressure on the skin capillaries as well as the lymphatics is too great or long-lasting, these organs then collapse. The result is time-dependent. High pressure for more than 2 hours produces irreversible damage. When the same pressures are applied for no longer than 5 minutes, there is no damage.[25] Prevention is the primary treatment. Multiple topical therapies are used if prevention has failed. Antipressure devices and specialised beds are also used. In terminal patients who are considered to be 2 weeks away from death, very little healing, if any, takes place in these wounds. Prevention involves relieving pressure, especially over bony prominences, maintaining skin integrity through cleanliness and keeping skin dry, improving nutritional status and promoting hydration, promoting patient movement and education of the patient and caregivers.[26]

In the dying patient, death is either preceded by progressive sedation or by delirium. More than one-third of dying patients experience some difficulties during their last 48 hours of life. There is frequently noisy and moist breathing, pain, and agitation and restlessness. Sublingual lorazepam and the continuous subcutaneous infusion of midazolam are used to treat terminal restlessness.[27]

THE TIME OF DEATH

In many traditions, the actual point of death is a time when the most beneficial and profound inner experiences can come about. Through repeated acquaintance with the process of death by practicing leaving the body in meditation, many inner paths provide training in the ability to let go at the time of death and also gain peace and spiritual realisation and transition at the time of death.[28-32] In some of these paths, an indication of the attainment of spiritual realisation during life and death is the fact that often the body of a realised soul does not begin to decay until long after death.

Death and the process of dying in modern life is a meeting point in many ways between the patient's spiritual tradition and the modern scientific tradition. The dying process is often managed by medical providers and by hospice workers and spiritual caregivers. Often it is only at the end of a person's life that all of these providers come together. And yet living and dying are very much interconnected within the frame of a given individual; the way that we live is often the way that we die. And the inclusion or exclusion of a spiritual life in living has a direct effect on dying.

These realities also have a great deal to do with the ability of medical providers to be present during the death process. Our ability to be present at death is a measure of our ability to be present during life.[33] It is often difficult to separate the two, for they are really a continuum. Anyone given a diagnosis of cancer immediately begins to think and feel about their own life in terms of dying and living. The continuum is an enumeration of a patient's ability to be. The living and the dying experience becomes a relationship between the patient and the provider; this relationship begins early in the medical relationship and is defined often by very early connections and understandings that evolve as part of the trust for and openness to each other. It does not matter what our beliefs are in this context. What matters is who we are.

In Daoism there are seven stages of being. The seventh stage refers to a return. For the sage, this means self-realisation and a return to the Dao – the source of the authentic self. For the individual who has not completely fulfilled his or her treasure (most of us), the seventh stage means death and the return of the lost self to the mysterious workings of the Dao. This is the primary way in which Chinese medicine and Daoism views life and death, but every religion and spiritual path has its own way of providing meaning. Especially at death, this meaning holds profound significance, and honoring and supporting that view of meaning is essential for providers. It provides a container for everyone involved to hold the death of their loved one.

The authenticity of an individual's life often becomes starkly apparent at the end of life. The memory of one's true nature is stored in the jing as a mandate from heaven that blows 'on the ten thousand things in a different way, so that each can be itself'. By fixing the will and turning inward, directing the mind inward to the jing, the depths of the self, one may rediscover heaven's commands and return the heart back into the world, fully expressed. With our destiny fulfilled, we may become a channel for the creative flow of the Dao, the very source of life and vitality. This is one way to look at death and the dying process. When something like this is experienced at the end of life it can be a glorious moment for all who are present.[34]

As Zhuangzi said: 'He who comprehends the greater destiny becomes himself a part of it. He who comprehends the lesser destiny resigns himself to the inevitable'. The implication here is that to the extent that we can become our true selves, we live on; and conversely to the extent that we do not become our true selves we construct our own demise. Therefore, death becomes a concept related to our own ability to comprehend the laws of nature and heaven. We live and die by becoming what we comprehend. For people who frequently witness death by providing service at the end of life, the process can be uplifted for the dying and their family by becoming in life all that we can be. Perhaps this is what is meant by 'healer heal thyself'. A healer who has expanded the comprehension of living to its fullest heals not only their own life but helps to heal the lives and deaths of their patients.

THE PROCESS OF DYING

The process of dying is explained in great detail in Tibetan teachings. These teachings were influenced by Ayurvedic tradition and Indian Buddhism, and in turn influenced the Daoist and Buddhist traditions of Chinese medicine. It is really very difficult to separate them from one another. In Tibetan medicine it is said that it is from the mind, which embodies the five elemental qualities, that the physical body develops. The

body is given a certain number of breaths and when these have been taken then it is time for the body to dissolve and the spirit to return to the 'clear light'. Many meditational practices can, in fact, slow the breath or allow the body to live without breath for periods of time in order to arrive at an auspicious time for death, thus ensuring a happy rebirth. The concept of reincarnation is not part of every religious tradition, and yet the Buddhism and Daoism that form the philosophical underpinnings of Chinese medicine are founded in the concept of reincarnation. For those of us steeped in the Western tradition of Christianity it is not difficult to maneuver within the two paradigms. It is important to understand and respect the philosophy surrounding the death experience and an afterlife in which our patients may believe.

The process of dying in Tibetan medicine is a complex and interdependent one, in which groups of related aspects of our body and mind disintegrate simultaneously. The following is taken from the *Tibetan Book of Living and Dying* by Sogyal Rinpoche,[35] which is in turn taken from the *Tibetan Book of the Dead*. As the internal winds disappear (not related to the concept of internal pathological wind in Chinese medicine), the bodily functions and the senses fail. The energy centers collapse, and without their supporting winds the elements dissolve in sequence from the grossest to the subtlest. The result is that each stage of the dissolution has its physical and psychological effect on the dying person, and is reflected by external, physical signs as well as inner experiences.

These stages of outer dissolution may take place extremely quickly and not very obviously. Modern drugs may mask the signs. But often we can at least see changes in breathing, changes in skin color, or a particular smell that seems to be related to the dying process. There is often a change in the state of mind of the dying person. Staying in contact with the patient and not separating from them is an important gift that can be for the patient, their family and for the practitioner.

In Tibetan medicine, the position for dying is called 'the sleeping lion', which is the posture in which Buddha died. The left hand rests on the left thigh; the right hand is placed under the chin, closing the right nostril. The legs are stretched out and very slightly bent. On the right side of the body are certain subtle channels that encourage the 'karmic wind' of delusion. This position blocks these channels and facilitates a person's recognition of the luminosity of sacredness or God or however we wish to speak of it when it dawns at death. It also helps the consciousness to leave the body through the aperture at the crown chakra, Baihui, since all other openings are blocked.

THE OUTER DISSOLUTION

First the senses dissolve, then the elements begin to dissolve. The earth element is first as the body begins to lose strength, feel heavy and pressed down. The cheeks sink and dark stains may appear on the teeth. The mind may be agitated and delirious but then sinks into drowsiness. These are signs that the earth is dissolving into water. The body loses control of bodily fluids. Incontinence and a discharge from the eyes may occur. The mouth and throat become dry. The nostrils cave in. There may be trembling and twitching. There may be a smell of death hanging over the body. Here the water element is dissolving into fire, which is taking over in its ability to support consciousness. There is a 'secret sign' at this juncture, and at each juncture ahead, where there may be a vision of a haze with swirling wisps of smoke.

The mouth and nose dry up completely. All of the body warmth begins to seep away, usually starting at the feet and moving upwards to the heart. A steamy heat may rise from the crown. The breath is cool or cold as it passes through the mouth and nose. The mind swings alternately between clarity and confusion. Family becomes unrecognisable. The individual who is dying may feel as though they are being consumed in fire. The fire element is dissolving in air. The secret sign at this juncture is of shimmering red sparks dancing above an open fire like fireflies.

As the air begins to dissolve, it becomes harder and harder to breathe. There may be rasping and rattling. The inhalation becomes shorter and the exhalation becomes longer. The eyes may roll upwards. There may be hallucinations, visions, and a replay of one's life. The inhalation becomes more and more shallow. At this point blood gathers and enters the channel of life in the center of the heart. Three drops of blood collect, one after the other, causing three long, final exhalations. Then breathing ceases. This is the end of the outer dissolution and modern medicine would proclaim the person dead because of a lack of vital signs. The inner process continues and can take any amount of time, but usually it is said to take the time to eat a meal – 20 minutes from the last breath. Remaining quiet during this time allows the inner dissolution to continue peacefully.

THE INNER DISSOLUTION

In the inner dissolution, where gross and subtle thought states and emotions dissolve, four increasingly subtle levels of consciousness are encountered. The process of death on these levels mirrors the process of conception but in reverse. At conception our consciousness, impelled by karma, is drawn in. The yang essence, which is described as white and blissful, rests in the chakra at the crown and at the top of the central channel. The yin essence, described as red and hot, rests in the chakra at Guanyuan (Ren 4). It is from these two essences that dissolution next evolves.

The white essence descends from the crown toward the heart. The awareness of the dying person becomes extremely clear and all thoughts arising from anger, 33 in all, come to an end. Then yin essence begins to rise through the central channel, as all thoughts arising from desire, 40 in all, ceases to function. There arises a state of bliss.

Red and white essences meet at the heart and consciousness becomes enclosed in them. The mind is free of all thoughts. The seven thought states resulting from ignorance and delusion are brought to an end. There is a slight consciousness again and a state is entered called 'the mind of clear light of death'. This consciousness is the innermost subtle mind, the real source of all consciousness. Being present and clear during this process of dying is an immense gift for family and providers.

THE PULSES

The pulses of Chinese medicine can be used to understand the quality and chronology of the death experience. The pulses of the left hand correspond fundamentally to the quality of function of the organ systems, which finds its basis in the kidney. The right hand pulses correspond to the digestive system. Weak or empty pulses on the left signify that the organ system has collapsed and this collapse suggests that the resources of jing, qi, and shen have been severely depleted and are compromised as guiding influences in life. The collapse of the organ system corresponds to the compromised function of Mingmen, which plays a key role in guiding the inherited constitution.

If the functioning of the digestive system, which guards the acquired constitution, collapses, then serious pathology cannot be far off. In this case, there may be superficial pounding in all positions. At the same time, there will be no depth to the pulse, indicating that the yang qi is dispersing. The emptiness indicates that the yin and the yang are at the terminal point of separation. When the yin is exhausted, the yang will float to the surface. This is exactly the dynamic of Hexagram 23 of the I Jing, the hexagram translated as 'splitting apart'. Heaven and Earth separate and nothing can be accomplished.

In Japanese Meridian Therapy, great attention is paid to the doyo, or the middle pulse. It is the stream within the tube of the stream of the radial pulse. The stomach qi is felt on the right in the upper middle position. It is also felt along both radial pulses in the center of the pulse tube. A healthy stomach pulse is the level at which you feel the pulse is strongest, and stronger than the yang above or the yin below. In hard and strong pulses, it is not possible to detect the middle pulse; the pulse has lost its resilience. Most often it is people with chronic illness who have this type of pulse. When this middle pulse is not present at all positions, it means that the digestive system is unable to provide the acquired qi necessary for rehabilitation of the organs. This indicates a serious injury if it is lacking in one or two positions. If the stomach qi pulse, or the doyo, is missing in every position, it is an indication that death is imminent. Terminal patients will not regain the middle pulse even with large amounts of drug therapeutics.

There are seven death pulses:

1. Swallow pecking feed. When the qi of the liver weakens or disappears, the patient will have this pulse.

2. Goldfish coming up for air. This is a frail pulse in which the heart qi is gone.
3. Scattered thread pulse. This pulse feels like a thick thread in which the fibers separate and become frayed. The stomach qi is gone.
4. Water dripping from the roof. 'Waiting for another drip' pulse is tardy and the stomach qi is gone.
5. Water boiling. Bubbles coming up from the bottom of a pan when the lung qi is missing.
6. Dragonfly flying just above the water. Feels like a dragonfly just flying over the surface of the water when the large intestine qi is gone.
7. Striking the stone pulse. Feeling the pulse feels like poking a stone. The kidney qi is gone.

All of these pulse qualities have in common the lack of the middle pulse. It is a very difficult challenge to treat these patients. The prognosis is very poor. Treatment is palliative and not for cure.

CONCLUSIONS

The sacred does all it can to nurture the unique seed that it has implanted within each of us. The only vested interest manifested is that this unique aspect of the Dao be expressed in the world. Life is the manifestation of this expression. When it is complete the soul returns to Oneness, or the Dao. The time of death is a sacred time full of mystery and joy. Following are some quotes from various philosophical paths demonstrating that no matter what one's path or religion is in this life, ultimately they are all the same.

Nothing is better for a man than to be without anything, having no asceticism, no theory, no practice. When he is without everything, he is with everything.
Sufi master al-Halláj

Behold I make all things new. I am alpha and omega, the beginning and the end.
John the Evangelist

As a mother at the risk of her life watches over her only child, so let everyone cultivate a boundlessly compassionate mind toward all beings.
The Buddha

We say release, and radiance, and roses, and echo upon everything that's known; and yet, behind the world our names enclose is the nameless: our true archetype and home.

Rainer Maria Rilke

Before the first word: silence. Before the first light: light.

Dov Baer of Mezritch

Blessedness opened its mouth of wisdom and said, 'Blessed are the poor in spirit, for theirs is the kingdom of heaven'.

Matthew 5:3

A man or a woman is said to be absorbed when the water has total control of him, and he no control of the water. A swimmer moves around willfully. An absorbed being has no will but the water's going. Any word or act is not really personal, but the way the water has of speaking or doing. As when you hear a voice coming out of a wall, and you know it is not the wall talking, but someone inside, or perhaps someone outside echoing off the wall. Saints are like that. They've achieved the condition of a wall, or a door.

Rumi

At the heart of any real intimacy is a certain vulnerability. It is hard to trust someone with your vulnerability unless you can see in them a matching vulnerability and know that you will not be judged. In some basic way it is our imperfections and even our pain that draws others close to us.

Rachel Naomi Remen, MD

I laugh when I hear that the fish in the water
  is thirsty.
You don't grasp the fact that what is most
  alive of all
Is inside your own house;
And so you walk from one holy city to the
  next with a
Confused look!
Kabir will tell you the truth: go wherever you
  like, to
Calcutta or Tibet;
If you can't find where your soul is hidden,
For you the world will never be real!

Kabir

References

1. Enck R. Medical care of terminally ill patients. Baltimore: Johns Hopkins University Press; 1994.
2. Curtis E. Common symptoms of patients with advanced cancer. J Palliat Care 1991; 7:25–29.
3. Harvey A. The principles and practice of medicine, 28th edn. London: Prentice-Hall; 1995.
4. Langstein HN. Mechanisms of cancer cachexia. Hematol/Oncol Clin North Am 1991; 5:103–123.
5. De Wys WD. Pathophysiology of anorexia and disturbances of taste in cancer patients. In: Frontiers in gastrointestinal cancers. New York: Elsevier; 1984.
6. Wadleigh RM. Dronobinol enhancement of appetite in cancer patients. Proc Am Soc Clin Oncol 1990; 9:331.
7. Saunders C. Principles of symptom control in terminal care. Med Clin North Am 1992; 66:1169–1183.
8. Reuben DB. Nausea and vomiting in terminal cancer patients. Arch Intern Med 1986; 146:2021–2023.
9. Loprinzi CL. Dose/response evaluation of megestrol acetate for the treatment of cancer anorexia/ cachexia: a Mayo Clinic and North Central Cancer Treatment Group Trial. Proc Am Soc Clin Oncol 1992; 11:378.
10. Carter RL. Pain and dysphagia in patients with squamous carcinomas of the head and neck: the role of perineural spread. J R Soc Med 1988; 75:598–606.
11. Lichter I. The last 48 hours of life. J Palliat Care 1990; 6:7–15.
12. Andrews MR. Dehydration in the terminal patient: perceptions of hospice nurses. Am J Hospice Care 1989; 6:31–34.
13. Zerwekh JV. Should fluid and nutritional support be withheld from terminally ill patients? Am J Hospice Care 1987; 4:37–38.
14. Wolfe SM Sources on concern about the Patient Self-Determination Act. New Engl J Med 1991; 325:1666–1671.
15. Hockley JM. Survey of distressing symptoms in dying patients and their families in hospital and the response to a symptom control team. BMJ 1988; 296:1715–1717.

16. Bruera EC. Continuous SC infusion for the treatment of narcotic bowel syndrome. Cancer Treat Rep 1987; 71:1121–1122.

17. Bruera EC. Hypodermolysis for the administration of fluids and narcotic analgesics in patients with advanced cancer. J Pain Symptom Manage 1990; 5:218–220.

18. Bruera EC. Delirium and severe sedation in patients with terminal cancer. Cancer Treat Rep 1987; 71:787–788.

19. Ferris FD. Pre-terminal delirium. A practical seminar on narcotic infusion. Toronto: Pain Management Group; 1990:25–28.

20. Cody M. Depression and the use of antidepressants in patients with cancer. Palliat Med 1990; 4:271–278.

21. Holland JC. Managing depression in the patient with cancer. CA Cancer J Clin 1997; 37:366–371.

22. Regnard C. Dyspnea in advanced malignant disease: a flow diagram. Palliat Med 1991; 5:56–60.

23. Reuben DB. Dyspnea in terminally ill cancer patients. Chest 1986; 89:234–236.

24. Regnard C. Urinary problems in advanced cancer. Palliat Med 1991; 5:344–348.

25. Bale S. Pressure sores in advanced disease. Palliat Med 1989; 3:263–265.

26. Hanson D. The prevalence and incidence of pressure ulcers in the hospice setting: analysis of two methodologies. Am J Hosp Palliat Care 1991; 8:18–22.

27. Fainsinger R. Symptom control during the last week of life on a palliative care unit. J Palliat Care 1991; 7:5–11.

28. Hixon L. Great Swan: meetings with Ramakrishna. Boston: Shambhala; 1992.

29. Kalu Rinpoche. Luminous mind: the way of the Buddha. Boston: Wisdom Publications; 1997.

30. Sri Aurobindo. The mind of light. New York: EP Dutton; 1971.

31. Almas AH. The pearl beyond price. Berkeley: Diamond Books; 1988.

32. Lu TP. Tai I Chin Hua Tsung Chih (The secret of the golden flower). Circa 850ACE.

33. Levine S. Meetings at the edge. Dublin: Gateway; 2002.

34. Wilber K. Grace and grit. Boston: Shambhala; 1993:398–405.

35. Sogyal Rinpoche. The Tibetan book of living and dying. San Francisco: Harper; 1993.

Chapter 14

Prevention

CHAPTER CONTENTS

Introduction   341

The epidemic   342

Solutions   343
   Reducing exposures   343
   Calorie restriction   346
   Water   347

Thoughts   348

Persistent chemical carcinogens   349

Detoxification and depuration   351
   Toxic screens   353
   Fasting   354
   Sauna therapy   355
   Salt baths   356
   Water therapy   356
   The lymph system   356
   Qi gong   357

Chinese herbal medicine   357

Discussion   358

> *The hottest place in hell in reserved for those who, in times of crisis, prefer to remain neutral.*
>
> *The Inferno*. Dante.

INTRODUCTION

The machinery of war is the basis of the chemical industry. It was during and since the First and Second World Wars, that 85 000 new chemicals have been produced, chemicals that were meant to have killing power and are now being used in other ways to manage life and change life as we know it. These chemicals, mostly petroleum-based, have changed agriculture, food production and preservation, pharmaceuticals and medicine, energy and fuel production, the industrial world, and, most of all, the environment.

This evolution of change is the culmination of a primarily White European way of thinking born during the Age of Enlightenment. It is the culmination described with amazing clarity by Vandana Shiva[1,2] and is part of the model that attempts to separate humankind from the world in which we live, a model that sees the environment as a tool for our own use, and a model that has convinced us that we are separate from the natural world, Mother Earth, the perennial cultures that are land-based, and from our own hearts. It is a mind-based culture that finds that certain losses are part of modern life and are acceptable.

Lonnie Jarrett, in *Nourishing Destiny*,[3] uses the word 'mind' to refer to a level of spirit that can connect the truth of the heart with the external world; it is the interface between inner truth and the external world. When the analytic capacity of the mind is separated from the truth of the heart, then the mind rules our lives instead of serving life. I would say that our current dilemma is emblematic of this split. It is emblematic of a way of life where the truth of the heart, which is love and compassion and the road less traveled, is no longer listened to or seen by the rampant thrust of the Western analytical mind, which is run by a version of scientific truth that takes one piece of life, the scientific question, out of all relationship to other life and calls the results of the double-blind randomised placebo study the scientific truth.

This limited way of viewing life has become the basis for much of the modern dilemma. In war, reason and purpose are given to pre-emptive strike. In medicine, antibiotics attack pathogens and chemotherapies kill cancer cells. In agriculture, the environment is remade by forcing huge acreages to grow one crop, whether it is environmentally practicable or not, by the addition of inputs that destroy the living soil and any creature that interrupts our goal. In industry, the focus is on profit-making and on convincing people that they need these products. The mechanism by which these products are made is run by petroleum and depends on petroleum for its sustenance and future. But the petroleum used to run the world is a non-renewable resource in the hands of short-sighted entrepreneurs who seem not to care about the impacts or the future. This destructive behavior demonstrates a split between mind and heart, knowing and denial that is the foundation for war and destruction. We are truly at a crossroads where the future is dependent upon the decisions and actions of today. Actions made from the heart carry hope. Actions made from greed and denial carry destruction. It is as simple as that. What is at stake is life, whole cultures of peoples, ecosystems, global weather, thousands of species, the global water system, peace, and the future.

THE EPIDEMIC

The problem statement put forth in the introduction of this book indicates that we are in the midst of a modern epidemic. There are probably two prongs to this epidemic, chronic viral infection and carcinogenic exposures. As with all epidemics, there are public health and political components based in the philosophical underpinnings of the culture in which the epidemic is happening. Currently the largest portion of chronic viral infection appears to be happening primarily in Africa and Asia. It is, however, truly a world epidemic, not only because it is impacting us all but because the epidemic in the developed world is hidden from sight; modern conventional medicine is rendering invisible the real impacts.

Conventional medicine does not have a great deal to offer chronic viral infection in terms of cure, and the public health problem of viral spread, whether it be HIV, hepatitis C virus (HCV), hepatitis B virus (HBV), or herpes simplex virus (HSV), to name a few, is not addressed, especially in the developing world where HIV and HCV/HBV are most rampant. The public health aspect of chronic viral infection is also a political issue. Chronic viral infection is happening worldwide and little is being done worldwide on a political basis. It has taken 20 years for antiretroviral therapies for HIV/AIDS to reach Africa, even though the health results are almost always the same no matter where one is in the world. But there are local nuances of the problem that require special interventions to address the philosophical and cultural underpinnings of the local area. An anthropocentric Western approach with Western medicine is inappropriate and may be as destructive as the infection it is trying to interpret and treat. The foundations of these epidemics are in poverty, environmental destruction, and the loss of land and the ability to make a living.[4]

We need to help one another. On a world scale, the political will to eradicate, or even control, chronic viral infection is not there. The extent of the problem is, therefore, largely invisible. When an epidemic is invisible, this means that the mind/heart connection is damaged in the onlookers.

The public health component of carcinogenic exposures evolves out of a similar milieu. The public, even the portion of the public already diagnosed with cancer, is not informed about how to reduce exposures to known carcinogenic substances. The political underpinnings of the public health systems in place today to protect citizens from disease dictate a milieu of ignorance. The implication is that if citizens knew the reality of the number and type of carcinogens to which they are exposed through water, food, air, pharmaceuticals, and others, they would not be willing to accept these exposures. This lack of acceptance would then lead to changes in how we live that would have unacceptable economic and philosophical impacts, especially in the corporate business world, the main purveyor of carcinogens.

Alongside these two prongs of the modern epidemic of cancer is the issue of promoting factors; those lifestyle factors that lay a foundation within an individual for the promotion of mutations caused by chronic viral infection or carcinogenic exposures. There seems to be an increase in the attention given to promoting factors (such as obesity, diabetes, alcoholism, improper diet, lack of exercise) and how we can change our lifestyle and thereby lessen our chance of getting cancer. Although these are very important aspects of cancer prevention, the truth is that, without carcinogens, promoting factors rarely cause cancer. Promoting factors will evolve into other diseases, like diabetes and cardiovascular disease. For these reasons alone, we should take care of ourselves. However, it is usually only when carcinogens are added to this environment that cancers occur. Very frequently no promoting environment exists within an individual diagnosed with cancer. That individual has taken excellent care of their mind, spirit and body and is still diagnosed with cancer.

Billions of dollars are being misspent in an ill-conceived effort against cancer. This effort is focused on treatment rather than prevention. Prevention means addressing and changing the causes of cancer; the main cause is an increasingly carcinogenic environment that we ourselves are creating by buying into the idea that anything that makes our lives easier must be good. Prevention does not mean the early detection stated by the National Cancer Institute (NCI).[5]

The changes needed to resolve the two linked modern epidemics of cancer and chronic viral infection will require public health and political solutions. In terms of chemical carcinogenic exposures, the 1940s philosophy of better living through chemicals has not borne the kind of fruit we were seeking. The road less traveled, referred to by Rachel Carson, is a road of natural living, in which every species has an equal opportunity to live, and every human being on earth has an equal opportunity to a healthy life. The only way that this can happen is through a clean environment, including air, water, and soil, and through global equal opportunity. The idea that there is an acceptable loss of life in order to continue to conduct business as usual simply does not compute. We are reaching critical mass, and the great cost we are paying for the path more easily traveled is becoming more and more evident.

SOLUTIONS

REDUCING EXPOSURES

A large section of each chapter has been dedicated to risk factors and causation of that particular cancer. Please refer back to each chapter for detailed information about prevention of recurrence and prevention of initial diagnosis for that cancer.

Part of the spirit line of Chinese medicine has always been prevention and, to the extent that we know, we teach the modern day issues of self-care to our patients and families. It seems obvious that one main approach should be reduction of exposure to carcinogens. Eating organically limits exposure to known carcinogenic pesticides. Avoiding food products from animals fed hormones, including beef and dairy produce, reduces the amount of hormone exposure, and this is important not only in breast cancer, but also in prostate and testicular, ovarian, and some other cancers. Drinking uncontaminated water is the main risk reduction action. Eliminating contaminated cosmetics and household products that are carcinogenic is tedious but very important. Finding alternatives can be dynamic and fun.

Food Choices

Vegetables and fruit

Box 14.1 lists the 12 most chemically-contaminated non-organically grown fruit and vegetables, and the 12 least chemically-contaminated. Washing may help reduce pesticide residues. However some pesticides are formulated to bind to the surface of the crop on which they are used and it may not be possible to wash them away. The recommendation is to wash all produce with soap and water and to eat organically as much as possible. Many pesticides are taken up into the plant and cannot be washed away. It is best to buy only organically grown crops of the fruit and vegetables in the first group, the 'dirty dozen'. Of all fruit and vegetables, spinach was found to be the most contaminated.

Fish

We look increasingly to the oceans for protein foods. Between 1950 and 1990, the world's oceanic fish catch increased from 19 million tons to 90 million tons. But since 1990 there has been no growth in the catch. For the first time in history, we cannot rely on the ocean fisheries for an expanding food supply. Nets are being dropped deeper and deeper to scoop up rarer species of fish. Areas not fished in the past are bringing species not seen before to Western tables. The smaller fish are being caught, leaving nothing for the larger species to eat. Future fish populations are being undermined as existing populations are being exhausted. Fish is not a renewable resource when the technology used to vacuum every last fish from the ocean is stressing many species to the point of extinction.

Currently, the United States governmental agency overseeing the fisheries (the US Fish and Wildlife Service) has recommended that people no longer eat freshwater fish in the United States. This points to an even greater problem. The freshwater fisheries are too contaminated now to allow fish caught in those waters to be eaten. Water is the lowest common denominator. Groundwater is a dynamic and moving entity that carries with it many of the contaminants from the vast areas around it into the watersheds. Even saltwater fish and mammals are contaminated, and in the last year the orca whales of Puget Sound in Washington State were listed endangered. The reason for the decline is partly through starvation from the loss of one of their principal food sources, salmon, through contamination and overfishing. The other cause of death is the PCB compounds absorbed from salmon and the other species that they eat, that live in Puget Sound, and which accumulate in their tissue. The quality of life in our waterways indicates the quality of life on our planet.

A number of studies show that farmed salmon accumulate PCBs from the fish meal they are fed. The meal is designed to contain large amounts of fish oil and is made largely from ground up small fish. PCBs concentrate in oils and fat. Farmed salmon not caught and, therefore, are subject to different restrictions than wild salmon. Currently, health guidance standards for PCB levels set for wild salmon in 1999 reflect that farm-raised salmon contain 500 times the concentration of PCBs than the wild standard. These levels were found in salmon tested in Washington, DC, Portland, Oregon, and San Francisco. The farmed salmon tested came from factory-scale farms in Canada, the USA, and Iceland.[6]

Alaska wild salmon is naturally low in PCBs. Eat only wild salmon and work to protect the wild

---

Box 14.1 Most and least chemically-contaminated non-organically grown fruit and vegetables

Most contaminated	Least contaminated
Apples	Asparagus
Pears	Kiwi
Bell peppers	Avocados
Potatoes	Mangos
Celery	Bananas
Red raspberries	Onions
Cherries	Broccoli
Spinach	Papaya
Imported grapes (from South America)	Cauliflower
Strawberries	Peas
Nectarines	Sweetcorn
Peaches	Pineapple

These lists are from the Environmental Working Group *FoodNews* website: www.foodnews.org.

runs of salmon in your locale. This includes working to re-establish habitats so that old runs can re-establish themselves. It is primarily the timber industry that has deforested lands around streams, reducing the shade necessary to maintain water temperatures and water quality for salmon to spawn successfully. The worldwide deforestation of all kinds of forests has led to changes in water quality, local weather patterns, the loss of indigenous species and local peoples who live off these forests. Think carefully about the options available to you in building a new house or improving an old house. There are many new renewable products available that are long lasting, fire proof, aesthetically beautiful, and do not destroy the environment.

It is also necessary for homeowners to change their lawn and gardening habits by eliminating the use of chemicals in their pest management and fertilising practices. These products enter the groundwater, which travels to local lakes and streams, and the contamination interrupts the life cycle of all species, including fresh water fish and salmon. Wash your car at a car wash and not on the street or in the driveway. Choose a car wash that states that the waste water is sent to the public water utility for cleaning before entering the water stream again. Learn integrated pest management techniques for your gardening. Think organic first and consider chemical applications a last resort.

Consider not eating ocean fish until a global entity is evolved that will work to establish worldwide standards of quality and quantity for all of the various fish. Today we eat fish from the Pacific Islands and SE Asia because we have fished out our own stocks. Once again, this is emblematic of a split between the heart and mind. No one in their right heart would continue in this way.

Meats

Grazing animals like cattle, bison, and sheep get all of their nutrients from pasture. Grass-fed beef, for example, are not raised on grain, animal by-products, synthetic hormones, or feed antibiotics. Grass farming is a win–win situation because it is healthier for the animals, healthier for farm families, healthier for the consumer, and healthier for the planet. Commercial feedlot cattle are raised on grass from 6 to 18 months and then they are sent to the feedlot to be 'finished'. Their feed is changed to grain, which marbles the flesh, makes the flesh more fatty, and also makes them gain weight – cattle are sold by weight. Their feed also contained until recently some unsavory ingredients including 'tankage'. Tankage included the ground up flesh, hooves, feathers, and bones of other animals, chicken or cattle manure, stale pastry, and ground cardboard.[7]

The animals' growth is further stimulated by synthetic hormones and antibiotics. An estimated 95% of feedlot cattle are being treated with growth-promoting hormones, like estrogen. Cattle lack a critical enzyme needed to metabolise starch. This diet must be introduced slowly and even then the animal may suffer from bloat, acidosis, laminitis, liver abscesses, telangiectasis, and sudden death syndrome, necessitating further treatment with antibiotics and other medications.[8] This combination of antibiotics, hormones, and other pharmaceuticals is absorbed into the human body when the meat is consumed.

The antibiotics that animals are fed are ingested by humans, and this exposure is spawning antibiotic-resistant bacteria. The percentage of antibiotic-resistant salmonella increased to 34% in 1996 from 1% in 1980.[9] Growth hormones increase the amount of insulin-like growth factor-1 (IGF-1) in cows' milk. Pasteurisation raises the levels higher.[10] IGF-1 is a risk factor for breast and gastrointestinal cancers.

It is not just antibiotics and hormones that are finding their way into our food. Grain fed to cattle is treated with pesticides. According to the Environmental Protection Agency, 90–95% of all pesticide residues are found in meat and dairy products, not in fruits, vegetables and grains.

Ruminant animals fed large amounts of grain produce meat and milk products that are less desirable for human health; they contain more 'bad' cholesterol and less 'good' cholesterol. The level of saturated fat is twice that in grass-fed animals. Eating less red meat should be the rallying call; it could also be 'eat less grain-fed meat'. Lean red meat lowers your cholesterol levels, and grass-fed animals are richer in omega-3 fatty acids, with 2–6 times more omega-3 fatty acids than grain-fed meats. Brain tissue relies on omega-3 fatty acids. The cardiovascular system also relies on omega-3s and there is much evidence that people who have higher levels of omega-3s are less vulnerable to cancer.[11]

Picking local grass-fed meats is a better choice. It supports the small organic farmer and supports local farmers in general, which supports the land in a way that may be invisible to you. Much of the beef, for example, used by the hamburger industry in the United States is imported from Brazil and other countries in South America. This beef is being raised on lands cleared from the tropical rainforests. The Amazon and tropical rainforests are the lungs of the world. When this land is cleared of trees we lose part of the global ecology in terms of cooling and water systems, oxygen, species, medicines, beauty, and our spiritual economy. All of this is done to clear land to raise cattle for fast-food burger retailers in the USA and their outlets in other countries.[12]

The tropical rainforests contain 80% of the world's species of land vegetation and account for much of the global oxygen supply. Half of the species on earth live in the moist tropical rainforests. Currently, one-quarter of our medicines derive from materials found in these rainforests. One hamburger produced from land obtained from forest clearance in India would, if the real costs were included in the price rather than subsidised, be $200.[13]

When the rainforests are removed huge amounts of carbon dioxide are pumped into the atmosphere through burning the trees and stumps. The status of the thin envelope that we call atmosphere surrounding the earth is intensely fragile. The addition of this huge load of carbon dioxide, a greenhouse gas, is a contributing threat to our ability to survive on the earth.[14] All of this is for the sake of paying 5¢ less for a hamburger in the burger wars, while parts of the world suffer from constant drought and starvation. This kind of insanity demonstrates the terrible sickness from which we are suffering.

At the same time, the amount of land needed to raise beef and other animals is much greater than that needed to raise vegetables and grains. There is a great deal of controversy about what is the proper diet for anyone, including the best diet to prevent cancer. It is purposeful that the subject has not been covered here. But it is appropriate to consider that 2.5 acres of land producing cabbage will meet the food energy needs of 23 people. The food

energy needs of only one person will be met when that same 2.5 acres is used to produce beef. There are many considerations to take into account when thinking about food, water, land availability, good diet, and the true daily requirements for health.

Eggs and poultry

Until quite recently all of our chickens and turkeys were 'pastured poultry'. Under this system they were allowed a period of rest during which the egg-layers could replenish much-needed minerals depleted from laying so many eggs. Layers usually laid about 200 eggs per year. Today they lay 300 eggs per year with caging, debeaking, vaccinations, medicated feed, and lights. These birds breathe large amounts of ammonia dust and fecal dust. They can become paralysed by 'cage fatigue' and are then ground up for other chickens to eat as 'spent hen meal'. People who work in chicken factories suffer a high rate of asthma and other respiratory diseases.

The antibiotics and other medications given to birds raised in these conditions lingers in their eggs long after traces are gone from their blood.[15] There are now studies underway to see if injecting the embryos of chickens and turkeys before they hatch produce heavier birds faster.

Free-range birds had 21% less total fat, 30% less saturated fat, and 28% fewer calories than conventionally raised chickens.[16] The breast meat from these birds was so lean that it was classified fat-free by the United States Department of Agriculture (USDA). The meat had 50% more vitamin A and 100% more omega-3 fatty acids. In eggs the pastured layers produced eggs that were 40% higher in vitamin A and 400% higher in omega-3 fatty acids. They also had 34% less cholesterol. When we buy and eat the eggs and flesh of animals raised as factory chickens and turkeys, we get what we deserve but they do not.

CALORIE RESTRICTION

The incidence of many cancers increases with age. Several studies have shown that calorie restriction in laboratory mice and monkeys leads to reductions of up to 50% in rates of cancer.[17] The protection may be due to an improved effect on the body's capacity to repair damaged DNA. Caloric restriction reverses an age-related decline in a certain type of DNA repair called base excision repair, giving older animals the same ability to repair damaged DNA as younger ones.[18] This ability corresponds to a reduced mutation frequency when these same animals are exposed to carcinogens.[19]

Calorie restriction also leads to a reduction in total blood cholesterol levels, blood pressure and glucose levels. These factors are promoting factors in terms of laying the terrain for a cancerisation environment. Other studies have shown that all types of calorie restriction produce significant reduction in prostate tumor growth in rats. There seems to be a shift in balance between antiangiogenic factors and angiogenic factors, like vascular endothelial growth factor and insulin-like growth factor-1.[20]

Intestinal tumorigenesis in male mice was also reduced by calorie restriction. The frequency of intestinal polyps was reduced by 57% when calorie intake was restricted by 40%.[21] Studies need to be done in humans to determine if the results of these animal studies can be extended to humans to prevent age-related diseases like cancer. Provision of all essential nutrients is a critical aspect of caloric restriction. This technique should not be considered in people who are anorexic or bulimic, in those suffering from starvation, or in those already diagnosed with advanced cancer. The nutritional needs of cancer patients are different from those who are well. The cancer itself increases the need for calories, and treatment with cytotoxic agents also increases caloric needs to rebuild tissues damaged or destroyed by toxic agents like chemotherapy. Patients with an advanced cancer may be in a cachexic state and fasting or calorie restriction would be contraindicated.

WATER

The hydrological cycle involves the movement of water from subterranean regions to the atmosphere and back again. There is evaporation from the oceans and other bodies of water and this evaporation is dynamic but somewhat nonenergetic. The evapotranspiration that occurs from vegetation, and especially from forests, is more dynamic and involves a higher vibratory matrix from resonances out of a living plant source. These additional qualities and energies are largely immaterial and almost homeopathic in substance. The constant dilution of these energies throughout the hydrological cycle lends efficacy to water as a healing medium.[21]

The water that rises from deep springs and aquifers carries the potency of these energies. The water that we drink from these sources is far more powerful and potent than the water that is treated multiple times and then issues from our taps. Water is a living substance that can energetically contribute to the quality of life.[22] When forests are depleted, and the land and soil quality is lessened, the quality of water is lessened. Water is not a self-contained isolated substance. It carries the characteristics of the medium or organism in which it resides and moves. Water is the universal solvent and has an extraordinary capacity to combine with more elements and compounds than any other molecule. When the vital quality of other elements and compounds is lowered through deforestation, contamination, devitalisation of the soil and everything it supports, then water is also devitalised.[23]

Fresh water has many qualities, which can be differentiated according to drinking quality. Distilled water is pure since it contains no other elements, but it is not alive and, as drinking water, is bad in quality. Rainwater contains some atmospheric gases but is also contaminated with many atmospheric contaminants. As drinking water it is poor in quality. Surface water from dams, rivers and reservoirs contains few trace elements or minerals and is poor in quality. Groundwater contains a greater quantity of minerals and is good in quality, if not contaminated. Seepage-spring water is similar to groundwater. True spring water is high in dissolved carbons and minerals and is the best in quality for drinking water. Artesian water is deep-lying water, which may be fresh or saline and can contain a variety of dissolved elements and gases. Artesian water is variable in quality.[21]

The quality of the ecosystems on earth, and especially of forests, and water quality are intimately connected to temperature, which is connected to human health. Temperature of breast tissue, for example, is related to breast cancer. The diurnal rhythm of temperature change in high-risk, precancerous or cancerous breast tissues is different. These breasts have a higher overall temperature than healthy ones.[22]

Cities with greater amounts of green space have lower temperatures and a lesser number of pathogens per cubic meter. For example, investigations determined that Paris contained 36 000 pathogenic bacteria per cubic meter, but the forest and open fields around Paris contained only 490 pathogenic bacteria per cubic meter. The rates for tuberculosis in London were found to be 1.9% in contrast to Paris where the rates were found to be 4.1%. London has 14% green space and Paris 4.5%. These findings were found in a 2-year study conducted in 1991–1993 and reported in *The Times* on December 14, 1993.[22] Eliminating trees has a direct effect on temperature. Eliminating trees also changes the quality and vitality of water. Trees are a storage unit for the earth's water. The complexity of a natural forest containing many different kinds of trees and many levels in the living structure of the forest is part of the recycling mechanism of living water, and, therefore, of life.[24]

THOUGHTS

In 1974 the world population was 4 billion. Today it is 6 billion. During the 1970s the world grain harvest was growing, but peaked in 1984 and has been falling ever since. The world's population growth is primarily in the poorest countries. These countries are those that are suffering from consistent drought, loss of water from their underground aquifers, problems like erosion, and destruction of agricultural land. Today more than a billion people do not have enough to eat and nearly one-third of children in the developing world are chronically hungry.[25] These are peoples whose cultures have been severely damaged by colonialism. This colonialism continues in a different form today.

For example, the Worldwatch Institute states: 'Higher meat consumption among the affluent frequently creates problems for the poor, as the share of farmland devoted to feed cultivation expands, reducing production of food staples. In the economic competition for grain fields, the upper classes usually win'. The number of landless peoples in Central America has multiplied four-

fold.[26] The tropical rainforests of Central America are being destroyed by multinational corporations for the production of grazing lands for cattle. The tightly concentrated distribution of economic power and the resultant use of resources benefit the wealthy and not the poor. Although the poor, unless they live in a toxic waste dump, are less at risk for cancer, they are at greater risk for an early death through starvation. The odd juxtaposition of dying young from war and starvation in the developing world and dying young from cancer in the developed world is emblematic of the strangeness of the world we have created. It is a world in which we all pay a heavy price.

The poor are almost always those peoples who have traditionally been land-based. As the monoculture system of modern agribusiness transplants the ancient and viable biodiverse techniques of perennial cultures, people who live with the land, as opposed to off the land, are being lost. Whole systems of knowledge about how to live on and with the land are being lost. The modern form of colonialism exports a way of life convincing local indigenous peoples, often by force, to accept the modern way of life.[27] This modern way of life is one in which the old viable systems of agriculture, based in that particular land, weather, and ecosystem, are thrown out, to be replaced by modern techniques, which require deforestation, seed which cannot be collected for next year's crop and, therefore must be purchased year after year, irrigation techniques, which destroy the local aquifers and water systems, and techniques that require chemical inputs, which must be purchased at great expense. These chemical inputs are all petroleum-based. The modern displacement of people off their lands, and the replacement of working non-destructive agricultural systems, which support people through valuable work and sustainable outputs, with a destructive one, is part of the cause of modern endemic and epidemic diseases.[28–32]

People who lose their land and their ability to sustain themselves are more susceptible to chronic diseases, poverty, and lack of education and the societal infrastructure necessary to organise viable societies. The disparity between those who are comfortable in the world and those who have no culture or way of sustaining themselves left is pulling us all down into the inferno. This disparity contributes to the destruction of the family and the community and contributes to women and children being enslaved. The sex trade industry is one form of enslavement that flourishes in poor countries where this kind of colonialism has destroyed the magnificent local cultures, and this is one basic cause of chronic viral infection in the world.

We are at an exquisitely sinister and potent crossroads in modern life where the viral infections unchecked in the developing world are being transmitted into the developed world, and the carcinogenic contamination of the developed world is insinuating itself into the developing world. The toxic soup of this admixture is a late sign that we are out of control and have lost all connection between the mind of external action and the heart of sacred internal truth. As the yin and yang separate, so does life.

> **Box 14.2   Some products containing known carcinogens**
>
> Menopause creams
> Nail treatments
> Hair regrowth treatments
> Powders containing talc
> Skin-coloring agents
> Depilatory creams
> Many sunscreens and tanning oils
> Many antiperspirants
> Many shampoos
> Eye and contact-lens care products
> Hair dyes
> Nail polish
> Eye makeup
> Facial moisturisers
> Anti-aging treatments

PERSISTENT CHEMICAL CARCINOGENS

The long list of carcinogens is getting longer by the day. Recently saccharin has been found, in an Italian study, to be carcinogenic not only in bladder cancer but also in lymphoma and leukemia. Saccharin is ubiquitous and it points again to the connection between chemicals, corporate interests, and politics. Saccharin has been a known carcinogen since the 1940s but remains for sale in the United States. It is the primary sugar substitute in all sugar-free products, including soft drinks. Stevia, a herb-based substitute, has been blocked by the saccharin lobby in Washington, DC, for decades, because of the money potentially lost by the saccharin industry. Where is the consumer in all of this? The Italian study was done outside the United States, the world's largest producer and consumer of saccharin. Several studies were done much earlier in Canada that also showed saccharin to be a carcinogen.

Although eliminating exposures to carcinogens is important, it also may be impossible. The chemical soup in which we all live is inside and outside of our own bodies. See Box 14.2. We are part of this environment and not separate from it. Unfortunately, it may not be enough to just avoid exposure. The Environmental Working Group

(www.ewg.org) has conducted many studies in the United States. One recent study sampled tap water in 28 American cities. The EWG found that the tap water in 28 of 29 midwestern cities contained atrazine, a known xenoestrogenic carcinogen. Atrazine was removed from Israeli agriculture and the rate of breast cancer in Israel decreased significantly (30%) over the next 10 years. Just by drinking tap water frequently we are re-exposed to a xenoestrogenic organochlorine known to cause breast cancer. Many chemical carcinogens have very long half-lives and persist for many years; DDT still persists in the environment. Reducing exposure has become very difficult. It is difficult to find a place on earth where there is a non-chemicalised and clean environment.

According to the EWG, the number of contaminants now found in the adult human body in the United States is on average between 70 and 90 of the 167 contaminants tested for. We do not know if all of the 85 000 new chemicals manufactured since the 1940s injure the body in any way, let alone through carcinogenicity. It is shocking to realise that only 1500 have been studied for any human health effect. No one knows how these chemicals might combine in the body and to what effect.[33]

We do know that as the rates of chemical use and exposure have been rising exponentially in the developed world, so have the rates for cancer, some to the point of being identified as epidemic. In the developed world, cancer is the only killing disease whose rates are on the rise. In terms of prevention of new diagnoses and recurrence, beyond reducing exposures the question becomes what to do. The current chemicals to which humans are exposed were never seen in China during past or recent times when classical theory was evolving. Is it possible to look at old and recent theory about cancer pathogenesis and at the biochemical analyses of modern chemical exposures to understand how we might rid the body of these potentially cancer-causing substances?

The organic farming community in the United States has been working with this problem and they have found that there are biological means by which soil can be decontaminated without removal of that soil. Generally, the main thrust of the mechanism for depuration of contaminated soil has been the introduction of various yeast cultures. These cultures eat and transform the damaging chemicals in the soil and render it clean again. The yeasts do not become contaminated themselves. This is what we are looking for and some work has begun in this immensely important arena. However, in the human body introducing a biological entity is problematic.[34]

Many traditions recognise that the human body constantly discharges toxins through the urine, stool, respiration, and sweat. These toxins are more traditionally body wastes from normal functioning and not toxins in terms of chemical exposures. However, some modern studies show that there is depuration of exogenous chemical toxins via these routes. Discharge traditionally also happens through mental activity, physical activity, menstruation, childbirth, and even lactation.[35–38] With regard to lactation, one way in which women can detoxify breast tissue is through breastfeeding. Unfortunately this occurs at the expense of the newborn.

This is indicative of the terrible binds in which modern women find themselves. Please read *Having Faith* by Sandra Steingraber, a fetal toxicologist with Cornell University. When placed in the context of modern production in manufacturing of energy and products, production which has by-products that are contaminating the environment including the human environment, how is the dilemma in which women find themselves any different than that of general manufacturing? Women produce offspring and milk to sustain their offspring. They are contaminating their offspring through endocrine disruptors and pesticides stored in their bodies. In this case it is seen as wrong and terribly sad that this is true. Why is it not considered equally wrong and sad that manufacturers of these same products that contaminate women and children are contaminating the earth? The truth is there is no difference. The cycle goes on and on.

Abnormal discharge occurs through diarrhea, frequent urination, abnormal emotions, and chronic restlessness. Signs exist on the continuum from normal to abnormal of chronic efforts to discharge. In fact, it is possible that many newer chronic illnesses like multiple sclerosis, chronic fatigue syndrome, multiple chemical sensitivity disorder, autism, Alzheimer's disease, amyotrophic lateral sclerosis (ALS), hyperactivity disorders, and so on, are all in some way related to ineffective efforts to discharge toxic chemicals.

The skin in particular can be a macrocosm for observation of ineffective discharge to chronic exposures. Skin markings in many traditional systems are indicators that the body is trying to discharge impurities or accumulations. Some of these skin signs include the following:

- skin tags, which are seen to be manifestations of blood and phlegm stasis
- white points, usually on the face, which are seen as phlegm stasis caused by an inability to properly digest dairy products
- brown skin markings, which are seen as manifestations of high carbohydrate and refined sugar consumption.

Accumulations represent the body's inability to discharge through normal functioning. Chronic sinus discharge, middle ear discharges, cysts in the breast or other tissue, fatty breasts or other organs, kidney stones, benign prostatic hypertrophy, and chronic vaginal discharges all can be symptoms of chronic deficiencies that can lead eventually to collapse. They are signs of localised toxins, and the localisation of toxins leads to the formation of a degenerative quality of cell. This sets the scene for a cancerisation or transformation to malignancy. Therefore, being able to recognise early the signs of a precancerous condition may be one way in which we can work to help our patients prevent cancer.

The toxins referred to in the above discussion are the result of a lifestyle that leads to the promotion of cancer. The promotion environment is a magnet for exogenous toxins and, at some point, the exogenous and the promoting environment become one. There really is no way to separate the two except in terms of the process of rectifying the promotional aspects. There are several signs of a pre-cancerous environment:

- calcified deposits as seen through conventional imaging techniques; these indicate blood stasis
- cysts anywhere in the body; for example ovaries, breasts, kidneys, liver; these indicate phlegm and blood stasis
- accumulations of mucus or fat around centrally located organs, like the liver, kidneys, gallbladder, pancreas; these indicate phlegm stasis
- skin tags anywhere on the body, but especially on the abdomen and the naso and muno areas; these indicate blood stasis
- a strong, dark color of long duration in the navel area after it is cupped for 3 minutes; this indicates systemic blood stasis
- dark areas localised on the tongue or vein distention or phlegm attachments over the veins under the tongue body; these indicate blood stasis when the veins are dark and swollen and phlegm stasis when the connective tissue is thick and white-grey and there is a lot of it
- a soft, soggy, slippery, choppy, wiry forceless pulse, a pulse lacking in a doyo position; these indicate a damp or phlegm stasis environment, or blood stasis, or specific organ injury depending on where the doyo is diminished or absent
- spider veins or angiomas in general, and especially when localiaed or concentrated over an area, for example, the trunk; these indicate blood stasis.

These are some of the many signs that can be seen in patients who may have an environment where cancer can evolve. Many of these signs can be addressed through traditional techniques of classical medicine. But what of the non-classical suppositions regarding chemical exposures and carcinogenicity? These suppositions occur within a context that is often latent and asymptomatic.

DETOXIFICATION AND DEPURATION

Detoxification is thought of as a two-step process. In phase one the concept is to render molecules of toxicity easy to pick or 'sticky'. A system of enzymes called cytochrome P-450 prepares leftover or toxic molecules of toxicity by activating them, or making them more sticky. These activated toxins are more dangerous than initially and, therefore, must be gotten out of the body quickly. Box 14.3 lists some common toxins.

Phase two refers to the timely appearance of molecules that can contain the toxins and carry them away. This phase is called conjugation; carrier molecules pick up and deactivate toxins and make them more soluble in the blood so that the kidneys can excrete them through the urine and so that bile can excrete them through the intestines. Two of the main carrier molecules are sticky because they are literally like sugar. Two other carrier molecules owe their stickiness to the same feature that makes garlic peels stick to your fingers – sulfur. Sulfur atoms have an adhesive function and methionine – an essential amino acid, which enters the body via food – is one of the principal ways that sulfur enters the body. This particular method for detoxification is primarily for heavy metals. It is unclear if this method can be modified to detoxify other types of chemicals, like organochlorine pesticides.[39]

An example of a toxin that can be 'discharged' through this detoxification method is lead. One symptom of chronic lead poisoning is seizure, which increases in incidence during northern summer months because the sunlight raises the vitamin D levels to affect the mobilisation of calcium and lead. Lead is treated as it enters the body as though it was calcium. Therefore, absorption is favored by calcium deficiency. This is why chronic lead poisoning shows up when the vitamin D levels are raised. To treat lead poisoning the body is supplied with adequate amounts of those substances naturally needed to carry out removal. Calcium is supplemented to displace the lead and prevent absorption. Vitamins B and C are

Box 14.3   Some toxins

PCBs are chemicals used as industrial insulators and lubricants. They were banned in 1976 but persist in the environment. They accumulate up the food chain and cause cancer and neurological injury. High levels have been found in all farm-raised salmon, almost all marine animals, humans, and around industrial sites.

Dioxins are by-products of PVC production, industrial bleaching, and incineration. They cause cancer in man, and persist for decades in the environment. They are endocrine disruptors and are still used today.

Furans are by-products of plastics production and industrial bleaching and incineration. They cause cancer in man, are persistent toxic chemicals, and are endocrine disruptors.

Heavy metals are neurotoxins and some are carcinogenic. Lead is found primarily in paint and from paint decay. Old lead pipes are also a common source of lead poisoning; many public water systems still have not replaced their lead pipes. Mercury exposure is primarily from canned tuna. Almost all fish are contaminated with mercury. Arsenic persists in the environment from pressure-treated lumber. Playground equipment made from wood has often been treated with arsenic. Arsenic also comes through contaminated drinking water, especially from contaminated wells where farm inputs have leached arsenic and other contaminants into the groundwater. Cadmium is released by pigments and bakeware.

Organochlorine pesticides and herbicides, like DDT, chlordane, atrazine, and so on, persist in the environment even though some have been banned. DDT still is found in drinking water and soil. It is still produced in the United States for export. It then returns to us in food imported from other parts of the world. These are cumulative toxins that persist. They cause cancer and many are endocrine disruptors, which act in different ways. Ultimately they affect the unborn, human or otherwise, and then manifest effects later on in the individual's lifecycle. One example is DES, a hormonal endocrine disruptor that is absorbed in utero but can cause cervical cancer much later in a young woman in her 20s.

Organophosphate insecticide metabolites are breakdown products of chlorpyrifos, malathion, and others. They are potent nervous system toxicants and carcinogens. They come via food in the form of residues.

Phthalates are plasticisers that cause birth defects in the male reproductive system. They are found in a wide range of cosmetic and personal care products. Many have recently been banned in Europe. They are endocrine disruptors and it is assumed that they may also be carcinogenic.

Volatile and semivolatile organic chemicals are industrial solvents and gasoline ingredients like xylene and ethyl benzene. They are neurotoxins and carcinogens.

Fluoride is a water additive that can protect teeth from decay. It is a known cause of bone cancer in young male children. Austria, Belgium, Denmark, Finland, France, Germany, Iceland, Italy, Luxembourg, Netherlands, Norway and Sweden have decided against fluoridating their public water supplies.

Nitrosamines are carcinogenic and are used as preservatives, particularly in pork meat products.

Coal-tar shampoos and hair products are carcinogenic. Formaldehyde is carcinogenic and is found in nail products and lotions.

Progesterone is a probable carcinogen and is found in many pharmaceuticals that are used as hormonal treatments.

Silica, found in many cosmetics, is a known carcinogen.

Talc is a known carcinogen and is found in female hygiene products and cosmetics and body powders. Talc is the carrier for fragrance in these products.

Chlorine bleach is a known carcinogen and is used to kill bacteria in the public water supply. Its carcinogenicity has been known for many years but it remains the main water purifier because it is cheap. The Food and Drug Administration (FDA) has set levels for chlorine in water but the known levels for safety are not known. Chlorine is one of the main carcinogens in terms of constant and ongoing exposure.

supplemented, along with reduced glutathione. In many ways this is similar to the classical treatment to move latent pathogenic factors to levels where they can be dispersed or drained. For example, ying and blood level LPFs are moved to the qi level for excretion through stool or urine. Qing hao (*Artemisia apiacea*) is traditionally the main herb used in this technique. It is combined with other herbs to affect the transition to a more active level.[40]

Sometimes lead and other heavy metal poisoning is so severe that chelating agents are required. DMSP is a main chelating agent. Chelating causes the loss of some nutritional elements like calcium, magnesium, and others. It is hard on the patient and should be used only when the patient is strong enough to be able to comfortably go through the detoxification process.[41] Part of the detoxification process becomes finding everything possible to optimise the overall health of the patient. Therefore, it is not a technique that should be used in a patient who has already been diagnosed with cancer.

The point of discussing the idea of detoxification and depuration is that this may be a major hope for preventing cancer. Living a lifestyle that eliminates the issues of promoting cancer cells is one part of prevention. But without avoiding exposure and depurating those exposures that have already occurred and may continue to occur because of the current status of our environment, we will still be at risk for cancer.

Treating chemical carcinogens as though they are latent pathogenic factors (LPFs) may be a valid approach. Modern natural agriculture has found ways to depurate the soil from chemical carcinogens. Chinese medicine and herbal medicine may have means whereby combining the classical theory of LPFs from wen bing xue with modern nature cures and modern laboratory analysis can depurate the soil of the human body. Certainly something needs to be done, and this kind of medicine and cure is already part of the spirit line of Chinese medicine.

TOXIC SCREENS

We are exposed to many toxins beyond heavy metals in the developed world, and these therefore form part of our discussion. Because air and water act as common denominators the spread of contaminants into the rest of the world is already happening and is assured. There are many tests already available that can be used to measure the levels of toxicity in individuals.

1. Stool tests.

    The gastrointestinal tract has a total surface area equal to the size of a tennis court. The gastrointestinal mucosa absorbs nutrients and excludes toxins. The GI tube is outside the body, and is one of only two sites in the body where the outside interfaces with the inside; the other is the lung. Perhaps this is why these two organs are coupled in Chinese medicine. They share a similarity in tissue, mucosal activity, a need for a wei qi component, and they share water metabolism as a function, and a membrane through which an inside/outside exchange can occur. The need for a system by which toxins and pathogens can be cleared is very important.

    Digestive strength, functionally and immunologically, is important in assessing the ability of any patient to detoxify. In conventional medical terms, bacterial growth in the colon helps break down fiber, and odorous stool can be an indication that bacterial growth is imbalanced or inappropriate. The secretory IgA will be increased in the presence of an infection or overgrowth of any flora. The secretory IgA will be decreased if this same overgrowth or infection is serious. Stool testing, therefore, can be a valuable aid in understanding if a patient is assimilating and absorbing nutrients on the one hand, and if the patient has a functionally adequate level of immunity on the other.

    There are many stool tests that evaluate the absorption of fats, immunoglobulin levels, and other absorption levels. Yeast screens and *Candida* screens may be helpful in evaluating the underlying foundations of spleen deficiency, which, if damaged, can lead to damp accumulations. Mucosal barrier screens can help us to understand the levels of wei qi and San Jiao function in the lower burner. When detoxifying, injuries to the GI tube and all of its functional components can lead to greater stress from toxins and a poorer ability to depurate. The hugeness of the spleen orb of activity in Chinese medicine affects all of the acquired qi. Maintaining and evaluating optimal function in this large arena is essential.

2. Oxidative stress can be tested with blood tests for lipid peroxides. High levels of oxidative stress can indicate toxins.

3. A heavy-metal screen can be done initially with hair analysis and then more accurately with urinalysis, both through Great Smokies Diagnostic Laboratory, NC.

4. Accu-Chem Laboratories (TX) provides a screen for PCBs of various kinds and for chlorine pesticides.

5. SpectraCell Laboratories (TX) provides a screen for antioxidant activity.

The Agency for Toxic Substances and Disease Registry (ATSDR) can help provide more information on this subject. The above screens are one place to start in the effort to understand what levels of chemical exposure need depuration in an individual. At this point in time, no one has devised a means for eliminating the multitude of chemical exposures to which we all have been subjected. However, there does seem to be theoretical overlap between Chinese medicine's theory of LPFs and other natural paradigms and their approach to detoxification.

FASTING

One ubiquitous form of detoxification across systems is fasting. Although there is little written material available on fasting or nature cure techniques in any era of Chinese medicine, it would seem more than possible that the Buddhist and Taoist practices as they relate to Chinese medicine had elements of fasting and what has been called nature cure. The Buddhists were the first in China to develop hospital settings for patients. These settings were often primarily retreats for rest and probably what we would call 'detoxification'. They were places for resting and recuperating from illness, somewhat like a sanatorium. They were possibly also sites for fasting, not unlike European spas.[42]

The benefits of fasting are broad-ranging. Fasting is used as a means of resting the gastrointestinal tract, the liver and kidneys and other organs. It is also used to allow the body a means by which self-produced wastes and other stored toxins can be released. An important element of detoxification is mobilising toxins from their storage sites. Often these sites are liver and fat. This occurs best and most efficiently during fasting.[43]

When fasting, certain biochemical changes take place that enable the body to fuel itself by burning up its fat reserves and conserving vital tissues. The body senses in a continued fast that it needs to preserve lean muscle mass and instead burn fat. Fats are broken down to fatty acids that can be used by the muscles, heart, and liver for energy. The brain, however, is the major burner of energy when the body is at rest, and the brain cannot be fueled by fatty acids; it requires glucose to fuel its activity. A special adaptation occurs in the fasting state whereby the brain can fuel itself with ketones instead of glucose. By the third day of a total fast, the liver starts generating a large quantity of ketones from the body's fat stores. As the level of ketones rises in the bloodstream, the brain and other organs begin to use these ketones as their major fuel supply, thus greatly diminishing the utilisation of glucose by the body. This significantly limits muscle wasting. This state is known as protein sparing and this state is preferred over a non-protein-sparing state accomplished by fasts that are not total.[44-46]

Fasting has been employed to treat chemical poisoning because of the powerful effect it has on accelerating the discharge of internal noxious wastes and toxins, particularly from fat tissue. A study done in Taiwan in 1984 involved patients who had ingested rice bran oil that had been contaminated with PCBs.[47] After a 7-day fast, dramatic relief was noted in symptoms. At the same time, there was an increased level of circulating xenobiotics in the participants' serum. Presumably the elevation in circulating toxins was due to the increased rate of lipolysis in fasting individuals, and fat-soluble PCBs were released from adipose tissue into the bloodstream at higher than normal rates. Once in circulation, PCBs are metabolised in the liver for elimination through bile or urine. If this change does not occur, they are redeposited in adipose tissue.

When the beneficial effects of the therapeutic fast have been investigated with various research parameters measuring organ function, it is found repeatedly that substantial improvements are seen in the autonomic nervous system, endocrine system, and adrenal function after the fast. And when done correctly and sometimes in combination with other techniques, like sweating, the release of xenobiotics was accomplished.[48]

Fasting and calorie restriction have a powerful effect on modulating free-radical production, repairing free-radical damage, and facilitating removal or detoxification of the products of free-radical damage, for example oxidative stress.[49] Fasting aids in the removal of other toxins, and has been shown to maintain the integrity of the cellular structure even at advanced stages.[50] Food restriction and fasting also decreases the rate of free-radical generation by reducing the rate of electron transport and oxygen utilisation. This may be the conventional science language equivalent of how damp phlegm knotted with toxin impedes the overall function of the wei qi and the San Jiao system.

As we place disease-causing stressors on our body throughout our lives, our cells can become weak and congested with cell-generated wastes. Eventually, as waste accumulates within the cell, it overtaxes the cell's detoxifying ability. This magnetises those LPFs and creates an environment where more and more waste is forced into the cellular wall, which marks the cell as aged and abnormal to immune surveillance. The immune system will begin its job of attacking the cell in an attempt to remove it. Many autoimmune diseases and cancers can be reversed if cellular detoxification through calorie restriction and fasting is implemented to reduce the load of metabolic wastes and toxins thereby allowing those cells to return to normal.[51,52]

Fasting can be used to reduce benign tumors. Nasal polyps, lipomas, ovarian cysts, fibroids, all respond well to fasting. Many benign tumors would be categorised as phlegm damp stasis accumulations and they most frequently occur in epithelial tissues or connective tissues. Most of these tissues have a mucosal lining that is secretory. Because of this they have a propensity for dampness and phlegm. This perhaps leads them to act as a magnet for damp phlegm accumulations; in fact, many naturally proliferative tissues are healthy phlegm damp structures. The primary environment in which dampness and phlegm evolves is one in which improper diet plays a part. This makes fasting an excellent means by which to treat them. Fasting gives the stomach/spleen axis a rest and a chance to rehabilitate function.

However, malignancies are less responsive to bodily control. They behave somewhat unpredictably and often grow faster than benign tumors. They tend not to follow the rules, and the body's normalisation strategies have been out of balance for some time and, therefore, have less influence over the cancer. Therefore, fasting with a cancer diagnosis is generally contraindicated. Fasting is primarily a technique that is best used in patients who are generally well, to detoxify and depurate some forms of toxins in order to regain balance and prevent cancer.

SAUNA THERAPY

Modified sauna therapy is also useful in detoxifying. A sauna chamber kept at low heat of 100–130°C allows patients to sit and sweat for a safer and longer period of time. It may be possible to sit in a regular high heat sauna for 10–20 minutes. In a lower heat sauna a 60-minute sweat can be induced. This allows the body's largest organ of elimination, the skin, to work to detoxify. One would think this level of discharge would be adequate to detoxify the Taiyang sphere of function. This may be considered to be a qi level detoxification. Dry skin brushing is usually done to remove old skin and open the pores. By adding herbal therapy to this scenario, could we postulate that we could actually disperse LPFs, in the form of chemical toxins, by activating the qi level with sweating and bringing blood level toxins to the qi level for dispersing with herbal techniques?

Patients who are blood deficient do not sweat easily. The level of deficiency in the yin aspect of the blood disallows normal sweating. It may be inappropriate to sweat these patients until foundational rehabilitation has been done to support sweating as a therapeutic cleansing tool.

Sauna therapy increases the rate of lipolysis in the adipose tissue throughout the body. When this occurs lipophilic xenobiotics are released into the bloodstream. Compounds in subcutaneous fat pads are mobilised both into the blood and out through perspiration. Because of this, the level of detoxification is deeper and may imply a level of flushing outward from the San Jiao aspect of the body. These questions are worthy of analysis.

SALT BATHS

The use of a salt bath that is at least 1% salt (1lb salt for every 12 gal water), drives a process of osmosis to take place. This means that a small amount of fluid will be drawn out through the skin and the minerals in the body fluids will naturally become a little concentrated. This concentration of minerals causes a slight rise in the alkalinity of the body fluids. A slight alkalinity is necessary for the proper functioning of all healthy cells including those cells that secrete enzymes. Most illnesses have at least part of the root in an acidic body condition or are encouraged by an acidic condition. The salt bath (along with diet) helps to bring the body back into an alkaline state.

The salt bath can also help to strengthen weak kidney function. Weak kidney function can lead to a more acidic environment because more frequent urination and the resulting loss of minerals through excretion leads to more acidity. Although salt baths do not directly depurate xenobiotics, they do aid in the overall environment and contribute to the ability of a patient to detoxify. Salt baths are not contraindicated in cancer patients.[53]

WATER THERAPY

The 'sacred waters' mentioned in the Bible refer to many uses of water. Colon therapy is one method of water therapy. Since many toxins are fat soluble, a primary storage unit is the liver, which is a fatty (more or less) organ. The fat in the liver acts as an insulator, among other things, for those toxins that cannot be immediately flushed from the body through stool or urine. Therefore, bile and its relationship to fat and the liver becomes the delivery mechanism for toxins via the colon. Colonic washing during discharge becomes a valuable tool for stimulating and enhancing the speed and the effect of the discharge. It also improves peristalsis and acts as a method for improving the function and detoxifying effect of the colon.

The Chinese herb product manufacturers, modern and ancient, have a long history of advertising the quality of their products based on the water used in production. Water is a living entity and, as such, contributes more greatly to health than we know. The water that we drink now in urban areas is contaminated with heavy metals, toxic chemicals including chlorine and fluoride, and often with parasites. It has been treated to the point that it is no longer a vital force, no longer containing a living charge as does spring water or water directly from an aquifer.[54,55]

Fresh pure alive water is a part of natural medicine. Water is a delivery means for nourishing the yin, flushing toxins (endogenous and exogenous), charging the vital force, and balancing all organ functions. Water taken orally as fluid nurturance has many of the same effects as water taken into the colon to stimulate bile flow and to wash the colon. Water that is pure cleanses and detoxifies.

Drinking alive and clean water is essential. Usually it is not possible. The cleanest source of water is derived through reverse osmosis filtering. It would be best to make a thorough study of the quality of your drinking water. If it is not clean, many water purification systems are available. Some are good; some are worthless. Generally, avoid tap water. Find a viable filtering system or purchase your water from a reliable source. If your water is chlorinated, place a dechlorination filter on your shower head and bathtub spout. These methods will only provide you with clean water but not with living water. For that, you must go to spring water.

THE LYMPH SYSTEM

In conventional terms the lymph system is part of the circulatory system and is a major organ of the immune system. One of its main jobs is to transport nutrients from the blood to each individual cell and to remove waste. Some of this waste is transported to the intestines via the lacteals, that part of the lymph system that empties into the small intestine. The numerous lymph nodes in the abdomen also become sites for waste and toxins. The San Jiao system may be a complex analog for the lymph system. Both are ubiquitous and complex, both have immune relationships. It seems safe to say that within the Chinese medicine paradigm, the San Jiao system is impacted when toxins are present. The fat cells of the greater omentum and the mesenterium are all part of the San Jiao. These special 'greasy membranes' may act as modules for decontaminating toxins.

All of the elements of detoxification already mentioned are important to overall San Jiao functioning. Additionally, it might be of value to include various forms of acupuncture and manual techniques, like lymph drainage techniques, to move and flush toxins from various types of tissue into the lymphatics and along for flushing. Visceral manipulation and lymphatic drainage may be potentiated by herbal medicine and acupuncture as a detoxification process.

QI GONG

The many flows that are part of qi gong therapy can be utilised specifically in relation to the above detoxification techniques. For example, a specific lung-oriented flow may enhance the detoxification process of sweating. Utilising a liver flow pattern might be useful to assist the liver. As a cancer prevention technique, the low-impact activities of tai qi chuan, qi gong, and yoga are all extremely beneficial; and all of these can be used by cancer patients. They are immensely helpful in surviving conventional treatment for cancer and in preventing recurrence, as well as preventing occurrence in the first place.[56,57]

CHINESE HERBAL MEDICINE

Herbal medicine has a long history of treating LPFs. Carcinogenic exposures are not part of the historical theoretical underpinnings of Chinese medicine but may be treatable by combining the techniques of different paradigms for detoxification with the herbal theory of clearing LPFs.

The words of Chinese medical theory that probably would refer to a modern carcinogenic chemical include fire, heat toxin, toxin, fu, and fu qi, among many. Looking at the traditional meaning of these words may give us some insight into how to combine paradigms with wen bing xue and the concept of the latent pathogen.

If the word fire is used as a starting point for a basis of carcinogenicity, then there may be some interesting characterisations that stem from this word. For example, we commonly think of some kind of transmutation of the yang qi when we think of fire. As a result of this transmutation there is damage to the fluids, local signs of heat leading to thicker secretions and turbidity and sometimes

bleeding. This word and its implied concepts of causation and treatment seem to work fairly well for the cancerisation process. However, in terms of LPF and a carcinogen acting as an LPF, it is talking usually about an end state rather than a preclinical condition. The clinical treatment of fire usually means clearing fire and nourishing yin. So yin becomes the key rather than heat or toxin. Can we say that chemicals like atrazine, for example, mainly cause injury to the yin? It doesn't seem so in practice.

The word or phrase 'heat toxin' refers to a process that arises from depression or suppression of a fire heat disease pathogen. Toxin is a word that is commonly used in relation to the old ideas of a toxin, like a toxin from a snakebite or spoiled food or stagnant water – in other words, biological toxins. At the same time, it also has elements central to it that may be useful to the discussion of how to get modern toxins, chemical rather than biological, out of storage in the human body. Many of the herbs used in yi du gong du realm of cancer treatment are antineoplastic in ways that are similar to modern chemotherapy. They are cold and bitter detoxifying herbs that create a certain amount of damage in order to clear a pathogen. They are so extreme that they close the circle by very nearly approaching the toxicity of the pathogen they are combating. This is 'slash and burn' theory and one from which we hope to extricate ourselves. Therefore, using treatment based on theory to treat a heat toxin may not be a good approach.

Looking at the six climatic factors could be useful. Is it possible that chemical exposures mimic climatic conditions? The heavy metal exposure of lead elicits certain symptoms not unlike summer heat or wind. Lead is a neurotoxin and is also carcinogenic, although little attention is paid to this last characteristic. If we look at organochlorine pesticides, which are stored in fat cells, it's another story. The signs and symptoms are latent. The effect of these chemicals is only partially known and we do not know how these chemicals combine and if the combinations are more problematic than the single exposure. It would be so much easier if the result of exposure were symptomatic in a more immediate sense. But only higher dose exposures are symptomatic. The constant but low-level exposure to which we are subjected is, as far as we know or can tell, asymptomatic.

We do know that many known carcinogens act in various ways. Xenoestrogenic effects from pseudoestrogens, like DDT, DDE, atrazine and others, have a very long half life. They stay in the body and accumulate in fat tissue. They metabolise more estrogen in the 'bad' form. This encourages the body to construct more estrogen receptors, making room for more estrogen, endogenous and exogenous, to attach to estrogen receptors. These pseudoestrogens, as one category of carcinogen, act like a fire toxin and a latent pathogenic factor.

Approaching chemical carcinogenicity may require a multipronged approach. Many chemicals act more or less like latent pathogens. The Shang han lun was the first text to mention the concept of LPF. The Wen bing tiao bian and San Jiao theory in various texts took the concept and fleshed it out giving treatment principles for releasing LPFs from the interior levels.

The terms that are used to describe these stuck embedded pathogens include:

- fu: a latent, dormant, deep-lying pathogen that is barely perceptible
- fu: same character for abdominal masses and lymph nodes
- fu qi: refers to a latent pathogen that can emerge later, long after the original exposure to the pathogen
- fu qi wen bing: refers to interior latent diseases caused by a pathogen that obstructs the qi mechanism; the pathogen lies dormant until a later season when it emerges or until another pathogen causes it to emerge to the surface.

The etiology of latent pathogens has two routes:

1. The pathogen enters the body, manifests a few brief signs and/or moves to the interior where it lies dormant.
2. A wind invasion with an acute pathogen that enters the body and is not expelled and sinks to the ying or blood level.

There are several predispositions for the above event. For example, a weak constitution, poor lifestyle habits, and diet, overwork, or overuse or improper use of treatment all can predispose an individual for an LPF. These predispositions are all promoting factors for cancer.

Looking only at organochlorine pesticides, we know that these molecules are fat soluble and lodge in the fat cells of the body, human or otherwise. Many of them have xenoestrogenic effects, which is one way in which they are carcinogenic because estrogens act as proliferation factors in certain types of hormonally-sensitive tissue. These effects are cumulative. If it is true that environmental exposures are the primary modern cause of cancers, then the xenoestrogenic effects of organochlorine pesticides are cumulative in the sense that there is a growing quantity of pathogen, and cumulative in the sense that the longer the time that the pathogen sits in the body the more damage it can do. It is hoped that you are beginning to see the links between the concept of the LPF and modern carcinogenic exposures that enter the body at all four levels and become very much like LPFs in the classical sense.

The consensus is that the more healthy the body is in an environment where these exposures occur, the better chance one has of surviving longer from the impacts of the exposures. Therefore, general good health is a strong anticancer factor in cancer prevention, even in people who are heavily exposed to carcinogens or in people who have a genetic risk for a given cancer. However, there seems to be a point at which the cumulative effect reaches its zenith and finally a triggering or induction phase is reached where a malignancy occurs.

This is not unlike the theory of LPFs. The pathogenic effect of the cumulative exposure emerges as a result of the body's own process. When the body reaches another imbalanced state either due to the pathogen itself or due to other chronic or acute events that destabilise the body balance, then an induction occurs within the imbalanced environment that triggers the malignancy. The switch is turned on. Treating the imblance is part of the cure, and releasing the latent pathogen is the other. If the LPFs can be released prior to advanced imbalance – the malignant state, then this is preventive medicine.

DISCUSSION

Latent pathogenic factors tend to be either heat, cold, or damp heat pathogens. These factors are assigned based on the presentation of the patient and this assumes a reaction or response at some time in the early pathology. Looking for fevers, chills, floating pulses or rapid pulses, and so on, may not be a help to us in terms of understanding how to clear chemicals in clinical treatment. However, conventional science research on these same exposures may help.

In the case, again, of organochlorine pesticides, we know how they act in terms of carcinogenesis. They act like normal estrogen and stimulate uncontrolled growth. Looking at these carcinogens as LPFs it may be that they are heat pathogens.

In terms of predispositions for these LPFs there are several predisposing and more constitutional issues:

1. People with a yin-deficient constitution are more prone because yin deficiency leads to empty heat, which then attracts inwardly unresolved pathogens.
2. Qi stasis generates heat and stasis and a chronic vicious cycle, which also leads to internal heat.
3. Spleen deficiency from dietary injuries both lead to dampness and phlegm. Dampness can attract or transform external pathogens to wind dampness, which can lead to damp heat in the interior. Damp heat in the interior can act as an LPF or attract an LPF. Heat or lingering heat combines easily with damp heat.

These predispositions help to explain how constitutional weaknesses that are emblematic of poor self-care can contribute to greater susceptibility to damage by LPFs and chemical exposures. Perhaps we can say that the nature of organochlorine pesticides is yang and a kind of heat toxin that remains asymptomatic until a cumulative breakpoint is reached and/or an imbalance acts as a trigger for a mutational process to begin. If the exposure is overwhelming, then this process is short. If it happens throughout a lifetime, then constitutional strength can serve to protect the individual for some time from the LPF and deeper injury.

It is important to identify the level of the LPFs. The possibilities are the qi level, and the ying and xue. The therapeutic principle is to vent the pathogenic qi to the exterior. If we are talking about the qi level, then the reference is to the lungs, spleen, gall bladder, urinary bladder, or intestines. In other words, to those organs that have an inside/ outside relationship and have a special type of epithelial tissue that enables them to meet with and mix the outside and inside.

If we are talking about the ying or xue level, we are referring to the constructive aspect that helps form the blood, which then circulates in the vessels to the organs and especially the deeper organs. This means the heart, kidney, and liver. Trapped heat in this level has traditionally manifested as mental disturbance, night sweats, agitation, and restlessness. The heart/kidney axis is disturbed with the liver caught in the middle. There are no lung or digestive symptoms in this presentation.

Within this schema, where exactly do pesticides lodge and accumulate? We are told that fat cells are the repository for these LPFs. If the fat is part of the San Jiao, then here we are back at the San Jiao. The San Jiao is ubiquitous and has a direct relationship with spleen, with lymph, with the ying, with the wei qi, and all of these are connected to the source qi at the kidney axis. Many of the functions of all of these functional units in Chinese medicine are related to the San Jiao. Fat cells in the omentum and the mesenterium are a storage system of sorts related to all of these functions. Never before, however, was the San Jiao asked to store organochlorine pesticides. Can we say that fat-soluble chemicals end up in the San Jiao? It used to be, before a very recent blood test became available, that a tiny amount of fat from the omentum was needed to study the levels of chemicals in the body.

The San Jiao is so ubiquitous that it is difficult to say that it is not at the qi or ying or blood level. Usually qi-level lingering heat pathogens present with low-grade fevers, chest constraint, intermittent sore throat, and insomnia. Perhaps this is as close as we can get to a lingering pathogen that is a pesticide. The wen bing school treats these conditions with herbs that 'out-thrust' internal lingering heat. Special herbs like dan dou chi (Sojae Semen preparatum; *Glycine max*; green soy beans), ge gen (Puerariae Radix; *Pueraria*), bo he (Menthae haplocalycis Herba; *Mentha haplocalyx*), xuan shen (Scrophulariae Radix; *Scrophularia*), and bai shao (Paeoniae Radix alba; *Paeonia lactiflora*) are used. These herbs have some sort of relationship with the special place that is between the wei level and the qi level. They are interlocutors, if you will.

Damp heat in the qi level usually presents with a feeling of heaviness, aching, chest oppression, and afternoon feverishness. Damp obstructs the clear yang, the ascending and descending functions are disturbed. There is aversion to cold due to yang obstruction by dampness. The spleen can be damaged if the original injury was by cold. Many iatrogenic injuries occur in this as a result of the cold nature of some pharmaceuticals. San ren tang is a formula of choice in this situation because it resolves damp heat and leads heat to the exterior.

In treating qi-level latent pathogenic heat factors it is important to tonify the zheng qi which is assumed deficient, in order to enable the body to move the pathogen exteriorly. In damp heat pathogens, it is best to chose tonic herbs that are neutral in temperature and also not too sweet, since the sweet nature of these herbs can contribute to dampness.

Another example is Yin qiao san, which is the primary formula to treat wind heat in the wei level. This formula can be modified to treat lung heat or heat in the qi level. The formula is specific to the respiratory system. Herbs are added to modify its effect. For example, jie geng (Platycodi Radix; *Platycodon grandiflorus*) can be added to open the qi mechanism of the lung. Sheng di huang (Rehmanniae Radix; *Rehmannia* unprepared root), mu dan pi (Moutan Cortex; *Paeonia suffruticosa* root cortex), and xuan shen (Scrophulariae Radix; *Scrophularia*) clear deficiency heat. To clear qi level heat one can add, dan zhu ye (Lophatheri Herba; *Lophatherum gracile*), and zhi mu (Anemarrhenae Rhizoma; *Anemarrhena*). To tonify the zheng qi one can use huang qi (Astragali Radix; *Astragalus membranaceus*) and xi yang shen (Panacis quinquefolii Radix; *Panax quinquefolium*).

Combining this approach for clearing qi-level latent heat pathogens during sweating might enhance the effect of the sweating in terms of releasing a chemical pathogen like an organochlorine pesticide. Lipolysis is increased during fasting, and sweating along with the releasing techniques for qi-level LPFs might help to potentiate the depuration of pesticides. By adding herbs that direct the formula to the San Jiao the formula can be made even more specific. Zhe bei mu (Fritillariae thunbergii Bulbus; *Fritillaria thunbergii*), for

example, is a herb that enters the San Jiao channel and may act as an envoy.

In wen bing xue, the method used to scatter and disperse a San Jiao qi aspect pathogen is multiple. The qi dynamic is diffused and phlegm heat is transformed and discharged. This is something that zhe bei mu does as one of its basic functions. The common formula used to treat a triple burner qi level pathogen is Wend an tang with modifications.

Another method for clearing a heat LPF at the ying level is to use a set of combined formulas that nourish the yin, clear deficiency heat, and clear deeper level heat pathogens that are otherwise difficult to clear. Two formulas generally are combined: Qing wen bai du yin plus Qing hao bie jia tang. In the latter formula qing hao (Artemisiae annuae Herba; *Artemisia annua*) goes deeply interior like a messenger herb and moves and vents the pathogen outward. It is almost like a chelating agent, in a sense. In Qing wen bai du yin, zhi mu (Anemarrhenae Rhizoma; *Anemarrhena*), and dan zhu ye (Lophatheri Herba; *Lophatherum gracile*) work together to clear heat from the qi level. Sheng di huang (Rehmanniae Radix; *Rehmannia* unprepared root), mu dan pi (Moutan Cortex; *Paeonia suffruticosa* root cortex), chi shao (Paeoniae Radix rubra; *Paeonia* lactiflora), and xuan shen (Scrophulariae Radix; *Scrophularia*) all clear ying level heat. Huang lian (Coptidis Rhizoma; *Coptis*) and huang qin (Scutellariae Radix; *Scutellaria baicalensis*) clear qi level heat and lian qiao (Forsythiae fructus; *Forsythia*) vents heat to the exterior. The combination of these herbs works to lift deep pathogens stuck in the ying and xue level to a higher and more exterior level in the body so that more common techniques can be used to clear them.

Qing wen bai du yin

zhi mu (Anemarrhenae Rhizoma; *Anemarrhena*)
dan zhu ye (Lophatheri Herba; *Lophatherum gracile*)
shui niu jiao (Bubali Cornu; *Bubalus* horn)
sheng di huang (Rehmanniae Radix; *Rehmannia* unprepared root)
mu dan pi (Moutan Cortex; *Paeonia suffruticosa* root cortex)

chi shao (Paeoniae Radix rubra; *Paeonia lactiflora* root)

xuan shen (Scrophulariae Radix; *Scrophularia*)

huang lian (Coptidis Rhizoma; *Coptis*)

huang qin (Scutellariae Radix; *Scutellaria baicalensis*)

lian qiao (Forsythiae fructus; *Forsythia*)

Qing hao bie jia tang

qing hao (Artemisiae annuae Herba; *Artemisia annua*)

sheng di huang (Rehmanniae Radix; *Rehmannia* unprepared root)

zhi mu (Anemarrhenae Rhizoma; *Anemarrhena*)

mu dan pi (Moutan Cortex; *Paeonia suffruticosa* root cortex)

During fasting these last two formulas combined may help to clear LPFs in the ying or blood level. Screens done pre- and post-fasting in combination with these formulas shows a greater depuration of pesticides than fasting alone. The percentage of increased clearing was 20% in two patients (out of two). Of course, this is too small a sample to draw conclusions. But it is perhaps intriguing enough and the need is great enough to continue with a larger group of people.

References

1. Shiva V. Staying alive. London: Zed Books; 1989.
2. Shiva V. Biopolitics. London: Zed Books; 1995.
3. Jarrett L. Nourishing destiny. Stockbridge: Spirit Path Press; 1998.
4. Sessions G. Ecocentrism and the anthropocentric detour. ReVision 1991; 13:3.
5. Epstein S. The politics of cancer revisited. USA: Eastridge Press: 1998.
6. Brown L. Fish farming may soon take over cattle ranching as a food source. Worldwatch Institute Issue Alert 9, October 3 2000.
7. Haapapuro ER. Review – animal waste used as livestock feed: dangers to human health. Prev Med 1997; 26:599–602.
8. Gillespie JR. Modern livestock and poultry production. Albany: Delmar Publishing; 1997:122.
9. Glynn MK. Emergence of multi-drug resistant *Salmonella enterica* serotype typhimurium D T 104 infections in the United States. N Engl J Med 1998; 338:1333–1338.
10. Epstein S. Unlabelled milk from cows treated with biosynthetic growth hormones. Int J Health Serv 1996; 26:173–185.
11. Simopoulos R. The omega diet. HarperCollins; 1999.
12. Rainforest Action Network. Seven things you can do to save the rainforest. Factsheet. 2000. Online. Available: www.ran.org.
13. Heitschmidt R. Ecosystems, sustainability, and animal agriculture. J Animal Sci 1996; 74:1395–1405.
14. Khalil M. Sources, sinks, and seasonal cycles of atmospheric methane. J Geophys Res 1983; 88:5131–5144.
15. Donoghue DJ. Modeling drug residue uptake by eggs: yokes contain ampicillin residues, even after drug withdrawal and nondetectability in the plasma. Poult Sci 1997; 76:458–462.
16. Kocamis H. Postnatal growth of broilers in response to in ovo administration of chicken growth hormone. Poult Sci 1999; 78:1216–1219.
17. American Federation of Aging Research. Clinical Immunology. 2002. Online: www.infoaging.org.
18. Spindler S. Short-term caloric restriction reverses expression of genes altered by aging. Proc Nat Acad Sci 2001; 98:10630–10635.
19. Mukherjee P. Calorie-restricted diets slow the growth of prostate tumors in rats. J NCI 1999; 91:489–491, 512–523.
20. Mai V. Calories restriction and diet composition modulate spontaneous intestinal tumorigenesis in APC(MIN) mice through different mechanisms. Cancer Prevention Fellowship Program, Division of Cancer Prevention, NCI. PMID: 12702556.
21. Coats C. The nature of water. In: Living energies: an exposition of concepts related to the theories of Viktor Schauberger. Bath: Gateway Books; 1996.
22. Jenny H. Kymatik/Cymatiks. ISBN 3-85560-009-0. Out of print.
23. Worldwatch Press Release. Falling water tables in China may soon raise food prices everywhere; 2000.
24. Schauberger V. Der Wald un Seine Bedeuntung. Tau Magazine 1992; 146:2.
25. Gardner G. Underfed and overfed: the global epidemic of malnutrition. Worldwatch Paper 150, Worldwatch Institute; 2000.
26. Institute for Policy Studies. Changing course: blueprint for peace in Central America and the Carribean. Washington, DC; 1984.
27. Shiva V. Stolen harvest: the hijacking of the global food supply. Cambridge, MA: Southend Press; 2000.

28. Worldwatch. Monoculture: the biological and social impacts; March/April, 1998.
29. Harden M. A case-control study of non-Hodgkin's lymphoma and exposure to pesticides. Cancer 1999; 85:1353–1360.
30. Lappe M. Against the grain: biotechnology and the corporate takeover of food. Common Courage Press; 1998.
31. Sessions G. Review of Conrad Bonifazi's 'The soul of the world'. Environmental Ethics 1981; 3:275–281.
32. Biehl J. Dialectics in the ethics of social ecology. In: Zimmerman M, ed. Environmental philosophy: from animal rights to radical ecology. Englewood Cliffs, NJ: Prentice-Hall; 1993.
33. Environmental Working Group. Body Burden. Online: www.ewg.org; 2005
34. Chirnside A. Bioremediation of pesticide contaminated soil utilising phanerochaete chrysosporium and a selective microbial consortium. Dissertation. Unpublished. 2003.
35. Rothman D, ed. Medicine and Western civilization. Rutgers University Press; 1995.
36. Grossinger R. Planet medicine: from stone age to post-industrial healing. Boulder: Shambhala; 1982.
37. Johari H. Dhanwantari. Healing Arts Press; 1998.
38. Kirchfield F. Nature doctors. Medicina Biologica; 1994.
39. Schware D. Evaluation of a detoxification treatment for fat stored xenobiotics. Med Hypothesis 1982; 9:265–282.
40. Ye Tian Shi. Wen Re Lun (Discussion of warmth and heat). 1766 ACE.
41. Schware D. Body burden reductions of PCBs, PBBs, and chlorinated pesticides in human subjects. Ambio 1984; 13:378–380.
42. Unschuld P. Medicine in China. Berkley: University of California Press; 1985.
43. Yashiro N. Clinico-psychological and pathophysiological studies on fasting therapy. Sapporo Med J (Japan) 1986; 55:125–136.
44. Yamamoto H. Psychophysiological study of fasting therapy. Psychotherapy and Psychosomatics (Switzerland) 1979; 32:229–240.
45. Owen O. Brain metabolism during fasting. J Clin Invest 1967; 46:1589–1595.
46. Salloum T. Fasting signs and symptoms: a clinical guide. Buckey Press; 1992.
47. Imamura M. A trial of fasting cure for PCB-poisoned patients in Taiwan. Am J Indust Med 1984; 5:147–153.
48. Tretjak Z. PCB reduction and clinical improvement by detoxification: an unexploited approach? Human Exp Toxic 1990; 9:235–244.
49. Mayne S. Dietary beta-carotene and lung cancer risk in US non-smokers. J NCI 1994; 86:33.
50. Yu BP. Influence on life-prolonging food restriction on membrane lipoperoxidation and antioxidant status. In: Simic MJ, Taylor KA, Ward, et al, eds. Oxygen radicals in biology and medicine. New York: Plenum Press; 1988:1067–1073.
51. Harmon D. Aging: a theory based on free radical and radiation chemistry. J Gerontol 1956; 11:298–300.
52. Bjorksten J. Crosslinkage theory of aging. J Am Geriatr Soc 1968; 16:408.
53. Vega Institute, California. The Vega salt bath.
54. Lechner P. The role of a modified Gerson therapy in the treatment of cancer. Aktuelle Ernahrungsmedisin 1989; 1:138–143.
55. Sauerbruch F. Die historiche Entierklung der operativen Behandlung der Lugentuberkulose. Zeitschift fur Tuberkulose 1930; 57:289–294.
56. Zhang Mingwu. Chinese Qigong Therapy. Shandong Science and Technology Press; 1988.
57. Takahashi M. Qigong for health. Japan Publications; 1986.

Further reading

Carson R. Silent spring. Houghton Mifflin; 1994.
Steingraber S. Having faith: an ecologist's journey to motherhood. Oxford: Perseus; 2001.

Appendix

Pinyin name	Pharmaceutical name	Scientific name	Common name
bai hua she	Agkistrodon	*Agkistrodon acutus*	—
ban mao	Mylabris	*Mylabris*	—
bing pian	Borneolum	*Dryobalanops aromatica*	Borneol
di long	Pheretima	*Pheretima*	Lumbricus
e jiao	Asini Corii Colla	*Equus asinus*	Donkey-hide gelatin
gui ban*	Testudinis Plastrum	*Chinemys reevesii*	Tortoise/turtle plastron
huo ma ren*	Cannabis Semen	*Cannabis sativa*	Cannabis seeds
ji nei jin	Gigeriae galli Endothelium corneum	*Gallus gallus domesticus*	Chicken gizzard lining
long gu	Fossilia Ossis Mastodi	—	Fossilised bone
long yi	Serpentis Periostracum	*Elaphe/Zaocys*	Snake slough
lu feng fang	Vespae Nidus	*Vespa*	Wasp/hornet nest
lu jiao	Cervi Cornu	*Cervus*	Deer antler
lu rong	Cervi Cornu pantotrichum	*Cervus nippon*	Deer velvet
mu li	Ostreae Concha	*Ostrea*	Oyster shell
quan xie	Scorpio	*Buthus martensii*	—
ru xiang	Olibanum	*Boswellia sacra*	Frankincense; gum olibanum
shan ci gu*	Cremastrae/Pleiones Pseudobulbus	*Cremastra/Pleione*	Orchid pseudobulbs
shi gao	Gypsum fibrosum	—	Calcium sulfate; gypsum
shui niu jiao	Bubali Cornu	*Bubalus*	Buffalo horn
tu bie chong	Eupolyphaga	*Eupolyphaga sinensis*	—
wu gong	Scolopendra	*Scolopendra subspinipes*	—
wu ling zhi	Trogopterori Faeces	*Trogopterus xanthipes*	Squirrel excrement
xue jie	Daemonoropis Resina	*Daemonorops draco*	Resina Draconis; dragon's blood

General Subject Index

A

abortions 201
abrin 199
ABVD 266, 268–9
AC 120–1, 128, 144
Accu-Chem Laboratories 354
acetaminophen 55, 248
aciclovir 292
acupuncture 71, 118, 146, 317, 322, 324, 334
acute lymphocytic leukemia (ALL) 284–5, 287–8
    classification of 287–8
    clinical features of 287
    etiology of 287
    prognosis for 288
    treatment of 288, 293
acute myelogenous leukemia (AML) 266, 284, 288–9, 315
    classification of 288
    clinical features of 288
    diagnosis of 288
    prognosis for 288
    treatment of 289, 293
acute non-lymphocytic leukemia 269
acute promyelocytic leukemia 14
adenocarcinomas 42, 57, 160–1, 188–9
    of cervix 178
    of ovary 197
adenosquamous carcinomas 178, 189
adenoviruses 5
adjuvant therapy 120, 217
adrenal glands 219, 259
Adriamycin 13, 24, 29–30, 111, 120, 122, 125, 127–8, 140, 266, 269
aflatoxins 232, 240–1
age
    and ALL 288
    and breast cancer 91

Agency for Toxic Substances and Disease Registry (ATSDR) 354
agrimony 49, 75, 80, 114, 174, 185, 222–3, 238, 275, 294
alcohol 227, 230
    and breast cancer 103
    and HRT 95
    and prostate cancer 156
alcoholism 234, 236
aldesleukin 219
alkaline phosphatase (AKP) 39, 233–4
alkylphenols 105
all-trans-retinoic acid 14
allogeneic BMT see bone marrow transplantation (BMT), allogeneic
allopurinol 290
aloe 23
aloe vera 73
alopecia 122
alpha fetoprotein (AFP) 196, 233, 246
alpha interferon 219, 290
alpha-1-globulin 233
alprazolam 99
altretamine 190, 198
Alzheimer's disease 350
    and HRT 95
Amazon rain forest 346
ambulation, impaired 315
amenorrhea 269
American Cancer Society 38, 67
amifostine 45
4-aminibiphenyl 216
aminoglutethimide 131
amitriptyline 100, 323
amphetamines 323
amphotericin-B 291
amygdalin 51
amyloid 95
amyotrophic lateral sclerosis (ALS) 350

analgesia, personally controlled 249
anastrozole 128, 165
anatomy
    in ovarian cancer 200–1
    in prostate cancer 157–8
Anderson Tumor Score System 265
androgens 131, 157, 308
    receptors 196
androstenedione 165, 189
anemias 137, 182, 192–3, 261, 287–9, 302–4, 307
    Chinese medicine 303–4
    conventional medicine 302–3
    diagnostic patterns for 304
    types of 303
anger 107
angiogenesis 158, 163
angiomas 351
animal fat 62–3
animal products 150
    avoidance of 138–9
Ann Arbor staging system 261, 265, 267
Ann Arbor–Cotswolds staging system 254
anorexia 20, 248, 306, 328, 347
    in breast cancer 131
    in colorectal cancer 64
    and dying 333–4
    in hepatocellular carcinoma (HCC) 234
    in lung cancer 38
    in ovarian cancer 204, 209
    in pancreatic cancer 230, 232, 237, 239
anthracyclines 111, 131, 288–9
antiandrogen therapy 165
antibiotics 86, 163, 304–5, 345
    side-effects of 257

antibodies 23
  abnormal 98
antibody-dependent cell-mediated
    cytotoxicity (ADCC) 232
anticonvulsants 232
antidepressants 87
antidiuretic hormone (ADH) 333
antiemetics 81, 145, 210–11, 309
antiestrogens 131, 163
antiferritin 234
antigens 5–6
  fetal 6
antihistamines 39
antihypertensive drugs 99
antioxidants, screen for 354
antitumor drugs 13
anxiety 30, 207, 317–19
  Chinese medicine 317–19
  clinical presentations of 318
  conventional medicine 317
  etiology of 318
  patterns of 318
anxiolytics 317
aphasia 141
apheresis 292
aplasia 284, 291
apoptosis 96, 197, 254–5, 261
appetite 84, 86, 249, 311
arachidonic acid 159
Aranesp 14
Aredia 132
argine vasopressin 38
Arimidex 128, 165
aromatase 100, 131, 166
arsenic 36, 284, 352
asbestos 36, 41–2, 65, 178, 191, 196,
    200, 218, 289
ascending colon 62
ascites 323, 327–8, 334
  Chinese medicine 327–8
  in hepatocellular carcinoma (HCC)
      232–3, 242–3
  in lymphomas 272
  in ovarian cancer 197, 199, 201
  patterns of 328
  in uterine cancer 188, 193
Ashwagandha 319
asparaginase 13, 288
aspartame 21
aspergillosis pneumonitis 291
aspirin 247
asthma 36, 346
astragalus 22–3
ataxia-telangiectasis 91
atelectasis 323–4
atenolol 99, 247
Ativan 208, 210
atrazine 101–2, 104, 279, 349, 352,
    357–8

atypical squamous cells of
    undetermined significance
    (ASCUS) 180–1
auramine 216
autism 350
autoantibodies 98
autoimmune hemolytic anemias 261
autologous bone marrow
    transplantation (ABMT) 199,
    263
autologous stem cell transplantation
    292–3
avastin 45
Ayurvedic formula 240, 245
Ayurvedic tradition 336
azaserine 230
Azimexon 13

B

baby food 104
bacillus Calmette–Guerin (BCG) 13,
    217, 224–7
  side-effects of 217
bacteria 104
  anaerobic 62, 64–5
  antibiotic-resistant 345
  Gram-negative 304
  Gram-positive 136, 304
  intestinal 96
  pathogenic 348
bacterial prostatitis 162
bag balm 124
balsam pear 240
bamboo, dried sap of 76, 310–11
bao gong 200
barium enemas 67
barley sprouts 55, 134, 136–7, 149,
    167, 205, 210, 237, 247–8, 306,
    311
beef 104
Benefit the Lung Decoction 51
benign prostatic hypertrophy (BPH)
    57, 156–7, 159, 161–2, 172
benzamides 309
benzene 284, 287
  hexachloride 104
benzidine 216, 230
benzo-α-pyrene 41
benzodiazepines 309
beta-carotene 42, 62, 156
beta-naphthylamine 230
beta2-microglobulin 67, 261
betel nut 183
Bethesda grading system 180
bi 316
  syndrome 317, 324
bicalutemide 165

bilateral orchiectomy 165
bile 63, 356
bilirubin 233–4, 246, 302
Binet system 289
biologic therapies 13–15
biological response modifiers (BRMs)
    23, 130
biological therapies, ovarian cancer
    199
biology
  of bladder cancer 216
  of lung cancer
    NSCLC 42–3
    SCLC 37
  of ovarian cancer 196–7
Birch, Stephen 201, 220, 258
bison 104, 345
bisphenol 105
bisphosphanates 132
black cohosh 97
bladder 219–20, 222, 359
  channel 158
bladder cancer 215–18, 349
  biology of 216
  case studies 226–7
  Chinese medicine 219–25
  diagnosis of 216
    differential 222–5
  epidemiology of 215–16
  pathology of 216
  staging for 216–17
  treatment of 217–18
blame 108
bleomycin 182, 262, 265–6, 268–70,
    334
blood 18–20, 183, 302, 308, 316
  activation of 25–6
  cell loss 29
  circulation 23–4
  and damp stasis 204–5
  deficiency 65, 295, 304
    in breast cancer 103, 114, 128
    in colorectal cancer 70–1
    in lymphomas 271, 277
    in pancreatic cancer 235
  dryness 129
  enrichment 274
  harmonisation 27
  heat 235, 296
  nourishment 30, 121
  and qi 304
  regulation 25
  stasis 28, 350–1
    in bladder/renal cancer 222–4
    in breast cancer 94, 99, 101,
        103, 109, 113–14, 116, 118,
        128, 137, 141
    in cervical cancer 181–3
    in colorectal cancer 64, 73

blood (Continued)
    in leukemia 293–4
    in lung cancer 49–50
    in lymphomas 276
    in ovarian cancer 201–4, 209
    in pancreatic cancer 235
    in uterine cancer 190
  in stools 64
  tests 43, 354
Bloom–Richardson score 143, 147
boar 104
bone, metastases 132
bone marrow 283, 287–9, 302
  failure 289
  harvesting 290–1
  restoration 30
  suppression 307–9
    Chinese medicine 308–9
    conventional medicine 307–8
  transplantation (BMT) 265–6, 284,
    288–90, 295
    allogeneic 290–1
    autologous (ABMT) 199, 263
Boost the Lungs Decoction 86
borage 97
borneol 188, 326
bosulfan 290
Bowen's disease 5
brachytherapy 148, 164, 182–3, 190,
  192
breast cancer 4–6, 89–154, 343, 347–8
  and age 91
  and alcohol 103
  and breast implants 98
  case studies 139–50
  chemoprevention of 98–9
  chemotherapy for 120–8
  Chinese medicine 107–10, 113–15
  and contraceptive pill 92–4
  detection of 111–12
  diagnostic procedures for 1123
  and dietary contaminants 101–2
  and dietary fat 101
  and endocrine disruptors 103
  epidemiology of 90
  etiology of 107
  and family history 90–1
  and food dyes 105
  and food packaging 105
  and food supply contamination
    104
  and HER-2/neu status 111
  and histologic grade 110–11
  hormonal therapies for 120–8
  and hormone replacement therapy
    94–6
  and hormone-receptor status 111
  and hyperinsulinemia 102–3
  invasive 107

breast cancer (Continued)
  and mammography 97–8
  and meat 105–6
  medication risks in 99–100
  metastatic 130–2
  non-invasive 106
  and nuclear emissions 102
  and nuclear grade 110–11
  and obesity 100–1
  and phytoestrogens 96–7
  prevention of 137–8
  principles of treatment of 115–29
  prognostic factors for 110
  and pseudoestrogens 103
  and radiation therapy 117–19
  and reproductive history 91–2
  risk factors for 90–106
  and sex hormones 105–6
  staging of 115
  surgery 115–17
  and tamoxifen 98–9
  and tumor size 110
  types of 106–7
breast self-examination (BSE) 97
breastfeeding 109, 350
breasts 351
  anatomy of 106
Brenner tumors 197
Bristol-Myers Squibb 94, 100
broccoli 4, 157
Broffman, Michael 150
Brunn's nests 216
Brussels sprouts 4
bubble gum 105
Buddhism 336, 354
bulimia 20, 64, 347
Burkitt's lymphoma 2, 5–6, 20, 263–4,
  270–1, 287
Burn creme 119, 145, 148
buserelin 165
busulfan 290–1

C

CA 15-3 111, 130
CA 19-9 67, 77, 81, 84, 231, 246
CA 27.29 111, 130, 140, 143, 146–7
CA 125 196, 198, 207, 211
cachectin 332
cachexia 131, 170, 237, 240, 244,
  332–3, 347
  and dying 333
cadmium 218, 352
calcified deposits 351
calcium 62–3, 65, 94, 159, 220, 247,
  351, 353
  di-glucarate 81
  excretion 137

calcium (Continued)
  serum 131
  sulfate 49
calorie restriction 346–7
cancer, epidemic of 342–3
Cancer Research Institute, New York
  171
candidiasis 210–11, 256, 291, 312, 333
cannabinoids 309
capecitabine 82
carbamazepine 82, 323
carboplatin 40–1, 45, 55, 190, 198, 203,
  207–9, 211–12, 310
carbuncles 273
carcinoembryonic antigen (CEA) 40,
  67, 77, 84, 130, 147, 196, 216,
  231, 246
carcinogens 8, 104–5, 343, 347
  environmental 7
  exposure to 342–3
    reduction of 343–6
  persistent 349–51
  products containing 349
carcinoma in situ (CIS) 6, 177, 216–17
cardamon 240
cardiomyopathy 269
cardiotoxicity 122
cardiovascular disease 46, 257, 343
care, integration of 15
carmustine 270, 293
L-carnitine 297
Carson, Rachel 90, 343
case studies
  bladder cancer 226–7
  breast cancer 139–50
  cervical cancer 191–3
  colorectal cancer 78–87
  in lung cancer 54–9
  lymphomas 277–80
  ovarian cancer 207–13
  pancreatic cancer 246–50
  prostate cancer 172–5
Casodex 165
castor oil 326
castration 165
cattle 345
cauliflower 4
causal factors 4–6
celiac axis block 232
celiac disease 264
central nervous system (CNS) 130,
  261, 287, 289
  and dying 334
cervical cancer 4–6, 20, 22, 177–88
  case studies 191–3
  Chinese medicine 183–8
  diagnosis of 180
  epidemiology of 177
  etiology of 178–9

cervical cancer (Continued)
 invasive 179–80
 natural history of 179
 pathology of 178
 prognosis of 181–2
 screening for 180
 staging of 181
 treatment of 182–8
cervical dysplasia 22, 159, 188
cervical intraepithelial neoplasia
 (CIN) 22, 159, 178–80
cervical malignancies 178
cervical neoplasia 178
cervicitis 184
cervix 178–80, 182, 190, 201
 adenocarcinomas of 178
CFP 128
chang feng 63–4
chelation therapy 138, 257
chemicals 341
 carcinogenic 5
 persistent 349–51
 petroleum-based 348
chemo arthritis 146
chemoembolisation 233–4
chemoprevention, of breast cancer
 98–9
chemoreceptor trigger zone 309
chemotherapy 12–13, 25, 28–9, 39,
 79–81
 adjuvant 44, 231
 in breast cancer 120–8
 in cervical cancer 182
 in colorectal cancer 74–6
 combination 40, 265
 continuous 30
 in gall bladder carcinoma 235
 in hepatocellular carcinoma (HCC)
 233–4
 high-dose 30–1, 263, 292–3, 295–6
 in Hodgkin's disease 266
 intrathecal 288
 issues caused by 313–14
 in leukemia 286
 in lymphomas 262
 and osteoporosis 94
 in ovarian cancer 198
 in pancreatic cancer 246
 and pregnancy 107
 side-effects of 276
 single-agent 40
 subcategories of 13
 symptoms of 120–1
 three combination 262
chest, retained fluids in 325
chickens 104, 346
 gizzard lining 80, 83, 85–7, 170,
 205, 247–8, 274, 278–9, 311
children, treating leukemia, in 297–8

Chinese medicine 15–17
 for anemias 303–4
 for anxiety 317–19
 for ascites 327–8
 in bladder cancer 219–25
 and bone marrow suppression
 308–9
 in breast cancer 107–10, 113–15
 categories of tumors in 17
 in cervical cancer 183–8
 in colorectal cancer 63–5
 diagnosis of 67–71
 diagnostic categories 166–72
 herbal 357–8
 in Hodgkin's disease 270–7
 in indolent lymphomas 255–60
 in leukemia 285–6, 293–8
 in liver cancer 240–4
 in lung cancer 45–54
 in lymphomas 270–7
 for mucositis 312–13
 for nausea 310–12
 for neutropenia 305–7
 in ovarian cancer 200–7
 and pain 323–4
 in pancreatic cancer 235–40
 and pathogenesis 17–22
 and pleural effusion 324–6
 in prostate cancer 158–60
 the pulses of 337–8
 in renal-cell carcinoma 219–25
 for stomatitis 312–13
 therapeutic principles of 22–5
 for thrombocytopenia 308–9
 treatment 25–32
 in prostate cancer 166–72
 rules of 30–1
 in uterine cancer 189
 and vomiting 310–12
Chinese raspberry 129
Chipsa Hospital, Tijuana 192
chlorambucil 269, 289
chloramphenicol 284
chlordane 104, 352
chlorine 352, 356
chlorpromazine 323
chlorpyrifos 352
CHOD-B/ESHAP/NOPP 262
cholecystectomy 144, 235
cholecystitis 234–5, 238
cholecystokinin (CCK) 231
cholelithiasis 234
cholesterol 99, 241–2, 246, 345–7
Chong channel
 in breast cancer 91, 93, 96, 99,
 101–3, 109, 129
 in leukemia 285
 in ovarian cancer 200–1, 203–4
 in prostate cancer 158, 160

CHOP 265, 275, 278
CHOP-Bleo 262
CHOP-R 262, 278
Christianity 336
chromoganin 37
chronic fatigue syndrome 257, 350
chronic lymphocytic leukemia (CLL)
 6, 261, 284–5, 289–90
 diagnosis of 289
 etiology of 289
 staging for 289
 subcategories of 290
 T-cell 290
 treatment of 289–90, 293
chronic myelogenous/myeloid
 leukemia (CML) 14, 284, 290–3
 categorisation of 290
 treatment of 293
chronic obstructive pulmonary
 disease (COPD) 334
ciclosporin 292
cilantro 240
cimetidine 100
cinnamon 240
cirrhosis 232–3, 236, 241–2, 245
CISCA 217
cisplatin 13, 40–1, 45, 182, 190, 198–9,
 203, 217, 265, 309–10
cladribine 290
classification
 acute lymphocytic leukemia (ALL)
 287–8
 acute myelogenous leukemia
 (AML) 288
Clavey, Steven 222
clear cell carcinoma 189, 197
clear heat 126, 360
clinical evaluation, lung cancer, SCLC
 39–40
clinical features
 of acute lymphocytic leukemia
 (ALL) 287
 of acute myelogenous leukemia
 (AML) 288
 of gall bladder carcinoma 234
 of hepatocellular carcinoma (HCC)
 232–3
 of lymphomas 261
 of non-Hodgkin's lymphoma
 (NHL) 264
 of pancreatic cancer 230
clinical presentation
 of anxiety 318
 in colorectal cancer 66–7
 in lung cancer
 NSCLC 43
 SCLC 37–8
 in renal-cell carcinoma 218
 in uterine cancer 189

Clomid 202
clomifene citrate 202
clotting 18–19
clove 310
clover sprouts 96
clumping 259
CMF 120, 125, 128, 130, 144–6
CNS leukemia, formula 297
coal-tar 352
cocaine 36, 46
cocoa butter 73–4
codeine 323
codonopsis 23
coffee 230
Cohen, Isaac 150
Colace 208
cold 316, 358
    attacking chest and lungs 325
    blood stasis 202
    phlegm 76
collagen 94
colon 62–3
    carcinomas 62
    therapy 356
colonialism 348–9
colonic polyposis 4
colonoscopy 67, 137
colony-stimulating factors (CSFs) 81,
        84, 125, 209, 278, 305, 308
colorectal cancer 4, 61–88
    case studies 78–87
    chemotherapy for 74–6
    Chinese medicine 63–5
    clinical presentation of 66–7
    diagnosis of 67
    epidemiology of 61–2
    and HRT 95
    later-stage 76–7
    pathogenesis of 62–5
    pathology of 65–6
    post-surgical formulae for 71–2
    prevention formula for 77–8
    radiation treatment of 72–4
    risk factors for 65
    screening for 67
    tumor types 66
colostomy 198
colposcopy 180–1, 188, 201
coma 59, 332
combined therapy 262, 268
complete blood count (CBC) 112, 266,
        307
computerised tomography (CT)
    in bladder cancer 216, 218
    in breast cancer 130
    in colorectal cancer 77, 84
    in lung cancer 39–40, 43
    in lymphomas 261, 266–8, 280
    in ovarian cancer 198, 208

computerised tomography (CT)
        (Continued)
    in pancreatic/hepatic cancers 230,
        233, 235
concurrent issues 301–29
cone biopsy/conisation 180, 182, 188
congee 240, 249–50
congestive heart failure (CHF) 334
conjugated linoleic acid 104
conjugation 351
connective tissue disorders 9
consolidation therapy 40
constipation 306, 309, 311–12
    in breast cancer 116, 127, 141–3
    chronic 65, 148, 167
    in colorectal cancer 76, 81
    and dying 334
    in ovarian cancer 206, 209, 211–12
    in pancreatic/hepatic cancers
        247–9
constraint disorder 319
constraint syndromes 321–2
consumption 322
contamination
    of eggs and poultry 346
    of fish 344–5
    of fruit and vegetables 344
    of meat 345–6
    of water 344
contraceptive pill 178
    and breast cancer 92–4
conventional medicine
    for anemias 302–3
    for anxiety 317
    for bone marrow suppression
        307–8
    for mucositis 312
    for nausea 309
    for neutropenia 304–5
    for stomatitis 312
    for thrombocytopenia 307–8
    for vomiting 309
Coombs' test 261
COP 289
COP-Bleo 262
CoQ10 81, 297
cord blood stem cells 291
core needle biopsy 112
coriander 240
corticosteroids 220, 288, 309, 333
cough 46, 48, 52
coumadin 140–1, 143
Courvoisier's sign 230
Cox inhibition 63
cricoid process 270
crisantaspase 13
Crohn's disease 65
cryosurgery 233
cryotherapy 182

cunkou 298
cupping 118
Cushing's syndrome 38
cyclic adenosine monophosphate
        (cAMP) 23
cyclin-dependent kinases (CDKs) 3
cyclophosphamide
    and breast cancer 120, 123, 125,
        140
    and leukemia 289–90, 293
    and lung cancer 40
    and lymphomas 262, 265, 269
    and ovarian cancer 198
    and uterine cancer 190
cystitis 171, 275, 293
    hemorrhagic 297
cysto-prostatectomy 217
cystoscopy 226
cysts 351, 355
cytarabine 13, 265, 288–9
cytochrome P-450 351
cytokines 292
cytomegalovirus (CMV) 260, 262
cytoreductive surgery 198
cytosine 289
cytotoxic therapy 25
cytotoxicity 29–30
Cytovene 292
Cytoxan 120, 140–1, 143, 198
dacarbazine 190, 266, 268
dactinomycin 190, 270

D

Dai channel 200
daidzen 96
damp 256, 316
    environment 256
    heat 250, 358, 360
        accumulation of 167–8, 184
        in breast cancer 101, 109, 145
        in cervical cancer 185
        in colorectal cancer 63–4, 67–8,
            78
        in liver gall bladder 242–3
        macerates flesh 316
    phlegm 64–5, 114, 179, 257, 355
        accumulation 20, 257
        stasis 46, 84
    stasis 122
        in lung 48–9
    toxin 186–7
dampness 31, 310, 321–2, 360
    in breast cancer 114
    in colorectal cancer 75
    drainage of 26
    in ovarian cancer 201, 204, 209,
        211

dampness *(Continued)*
  in pancreatic cancer 236
  and phlegm accumulation 20,
    257
  in prostate cancer 158–9, 166–7
  in uterine cancer 190–1
Dan Tian 220
Dao 335–6, 338
Daoism 335–6
darbapoeitin alfa 14
daunorubicin 289
DDE/DDT 21, 101–4, 147–8, 255, 279,
    352, 358
death 331–40
  pulses 338
  rattle 333
  the time of 335–6
  Western approach to 331–3
Decadron 208, 210
Decoction for Invigorating Yang 141
decubitus ulcers 335
deep vein thrombosis 99
deer antler 22, 138–9, 143, 308
deer velvet 26, 307
deficiency fire 145
deficiency heat 49–50
  symptoms 126
deglycyrrhised licorice (DGL) 245
dehydration, and dying 333–4
dehydroepiandrosterone 165
delayed impotence (ED) 164–5
delirium 334–5
Depo-Provera 93, 219
depression 30, 140, 146, 207, 227,
    319–22
  and dying 334
  etiology of 319
  symptoms of 320
depressive liver fire 136–7
depuration 257, 350–3, 361
descending colon 62
Desogen 93
detection, breast cancer 111–12
detoxification 351–3
DEXA scan 137–8
dexamethasone 145, 206, 208, 210,
    262, 265, 309, 323
DHAP 265
diabetes 21, 46, 64, 94, 100, 103, 230,
    236, 240, 257, 343
diagnosis 8–11
  in acute myelogenous leukemia
    (AML) 288
  in bladder cancer 216
  in cervical cancer 180
  in chronic lymphocytic leukemia
    (CLL) 289
  in colorectal cancer 67
  in gall bladder carcinoma 235

diagnosis *(Continued)*
  in hepatocellular carcinoma (HCC)
    233
  in lung cancer, NSCLC 43–4
  in lymphomas 261
  in non-Hodgkin's lymphoma
    (NHL) 264
  in pancreatic cancer 230–1
  in prostate cancer 161–2
  in renal-cell carcinoma 218
  in uterine cancer 189
diagnostic patterns, anemia 304
diagnostic procedures, breast cancer
    1123
diarrhea 310, 312, 350
  in breast cancer 124
  in cervical cancer 188
  chronic 73
  in colorectal cancer 77, 84
  in ovarian cancer 206, 209
  in pancreatic cancer 239
diazepam 99, 323
2,4-dichlorophenoxyacetic acid (2,4-D)
    255, 264
dieldrin 104
diet
  and bladder/renal cancer 227
  and colorectal cancer 62
  and non-Hodgkin's lymphoma
    (NHL) 257
  and ovarian cancer 202
  and prostate cancer 156, 159
  as a risk factor 42, 230
dietary contaminants, and breast
    cancer 101–2
dietary fat 218, 230
  and breast cancer 101
diethylstilbestrol (DES) 105, 166, 352
differential diagnosis
  in bladder cancer 222–5
  in renal-cell carcinoma 222–5
diffuse intra-arterial coagulopathy
    (DIC) 140–3, 161
  formula 296
Diflucan 291
digestive fire 65
digital rectal examination (DRE) 67,
    77, 157, 161–2, 164
digoxin 269
dihydrotestosterone (DHT) 156, 231
dilatation and curettage (D&C) 189
dimethylbenz-α-anthracene 41
diosgenin 92
dioxins 352
diphenhydramine 39
  hydrochloride 248
diptheria 199
disharmony, of qi, blood and
    emotions 18–20

disseminated intravascular
    coagulopathy (DIC) 24, 288
dissolution, outer and inner 337
diuretics 125
DNA ploidy 11
docetaxel 111, 131, 208
donkey-hide gelatin 143, 186, 308
dosage 32
Dow Corning 98
Down's syndrome 284, 287
doxazosin 163
doxorubicin 13, 289
  and bladder cancer 217
  and breast cancer 111, 120, 131
  and hepatocellular carcinoma
    (HCC) 233
  and lung cancer 40
  and lymphomas 262, 265–6,
    268–70
  and prostate cancer 166
  and uterine cancer 190
doyo 59, 192, 338, 351
dragon's blood 114
drugs
  analgesic 323, 334
  antiadrenal 13, 128
  antibiotic 86, 163, 304–5, 345
  anticonvulsant 232, 323
  antidepressant 87, 323
  antiemetic 76, 81, 145, 210–11, 309
  antihypertensive 99
  antitumor 13
  anxiolytic 323
  diuretic 324
  dose-intense delivery of 30
  opioid 333–4
  sulfa 104
drum distention 327
dry mouth 311
Du 158
  channel 285
ductal adenocarcinoma 230
ductal carcinoma in situ (DCIS) 6, 143
  types of 106
Duncan's syndrome 264
duodenal obstruction 231
dying 331–40
  and anorexia 333
  and cachexia 333
  central nervous system (CNS) in
    334
  and constipation 334
  and dehydration 333–4
  and depression 334
  and dyspnea 334
  general symptoms of 333–5
  and nausea 333
  and pressure sores 335
  process of 336–7

dying (*Continued*)
    and urinary incontinence 334–5
    and vomiting 333
dysfibrinogenemia 233
dyshydrosis 43
dyspareunia 183
dysphagia 140, 333
dysplasia 66, 179
dyspnea 326
    and dying 334
dysuria 216

E

Early Breast Cancer Trial 120
edema 107, 188, 193, 207, 240, 260, 334
Efudex 182
eggs, contamination of 346
Eight Corrections Powder 222
Eight Extra Meridians 200–1
Eight Extraordinary Channels 200, 285
ejaculation 158
ejection fraction 128–9
Elavil 100
electrolytic disturbances 9
emesis, types of 309
emotional constraint 321–2
    deficiency/excess 322
emotions 18–20
empty fire flaring 313
endocrine disruptors 102
    and breast cancer 103
endocrine syndromes 10
endometrial cancer 188
endometriosis 197
endometrium 178, 180
endoscopic retrograde cholangiopancreatography (ERCP) 230–1
endrin 104
enophthalmos 43
enterococci 304
enterocytes 62
enterolactone 96
environment, pre-cancerous 351
Environmental Protection Agency (EPA) 41, 104, 345
Environmental Working Group 5, 104, 349
epidemic, cancer 342–3
epidemiology
    of bladder cancer 215–16
    of breast cancer 90
    of cervical cancer 177
    of colorectal cancer 61–2
    of Hodgkin's disease 267

epidemiology (*Continued*)
    of leukemia 284
    of lung cancer 35–6
    of non-Hodgkin's lymphoma (NHL) 263–4
    of ovarian cancer 195
    of pancreatic cancer 229–30
    of prostate cancer 156
    of renal-cell carcinoma 218
Epo 209
Epstein–Barr virus (EBV) 4–5, 20, 264, 267, 285
equol 96
Er Xian Tang 259
erectile dysfunction 174
erythema 107
erythrocytosis 233
erythropoietin 302, 308
ESHAP 265
esophageal cancer 4–5, 20
esophagitis 45
Estrace 94
estradiol 92, 94, 96, 105, 143, 156, 189
    receptors 133
Estradurin 166
estramustine 166
    phosphate 166
estriol 92, 94, 96
estrogen 308, 345, 358–9
    and lymphomas 255
    bioavailability of 143
    and breast cancer 91–100, 103, 110, 113, 133, 138–9, 142
    cascade 138
    and cervical cancer 178, 183
    deprivation 131
    and ovarian cancer 196
    and prostate cancer 166
    receptors 358
        and breast cancer 96, 102–3, 105–7, 111, 133, 143
        and cervical/uterine cancers 178, 189
        and ovarian cancer 196, 200
    replacement therapy (ERT) 94
    and uterine cancer 188–9, 191
estrone 92, 94, 96, 189
    receptors 133
ethinyl estradiol 82, 92, 166
ethyl benzene 352
etiological agents 7
etiology
    of acute lymphocytic leukemia (ALL) 287
    of anxiety 318
    of breast cancer 107
    of cervical cancer 178–9
    of chronic lymphocytic leukemia (CLL) 289

etiology (*Continued*)
    of depression 319
    of leukemia 284, 286
    of non-Hodgkin's lymphoma (NHL) 263–4
    of ovarian cancer 195–6
    of pancreatic cancer 229–30
    of prostate cancer 156–7
etoposide 13, 40–1, 45, 166, 265
Eulexin 165
excision 106–7
    repair 347
excrement 26, 114, 224
exercise, lack of 46, 160
exhaustion 21
exterior pernicious influences (EPIs) 21, 98, 258, 305
external pathogens 21–2, 101

F

familial polyposis 65–6
family history, and breast cancer 90–1
Fanconi syndrome 284
fasting 354–5
fat, accumulation 351
fecal occult blood tests 67
Femara 128
fennel seed 25, 27, 212, 247
fentanyl 192, 249, 323
fenugreek 136, 149, 240
ferritin 234
fertilisers 289
fertility, reduction in 269
fetal toxin 285
α-fetoprotein 6
fever 261
fiber 62, 65
fibrates 100
fibrinogen 24
fibroids 355
fibrosis 270
filgrastim 14, 209, 291, 305
finasteride 162–3, 165
fine needle aspiration (FNA) 8, 10, 43, 112, 230, 233, 261, 264
fire 108, 318, 357
    poisons 20–1, 63, 91, 94, 101, 107, 109, 113–14, 128
    toxins 98, 102–3, 358
fish, contamination of 344–5
Five Phase cycle 21, 92, 100, 122, 259
Five Phase Theory 19, 65, 236
Flagyl 99
flare 131
flat condylomas 179
flax seeds 96
flax-seed oil 144

flow, maintenance 26
floxuridine 219, 233
fluconazole 291
fludarabine 289–90
fluid stasis 116
fluorescent in situ hybridisation
        (FISH) 289
fluoride 352, 356
fluorouracil (5-FU)
    and breast cancer 120, 123–5
    and cervical cancer 182
    and colorectal cancer 63, 74–5,
        80–2
    and gall bladder carcinoma 235
    and pancreatic cancer 231–2
    and renal-cell carcinoma 219
    side-effects of 74, 80, 123
    and uterine cancer 192
fluorscopic endoscopy 38
fluoxetine 100
fluoxymesterone 131
flutamide 165–6
folic acid 246, 297, 312
follicle stimulating hormone (FSH)
        130
follicular lymphomas see lymphomas,
        follicular
Food and Drug Administration (FDA)
        93, 95, 98, 105, 352
food dyes, and breast cancer 105
food packaging, and breast cancer
        105
food stasis 109
food supply contamination, and
        breast cancer 104
formaldehyde 352
formulas
    for AC regimen 122–3
    advanced stage 126–7
    Ayurvedic 240, 245
    for bacillus Calmette–Guerin
        (BCG) 224–5
    for bone marrow suppression 308
    botanical 245
    for chemotherapy 275, 308–9
    for CMF regimen 123–4
    for CNS leukemia 297
    for combined therapy 275
    constitutional patterns of 132–7
    for diffuse intra-arterial
        coagulopathy (DIC) 296
    early stage 126
    for hemorrhage 296
    for hemorrhagic cystitis 297, 314
    for leucocytopenia 296
    for local application 188
    for pancreatitis 314
    for pericarditis 297
    postoperative 52

formulas (Continued)
    pre- and post-surgical 71–2,
        116–17
    preoperative 51–2
    for prevention 53–4
        in colorectal cancer 77–8
        in lymphomas 276
    for radiation treatment 52–3, 119,
        148, 183–4, 275
    for skin rashes 314
    and staging 125–8
    sterile 295
    Taichung Medical College 138
    for tamoxifen 129
    for Taxol regimens 124–5
    for thrombocytopenia 296, 308
    for toxic hepatitis 313
    for toxic myocarditis 297, 313
    for toxic nephritis 314
Formulas to Aid the Living 259
fossilised bone 129, 274, 276, 279
fossilised teeth 297
Four Gentlemen Decoction 48, 50
frankincense 27, 114, 324
French–American–British (FAB)
        Cooperative Working Group
        287–8
fright 107
fruit, contamination of 344
fu 84, 256, 357–8
fu qi 256, 357–8
fu qi wen bing 256, 358
fu zheng 125–6
    therapy 23, 296
Furacin 99
furans 352
furazolidone 99
Furhman system 218
Furoxone 99

G

gall bladder 19, 135, 137, 230, 321,
        351, 359
    channel 149
    qi 71
gall bladder carcinoma 234–5
    clinical features of 234
    diagnosis of 235
    natural history of 234
    pathology of 234
    staging for 235
    treatment of 235
gamma interferon 219
gamma knife irradiation 118
ganciclovir 292
garlic 183
gastric acid 136

gastric lymphoma 272
gastrin-releasing peptide 37
gastroesophageal reflux (GERD)
        208–9
gastrointestinal disturbances 9
gefitinib 57, 131
gemcitabine 45, 80–1, 131, 198, 212,
        231
    side-effects of 80
Gemzar 198, 212–13
gender, in society 92
gene therapy 199
genetic factors
    and leukemia 284
    and prostate cancer 157
genistein 84–5, 96, 124, 157, 168, 239
Gerota's fascia 219
Gerson therapy 192–3
giardia 99
ginger tea 306
ginseng 23, 212
    American 51
    red Chinese 84–5
    white 22, 50, 55, 84–7, 134, 141,
        170, 212, 239
glassy-cell carcinoma 178
Gleason score 161, 164, 172
globe artichoke 245
glucose 102, 138, 246, 354
glutamine 312
glutathione 62, 81, 353
    transferases 199
glycoproteins 162
glycyrrhetic acid 23
Gofman, John 97
goitre 25
golden rod 184
gonadotropins 131
goserelin 165, 190
gotu kola 146
graft failure 291
graft-versus-host disease (GVHD)
        291–2
grains 104, 144, 157
granulocyte colony stimulating factor
        14, 291
granulocyte macrophage colony
        stimulating factor 14, 307
granulocytes 125, 302
granulocytopenia 125, 204, 209, 288,
        293
Great Smokies Diagnostic Laboratory
        354
great void 317
green tea 143–4, 157, 278, 313
growth factors 3
    receptors 3
gu qi 63, 303
gu zhang 327

guaiac 67
Guang An Men Hospital, Beijing 27, 53
gulls 103
gum olibanum 27, 114, 324
gums, bleeding 306
gynecology 320
gynecomastia 100, 165, 233
gypsum 49

H

hair-coloring agents 289
hairy cell leukemia 290
hairy leukoplakia 312
Haldol 100
haloperidol 100, 323
Halotestin 131
Halsted radical mastectomy 115
hand/foot syndrome 124
hara signs 146
hardness, softening of 26
harmonisation, stomach/spleen 26
Hashimoto's thyroiditis 96, 264
heart 200, 317, 359
    and anxiety 318
    blood deficiency 318–19
    disease 94, 100
    fire 318
    qi 101
        deficiency 318
        stasis 92, 318
    shen 318
heart/kidney axis 274, 278–9, 317, 359
heat 316, 358
    accumulation 202
    attacking chest and lungs 325
    damage to lung and body fluids 315–16
    deficiency 310
    internal 326
    toxins 24–5, 99, 260, 357
        accumulation of 202
    yin-deficient 159, 305
heavy metals 352–3
    screen for 354
hematocrit 303
hematopoiesis 10, 253, 287, 293
hematopoietic growth factors 14
hematuria 174, 216, 222, 226, 244
hemiplegia 141
Hemoccult SENSA 67
HemoQuant 67
hemorrhage, formula 296
hemorrhagic cystitis, formula 297, 314
hemostatics 201
heparin 241

hepatitis B (HBV) 4, 232, 236, 241, 244, 260, 342
hepatitis C (HCV) 4–5, 232, 236, 241, 342
    treatment for 244–6
hepato-cellular cancer 4
hepatocellular carcinoma (HCC) 232–4, 241
    chemotherapy for 233–4
    clinical features of 232–3
    diagnosis of 233
    pathology of 232
    staging for 233
    treatment of 233–4
    see also liver cancer
hepatoma 6
hepatomegaly 233, 243, 289
hepatosplenomegaly 287
heptachlor 104
herbal Chinese medicine 357–8
herbal formulas, criteria for customisation 29
herbicides, organochlorine 352
herbs
    analgesic 323–4
    antineoplastic 31, 213, 223, 238–9, 242–4, 249, 270–3, 275
    antiviral 245
    blood-cracking 238, 271
    blood-heat-clearing 271–2, 307
    blood-nourishing 207, 310
    blood-regulating 114, 183, 203, 271, 275
    breast 114–15
    calm-the-spirit 142
    for chemotherapy 273
    clear-heat-and-toxin 24–5, 127, 137, 145, 272, 278
    contamination of 31–2, 305–6
    cooling 248
    detoxifying 31
    drain-damp 129, 185, 225
    eliminating 31
    envoy 278
    fire-poison 22
        in breast 114–15
    fluid-draining 325
    fu-zheng 27
    heat-clearing 271
    immunomodulating 249
    kidney-yang-tonic 306–7
    messenger 272, 360
    pacify-wind 136
    phlegm-resolving-breast 114
    phlegm-transforming 25, 212, 273
    qi-regulating 128, 212
    qi-tonic 31, 117, 127, 171, 238, 305–7
    release-the-exterior 149

herbs (Continued)
    soften-hard-mass-breast 115
    to treat infections 307
    tonic 22, 31, 306–7, 360
    toxic-heat-clearing 307
    toxin-clearing-breast 114–15
    warming-transform-cold-phlegm 136
    wine-prepared 270, 272
    yang-tonic 275
    yin-nourishing 123, 145, 171, 207, 244, 274–5, 307, 312
Herceptin 3, 111, 113, 120, 128, 130–1
hernia 208–9, 212
Herpes simplex virus (HSV) 3–4, 20, 178–9, 183, 260, 312, 333, 342
Hexalen 190, 198
high-intensity focused ultrasound (HIFU) 163
Hiroshima 97, 102, 284–5
histologic grade 11
    and breast cancer 110–11
HIV 258, 264, 267, 342
    and CIN 178–9
HIV/AIDS 260, 331, 342
Hodgkin's disease 5, 14, 266–76
    chemotherapy for 266
    Chinese medicine 270–7
    diagnosis of 266
    epidemiology of 267
    histologic types of 267
    and leukemia 284, 286
    staging for 267–8
    subtypes of 266
    treatment of 265, 268–77, 293
    see also lymphomas; non-Hodgkin's disease
hoelen 23
honey 240
hormonal therapy 12–13
    in breast cancer 120–9
    side-effects of 131, 166
hormone refractory prostate cancer 166
hormone replacement therapy, and breast cancer 94–6
hormones 345
horn 138, 224, 294, 296, 360
Horner's syndrome 43
hornet nest 114, 224, 273
host resistance 10
hsi fan 240
human chorionic gonadotropin (HCG) 196
human leukocyte antigen (HLA) 290
human papilloma virus (HPV) 4–5, 20, 22, 178–9, 183, 186, 188, 191, 260

human T-cell lymphotrophic virus (HTLV)-1 264
hun 158, 160
huo xue therapy 23
hydralazine 99
Hydrea 290
hydroxycarbamide 290
hydroxyurea 182
hydroxyzine 323
hyperactivity disorders 350
hypercalcemia 42–3, 131–2, 197, 233, 333
hypercholesterolemia 233
hypercoagulability syndrome 46, 161
hypereosinophil syndrome 287
hyperestrinism 189
hyperinsulinemia 46, 138, 156
    and breast cancer 102–3
hyperpigmentation 122
hyperplasia 189
hypertension 94
hyperthermia 163
hypoalbuminemia 66
hypochondrium 149, 246, 325–6
hypoglycemia 233
hypokalemia 66, 327
hyponatremia 38, 327
hypoproteinemia 66
hypothermia 58
hypothyroidism 137–8, 266, 269
hypovolemia 327
hypoxia 302
hysterectomy 130, 182–3, 190, 198, 207

I

ifosfamide 41, 45, 182, 190, 265, 297
ileitis 65
IM8262–302 207
imipramine 323
immune deficiency 284
immune system 126
immunity, lowered 19
immunoglobulin (Ig) 254, 292, 353
immunologic factors, in leukemia 284–5
immunoproliferative small intestinal disease (IPSID) 262
immunosuppression 295
immunotherapy 196, 219
implants 97
impotence 164
incontinence 164, 174
    urinary 334–5
induction therapy 40, 45
infections 10
infertility 189, 269

infiltrating ductal carcinoma (DIC) 107
inflammatory bowel syndrome 65
inflammatory carcinoma of the breast (IBC) 107
inguinal lymphadenopathy 277
insomnia 23, 125, 207, 359
insulin 62
insulin-like growth factor 1 (IGF-1) 62, 106, 345, 347
interferon 13–14, 163, 199, 233, 245, 263
    α 244
    α-2a 233
interior damp-heat stasis 236–7
interleukin 13
    2 14, 199, 219, 290
    6 196
    10 196
    12 163
International Association for the Study of Lung Cancer (IASLC) 37
International Bone Marrow Transplant Registry 290
International Federation of Gynecology and Obstetrics (FIGO) 180–1, 190, 198
International Index 254
International Medical Research, Inc 171
intestinal tumorigenesis 347
intestines 84, 359
intra-arterial infusion (IAC) 233
intravaginal radiation 190
intravesical therapy 217, 224–5
invasive breast cancer 107
invasive carcinoma 181
    in cervical 179–80
inversion fire 109
iodine 273
    125 232
ionising radiation, biological effects of 12
Iressa 40, 45, 57, 131
iron 312
isoflavones 96

J

Jade Screen 258
Jarrett, Lonnie 160, 342
jaundice 230–2, 234, 236–7, 246, 248, 328, 332
jejunum 20
Jewett ABCD system 163
Jewett–Marshall system 217
Ji Shang Feng 259

jin 220–1
    withered and blood parched 303
Jin Gui Yao Lue 258
Jin Gui Yi 169
jin ku xue zao 304
jin ye 19–20, 136, 303, 326
    loss 305
jing 317, 336, 338
    in bladder/renal cancer 220–1
    in leukemia 285
    in lymphomas 256
    in ovarian cancer 200–1
    in prostate cancer 158, 160
jinye 325
Jueyin 92–3, 107, 126, 169
jujube 122–3, 325

K

K6 201
Kaiser Permanente Hospitals 119
kale 4
Kaposi's sarcoma 14
karma 337
Kava 319
kelp thallus 26, 115, 271–2, 274
ketoconazole 166
ketones 354
kidney 96, 99, 103, 200, 219, 222, 303, 359
    channel 158
    deficiency 167, 186–7, 223
        early stage 168–9
    fire 68, 129, 200
    function 356
    jing 220, 285
    qi 38, 129, 159, 221, 257
        deficiency 55, 221, 320
        nourishment 124
    yang 76, 84, 158, 192–3, 220–1, 223, 257
        deficiency 250
            in breast cancer 91, 109, 132
            in cervical cancer 186–7
            in colorectal cancer 64–5, 69, 83, 87
            in lung cancer 50–1, 58
            in ovarian cancer 223–4
            in pancreatic cancer 239
            in uterine cancer 192
        nourishment 124
        tonic 143
        warmth and tonification 26, 175
    yin 38, 192–3, 221, 223, 285, 315
        deficiency 316, 328
            in breast cancer 91, 103, 108–9, 132–3, 145–6, 148

kidney (Continued)
  in colorectal cancer 69–70, 78
  in leukemia 293–4
  in lung cancer 55
  in ovarian cancer 205–6
  in uterine cancer 192
  nourishment 124
  tonification 26
  ying 91
kidneys 38, 221, 258–60, 317, 327, 351
  and anxiety 318
  tonification of 27
Klinefelter's syndrome 284
knotted qi 319
knotted toxin 203–7, 236, 260
Ko cycle 135, 159, 236, 241, 321
konjac 273

L

lactate dehydrogenase (LDH) 39, 196, 261
lactation 350
laetrile 54
laminaria 23
lamivudine 245
Lamson, Davis 119
laparoscopy 201, 233
laparotomy 207
large intestine 158, 316
large-cell carcinoma 42
laser therapy 182
latent liver heat, and liver qi stasis 136–7
latent pathogenic factors 20–1, 353, 355, 358–61
  in breast cancer 96, 98, 101–3
  in cervical cancer 179
  etiology of 256
  in hepatocellular carcinoma (HCC) 241
  in herbal medicine 357–8
  in leukemia 285, 293
  in lymphomas 255–60, 264, 270, 272–4, 276–9
  in pancreatic cancer 236
  predisposition to 256–8
latent virus 285
laxative 79
lead 21, 351–3, 357
legumes 144, 157
lemon grass 319
lentinus 23
letrozol 128
leucocytopenia, formula 296
leucovorin 74, 82
leukapheresis 292

leukemia 2, 5, 38, 253, 260, 266, 274, 283–300, 349
  acute 286
  chemotherapy for 286
  Chinese medicine 285–6, 293–8
  chronic 5, 286
  complications of 296–7
  epidemiology of 284
  etiology of 284, 286
  external triggers of 285–6
  genetic factors in 284
  immunologic factors in 284–5
  and latent pathogenic factors 285
  and physiological imbalances 285
  symptoms of 286
  treating children with 297–8
  and twins 284, 287
  viral factors in 284
leukemia cutis 288
Leukine 14, 305
leukocytes 305
leukopenia 124, 131, 237
leukorrhea 188–9
leuprolide 13, 165
levamisole 13, 74
li stasis 327
licorice root 26, 48, 50, 53, 125, 127, 168, 171, 185, 187, 203–6, 237–9, 242, 244–5, 247, 275, 294–6, 308, 313, 326, 328
Lieque 201
lignans 96
lignum sappan 175
lindane 104
Ling Shu 258
lipolysis 355, 360
lipomas 355
lipomatosis 4
listening 207
listeriosis 262
liver 19, 96, 99, 103, 135, 283, 289, 321, 327, 351, 356, 359
  and anxiety 318
  blood stasis 241
  cancer 5, 84
    Chinese medicine 240–4
    and HRT 95
    see also hepatocellular carcinoma (HCC)
  channel 107, 158, 185
  function tests 112
  metastases 131
  qi 71, 92, 100–1, 159, 227
    circulation 126
    constraint 179
    stasis 322, 327
      in breast cancer 92, 101, 108–9, 128, 147–9
      with constraint 133–4

liver (Continued)
    in hepatocellular carcinoma (HCC) 241
    and latent liver heat 136–7
    in pancreatic cancer 236
    in prostate cancer 159, 169–70
    with spleen deficiency 134–5, 159
  regrowth of 85
  shen 158
  tonification 27
  transplantation 234
  yang 136, 145
  yin 136, 223
    deficiency 316, 328
      in breast cancer 103, 108, 133, 145–6, 148
      in colorectal cancer 69–70, 78
      in hepatocellular carcinoma (HCC) 241
      in leukemia 293–4
      in ovarian cancer 205–6
    nourishment 124
    tonification 26
liver/kidney axis 316
lobular carcinoma in situ (LCIS) 6, 106–7
loofah 114, 134, 137
loop electrosurgical excision procedure (LEEP) 181–2
lorazepam 208, 309, 335
lovastatin 166
lower jiao 325
  in bladder/renal cancer 225
  in breast cancer 99, 103, 127, 135
  in cervical cancer 185
  in colorectal cancer 63, 68, 71–2
  in ovarian cancer 211
  in prostate cancer 158, 166
  stasis 209
lu 7 201
lumbricus 141
lumpectomy 112, 116, 119, 144, 148
lung 316
  heat 47–8
  phlegm heat 58
  qi 92, 101, 219, 221, 297, 316
    deficiency 55, 58, 325
    stasis 92, 116
  wind heat 58
  yin, deficiency 55, 58, 260
lung cancer 35–60
  biology of
    NSCLC 42–3
    SCLC 37
  case studies 54–9
  Chinese medicine 45–54

lung cancer (Continued)
　clinical evaluation, in SCLC 39–40
　clinical presentation
　　in NSCLC 43
　　in SCLC 37–8
　diagnosis, in NSCLC 43–4
　diagnostic patterns of 47–54
　　blood stasis with deficiency
　　　heat and pathogenic heat
　　　49–50
　　lung heat with yin deficiency
　　　heat 47–8
　　phlegm/damp stasis in the
　　　lung 48–9
　　spleen and kidney yang
　　　deficiency 50–1
　epidemiology of 35–6
　etiology of 46
　natural history, in SCLC 39
　pathology, in SCLC 37
　prognostic factors, in SCLC 40
　risk factors 35–6
　　in NSCLC 41–2
　screening tools, in SCLC 38–9
　stage III disease 45
　staging
　　in NSCLC 44
　　in SCLC 39
　treatment
　　in NSCLC 44–5
　　in SCLC 40–1
　types of 36
lungs 19, 51, 258–60, 359
　and anxiety 318
luo channels 142
Lupron 13, 165, 190
Luschka's ducts 234
luteinising hormone (LH) 130
luteinising hormone-releasing
　　hormone (LHRH) 128, 165
lycopene 156
lymph 359
　system 356–7
lymph node biopsy 261
lymph nodes 106, 143, 197, 258, 261,
　　264, 283, 289
　swollen 127–8
lymphadenopathy 25, 260, 266, 287,
　　289
lymphedema 118, 144, 212, 324
lymphoblasts 287
lymphocytes 254, 289
　proliferation 290
lymphocytic leukemia 5
lymphomagenesis model 255
lymphomas 4, 253–82, 286, 349
　abdominal 271
　case studies 277–80
　chemotherapy for 262

lymphomas (Continued)
　Chinese medicine 270–7
　clinical features of 261
　diagnosis of 261
　early stage 270, 272
　follicular 255, 261–2
　　natural history of 260–1
　gastric 272
　indolent 254–63
　　biology of 254–5
　　Chinese medicine 255–60
　large-cell 273
　late stage 272–3
　MALT 262
　mantle-cell 262–3
　metastases 273
　prognosis for 261
　radiation therapy for 262
　spleen 262
　staging for 254, 261, 271
　thymus gland 272–3
　treatment of 262–3, 270–7, 293
　types of 254
　　low-grade 261–2
　see also Hodgkin's disease; non-
　　Hodgkin's lymphoma
lymphoproliferative syndrome 264
lymphosarcoma 273
Lynch syndrome 65, 196

M

m-BACOD 265
Ma Shocun 317
magnesium 246, 353
magnetic resonance imaging (MRI)
　in breast cancer 97, 112, 130,
　　148
　in hepatocellular carcinoma (HCC)
　　233
　in lung cancer 39–40, 43
maintenance therapy 40
malar flush 306
malathion 352
malignant melanoma 5
malnutrition 188, 239–40
malt 55, 134, 136–7, 149, 167, 205, 210,
　　237, 247–8, 306, 311
mammography 111
　and breast cancer 97–8
management, of abnormal smears
　　180–1
mantle-cell lymphoma 254
maple syrup 240
maraschino cherries 105
Marcia Rivkin Breast and Ovarian
　　Cancer Study 148
marijuana 36, 46

markers 111
　in pancreatic cancer 231
mastectomy 106, 119, 144
　bilateral 107
　and pregnancy 107
　radical 115–16
　segmental 116
mastitis 134, 147
Mayo Clinic 240
meat
　and breast cancer 105–6
　contamination of 345–6
mechlorethamine 266, 268–9, 284
medicated leaven 75, 80, 122, 170,
　　205, 212, 237, 246, 248, 311, 328
medication risks, and breast cancer
　　99–100
medroxyprogesterone acetate 190
medullary carcinoma 107
Megace 131, 140
megakaryocytes 302
megakaryocytopoiesis 302
megestrol 128, 130, 140, 143, 165
　acetate 131, 333
meiosis 43
melanoma 5–6
melphalan 284
menopause 90, 92, 95, 97, 100, 148,
　　316
menstruation 91–2, 100, 142
meperidine 323
mercaptopurine 288
mercury 104, 352
Meridian Therapy 338
mesenterium 356
Mesna 123, 265, 297
mestranol 92
metabolic disturbances 9
metastases 6
　bone 132
　in breast cancer 107, 127–8, 130–2,
　　139–40
　in colorectal cancer 66
　liver 57
　lung 85
　in lung cancer
　　NSCLC 44–5
　　SCLC 39–40
　in lymphomas 273
　occult 40
　in pancreatic cancer 230
　in prostate cancer 161, 165–6
　in renal-cell carcinoma 218–19
　sites of 8
metastatic melanoma 14
methadone 323
methionine 351
methotrexate 120, 123, 125, 130, 163,
　　217, 265, 269, 288, 291–2

methylprednisolone 265
metoclopramide 309
metronidazole 99
Mexican wild yam 92
midazolam 335
middle burner 76
middle jiao 27, 304, 310, 320, 325, 327
    in bladder/renal cancer 219, 221
    and blood 303
    in breast cancer 100, 103, 123,
        134–5, 142, 145, 149
    in colorectal cancer 1, 63–4, 69, 71,
        75, 77, 84–6
    deficiency 313
    in leukemia 256–7, 272, 275
    in lung cancer 46, 51, 59
    in ovarian cancer 205–6, 210, 212
    in pancreatic/hepatic cancers
        235–6, 242, 247–8
    in prostate cancer 159, 169
    tonic 48
middle pulse 59
milk 216
milk thistle 245
millet sprouts 311
Millstone I reactor 102
MIME 265
Mingmen 149, 159, 187, 220–1,
    259–60, 338
mirex 104
miso 96, 250
mitomycin 45, 217, 231, 233, 269
mitoxantrone 262
mobilisation 290–1
monoamine oxidase 319
monoclonal antibodies 15
monocyte macrophage CSF 14
monocytes 302
MOPP 266, 268–9, 275, 284
morphine agonists 323
moxibustion 118, 146, 324
mucositis 124, 312–13
    Chinese medicine 312–13
    conventional medicine 312
mucus 46, 64
    accumulation 351
MUGA-scan 128, 137
mugwort floss 114
multiple myeloma 98
    treatment of 293
multiple organ failure 332
multiple sclerosis 350
multipotential CSF 14
mun 326
mungbean sprouts 96
mushrooms 23
MVAC 217
    side-effects of 218
myasthenia gravis 315

mycotoxins 232
myeloablation 290
myelocytes 302
myelodysplastic syndrome 266, 269
myeloma 5
myelopoiesis 302
myelosuppression 307–8
    in bladder cancer 217
    in breast cancer 124–5, 143
    in colorectal cancer 83
    in leukemia 291, 295
    in lung cancer 55
    in lymphomas 275
    in ovarian cancer 203, 209
Myleran 290
myocardial infarction 269
myometrium 190
myrrh 27, 114, 135, 149, 238, 248, 324

N

nabilone 309
Nagasaki 97, 102, 284–5
nalbuphine 323
2-naphthylamine 216
narcotic bowel syndrome 334
nasopharyngeal cancer 6
National Breast Center of Australia
    91
National Cancer Institute (NCI) 93,
    97–9, 180, 240, 263, 343
National Institutes of Health 25, 93
natural history
    of cervical cancer 179
    of follicular lymphoma 260–1
    of gall bladder carcinoma 234
    of lung cancer, SCLC 39
    of prostate cancer 160–1
natural killer cells 14
    in bladder/renal cancer 222
    in breast cancer 122, 126, 145
    in cervical cancer 184
    in colorectal cancer 69, 75, 84, 87
    in leukemia 290
    in ovarian cancer 196, 207
    in pancreatic/hepatic cancer 239,
        242, 248
    in prostate cancer 168
nausea 32, 309–12
    in breast cancer 122, 124–5, 145
    Chinese medicine 310–12
    in colorectal cancer 67, 75–6, 81, 84
    conventional medicine 309
    and dying 333
    in hepatocellular carcinoma (HCC)
        234
    in ovarian cancer 204, 208–12
    prevention of 86

Navelbine 120, 128, 131
NB-70K 196
necrosis 126, 188, 249, 266, 270, 305
Neijing 315, 321
neoadjuvant chemotherapy for
    217
neoplasms 1–2
    endocrine 4
    presentation modes of 6
Neulasta 14, 209
Neupogen 14, 125, 209, 291, 305
neuroblastoma 6
neuromuscular disorders 9
neutropenia 122, 131, 212, 287, 291,
    304–8
    Chinese medicine 305–7
    conventional medicine 304–5
neutropenic fevers 127, 193, 304–7
neutrophils 302, 304
Nevin & Moran system 235
nicotine 36, 227
night sweats 261
nightshade 245
nitrates 63, 289
nitrites 21, 104
nitrofurazone 99
nitrosamines 41, 104, 230, 234, 352
nodules, dispelling of 26
Nolvadex 98, 198
nolylphenol 105
non-Hodgkin's lymphoma (NHL) 14,
    254–66, 269
    B-cell 254–5, 261–2
    clinical features of 264
    diagnosis of 264
    epidemiology of 263–4
    etiology of 263–4
    high-grade 263–6
    indolent 254–63
    intermediate 263–6
    staging for 265–6
    symptoms of 264
    T-cell 254
    treatment of 262–3, 265–6
    see also Hodgkin's disease;
        lymphomas
non-invasive breast cancer 106–7
non-small-cell lung cancer 41–5
    biology of 42–3
    clinical presentation of 43
    diagnosis of 43–4
    risk factors for 41–2
    stage III disease 45
    stage IV disease 45
    staging for 44
    subtypes of 42
    treatment of 44–5
non-steroidal anti-inflammatory drugs
    (NSAIDs) 63

norethindrone 82
Norplant 93
Norvasc 247
novantrone 166
nu zi bao 200
nuclear emissions, and breast cancer
    102
nuclear grade 11
    and breast cancer 110–11
nuclear transcription factors 3
nucleosides 289
nulliparity 90
nutmeg seeds 69, 75, 83, 85
nutritional therapy 246
nuts 104

O

obesity 218
    and breast cancer 100–1
    and uterine cancer 189, 191
oleic acid 159
omega-3 fatty acids 63, 81, 104, 157,
    345–6
omenectomy 198
omentum 356, 359
oncogenes 2–3, 37, 111, 158, 190,
    196–7, 216, 231, 264
Oncovin 266, 284
oncoviruses 4
ondansetron 206, 208, 309
oophorectomy 120, 131, 190, 197
open biopsy 8
open breast biopsy 112
opposed hormonal therapy (HRT)
    94–5
    side-effects of 95
oral contraceptives see contraceptive
    pill
oral decoction 184
oral erythema multiforme 312
orca whales 344
orchiectomy 165
organ agitation 319
    etiology and pathology of 320–1
organochlorines 5, 21, 101, 103, 255,
    257–8, 351–2
organophosphate insecticides 352
Ortho-Novum 82
orthopnea 52, 58
osteogenic sarcoma 5
osteopenia 132, 137
osteoporosis 94–6, 132
ovarian cancer 4, 99, 195–214, 343
    anatomy of 200–1
    biological therapies for 199
    biology of 196–7
    case studies 207–13

ovarian cancer (Continued)
    Chinese medicine 200–7
    epidemiology of 195
    etiology of 195–6
    and HRT 95
    pathogenesis of 196–7
    pathology of 197, 201–2
    patterns for 202–7
    physiology of 200–1
    and pregnancy 200
    prevention of 207
    screening for 196
    staging for 197–8
    treatment of 198–9
    tumor markers 196–7
ovarian papillary serous carcinoma
    189
ovaries 200, 351
oxaliplatin 82–3
oxycodone 248, 323
Oxycontin 248–9
oxygenation 183
oyster shell 26, 115, 128–9, 134, 271–2,
    274, 278–9

P

paclitaxel 40, 45, 55, 111, 131, 166, 190,
    198, 203, 207–8, 314–15
Paget's disease 107, 132
pain 192, 243, 248, 321
    abdominal 311
    cancer-related syndromes
        322–4
    Chinese medicine 323–4
    control of 55, 232, 249
    management of 248
    neuropathic 322
    nociceptive 322
    prevention of 26–7, 224
    reduction of 76
painful urinary dysfunction (PUD)
    122, 243
palpation 113
pamidronate 132
Pancoast's syndrome 43
pancreas 19, 205, 235, 351
pancreatic cancer 229–32
    case studies 246–50
    chemotherapy in 246
    Chinese medicine 235–40
    clinical features of 230
    diagnosis of 230–1
    epidemiology of 229–30
    etiology of 229–30
    markers for 231
    metastases 230
    pathology of 230

pancreatic cancer (Continued)
    staging for 231
    treatment of 231–2
pancreatitis 230, 236
    formula for 314
pancreatoduodenectomy 231
pancytopenia 293
Pap (Papanicoloau) smears 22, 43,
    177, 179–81, 189, 191
paracentesis 327
paraneoplastic syndromes 38
parenteral hydration 333
paresthesia 140
parotid gland 270
passive smoking 41
pathogenesis 17–22
    etiological factors in 18–22
    in ovarian cancer 196–7
    in prostate cancer 158–60
pathogenic heat 49–50, 293
pathogens, external 21–2
pathology
    of bladder cancer 216
    of cervical cancer 178
    of colorectal cancer 65–6
    of gall bladder carcinoma 234
    of hepatocellular carcinoma (HCC)
        232
    of lung cancer, SCLC 37
    of ovarian cancer 197, 201–2
    of pancreatic cancer 230
    of prostate cancer 160–1
    of renal-cell carcinoma 218
pathophysiology 1–34
patterns, for ovarian cancer 202–7
PC-SPES 171
pegfilgrastim 14, 209
pelvic exenteration 182
penis 157
pentamidine 292
pentazocine 323
pentostatin 290
pepsin 136
peptides 196
pericarditis 266, 269
    formula for 297
pericardium 149, 160
    channel 107
perineum 164
peripheral blood progenitor (PBP)
    cells 293
peripheral blood stem cells (PBSC)
    199
peripheral neuropathy 84, 125, 314–17
peristalsis 71–2, 210, 247, 356
peritoneal mesotheliomas 197
peritoneum 199
peritonitis 333
    bacterial 327

peroxides 354
pesticides 101–2, 104, 108, 287, 289,
    345, 361
    organochlorine 351–2, 357–9
    screen for 354
petroleum 342
    products 218, 230, 341
phagocytosis 23
    in breast cancer 117, 122, 124, 126,
        145
    in cervical cancer 185
    in colorectal cancer 69–70, 81, 84,
        87
    in lung cancer 48, 51–2
    in ovarian cancer 212
    in uterine cancer 193
phenacetin 216
phenothiazines 309, 323
phenotypic markers 2
phenylbutazone 284
phenytoin 291, 323
Philadelphia syndrome 290
phlegm 321–2, 325
    fire 318
    heat 45–6, 128, 235, 257
    heated/hot 76, 273
    in lymphomas 258–9, 271
    nodules 274
    in ovarian cancer 201
    stasis 350–1
        in breast cancer 101, 103, 114,
            128
        in colorectal cancer 65
        damp 113, 355
        in lung 48–9
        in ovarian cancer 202
    transformation 26, 126, 278
    treatment of 274
    tumors 75
        damp 190
    in uterine cancer 190–1
phthalates 352
physiological abnormalities 6–8
physiology, ovarian cancer 200–1
phytoestrogens, and breast cancer
    96–7
pi 235
Pi Wei Lun 235
pitchblende mining 36
pituitary gland 138
plastron 27, 129, 135, 170, 244, 274,
    279, 294–5, 307
platinum 203, 207
pleural effusion 39, 55, 199, 324–7
    Chinese medicine 324–6
    patterns for 325–6
plum pit qi 319–20
    etiology and pathology of
        319–20

pneumonia 49, 324, 332
    bacterial 58
    pneumocystis 262, 292
pneumonitis 266, 270, 290
podophyllotoxins 13
poliomyelitis 315
polyA-polyU 13
polychlorinated biphenyls (PCBs)
    344, 352, 354
polycyclic aromatic hydrocarbons 41
polycystic ovarian syndrome (POS)
    189
polyestradiol phosphate 166
polyporus 23
polyps 65–6, 355
    adenomatous 62–3, 65
    neoplastic 65–6
    non-neoplastic 65
polysaccharides 23, 184
polyurethane foam 98
polyuria 168
pork 104
porphyria cutanea tarda 233
positron emission tomography (PET)
    97, 112, 130, 146
potassium 220–1
poultry, contamination of 346
poverty 348–9
prana 303
Pravacol 100
pravastatin 100
prediabetes 103
prednisolone 323
prednisone 13, 128, 130, 262, 265–6,
    284, 288–9, 292
pregnancy 90, 92
    and ovarian cancer 200
preinvasive carcinoma 181
preinvasive lesions 180–1
preleukemia 286
Premarin 94–5
premenstrual syndrome (PMS) 130
prescription, writing of 28–30
pressure sores, and dying 335
prevention 32, 128–9, 341–62
    in breast cancer 137–8
    in ovarian cancer 207
prevention formula, colorectal cancer
    77–8
procarbazine 262, 266, 269–70, 284
Procrit 13, 125
proctosigmoidoscopy 67
progesterone 92, 94–5, 183, 308, 352
    receptors 107, 111, 143, 189, 196
progestins 13, 92–5, 105, 128, 131, 219,
    323
prognosis
    for acute lymphocytic leukemia
        (ALL) 288

prognosis (Continued)
    for acute myelogenous leukemia
        (AML) 288
    for cervical cancer 181–2
    for lymphomas 261
    for uterine cancer 189–90
prognostic factors
    in breast cancer 110
    in lung cancer, SCLC 40
prolactin 100
Proleukin 219
prolymphocytic leukemia 290
ProMACE-CytaBom 265
Proscar 162, 165
prostaglandins 63, 159
prostate, anatomy of 157–8
prostate cancer 6, 13, 58–9, 155–76,
    343
    anatomy of 157–8
    case studies 172–5
    Chinese medicine 158–60
    diagnosis of 161–2
    epidemiology of 156
    etiology of 156–7
    and genetics 157
    hormone refractory 166
    increased/decreased risk of 157
    metastases 161, 165–6
    natural history of 160–1
    pathogenesis of 158–60
    pathology of 160–1
    radiation therapy in 164–5
    screening for 162–3
    stage C 165
    staging for 163
    treatment of 163–6
    treatment principles in 171–2
    and watchful waiting 163–4
Prostate Cancer Intervention vs.
        Observation Trial (PIVOT) 162
Prostate, Lung, Colon, Ovarian
        Cancer (PLCO) study 162
prostate specific antigen (PSA) 57–8,
    160–5, 172
prostatic adenocarcinoma 158
prostatic adenosis 159
prostatic intraepithelial neoplasia 158
protein kinase C (PKC) 62
proto-oncogenes 2–3
Provenge 166
Prozac 100
pseudoestrogens 21, 104–5, 358
    and breast cancer 103
pseudomyxoma peritonei 197
PSOC 1702 208
psychoneuroimmunology 108
ptosis 43
Puget Sound 344
pulmonary complication 269

pulses 24, 351
  in Chinese medicine 337–8
pumpkin seeds 96, 157
pus 107, 145, 270, 273–4

Q

qi 18–21, 23, 27, 303, 308, 316, 338,
    353, 355, 360
  in bladder/renal cancer 223
  blockage 107
  and blood 304
    deficiency 206–7
    stasis 202, 237–8, 241–2
  in breast cancer 116
  in cervical cancer 183
  circulation 66, 76, 84
  deficiency 22, 304–6, 310
    in breast cancer 118, 128
    in colorectal cancer 65, 70–1, 73
    in leukemia 294–5
    in lung cancer 46
    in lymphomas 271, 274, 277
    in ovarian cancer 207
    in prostate cancer 170–1
    in uterine cancer 193
  disharmony 326
  heat 360
  injury 45
  knotted 126
  in leukemia 285–6
  lower sea of 220
  lung 86
  in lung cancer 51
  in lymphomas 258, 270
  movement 31, 110, 274
  normal 23
  in prostate cancer 158
  regulation 25, 76
  scattering 317
  source 27, 102
  stagnant 202
  stasis 64, 116, 133, 147, 150, 257, 359
  tonification 30, 72, 121, 125, 276,
    278
  transformation 220
  weak 31
qi gong therapy 357
qing re therapy 24
quadrantectomy 116
quercitin 4, 184

R

radiation 21, 36, 182
  cranial 288
  in Hodgkin's disease 266

radiation (Continued)
  intraoperative 232
  intravaginal 190
  and leukemia 284, 287
  side-effects of 52–3, 276
radiation enteritis 171
radiation therapy 11–12
  in breast cancer 117–19
  in cervical cancer 182–3
  contraindication for 117
  in gall bladder carcinoma 235
  in hepatocellular carcinoma (HCC)
    234
  in Hodgkin's disease 268
  in lymphomas 262
  in ovarian cancer 199
  in prostate cancer 164–5
radiation treatment 28
  in colorectal cancer 72–4
radiation vaginitis 184
radical cystectomy 217
radical nephrectomy 219
radical prostatectomy 164
radiotherapy 39, 217, 231
radon 36
Rai system 289
raloxifene 128
ranitidine 208
recombinant bovine growth hormone
    (rBGH) 105–6
recombinant immunoblot assay
    (RIBA) 244
rectal bleeding 66
rectal cancer 73
Rectify Qi and Loosen the Intestine
    Decoction 71–2
rectosigmoid colon 66
rectum 61, 66, 157
red blood cells 303–4, 308
  in breast cancer 113, 122–3, 125
  in colorectal cancer 70, 75–6, 84
  in leukemia 285
  in ovarian cancer 211–12
  in pancreatic/hepatic cancer 239,
    248–9
  in prostate cancer 171, 174
  in uterine cancer 193
red dye 3 105
red ginseng 84–5
red jujube 55, 75–6, 243, 249, 276
Reed–Sternberg cells 266–7
ren 158, 160, 200–4
Ren channel
  in breast cancer 91, 93, 96, 99,
    101–3, 109, 129
  in leukemia 285
Ren mai 113
renal cell carcinoma 14
renal failure 327

renal toxicity 123–4
renal-cell carcinoma
  Chinese medicine 219–25
  clinical presentation of 218
  diagnosis of 218
  differential diagnosis of 222–5
  epidemiology of 218
  metastases 218–19, 223–4
  pathology of 218
  staging for 218–19
  treatment of 219
reproductive history, and breast
    cancer 91–2
resection 62
  in NSCLC 44
reserpine 99
Resina Draconis 114
restlessness 306, 350
  terminal 335
retention enema 73–4, 188
reticuloctopenia 287
retinoblastoma 4
retinoic acid syndrome 14
retinoids 14, 163, 308
retinol 14
  carbohydrates 103
retroviruses 284
reverse transcriptase 284
rheumatoid arthritis 98
ribavirin 233, 244
Richter's syndrome 290
ricin 199
Rinpoche, Sogyal 336
risk factors 343
  for breast cancer 90–106
  for colorectal cancer 65
  for lung cancer 35–6
Rituxan 262–3, 265, 278
rituximab 262–3
RNA viruses 284
Robson's staging system 218
rotating delivery of excitation off-
    resonance (RODEO) scans 97,
    112
ruan jian therapy 25
rubber 289
Rye classification 267

S

S-phase fraction 11
saccharin 216, 349
sage 240
Sahoyang 325
St John's wort 319
salicylic acid 184
saline implants 98
salmon 104, 344–5

salmonella 345
salpingo-oophorectomy 190, 198, 207
salt 240
    baths 356
salvage therapy 40–1, 131, 171, 212,
    265
San Jiao 303, 353, 355–7, 359
    in bladder/renal cancer 219–21
    in colorectal cancer 63
    function 325
    in gall bladder carcinoma 235
    in lymphomas 258–60
    in prostate cancer 159, 169
    theory 358
sarcomas 23, 188
sargramostim 14, 305
saturated fat 62–3, 65
sauna therapy 355
saw palmetto 171
scleroderma 98
sclerosis 315
screening
    in cervical cancer 180
    in colorectal cancer 67
    in ovarian cancer 196
    in prostate cancer 162–3
screening tools, for SCLC 38–9
seaweeds 144, 273
segmental mastectomy 116
seizures 82, 86, 291, 351
selective estrogen receptomodulators
    (SERMs) 98
selenium 62–3, 81, 166
self-breast examination (SBE) 111
semen 157–8
senna leaf 248, 311
sentinel node biopsy 112
septic shock 332
serotonin 309
    receptor antagonists 309
serous carcinoma 189, 208
serum glutamic oxaloacetic
    transaminase (SGOT) 39
sex, during menses 201
sex hormones, and breast cancer
    105–6
sex-hormone-binding globulin
    (SHBG) 156
Shang Han Lun 358
Shang Han Za Bing Lun 255
Shaoyang channel 317
Shaoyang stage heat 273
Shaoyang unit 258
sheep 345
shen 160, 304, 317, 338
    cycle 236, 321
Sheng Ji Zong Lu 325
Shiva, Vandana 341
Shuangzi powder 188

sialic acid protein 196
Siberian ginseng 23, 319
Sichuan pepper 56
side-effects 45
    of antiemetics 309
    of bacillus Calmette–Guerin (BCG)
        217
    of fluorouracil (5-FU) 74
sigmoid colon 62
signal transducers 3
silica 352
silicone 98
    gel implants 98
Sjögren's syndrome 264
skin 350
    rashes formula 314
    tags 351
sleep 108, 127, 144, 192, 204, 256
    deprivation 279
small intestine 158
small lymphocytic lymphomas 261
small-cell carcinomas 178, 197
small-cell lung cancer 4, 29, 36
    biology of 37
    clinical evaluation of 39–40
    limited/extensive classification of
        39
    natural history of 39
    pathology of 37
    prognostic factors for 40
    screening tools for 38–9
    staging for 39
    treatment of 40–1
    types of 37
smears, abnormal 180–1
smoking 35–9, 42, 57, 178, 221, 226–7
    cigarette 41–2, 45–6, 216, 230
    passive 41
snake slough 270–1
sodium 220–1
soil, decontamination of 350
solvents 352
somatostatin 231
soy 84, 96–7, 99, 157
    fermented 250
SpectraCell Laboratories 354
spider angiomas 233
spider veins 351
spinach 344
spironolactone 99
spleen 19, 303, 316, 325, 327, 359–60
    and anxiety 318
    in breast cancer 100, 135
    in colorectal cancer 63–4, 84
    deficiency 310, 359
        in breast cancer 100, 103, 109,
            114, 133–5, 145, 148
        in cervical cancer 179, 186–7
        in colorectal cancer 65

spleen (Continued)
    with damp accumulation 242
    in lymphomas 257
    in ovarian cancer 202, 209
    in pancreatic/hepatic cancer
        223
    in prostate cancer 159, 167
    invigoration 27
    in leukemia 283, 289
    in lymphomas 258–60, 274,
        278–9
    in ovarian cancer 205
    in pancreatic/hepatic cancer 235,
        243
    pulse 59
    qi 64, 71, 159, 206, 210, 223, 257,
        297
        deficiency 166–7, 235, 304,
            320
        injury 122
    sho 174
    tonic 85
    yang 76, 84, 206, 221, 257
        deficiency
            in bladder/renal cancer
                223–4
            in cervical cancer 186–7
            in colorectal cancer 64, 69,
                83
            in lung cancer 50–1
            in pancreatic/hepatic cancer
                235, 239, 250
            in uterine cancer 192
    yin, deficiency 64, 192, 235
spleen/liver axis 257
spleen/stomach axis 316
spleen/stomach stasis 313
splenectomy 266, 289–90
splenomegaly 233, 261, 289, 308
spontaneous bleeding 24
Spring Wind Burn Creme 119, 145,
    148
Spring Wind herbs 119
sputum culture 38
squamous cell carcinomas 42, 178
squamous intraepithelial lesion (SIL)
    180–1
squash 104
staging 11, 106
    for bladder cancer 216–17
    for breast cancer 115
    for cervical cancer 181
    for chronic lymphocytic leukemia
        (CLL) 289
    and formulas 125–8
    for gall bladder carcinoma 235
    for hepatocellular carcinoma
        (HCC) 233
    for Hodgkin's disease 267–8

staging (Continued)
  for lung cancer
    NSCLC 44
    SCLC 37, 39
  for lymphomas 254, 261
  for non-Hodgkin's lymphoma
    (NHL) 265–6
  for ovarian cancer 197–8
  for pancreatic cancer 231
  for prostate cancer 163
  for renal-cell carcinoma
    218–19
  TNM system of 11, 44, 115
  for uterine cancer 189–90
stagnation 305
standard American diet (SAD) 96,
  144
staphylococci 304
stasis 310, 318
  removal of 26
  spleen/stomach 313
statins 100
Steingraber, Sandra 104, 350
stem cell transplants 291–2
  complications of 291
stereotactic biopsy 112
stereotaxic needle localisation 10
sterility 266
steroids 206, 232, 257, 260, 323
Stevia 349
Stilphostrol 166
stomach 19, 100, 135, 316
  channel 107
  cold 312
  heat 109, 312
  pacification 27
  qi 109, 209–10, 338
    rebellious 135
  yin 206
stomach/spleen axis 76, 149, 315–16,
  355
stomach/spleen deficiency 316
stomach/spleen disharmony 205–6,
  310
stomatitis 312–13, 333
  Chinese medicine 312–13
  conventional medicine 312
stool tests 353–4
streptococci 304
stress, chronic 159
stroke 140–2
strontium-89 166
strontium-90 102
styrene 105
Su Wen 221, 315
sucrose 103
sulfur 351
super-infections 304
superior vena cava syndrome 261
suppositories 73–4, 183, 188

surgery 11
  in breast cancer 115–17
suspended fluids 324
sweating 306, 350, 355, 360
symptoms
  B 273
  in leukemia 286
systemic lupus erythematosus 98

T

T-cell acute lymphoblastic lymphoma
  (T-ALL) 263–4
Tagamet 100
tai qi chuan 357
Taichung Medical College, formula
  138
Taiyang 355
  layer 256
  organs 222
  stage 225
talc 178, 188, 191, 196, 200, 352
tamoxifen 13
  and breast cancer 97–9, 109, 120,
    128, 130–1, 139–40, 143, 146
  formula for 129
  and ovarian cancer 198, 208
  and pancreatic cancer 231
  and prostate cancer 165
  side-effects of 99, 129, 140, 146
  and uterine cancer 189
tampons 178, 183, 187–8, 196, 202
tangkuei tail 26, 68
tankage 345
Taoism 354
taraxacum 23
Taxatere 111, 120
Taxol 314
  and bladder cancer 217
  and breast cancer 111, 120, 124–5,
    128, 131
  and lung cancer 41, 55
  and ovarian cancer 198, 203,
    207–9, 211–12
  and prostate cancer 166
  and uterine cancer 190
Taxotere 208
Tegretol 82
tempeh 96
Ten Herb Tonify the Great Decoction
  117
Ten Thousand Brights cream 119
terazosin 163
testes/testicles 158, 169, 287
testicular cancer 5–6, 343
testosterone 13
  and bladder/renal cancer 220
  and breast cancer 94–5, 100, 105,
    138–9

testosterone (Continued)
  and pancreatic cancer 231
  and prostate cancer 156–7, 159,
    165–6
thirst 306
thoracentesis 39, 56, 324
thoracic irradiation, in SCLC 41
thoracotomy 44
Three Mile Island 102
three-dimensional conformal
    radiation therapy (D-CRT) 164
thrombocytopenia 124, 131, 143, 166,
    182, 209, 212, 261, 287–9, 297,
    307–9
  Chinese medicine 308–9
  conventional medicine 307–8
  formula for 296
thrombocytosis 58
thromboembolism 131, 208
thrombopoietin 293, 308
thrush see candidiasis
thyme 240
thymus gland 272–3
Tibetan medicine 336
TNM system 11, 62, 115, 163, 217–18,
    231, 233, 235
tobacco 35–6, 41, 46, 218
  chewing 216
tofu 96
tomato 157
tongue 113
topoisomerase II 96
topotecan 198
total body irradiation (TBI) 290
total lymphoid irradiation (TLI) 262
total parenteral nutrition (TPN) 239
toxaphene 104
toxic heat 45, 222
  pathogens 20–1
toxic hepatitis, formula 313
toxic myocarditis, formula 297, 313
toxic nephritis, formula 314
toxicity, cardiac 293
toxins 352, 357
  accumulation 185
    in colorectal cancer 68–9
  clear and heat 26
  dissolution of 26
  internal stasis of 169–70
  localised 350
  screens for 353–4
  stasis 203–4
tranquilisers 99
transaminases 233, 291
transcutaneous electrical nerve
    stimulation (TENS) 323
transitional cell carcinoma (TTC) 226
transparenteral nutrition 333
transrectal ultrasonography (TRUS)
    161, 163

transurethral bladder resection (TURBT) 217, 226
transurethral incision of the prostate (TUIP) 163
transurethral microwave therapy (TUMT) 163
transurethral needle ablation (TUNA) 163
transurethral resection of the prostate (TURP) 163
transvaginal ultrasound 196
transverse rebellion 135
trastuzumab 3, 13, 111
treatment 25–32
  of acute lymphocytic leukemia (ALL) 288
  of acute myelogenous leukemia (AML) 289
  of bladder cancer 217–18
  of breast cancer 115–29
  of cervical cancer 182–8
  of chronic lymphocytic leukemia (CLL) 289–90
  of gall bladder carcinoma 235
  of hepatitis C (HCV) 244–6
  of hepatocellular carcinoma (HCC) 233–4
  of Hodgkin's disease 265, 268–77
  of late-stage colorectal cancer 76–7
  of lung cancer
    NSCLC 44–5
    SCLC 40–1
  of lymphomas 262–3, 270–7
  of non-Hodgkin's lymphoma (NHL) 262–3, 265–6
  of ovarian cancer 198–9
  palliative 76
  of pancreatic cancer 231–2
  principles of 11–15, 115–29
  of prostate cancer 163–6, 171–2
  of renal-cell carcinoma 219
  rules of 30–1
  of side-effects 276
  of uterine cancer 190–1
trichomonas 99
tricyclic antidepressants 232
triglycerides 246
trihalomethane 216
trimethoprim-sulfamethoxazole 292
Trousseau's sign 230
Trousseau's syndrome 42
True Qi 258
tuberculosis 36, 52, 286, 348
tubular adenomas 66
tubular carcinoma 107
tui na 118
tumor lysis syndrome 265
tumor markers, ovarian cancer 196–7

tumor necrosis factor (TNF) 333
tumor regression 183
tumor size 11
  and breast cancer 110
tumor suppressor genes 4, 37
tumors
  categories in Chinese medicine 17
  in colorectal cancer 66
  testicular 5
turbid 159
  yin 166
turbidities 219
turkeys 104, 346
twins, and leukemia 284, 287
Tylenol PM 248
tyrosine kinase 3, 96, 158

U

ulcerative colitis 65, 234
ultrasound 230, 233, 235
ultraviolet light exposure 156
United States Department of Agriculture (USDA) 346
United States Fish and Wildlife Service 344
University College San Francisco Medical Center 97, 99
upper jiao 19, 323, 325
  in breast cancer 99, 101, 103
  heat 58
  in lung cancer 51–2
  in ovarian cancer 209
  qi 209
  in renal-cell carcinoma 219
ureters 158
urethra 157, 169
uric acid 290
urinalysis 137
urinary incontinence, and dying 334–5
urinary tract problems, and HRT 95
urine 157, 350
  odor of 147
uterine cancer 99, 188–91
  Chinese medicine 189
  clinical presentation of 189
  diagnosis of 189
  and estrogen 188–9
  prognosis for 189–90
  staging for 189–90
  treatment of 190–1
uterine cervix 6
uterine papillary serous carcinoma 189
uterine sarcomas 190
uterus 190–1, 200
  retroverted 202

V

vagina 178, 180, 183
vaginal bleeding 189
vaginal cancer 105
vaginal douche 184
vaginitis 184
vancomycin 304
vasectomy 156
vegetables, contamination of 344
venison 104
veno-occlusive disease (VOD) 327
verrucous carcinoma 178
Veterans Administration Lung Cancer Study Group (VALCSG) 39
Vicodin 55
villous adenomas 66
vinblastine 219, 266, 268
vincristine 13, 40, 190, 262, 265–6, 284, 288–9
vindesine 45
vinorelbine 45, 131
viral factors, in leukemia 284
viral infection 342–3
  epidemic of 342–3
  reducing exposure to 343–6
viruses 5
  latent 285–6
vitamin A 14, 156, 216, 246
vitamin B 351
vitamin B_6 124
vitamin B_{12} 124, 246, 312
vitamin C 42, 62, 81, 246, 351
vitamin D 14, 62–3, 81, 156, 351
vitamin E 62–3, 73–4, 166, 246
  succunate 81
vitamin K 247
vomiting 122, 124, 209–10, 232, 234, 309–12
  Chinese medicine 310–12
  conventional medicine 309
  and dying 333
von Hippel–Lindau disease 218

W

Waldenstrom's lymphoma 254
walnut twigs 272
walnuts 272
warm disease theory 255
wasp nest 114, 224, 273
watchful waiting, in prostate cancer 163–4
water 347–8
  contamination of 344, 349
  edema 38
  metabolism 65
  therapy 356

water-melon powder 313
wei 121, 200, 210, 244, 259, 270, 316,
    360
  bi 315
  harmonisation 30
  qi 18–19, 303, 315, 353, 355, 359
    in bladder/renal cancer 221–2
    in breast cancer 108
    deficiency 73, 274, 277
    in lung cancer 46
    in lymphomas 256–9
    in ovarian cancer 200
  suo 315–16
  syndrome 316–17
wen bing 359
  theory 255
  xue 353, 357, 360
Wen bing tiao bian 358
Whipple resection 231, 236
white blood cells 304–6
    in breast cancer 117, 121–6, 129,
      145, 150
    in cervical cancer 183–5
    in colorectal cancer 69–70, 75–6,
      81, 84
    in leukemia 283, 285, 287–8, 290
    in lymphomas 279
    in ovarian cancer 207, 211–12
    in pancreatic/hepatic cancer 239,
      242, 248–9
    in prostate cancer 168, 171, 174
    in uterine cancer 193
White Snake Six Ingredient Pill 222–3
whole abdominal radiation (WAR)
    199
wilting impediment syndrome 315
wind 63, 316
  bi 142
    damp 270
  dispelling 273
  heat 63–5, 256
  internal 141
  pathogen 65, 256
Working Formulation 263, 265
World Health Organization (WHO)
    95, 322
Worldwatch Institute 348

X

X-ray therapy 41, 45, 118–19, 146, 148,
    163
  side-effects 52–3
X-rays 10, 43, 97, 267–8
  chest 38, 77, 112, 130, 218, 261, 266
Xanax 99
Xeloda 82
xenobiotics 21, 354–6

xenoestrogens 349, 358
  in breast cancer 100, 108, 110, 147
  in cervical cancer 178
  in non-Hodgkin's lymphoma
    (NHL) 255
  in ovarian cancer 196
  in uterine cancer 191
Xiao Yan San pattern 236
xu lao 304
xuan yin 324–5
xue 359–60
xylene 352

Y

yang 21, 308, 316–17, 338, 349, 359–60
  ascending 129
  in bladder/renal cancer 221
  in breast cancer 102, 108, 116, 135,
    137
  deficiency 310, 320, 325
    in breast cancer 127–8, 141
    in colorectal cancer 85
    in lymphomas 259
    in prostate cancer 159
    symptoms 127
  essence 337
  floating 128
  hyperactive 159
  invigoration 125
  in leukemia 285, 297–8
  in lung cancer 51
  meridians 201
  in ovarian cancer 200
  in prostate cancer 159
  qi 221, 259, 317, 338, 357
  sunken 166, 304
  tonic 30, 81, 121, 212
  young 297–8
Yangming 107, 316–17
  channel 142, 324
ye fluids 220–1
yeast, depuration by 350
yi du gong du therapy 25, 357
yin 19, 21, 31, 303, 308, 316–17, 338,
    349, 355
  in bladder/renal cancer 221
  in breast cancer 102, 125, 135–6
  in colorectal cancer 64
  deficiency 306, 326, 359
    in breast cancer 94, 108, 118,
      127–9
    in cervical cancer 179, 183
    in colorectal cancer 73
    heat 47–8, 99
      toxin 238–9
    in leukemia 296
    of liver and kidney 243–4

yin (Continued)
    in lung cancer 45–6, 59
    in lymphomas 256–7
    in ovarian cancer 207
    in pancreatic cancer 235
    in prostate cancer 159, 170–1
    in uterine cancer 193
  in leukemia 285–6, 297–8
  in lung cancer 45, 51
  in lymphomas 273
  meridians 201
  nourishment 30, 121, 276, 356–7,
    360
  organs 64
  in ovarian cancer 200
  in prostate cancer 159
  tonic 125
  wei 113
  young 297–8
ying 20, 303, 353, 359–60
  in breast cancer 98, 121
  harmonisation 30
  heat 360
  in hepatocellular carcinoma (HCC)
    244
  in lymphomas 258–9
  in ovarian cancer 200, 210
  in pancreatic cancer 235
yoga 357
yuan qi 91, 102, 200, 220–1, 258, 315

Z

zang du 63–4
zang fu 20, 63, 112, 200, 220, 258, 297,
    317
  deficiencies 19–21
  function 28
  restoration 30
  yin 123
zang organs 318
Zantac 208
zedoary 114, 185–6, 193, 224, 326, 328
Zhang Jing Yue 315
Zhang Zhong Jing 102, 255
zheng qi 19, 23, 27, 303, 360
  in lung cancer 51, 59
  in lymphomas 258
  in ovarian cancer 205
Zhu Bing Yuan Hou Lun 258
Zhu Dan Xi 108
zigong 200
zinc 159
  picolinate 246
Zofran 206, 208, 210
Zoladex 165, 190

Pharmaceutical Name Index

A

Achyranthis bidentatae Radix 185, 225, 328
Aconiti Radix preparata 26, 175, 187
Actinidiae chinensis Radix 238
Adenophorae Radix 271
Agkistrodon 57, 140
Agrimoniae Herba 49, 75, 80, 114, 174, 185, 222–3, 238, 275, 294
Akebiae Caulis 297, 314
Akebiae Fructus 49, 127, 139, 149, 167, 173, 238, 249, 271, 296
Albiziae Cortex 85, 87, 141, 146
Alismatis Rhizoma 48, 70, 122–4, 129, 168, 173, 185, 187, 204, 225, 239, 242, 244, 246, 308
Allii macrostemi Bulbus 59, 86, 127, 134
Allii sativi Bulbus 183
Alpiniae oxyphyllae Fructus 76, 168, 173, 314
Amomi Fructus 86, 210
Amorphophalli Rhizoma 273
Anemarrhenae Rhizoma 49, 69, 73, 80, 119, 187, 238, 243–4, 294, 307–8, 311, 360–1
Angelicae dahuricae Radix 134–5, 141, 149, 324
Angelicae pubescentis Radix 26
Angelicae sinensis radicis Cauda 26, 68
Angelicae sinensis Radix 26, 70, 71–2, 76, 79, 116–17, 126–7, 134, 136, 138–9, 167, 169, 173, 185–7, 203, 210, 222–3, 246–7, 270–1, 274–6, 278–9, 294–6

Aquilariae Lignum resinatum 169
Arctii Fructus 273
Arecae Pericarpium 242, 247
Arecae Semen 183
Arisaematis Rhizoma preparatum 72, 114, 141, 146, 271, 276
Armeniacae Semen 53, 86
Armeniacae Semen amarum 48, 50, 326
Arnebiae Radix 139, 183–4, 188, 245, 274, 278–9
Artemisiae annuae Herba 272, 278, 295, 360–1
Artemisiae argyi Folium 114
Artemisiae scopariae Herba 167, 173, 244–5, 313
Asini Corii Colla 143, 186, 308
Asparagi Radix 47, 73, 75, 117, 119, 122, 174–5, 243, 274–5, 279, 307, 311
Asteris Radix 48, 86
Astragali Radix 26, 50–3, 55, 70–2, 75–7, 79–80, 84–7, 116–17, 122–4, 126–7, 134, 138, 141, 143–5, 168, 173–5, 184, 186–7, 193, 203, 206, 210, 212, 223–4, 239, 245, 247, 249, 271–2, 274–6, 278, 294–7, 306–8, 311, 313, 328, 360
Atractylodis macrocephalae Rhizoma 26–7, 48, 69–70, 72, 76, 78, 83, 85, 87, 122–3, 125, 134, 136, 138, 141, 167–8, 170, 175, 184–7, 203–6, 237–9, 241–2, 275–6, 294–6, 308
Aucklandiae Radix 75–6, 274, 279, 311, 324
Aurantii Fructus 139, 325
Aurantii Fructus immaturus 128, 212

B

Bambusae Caulis in taeniam 51, 75, 145
Bambusae Succus 76, 310–11
Baphicacanthis Radix 171, 183, 245, 273
Benincasae Exocarpium 326
Bidentis bipinnatae Herba 273
Bidentis pilosae Herba 273
Biotae Semen 59, 141, 276
Bistortae Rhizoma 49, 188
Borneolum 188, 326
Bruceae Fructus 125
Bubali Cornu 224, 294, 296, 360
Bupleuri Radix 72, 126, 134, 137–8, 173, 203, 241, 272–3, 325

C

Cannabis Semen 79, 204, 239, 306, 311
Carthami Flos 26, 68, 141, 175, 294, 296
Caryophylli Flos 249, 310
Cassiae Semen 271
Centellae Herba 146
Cervi Cornu 138–9, 143, 308
Cervi Cornu pantotrichum 26, 307
Chebulae Fructus 69, 83
Chelidonii Herba 238, 311
Chrysanthemi Flos 171
Chuanxiong Rhizoma 26–7, 71, 79, 84, 124, 134–5, 139, 149, 204, 247, 274, 276, 294, 316, 324
Cimicifugae Rhizoma 72, 187, 223
Cinnamomi Cortex 26, 127, 186
Cinnamomi Ramulus 26, 175, 249
Cirsii Herba 224, 297, 308, 314

Cirsii japonici Herba sive Radix 224, 297, 314

Cistanches Herba 26, 125, 186, 311, 314

Citri reticulatae Pericarpium 25–7, 48, 50, 71–2, 75, 79, 126, 133, 137, 149, 169, 212, 271–2, 275–6, 311, 326, 328

Citri reticulatae viride Pericarpium 25, 128, 133, 137, 139

Citri sarcodactylis Fructus 86, 210, 297, 311

Clematidis Radix 204, 225, 323

Codonopsis Radix 26–7, 48, 69, 72, 76–7, 83–4, 87, 123–5, 146, 149, 168, 173–4, 186–7, 193, 203, 205–6, 212, 224, 239–40, 242, 245, 272, 275, 278, 295–6, 307–8, 311

Coicis Semen 48, 53, 68–9, 76, 80, 83, 85, 127, 167, 170, 173–4, 184, 204, 223–4, 237, 240, 242–3, 249, 274, 278–9, 314, 326, 328

Coptidis Rhizoma 183, 210, 245, 297, 310, 312–13, 360–1

Cordyceps 50, 86, 193, 307

Coriolus 308

Corni Fructus 26–7, 50–1, 129, 223, 274, 279, 297, 308, 313–14

Corydalis Rhizoma 27, 59, 79, 134, 224, 238, 248, 311, 324

Crataegi Fructus 134, 166, 245, 311

Cremastrae Pseudobulbus 53, 115, 117, 126, 139, 174, 203, 274, 326

Curcumae longae Rhizoma 223

Curcumae Radix 27, 114, 123, 126, 138, 167, 170, 173, 185, 204, 224, 237, 241, 243, 246, 275–6, 313–14, 323

Curcumae Rhizoma 114, 185–6, 193, 224, 326, 328

Cuscutae Semen 26–7, 78, 125, 186, 275, 296

Cyperi Rhizoma 25, 27, 71, 79, 139, 276, 326

D

Daemonoropis Resina 114

Dendrobii Herba 47, 49, 52, 59, 125–6, 187, 206, 238, 243–4, 295, 297, 306, 311

Desmodii styracifolii Herba 314

Dianthi Herba 167, 173, 185, 225

Dictamni Cortex 247, 314

Dioscoreae bulbiferae Rhizoma 114, 272, 274

Dioscoreae hypoglaucae Rhizoma 314

Dioscoreae Rhizoma 26, 48, 119, 129, 168, 185, 203, 205, 244, 246, 271, 274–5, 279, 308–9, 311

Draconis Dens 297

Drynariae Rhizoma 55, 84, 124, 204, 316

E

Eckloniae Thallus 26, 115, 271–2, 274

Ecliptae Herba 26, 143, 186, 188, 223, 245

Ephedrae Herba 306

Epimedii Herba 26, 168, 173, 275, 295, 307–8

Eriobotryae Folium 51–3, 114

Eucommiae Cortex 27, 123

Eupatorii Herba 247

Euphorbiae pekinensis Radix 325–6

Eupolyphaga 183, 203–4, 212, 271

Euryales Semen 48, 242, 309, 311

Evodiae Fructus 69, 122–3, 210, 310

F

Foeniculi Fructus 25, 27, 212, 247

Forsythiae fructus 144, 174, 183, 270, 273, 306, 360–1

Fossilia Dentis Mastodi 297

Fossilia Ossis Mastodi 129, 274, 276, 279

Fraxini Cortex 312

Fritillariae cirrhosae Bulbus 26, 47–8, 50–3, 55, 86, 114, 126, 134, 139, 271–2, 276

Fritillariae thunbergii Bulbus 26, 79, 114, 134, 238, 271, 360

G

Ganoderma 84, 119, 124, 143, 171, 212, 249, 308

Gardeniae Fructus 137, 139, 185, 225, 241, 243–4, 270

Gastrodiae Rhizoma 297

Genkwa Flos 86, 325

Gentianae macrophyllae Radix 246

Gentianae Radix 185, 323

Gigeriae galli Endothelium corneum 80, 83, 85–7, 170, 205, 247–8, 274, 278–9, 311

Ginseng Radix 50, 55, 84–7, 134, 138, 141, 170–1, 203, 212, 239, 250, 276, 279, 294–7, 308, 313–14

Gleditsiae Spina 114, 135, 144, 149, 174

Glehniae Radix 47, 51–3, 55, 73, 119, 122–4, 170, 184, 187, 204–5, 238, 244, 275, 294, 306, 309, 312, 326

Glycyrrhizae Radix 26, 48, 50, 53, 71–2, 78, 125, 127, 168, 171, 185, 187, 203–6, 237–9, 242, 244–5, 247, 275, 294–6, 308, 313, 326, 328

Gypsum fibrosum 49

H

Hedyotis diffusae Herba 47, 49–53, 55, 73, 75–6, 80, 84–5, 117, 174, 183–4, 186–7, 193, 203–4, 238, 241–3, 249, 275–6, 295, 307, 314, 328

Herba Capsellae 297, 314

Herba Duchesneae indicae 115, 222–3

Herba Euphorbiae humifusae 273, 278

Herba Gynostemmatis 47, 52, 126, 170, 184–5, 187, 205, 238, 243–4, 295–6

Herba Humuli scandentis 297, 314

Hordei Fructus germinatus 55, 134, 136–7, 149, 167, 205, 210, 237, 247–8, 306, 311

Houttuyniae Herba 47, 49, 51, 55

Hyperici japonici Herba 245

I

Imperatae Rhizoma 26, 49, 114, 123, 222–4, 238, 275, 297, 311, 314

Indigo naturalis 294

Inulae Flos 75, 210, 326

IsatidisRadix 171, 183, 245, 273

J

Juglandis Semen 272

Jujubae Fructus 55, 75–6, 122–3, 243, 249, 276, 325

Junci Medulla 225

K

Kaki Calyx 122–3, 129, 310–11

Kansui Radix 325

L

Lablab Semen album 76, 210
Ledebouriellae Radix 141, 270
Lepidii Semen 55, 59, 325
Ligustici Rhizoma 26
Ligustri lucidi Fructus 26–7, 70, 73, 77, 80, 119, 122–5, 131, 146, 149, 168, 173–5, 186, 193, 206, 212, 223, 239, 275, 278, 295–6, 309
Lilii Bulbus 47, 52, 55
Linderae Radix 71, 79, 123, 311
Liquidambaris Fructus 326
Lithospermi Radix 139, 183–4, 188, 245, 274, 278–9
Lobeliae chinensis Herba 114, 238, 242
Longan Arillus 187, 274, 278–9
Lonicerae Caulis 138, 183
Lonicerae Flos 49, 51, 53, 68, 117, 119, 126–7, 134, 144, 146, 174, 183–5, 238, 270, 272, 274–5, 279, 294–5, 307, 313
Lophatheri Herba 225, 360
Luffae Fructus Retinervus 114, 134, 137
Lycii Cortex 186, 193, 270, 272, 326
Lycii Fructus 26–7, 47, 50, 52–3, 55, 70, 73, 75, 78, 122–5, 168, 170, 175, 184, 187, 206, 224, 275, 295–6, 308
Lygodii Spora 167, 170, 173
Lysimachiae Herba 222

M

Magnoliae officinalis Cortex 71, 79, 312
Massa medicata fermentata 75, 80, 122, 170, 205, 212, 237, 246, 248, 311, 328
Menthae haplocalycis Herba 72, 139, 359
Mori Cortex 86, 325–6
Morindae officinalis Radix 125
Moutan Cortex 25, 27, 119, 129, 134, 137, 144, 168, 170, 173–4, 185, 187, 223–4, 244, 275–6, 294, 297, 306–8, 314, 360–1
Mylabris 114, 183
Myristicae Semen 69, 75, 83, 85
Myrrha 27, 114, 135, 149, 238, 248, 324

N

Nelumbinis Nodus rhizomatis 224, 238, 297, 311, 314

Nelumbinis Semen 311
Notoginseng Radix 26, 117, 122–3, 125, 143, 174, 206, 222, 224, 295–7, 313, 326

O

Olibanum 27, 114, 324
Ophiopogonis Radix 47, 49, 51–3, 55, 73, 75, 122–3, 125–6, 168, 170, 186–7, 204–6, 224, 238, 243, 274–5, 279, 294, 296, 307, 309, 312, 326
Origani vulgaris Herba 237, 244
Ostreae Concha 26, 115, 128–9, 134, 271–2, 274, 278–9

P

Paeoniae Radix alba 27, 68, 70, 71–2, 76, 79, 87, 117, 126, 131, 138–9, 141, 174, 185–6, 224, 245, 271–2, 274, 359
Paeoniae Radix rubra 26–7, 49, 127, 134, 167, 203–4, 238, 241, 270–1, 274, 294, 297, 308, 323, 325, 360–1
Panacis quinquefolii Radix 50, 52, 122, 170, 210, 224, 248, 294–5, 306, 323, 360
Paridis Rhizoma 86–7, 146, 149, 174, 184–5, 212, 249, 274
Patriniae Herba 68–9, 79–80, 132
Perillae Fructus 326
Persicae Semen 26, 68, 167, 294, 296, 328
Peucedani Radix 48
Pharbitidis Semen 328
Phaseoli Semen 225, 297, 314
Phellodendri Cortex 26, 68, 70, 80, 183, 185, 187–8, 225, 314
Pheretima 141
Phragmitis Rhizoma 210
Phyllanthi amari Herba 245
Pinelliae Rhizoma preparatum 26, 48, 75, 80, 122–3, 139, 205, 210, 212, 271–2, 306, 310, 325–6
Plantaginis Semen 48, 185, 204, 225, 242–3, 297, 314
Platycladi Cacumen 79
Platycodi Radix 26, 51, 53, 127, 134–5, 149, 270, 325, 360
Pleiones Pseudobulbus 53, 115, 117, 126, 139, 174, 203, 274, 326
Podophylli Rhizoma 114
Polygalae Radix 127, 276

Polygonati odorati Rhizoma 50–1, 53, 55, 75, 168, 170, 173, 184, 187, 244, 295, 311, 326
Polygonati Rhizoma 122–4, 206, 245, 276, 297, 309, 313
Polygoni avicularis Herba 222
Polygoni chinensis Herba 183
Polygoni cuspidati Rhizoma 245
Polygoni multiflori Radix preparata 73, 122–4, 186, 295–6, 308, 310–11
Polyporus 48, 52–3, 55, 59, 75, 86, 117, 119, 167, 170, 174, 184–6, 193, 204, 206, 212, 222, 224, 237, 239, 242–3, 275, 297, 313–14, 328
Poria 26, 48–53, 59, 69–70, 72, 75, 77, 80, 83, 85, 87, 117, 119, 122–4, 126, 129, 134, 138–9, 145, 167–8, 170, 173, 184–5, 187, 203, 205–6, 210, 212, 222, 224, 237–9, 240–2, 249, 271–2, 275–6, 294–7, 308, 313–14, 325–6, 328
Poriae Sclerotium pararadicis 141–2, 249
Portulacae Herba 68, 80
Prunellae Spica 114, 117, 126–7, 139, 149, 271–2, 274
Pseudostellariae Radix 26, 49–53, 70, 75, 77, 85, 117, 119, 124, 126, 167–8, 170, 174–5, 184–5, 187, 204, 206, 224, 237–8, 248, 275–6, 294–5, 297, 307, 311, 313
Psoraleae Fructus 55, 69, 77, 80, 83, 85, 87, 123–5, 168, 173, 187, 204, 212, 239, 296, 307, 312
Puerariae Radix 240, 306–7, 359
Pyrrosiae Folium 169, 225, 296

R

Rabdosiae rubescentis Herba 168, 171, 173–4
Ranunculi japonici Radix 114
Ranunculi ternati Radix 272
Raphani Semen 210, 249, 328
Rehmanniae Radix 173, 186, 223–4, 271–2, 274, 279, 297, 306–7, 311, 314, 360–1
Rehmanniae Radix preparata 70, 73, 75, 80, 86–7, 123, 125–6, 129, 134, 139, 168, 187, 206, 239, 244–5, 276, 294–6, 308, 311
Resina Draconis 114
Rhei Radix et Rhizoma 49, 141, 210, 237, 239, 243, 248, 270, 296, 306, 311, 326
Rhizoma Bolbostemmae 273
Rosae laevigatae Fructus 129

Rubi Fructus 129
Rubiae Radix 138, 296

S

Salicis babylonicae Ramulus 308
Salviae miltiorrhizae Radix 26–8, 53, 70, 76, 84–5, 119, 122, 124–5, 167, 170, 173, 184, 203–4, 212, 222–3, 238, 245, 248, 271–2, 275, 294, 296–7, 313–14, 316
Sanguisorbae Radix 68, 80, 123, 143
Sappan Lignum 175
Sargassum 26, 115, 127, 204, 241, 271–4
Sargentodoxae Caulis 76
Schisandrae Fructus 50, 75, 86, 129, 131, 245, 274, 279, 295, 297, 313
Schizonepetae Herba 141
Scolopendra 136
Scorpio 136
Scrophulariae Radix 126, 128, 134, 186, 271–4, 278–9, 294–5, 297, 307, 311, 313, 359, 360–1
Scutellariae barbatae Herba 47, 55, 73, 75–6, 114, 126, 184, 237–8, 242, 328
Scutellariae Radix 47, 55, 144–5, 171, 183–5, 241, 243, 245, 274, 278–9, 314, 325, 360–1
Sellaginellae doederleinii Herba 131
Semiaquilegiae Radix 114, 169
Senecionis scandens Herba 245
Sennae Folium 248, 311
Serenoae repens Fructus extractum 171

Serpentis Periostracum 270
Setariae Fructus germinatus 311
Sinapis Semen 138, 271
Smilacis glabrae Rhizoma 184–5, 223, 249, 273, 307
Sojae Semen preparatum 359
Solani lyrati Herba 49, 139, 170, 222–3, 237, 239, 241, 243–5, 249, 313–14, 328
Solani nigri Herba 84, 115, 124, 183, 187, 222–4, 328
Solidaginis virgaureae Herba 184
Sophorae flavescentis Radix 183, 314
Sophorae Flos 68, 80, 84–5
Sophorae tonkinensis Radix 222–3, 273, 278
Sparganii Rhizoma 114, 135, 149, 167, 173, 203, 224
Spatholobi Caulis 26, 55, 75, 84, 117, 122–5, 175, 187, 193, 212, 239, 275, 294, 296, 308–12

T

Taraxaci Herba 114, 119, 126–7, 134, 137, 139, 149, 183, 245, 271, 308
Testudinis Plastrum 27, 129, 135, 170, 244, 274, 279, 294–5, 307
Tetrapanacis Medulla 185, 222, 224, 326
Thlaspi Herba 68, 79, 132
Toosendan Fructus 238
Tremella 308
Trichosanthis Fructus 26, 55, 72, 114, 117, 126–7, 134, 136–8, 149, 325

Trichosanthis Radix 26, 79, 114, 127, 134, 175, 271, 273–4, 279, 326
Trichosanthis Semen 47, 49, 76, 85, 114, 174, 204, 237–8, 243, 311
Trigonellae Semen 135, 149
Trogopterori Faeces 26, 114, 224
Typhae Pollen 224, 314
Typhonii Rhizoma 141

U

Uncariae Ramulus cum Uncis 297

V

Vaccariae Semen 27, 114, 139, 167, 169
Vespae Nidus 114, 224, 273
Violae Herba 127, 134, 188, 294

W

Wedeliae Herba 273
Wikstroemiae indicae Radix 128

Z

Zanthoxyli Pericarpium 56
Zanthoxyli Semen 55, 325
Zingiberis Rhizoma 75
Zingiberis Rhizoma recens 26, 210
Zingiberis Rhizomatis Cortex 326
Ziziphi spinosae Semen 187, 295

Pinyin Name Index

A

ai ye 114

B

ba ji tian 125
ba jiao lian 114
ba yue zha 49–50, 127, 139, 149–50,
    167–8, 173, 238, 249, 271,
    296
Ba zhen tang 70, 117, 128, 136, 222
bai bian dou 76–7, 210
bai he 47, 52, 55–6
Bai he gu jin tang 140
bai hua she 57, 140
bai hua she she cao 47, 49–56, 73–7,
    80, 84–5, 117, 174–5, 183–7, 193,
    203–4, 238–9, 241–3, 249, 275–6,
    295, 307, 314, 328
bai jiang cao 68, 79, 132
bai jie zi 138, 271
bai mao gen 26, 49, 114, 123–4,
    222–5, 238–9, 275, 297, 311,
    314
bai mao teng 49–50, 170, 222–3, 237,
    239, 241–2, 243–5, 249, 313
bai mu er 308
bai qu cai 238, 311
bai ren shen 50–1, 55, 86–7, 134,
    141–2, 170–1, 212, 239
bai shao 27, 68, 70, 71–2, 76–7, 79, 87,
    117, 126, 131, 138–9, 141–2, 174,
    185–6, 224, 245, 271–2, 274,
    359
Bai she liu wei wan 222–3
bai xian pi 247–8, 314
bai ying 50, 328
bai zhi 134–6, 141–2, 149, 324

bai zhu 26–7, 48, 69–70, 72, 76–8,
    83–5, 87, 122–5, 134, 136, 138,
    141–2, 167–8, 170, 175, 184–7,
    203–6, 237–9, 241–2, 275–6,
    294–6, 308
bai zi ren 59, 141–2, 276
Bai zi yang xin tang 319
ban bian lian 114, 238–9, 242
ban lan gen 171, 183, 245, 273
ban mao 114, 183
ban xia 206, 272
Ban xia hou pou tang 320
ban zhi lian 47, 55–6, 73–7, 114, 126–7,
    184–5, 237–9, 242, 328
Bao he wan 27
bei sha shen 47, 51–3, 55, 73, 119,
    122–5, 170, 184, 187, 204–5, 238,
    244, 275, 294, 306, 309, 312, 326
bi xie 314
bian xu 222
bing lang 183
bing pian 188, 326
bo he 72, 139, 359
Bu fei tang 51–2, 86–7
bu gu zhi 55–6, 69, 77, 80–1, 83–5, 87,
    123–5, 168, 173, 187, 204, 212,
    239, 296, 307, 312
Bu yang huan wu tang 141
Bu zhong yi qi tang he Bai he gu jin
    tang jia jian 50
Bu zhong yi qi tang 72, 79, 173
Bu zhong yi qi tang jia wei 313
Bu zhong yi qi wan jia jian 166–7

C

cao he che 49, 188
ce bai ye 79
chai hu 72, 126, 134–5, 137–8, 173,
    203, 241–2, 272–3, 325

Chai hu shu gan san 169
Chai zhi ban xia tang jia jian
    325
che qian zi 48, 185–6, 204–5, 225,
    242–3, 297, 314
chen pi 25–7, 48, 50–1, 71–2, 75–6, 79,
    126, 133, 137, 149–50, 169, 212,
    271–2, 275–6, 311, 326, 328
Chen xiang san jia jian 169
chen xiang 169
chi shao 26–7, 49, 127, 134–5, 167–8,
    203–5, 238, 241–2, 270–1, 274,
    294, 297, 308, 323, 325,
    360–1
chi xiao dou 225, 297, 314
Chin wan hung 119
chong lou 86–7, 146, 149–50, 174–5,
    184–6, 212–13, 249, 274
chuan bei mu 26, 47–8, 50–6, 86,
    114, 126, 134, 139, 271–2,
    276
Chuan bei pi pa lu 86
chuan jiao 56
chuan lian zi 238
chuan shan jia 50, 150
chuan xiong 26–7, 71, 79, 84, 124–5,
    134–6, 139, 149, 204, 247, 274,
    276, 294, 316, 324

D

da fu pi 242, 247–8
da huang 49–50, 141–2, 210–11, 237,
    239, 243, 248–9, 270, 296, 306,
    311, 326
da ji 224–5
da ji gen 297, 314
da suan 183
da zao 122–3, 325
dan dou chi 359

dan shen 26–8, 53, 70, 76–7, 84–5, 119, 122, 124–5, 167–8, 170, 173, 184, 203–5, 212, 222–3, 238, 245, 248–9, 271–3, 275, 294, 296–7, 313–14, 316
dan zhu ye 225, 360
dang gui 26, 70, 71–2, 76–7, 79, 116–17, 126–7, 134, 136, 138–9, 167, 169, 173–4, 185–8, 203, 210, 222–3, 246–7, 270–1, 274–6, 278–9, 294–6
Dang gui bu xue tang 70, 77, 135
dang gui wei 26, 68
Dang gui xiao yao san 143
dang shen 26–7, 48, 69, 72, 76–7, 83–5, 87, 123–5, 146, 149–50, 168, 173–4, 186–7, 193, 203, 205–6, 212, 224, 239–40, 242, 245, 272, 275, 278, 295–6, 307–8, 311
deng xin cao 225
di er cao 245
di gu pi 186, 193, 270–2, 326
di jin cao 273, 278
di long 141–2
di yu 68, 80, 123–4, 143
ding xiang 249–50, 310
Ding zhi wan 319
dong chong xia cao 50–1, 86, 193, 307
dong gua pi 326
dong kui zi 169
dong ling cao 168, 171, 173–4
du huo 26
du zhong 27, 123–4

E

e jiao 143, 186, 308
e zhu 114, 185–8, 193, 224, 326, 328

F

fan xie ye 248–9, 311
fang feng 141–2, 270
Fei liu ping 54
Fei liu ping (gao) 53
Fei liu ping jia jian 59
fo shou 86, 210, 297, 311
fu ling 26, 48–53, 59, 69–70, 72, 75, 77, 80–1, 83–5, 87, 117, 119, 122–6, 129, 134, 138–9, 145, 167–8, 170, 173, 184–5, 187, 203, 205–6, 210, 212, 222, 224, 237–9, 240–2, 249, 271–2, 275–6, 294–7, 308, 313–14, 325–6, 328
fu pen zi 129
fu shen 141–2, 249
Fu zheng qu xie 23

Fu zheng zeng xiao fang 175
fu zi 26, 175, 187–8
Fu zi li zhong tang 250, 313

G

gan cao 26, 48, 50, 53, 125, 127, 168, 171, 185, 187–8, 203–6, 237–9, 242, 244–5, 247, 275, 294–6, 308, 313, 326, 328
gan jiang 75
Gan mai da zao tang 306, 320
gan sui 325
gao ben 26
ge gen 240, 306–7, 359
Ge xia zhu yu tang 202
gou qi zi 26–7, 47, 50, 52–3, 55–6, 70, 73, 75, 78, 122–5, 168, 170–1, 175, 184, 187–8, 206–7, 224, 275, 295–6, 308
gou teng 297
gu sui bu 55–6, 84, 124–5, 204, 316
gua lou ren 47, 49–50, 76–7, 85, 114, 174–5, 204–5, 237–9, 243, 311
gua lou shi 26, 55–6, 72, 114, 117, 126–7, 134, 136–8, 149–50, 325
Gua lou xiao yao tang 138
guang jin qian cao 314
gui ban* 27, 129, 135–6, 170–1, 244, 274, 279, 294–5, 307
Gui pi tang 117, 143, 186
gui zhen cao 273
gui zhi 26, 175, 249–50
Gui zhi fu ling wan 143

H

hai jin sha 167, 170, 173
hai zao 26, 115, 127, 204–5, 241, 271–4
han lian cao 26, 143, 186, 188, 223, 245
he huan pi 85, 87, 141–2, 146
he shou wu 73, 122–5, 186, 295–6, 308, 310–11
he zi 69, 83–4
Hei xiao yao san 136–7
hong da zao 55–6, 75–7, 243, 249, 276
hong hua 26, 68, 141–2, 175, 294, 296
hong ren shen 84–5
hong teng 76–7
hou po 71, 79, 312
hu lu ba 135, 149
hu tao ruo 272
hu zhang 245
Huai hua di yu tang jia jian 68
huai hua 68, 80, 84–5
huai niu xi 185, 225, 328
huang bai 26, 68, 70, 80, 183, 185, 187–8, 225, 314

huang jing 122–5, 206–7, 245, 276, 297, 309, 313
huang lian 183, 210, 245, 297, 310, 312–13, 360–1
Huang lian e jiao tang 318
Huang lian jie du pian 313
huang qi 26, 50–3, 55, 70–2, 75–7, 79–81, 84–7, 116–17, 122–7, 134, 138, 141–5, 168, 170–1, 173–5, 184, 186–7, 193, 203, 206–7, 210–12, 223–4, 239, 245, 247–9, 271–2, 274–6, 278, 294–7, 306–8, 311, 313, 328, 360
huang qin 47, 55–6, 144–5, 171, 183–5, 241–2, 243, 245, 274, 278–9, 314, 325, 360–1
huang yao zi 114, 272, 274
huo ma ren* 79, 204–5, 239, 306, 311
huo tan mu 183
Huo xue qu yu 23, 161

J

ji cai 297, 314
ji nei jin 80–1, 83–7, 170, 205, 247–9, 274, 278–9, 311
Ji sheng qi wan jia jian 328
ji xue cao 146
ji xue teng 26, 55, 75, 84, 117, 122–5, 175, 187–8, 193, 212, 239, 275, 294, 296, 308–12
Jian bu hu qian wan 316
jiang huang 223
jiao gu lan 47, 52, 126–7, 170, 184–5, 187, 205–6, 238–9, 243–4, 295–6
jiao mu 55–6, 325
jie geng 26, 51–4, 127, 134–6, 149, 270–1, 325, 360
jin qian cao 222
jin yin hua 49, 51, 53, 68, 117, 119, 126–7, 134, 144–6, 174, 183–5, 238–9, 270, 272, 274–5, 279, 294–5, 307, 313
jin ying zi 129
jing da ji 325–6
jing jie 141–2
jiu jun da huang 270
ju hua 171
ju ruo 273
ju ye zong 171

K

ku shen 183, 314
ku xing ren 48, 50–1, 326
kun bu 26, 115, 271–2, 274

L

lai fu zi 210, 249, 328
Li qi kuan chang tang 71
Li qi kuan chang tang jia jian 79
Li zhong tang 249–50
lian qiao 144–5, 174, 183, 270, 273, 306, 360–1
lian zi 311
Liang di tang ji nei bu wan jia jian 186
Liang ge san 313
ling zhi 84, 119, 124–5, 143, 171, 212, 249, 308
Liu jun zi tang jia jian 48
Liu wei di huang tang 144
Liu wei di huang wan 81, 113, 117, 133, 143, 145, 175, 187, 223
Liu wei di huang wan jia jian 328
liu zhi 308
long chi 297
long dan cao 185–6, 323
Long dan xie gan jia jian 185
long gu 129, 274, 276, 279
long kui 84, 115, 124–5, 183, 187–8, 222–4, 328
long yan rou 187, 274, 278–9
long yi 270–1
lu cao 297, 314
lu feng fang 114, 224, 273
lu gen 210–11
lu jiao 138–9, 143, 308
lu lu tong 326
lu rong 26, 307

M

ma chi xian 68, 80
ma huang 306
ma lan jin 273
mai dong 47, 49, 51–3, 55–6, 73, 75, 122–7, 168, 170, 186–7, 204–7, 224, 238, 243, 274–5, 279, 294, 296, 307, 309, 312, 326
mai ya 55–6, 134, 136–7, 149–50, 167, 205, 210, 237, 247–9, 306, 311
mao gen 114
mao zhua cao 272
mo yao 27, 114, 135–6, 149, 238, 248–9, 324
mu dan pi 25, 27, 119, 129, 134, 137, 144–5, 168, 170, 173–4, 185, 187, 223–5, 244, 275–6, 294, 297, 306–8, 314, 360–1
mu li 26, 115, 128–9, 134, 271–2, 274, 278–9

mu tong 50, 297, 314
mu tou hui 68–9, 80
mu xiang 75–7, 274, 279, 311, 324

N

nan sha shen 271–2
niu bang zi 273
nu zhen zi 26–7, 70, 73, 77, 80–1, 119, 122–5, 131, 146, 149, 168, 173–5, 186, 193, 206–7, 212, 223, 239, 275, 278, 295–6, 309

O

ou jie 224–5, 238–9, 297, 311, 314

P

pei lan 247
pi pa ye 51–3, 114
Ping wei san 27
pu gong ying 114, 119, 126–7, 134, 137, 139, 149–50, 183, 245, 271, 308
pu huang 224, 314
pu huang tan 224–5
pu yin gen 128

Q

qian cao gen 138, 296
qian hu 48
qian li guang 245
qian niu zi 328
qian shi 48–9, 242, 309, 311
qin jiao 246
qin pi 312
qing dai 294
Qing gan zhi li tang 185
qing hao 272, 278, 295, 353, 360–1
Qing hao bai du yin 278
Qing hao bie jia tang 278, 360
Qing long yi jiu 272
qing pi 25, 128, 133–4, 137, 139
Qing re bu qi tang 313
Qing re jie du 24
Qing wen bai du yin 360
Qing zai jiu fei tang 52
Qing zao jiu fei tang 316
Qing zao jiu fei tang jia jian 47
Qing zhi si wu tang 139
qu mai 167, 173, 185–6, 225
quan xie 136

R

ren dong teng 138, 183
ren shen 138, 142, 171, 203, 250, 276, 279, 294–7, 308, 313–14
rou cong rong 26, 125, 186, 311, 314
rou dou kou 69, 75, 83–5
rou gui 26, 127–8, 186–8
ru xiang 27, 114, 324
Ruan jian san jie 25

S

san leng 114, 135–6, 149, 167–8, 173, 203, 224
san qi 26, 117, 122–5, 143, 174–5, 206–7, 222–4, 295–7, 313, 326
San ren tang 360
sang bai pi 86, 325–6
sha ren 86, 210
sha shen 56, 205–6, 239
Sha shen mai dong tang 316
Sha shen mai dong tang he Xie bai jia jian 326
shan ci gu* 53–4, 115, 117, 126, 139, 174–5, 203, 274, 326
shan dou gen 222–3, 273, 278
shan yao 26, 48, 119, 129, 168, 185, 203, 205, 244, 246, 271, 274–5, 279, 308–9, 311
shan zha 134–5, 166–7, 245, 311
shan zhu yu 26–7, 50–2, 129, 223, 274, 279, 297, 308, 313–14
she mei 115, 222–3
Shen ling bai zhu san 69
Shen ling bai zhu tang 316
shen qu 75–6, 80–1, 122, 170, 205, 212, 237, 246, 248–9, 311, 328
sheng di huang 173, 186, 223–5, 271–2, 274, 279, 297, 306–7, 311, 314, 360–1
sheng jiang 26, 210
sheng jiang pi 326
sheng ma 72, 187–8, 223
Shi chuan da bu tang 117
Shi chuan da bu wan 117
shi di 122–4, 129, 310–11
shi gao 49
shi hu 47, 49, 52, 59, 125–7, 187, 206–7, 238–9, 243–4, 295, 297, 306, 311
shi shang bai 131
shi wei 169, 225, 296
Shi zao tang 325

shu di 70, 73, 75, 80–1, 86–7, 123–7, 129, 134–5, 139, 168, 187–8, 206–7, 239, 244–5, 276, 294–6, 308, 311
Shu gan wan 133, 169, 322
shu yang quan 139, 314
shui niu jiao 224, 294, 296, 360
si gua luo 114, 134, 137
Si jun zi tang 27, 48, 50, 77, 84–5, 124–5, 135, 142, 145, 168, 186–7, 203, 205–7, 224, 238–9, 242, 275, 306
Si jun zi tang he Wu ling san jia jian 328
Si miao wan 316
Si shen wan jia jian 69
su mu 175
su ya 311
su zi 326
suan zao ren 187–8, 295
Suan zao ren tang 318–19

T

tai zi shen 26, 49–53, 70, 75, 77, 85, 117, 119, 124–5, 126–7, 167–8, 170, 174–5, 184–5, 187, 204–7, 224, 237–9, 248–9, 275–6, 294–5, 297, 307, 311, 313
Tao hong si wu tang jia jian 68
tao ren 26, 68, 167–8, 294, 296, 328
teng li 238
tian dong 47, 73, 75, 117, 119, 122, 174–5, 243, 274–5, 279, 307, 311
tian hua fen 26, 79, 114, 127, 134–5, 175, 271, 273–4, 279, 326
tian kui zi 114, 169
tian ma 297
tian nan xing 72, 114, 141–2, 146, 271, 276
Tian wang bu xin tang 318–19
ting li zi 55–6, 59, 325
tong cao 185–6, 222, 224–5, 326
tu bei mu 273
tu bie chong 183, 203–4, 212–13, 271
tu fu ling 184–6, 223, 249, 273, 307
tu si zi 26–7, 78, 125, 186, 275, 296
tu yin chen 237, 244

W

wang bu liu xing 27, 114, 139, 167, 169
wang jiang nan 271

wei ling xian 204, 225, 323
Wen jing tang 202
Wend an tang 360
wu gong 136
wu ling zhi 26, 114, 224
wu wei zi 50–1, 75, 86, 129, 131, 245, 274, 279, 295, 297, 313
wu yao 71, 79, 123–4, 311
wu zhu yu 69, 122–4, 210, 310

X

Xi gua shuang 313
Xi jiao tang he hua ban tang 294
xi yang shen 50–2, 122–3, 170, 210–11, 224, 248–9, 294–5, 306, 323, 360
xia ku cao 114, 117, 126–7, 139, 149–50, 271–2, 274
xian feng cao 273
xian he cao 49, 75, 80–1, 114, 174, 185–6, 222–3, 238, 275, 294
xiang fu 25, 27, 71, 79, 139, 276, 326
Xiang fu xuan fu hua tang jia jian 326
Xiang sha liu jun zi tang 27, 144
xiao hui xiang 25, 27, 212, 240, 247
xiao ji 224, 297, 308, 314
Xiao yao 202
Xiao yao san 27, 72, 133, 148, 169, 227, 236, 318, 322
xie bai 59, 86, 127, 134–5
xing ren 53–4, 86
xuan fu hua 75, 210, 326
xuan shen 126, 128, 134, 186, 271–4, 278–9, 294–5, 297, 307, 311, 313, 359, 360–1
Xue fu zhu yu tang 202
xue jie 114

Y

ya dan zi 125
yan hu suo 27, 59, 79, 134, 224, 238, 248–9, 311, 324
Yang xin tang 319
Yi du gong du 25
yi ren 48, 53, 68–9, 76–7, 80, 83–5, 127, 167, 170, 173–5, 184–5, 204–5, 223–4, 237, 240, 242–3, 249, 274, 278–9, 314, 326, 328
yi zhi huang hua 184
yi zhi ren 76–7, 168, 173, 314
yin chen hao 167, 173, 244–5, 313
Yin qiao hong jiang jie du tang 202
Yin qiao san 360

yin yang huo 26, 168, 173, 275, 295, 307–8
You gui wan 174, 315
You gui yin 87, 132, 212
You gui yin jia jian 212
yu jin 27, 114, 123–4, 126, 138, 167–8, 170, 173, 185, 204–5, 224, 237, 241, 243, 246, 275–6, 313–14, 323
yu xing cao 47, 49–51, 55–6
yu zhu 50–3, 55–6, 75, 168, 170, 173, 184, 187, 244, 295, 311, 326
yuan hua 86, 325
yuan zhi 127, 276
yun zhi 308

Z

zao ci 136
zao jiao ci 114, 135, 144–5, 149, 174
ze xie 48, 70, 122–5, 129, 168, 173, 185–7, 204–5, 225, 239, 242, 244, 246, 308
Zha mei yi wei tang jia jian 53
zhe bei mu 26, 51, 79, 114, 134, 238, 271, 360
zhen zhu cao 245
Zhi bai di huang wan 70
zhi bai fu zi 141
Zhi bai huang tang 313
zhi ban xia 26, 48, 75, 80–1, 122–4, 139, 205, 210, 212, 271–2, 306, 310, 325–6
zhi gan cao 71–2, 78
zhi huang qi 173–4
zhi ke 139, 325
zhi mu 49, 69–70, 73, 80–1, 119, 187, 238–9, 243–4, 294, 307–8, 311, 360–1
zhi shi 128, 212
zhi zi 137, 139, 185–6, 225, 241–2, 243–4, 270
zhu li 76, 310–11
zhu ling 48, 52–3, 55–6, 59, 75, 86, 117, 119, 167–8, 170, 174–5, 184–7, 193, 204–7, 212, 222, 224, 237, 239, 242–3, 275–6, 297, 313–14, 328
zhu ru 51–2, 75–6, 145
zi cao 139, 183–4, 188, 245, 274, 278–9
zi hua di ding 127, 134, 188, 294
zi wan 48, 86
Zui gui yin 140
Zuo gui wan 315
Zuo gui yin 56, 132, 140

Scientific Name Index

A

Achyranthes bidentata 185, 225, 328
Aconitum carmichaelii 26, 175, 187
Actinidia chinensis 238
Adenophora 271
adenovirus 291
Aegle marmelos 240
Agkistrodon acutus 57, 140
Agrimonia pilosa var. japonica 49, 75,
    80, 114, 174, 185, 222–3, 238,
    275, 294
Akebia 49–50, 127, 139, 149, 167, 173,
    238, 249, 271, 296–7, 314
Albizia 85, 87, 141, 146
Alisma 48, 70, 122–4, 129, 168, 173,
    185, 187, 204, 225, 239, 242, 244,
    246, 308
Allium macrostemon 59, 86, 127, 134
Allium sativum 183
Alpinia oxyphylla 76, 168, 173, 314
Amomum 86, 210
Amorphophallus 273
Amorphophallus rivieri 273
Amorphophallus sinensis 273
Anemarrhena 49, 69, 73, 80, 119, 187,
    238, 243–4, 294, 307–8, 311,
    360–1
Angelica 26
Angelica dahurica 134–5, 141, 149, 324
Angelica sinensis 26, 68, 70, 71–2, 76,
    79, 116–17, 126–7, 134, 136,
    138–9, 167, 169, 173, 185–7, 203,
    210, 222–3, 246–7, 270–1, 274–6,
    278–9, 294–6
Aquilaria 169
Arctium lappa 273
Areca catechu 183, 242, 247
Arisaema erubescens 72, 114, 141, 146,
    271, 276

Arnebia 139, 183–4, 188, 245, 274,
    278–9
Artemisia annua 272, 278, 295, 360–1
Artemisia apiacea 353
Artemisia argyi 114
Artemisia capillaris 167, 173, 244–5, 313
Artemisia scoparia 167, 173, 244–5, 313
Asparagus 47, 73, 75, 117, 119, 122,
    174–5, 243, 274–5, 279, 307, 311
Aspergillus 232, 241, 291, 305
Aster tataricus 48, 86
Astragalus 70
Astragalus membranaceus 26, 50–3, 55,
    70–2, 75–7, 79–80, 84–7, 116–17,
    122–4, 126–7, 134, 138, 141,
    143–5, 168, 173–5, 184, 186–7,
    193, 203, 206, 210, 212, 223–4,
    239, 245, 247, 249, 271–2, 274–6,
    278, 294–7, 306–8, 311, 313, 328,
    360
Astragalus mongolicus 23
Atractylodes macrocephala 26–7, 48,
    69–70, 72, 76, 78, 83, 85, 87,
    122–3, 125, 134, 136, 138, 141,
    167–8, 170, 175, 184–7, 203–6,
    237–9, 241–2, 275–6, 294–6, 308
Azadirachta indica 240

B

Bambusa 76, 310–11
Baphicacanthus 171, 183, 245, 273
Basidiomycetes 13
Benincasa hispida 326
Bidens bipinnata 273
Bidens pilosa 273
Biota 59, 141, 276
Biota orientalis 79
Bolbostemma paniculatum 273
Borago 97

Boswellia sacra 27, 114, 324
Brucea 125
Bubalus 224, 294, 296, 360
Bupleurum 72, 126, 134, 137–8, 173,
    203, 241, 272–3, 325
Buthus martensii 136

C

Caesalpinia sappan 175
Candida 291, 353
Cannabis sativa 79, 204, 239, 306, 311
Capsella 297, 314
Carthamnus tinctorius 26, 68, 141, 175,
    294, 296
Cassia 248, 271, 311
Cassia occidentalis 271
Centella asiatica 146
Cervus 139, 143, 308
Cervus nippon 26, 307
Chelidonium 238, 311
Chinemys reevesii 27, 129, 135, 170,
    244, 274, 279, 294–5, 307
Chrysanthemum 171
Cimicifuga 72, 187, 223
Cimicifuga racemosa 97
Cinnamomum 188
Cinnamomum cassia 26, 127, 175, 186,
    249
Cinnamomum tamala 240
Cirsium 224, 297, 308, 314
Cirsium japonicum 224, 297, 314
Cistanche 26, 125, 186, 311, 314
Citrus aurantium 128, 139, 212, 325
Citrus reticulata 25–7, 48, 50, 71–2, 75,
    79, 126, 128, 133, 137, 139, 149,
    169, 212, 271–2, 275–6, 311, 326,
    328
Citrus sarcodactylis 86, 210, 297, 311
Clematis chinensis 204, 225, 323

Codonopsis pilosula 26–7, 48, 69, 72, 76–7, 83–4, 87, 123–5, 146, 149, 168, 173–4, 186–7, 193, 203, 205–6, 212, 224, 239–40, 242, 245, 272, 275, 278, 295–6, 307–8, 311

Coix lacryma-jobi 48, 53, 68–9, 76, 80, 83, 85, 127, 167, 170, 173–4, 184, 204, 223–4, 237, 240, 242–3, 249, 274, 278–9, 314, 326, 328

Commiphora myrrha 27, 114, 135, 149, 238, 248, 324

Coptis 183, 210, 245, 297, 310, 312–13, 360–1

Cordyceps 50, 86, 193, 307

Coriolus versicolor 308

Cornus officinalis 26–7, 50–1, 129, 223, 274, 279, 297, 308, 313–14

Corydalis yanhusuo 27, 59, 79, 134, 224, 238, 248, 311, 324

Corynebacterium parvum 13

Crataegus 134, 166, 245, 311

Cremastra 53, 115, 117, 126, 139, 174, 203, 274, 326

Curcuma longa 27, 114, 123, 126, 138, 167, 170, 173, 185, 204, 223–4, 237, 241, 243, 246, 275–6, 313–14, 323

Curcuma zedoaria 114, 185–6, 188, 193, 224, 326, 328

Cuscuta 26–7, 78, 125, 186, 275, 296

Cymbopogon citratus 319

Cynara scolymus 245

Cyperus rotundus 25, 27, 71, 79, 139, 276, 326

cytomegalovirus (CMV) 291

D

Daemonorops draco 114

Daphne genkwa 86, 325

Dendranthema morifolium 171

Dendrobium 47, 49, 52, 59, 125–6, 187, 206, 238, 243–4, 295, 297, 306, 311

Desmodium styracifolium 314

Dianthus 167, 173, 185, 225

Dictamnus 247, 314

Dimocarpus longan 187, 274, 278–9

Dioscorea bulbifera 114, 272, 274

Dioscorea floribunda 92

Dioscorea hypoglauca 314

Dioscorea opposita 26, 48, 119, 129, 168, 185, 203, 205, 244, 246, 271, 274–5, 279, 308–9, 311

Diospyros kaki 122–3, 129, 310–11

Dolichos lablab 76, 210

Drynaria 55, 84, 124, 204, 316

Dryobalanops aromatica 188, 326

Duchesnea indica 115, 222–3

E

Ecklonia kurome 26, 115, 271–2, 274

Eclipta prostrata 26, 143, 186, 188, 223, 245

Elaphe 270

Elaphe carinata 271

Elaphe taeniura 271

Eleutherococcus senticosus 23, 319

Ephedra 306

Epimedium grandiflorum 26, 168, 173, 275, 295, 307–8

Epstein–Barr virus (EBV) 4

Equus asinus 143, 186, 308

Eriobotrya japonica 51–3, 114

Escherichia coli 304

Eucommia ulmoides 27, 123

Eupatorium fortunei 247

Euphorbia humifusa 273, 278

Euphorbia kansui 325

Euphorbia pekinensis 325–6

Eupolyphaga sinensis 183, 203–4, 212, 271

Euryale 48, 242, 309, 311

Evodia 69, 122–3, 210, 310

F

Ficus racemosa 240

Foeniculum vulgare 25, 27, 212, 247

Forsythia 144, 174, 183, 270, 273, 306, 360–1

Fraxinus 312

Fritillaria cirrhosa 26, 47–8, 50–3, 55, 86, 114, 126, 134, 139, 271–2, 276

Fritillaria thunbergii 26, 51, 79, 114, 134, 238, 271, 360

G

Gallus gallus domesticus 80, 83, 85–7, 170, 205, 247–8, 274, 278–9, 311

Ganoderma 84, 119, 124, 143, 171, 212, 249, 308

Ganoderma lucidum 23

Gardenia 137, 139, 185, 225, 241, 243–4, 270

Gastrodia elata 297

Gentiana 185, 323

Gentiana macrophylla 246

Ginkgo biloba 319

Gleditsia 114, 135–6, 144, 149, 174

Glehnia 47, 51–3, 55, 73, 119, 122–4, 170, 184, 187, 204–5, 238, 244, 275, 294, 306, 309, 312, 326

Glycine max 84, 96–7, 99, 359

Glycyrrhiza 26, 48, 50, 53, 125, 127, 168, 171, 185, 187, 203–6, 237–9, 242, 244–5, 247, 275, 294–6, 308, 313, 326, 328

Glycyrrhiza glabra 23, 245

Glycyrrhiza uralensis 23, 71–2, 78

Grifola 48, 52–3, 55, 59, 75, 86, 117, 119, 167, 170, 174, 184–6, 193, 204, 206–7, 212, 222, 224, 237, 239, 242–3, 275, 297, 313–14, 328

Gymnema sylvestre 240

Gynostemma 47, 52, 126, 170, 184–5, 187, 205, 238, 243–4, 295–6

H

Helicobacter pylori 99, 262, 264

herpes simplex virus (HSV) 4, 291

herpes zoster 291

Hordeum vulgare 55, 134, 136–7, 149, 167, 205, 210, 237, 247–8, 306, 311

Houttuynia 47, 49, 51, 55

human papilloma virus (HPV) 4

Humulus scandens 297, 314

Hypericum 245

Hypericum perforatum 319

I

Imperata cylindrica 26, 49, 114, 123, 222–4, 238, 275, 297, 311, 314

Indigofera tinctoria 294

Inula 75, 210, 326

Isatis 171, 183, 245, 273

J

Juglans 272

Juncus effusus 225

K

Klebsiella 304

L

Laminaria 25

Ledebouriella 141, 270

Lepidium 55, 59, 325
Ligusticum 26
Ligusticum wallichii 26–7, 71, 79, 84, 124, 134–5, 139, 149, 204, 247, 274, 276, 294, 316, 324
Ligustrum lucidum 26–7, 70, 73, 77, 80, 119, 122–5, 131, 146, 149, 168, 173–5, 186, 193, 206, 212, 223, 239, 275, 278, 295–6, 309
Lilium 47, 52, 55
Lindera 71, 79, 123, 311
Linum 96
Liquidambar formosana 326
Lithospermum 139, 183–4, 188, 245, 274, 278–9
Lobelia chinensis 114, 238, 242
Lonicera 49, 51, 53, 68, 117, 119, 126–7, 134, 144, 146, 174, 183–5, 238, 270, 272, 274–5, 279, 294–5, 307, 313
Lonicera japonica 25, 138, 183
Lophatherum gracile 225, 360
Luffa cylindrica 114, 134, 137
Lycium 186, 193, 270, 272, 326
Lycium chinensis 26–7, 47, 50, 52–3, 55, 70, 73, 75, 78, 122–5, 168, 170, 175, 184, 187, 206, 224, 275, 295–6, 308
Lygodium japonicum 167, 170, 173
Lysimachia 222

M

Magnolia officinalis 71, 79, 312
Melia toosendan 238
Mentha haplocalyx 72, 139, 359
Momordica charantia 240
Morinda officinalis 125
Morus alba 86, 325–6
Mylabris 114, 183
Myristica fragrans 69, 75, 83, 85

N

Nelumbo nucifera 224, 238, 297, 311, 314

O

Oldenlandia 25, 47, 49–53, 55, 73, 75–6, 80, 84–5, 117, 174, 183–4, 186–7, 193, 203–4, 238, 241–3, 249, 275–6, 295, 307, 314, 328

Ophiopogon 47, 49, 51–3, 55, 73, 75, 122–3, 125–6, 168, 170, 186–7, 204–6, 224, 238, 243, 274–5, 279, 294, 296, 307, 309, 312, 326
Origanum vulgare 237, 244
Ostrea 26, 115, 128–9, 134, 271–2, 274, 278–9

P

Paeonia lactiflora 26–7, 49, 68, 70, 71–2, 76, 79, 87, 117, 126–7, 131, 134, 138–9, 141, 167, 174, 185–6, 203–4, 224, 238, 241, 245, 270–2, 274, 294, 297, 308, 323, 325, 359–1
Paeonia suffruticosa 25, 27, 119, 129, 134, 137, 144, 168, 170, 173–4, 185, 187, 223–4, 244, 275–6, 294, 297, 306–8, 314, 360–1
Panax ginseng 50, 55, 84–7, 134, 138, 141, 170–1, 203, 212, 239, 250, 276, 279, 294–7, 308, 313–14, 319
Panax notoginseng 26, 117, 122–3, 125, 143, 174, 206, 222, 224, 295–7, 313, 326
Panax quinquefolium 50, 52, 122, 170, 210, 224, 248, 294–5, 306, 323, 360
Paris 86–7, 146, 149, 174, 184–5, 212, 249, 274
Patrinia 68–9, 79–80, 132
Perilla frutescens 326
Peucedanum 48
Pharbitis 328
Phaseolus calcaratus 225, 297, 314
Phellodendron 26, 68, 70, 80, 183, 185, 187–8, 225, 314
Pheretima 141
Phragmitis communis 210
Phyllanthus amarus 245
Phyllostachys nigra 51, 75, 145
Pinellia ternata 26, 48, 75, 80, 122–3, 139, 205, 210, 212, 271–2, 306, 310, 325–6
Piper methysticum 319
Plantago 48, 185, 204, 225, 242–3, 297, 314
Platycodon grandiflorus 26, 51, 53, 127, 134–5, 149, 270, 325, 360
Pleione 53, 115, 117, 126, 139, 174, 203, 274, 326
Pleurotos pulmonarius 13
pneumocystis 291
Podophyllum peltatum 13
Podophyllum pleianthum 114
Polygala 127, 276

Polygonatum 122–4, 206, 245, 276, 297, 309, 313
Polygonatum odoratum 50–1, 53, 55, 75, 168, 170, 173, 184, 187, 244, 295, 311, 326
Polygonum aviculare 222
Polygonum bistorta 49, 188
Polygonum chinense 183
Polygonum cuspidatum 245
Polygonum multiflorum 73, 122–4, 186, 295–6, 308, 310–11
Polyporaceae 207
Polyporus 48, 52–3, 55, 59, 75, 86, 117, 119, 167, 170, 174, 184–6, 193, 204, 206, 212, 222, 224, 237, 239, 242–3, 275, 297, 313–14, 328
Poria 23, 142
Poria cocos 26, 48–53, 59, 69–70, 72, 75, 77, 80, 83, 85, 87, 117, 119, 122–4, 126, 129, 134, 138–9, 141–2, 145, 167–8, 170, 173, 184–5, 187, 203, 205–6, 210, 212, 222, 224, 237–9, 240–2, 249, 271–2, 275–6, 294–7, 308, 313–14, 325–6, 328
Portulaca 68, 80
Prunella vulgaris 25, 114, 117, 126–7, 139, 149, 271–2, 274
Prunus 26, 68, 167, 294, 296, 328
Prunus armeniaca 48, 50, 53–4, 86, 326
Pseudomonas 199, 304
Pseudomonas aeruginosa 304
Pseudostellaria heterophylla 26, 49–53, 70, 75, 77, 85, 117, 119, 124, 126, 167–8, 170, 174–5, 184–5, 187, 204, 206, 224, 237–8, 248, 275–6, 294–5, 297, 307, 311, 313
Psoralea 55, 69, 77, 80, 83, 85, 87, 123–5, 168, 173, 187, 204, 212, 239, 296, 307, 312
Pterocarpus marsupinum 240
Pueraria 240, 306–7, 359
Pyrrosia 169, 225, 296

R

Rabdosia 168, 171, 173–4
Ranunculus japonicus 114
Ranunculus ternatus 272
Raphanus sativus 210, 249, 328
Rehmannia 70, 73, 75, 80, 86–7, 123, 125–6, 129, 134, 139, 168, 173, 186–7, 206, 223–4, 239, 244–5, 271–2, 274, 276, 279, 294–7, 306–8, 311, 314, 360–1
Rheum 49, 141, 210, 237, 239, 243, 248, 270, 296, 306, 311, 326
Rosa laevigata 129

Rubia cordifolia 138, 296
Rubus chingii 129

S

Salix babylonica 308
Salvia miltiorhiza 26–8, 53, 70, 76, 84–5,
        119, 122, 124–5, 167, 170, 173,
        184, 203–4, 212, 222–3, 238, 245,
        248, 271–2, 275, 294, 296–7,
        313–14, 316
Sanguisorba 68, 80, 123, 143
Sargassum 26, 115, 127, 204, 241,
        271–4
Sargentodoxa cuneata 76
Saussurea 75–6, 274, 279, 311, 324
Schisandra 50, 75, 86, 129, 131, 245,
        274, 279, 295, 297, 313
Schizonepeta 141
Scolopendra subspinipes 136
Scrophularia 126, 128, 134, 186, 271–4,
        278–9, 294–5, 297, 307, 311, 313,
        359, 360–1
Scutellaria baicalensis 47, 55, 144–5,
        171, 183–5, 241, 243, 245, 274,
        278–9, 314, 325, 360–1
Scutellaria barbata 25, 47, 55, 73,
        75–6, 114, 126, 184, 237–8, 242,
        328
Selaginella doederleinii 131
Semiaquilegia adoxoides 114, 169
Senecio scandens 245
Serenoa repens 171
Setaria italica 311
Silybum 245
Sinapis 138, 271
Smilax glabra 184–5, 223, 249, 273,
        307

Solanum lyratum 49, 139, 170, 222–3,
        237, 239, 241, 243–5, 249,
        313–14, 328
Solanum nigrum 84, 115, 124, 183,
        187–8, 222–4, 328
Solidago 184
Sophora 68, 80, 84–5
Sophora flavescens 25, 183, 314
Sophora subprostrata 25
Sophora tonkinensis 222–3, 273,
        278
Sparganium 114, 135, 149, 167, 173,
        203, 224
Spatholobus suberectus 26, 55, 75, 84,
        117, 122–5, 175, 187, 193, 212,
        239, 275, 294, 296, 308–12
Staphylococcus aureus 304
Streptococcus pneumoniae 291
Streptomyces 122
Syzygium aromaticum 250, 310
Szygium cumini 240

T

Taraxacum mongolicum 25, 114, 119,
        126–7, 134, 137, 139, 149, 183,
        245, 271, 308
Terminalia chebula 69, 83
Tetrapanax papyriferus 185, 222, 224,
        326
Thlaspi 68, 79, 132
Tinospora cordifolia 240
toxoplasma 291
Tremella 308
Trichosanthes 26, 47, 49, 55, 72, 76, 79,
        85, 114, 117, 126–7, 134, 136–8,
        149, 174–5, 204, 237–8, 243, 271,
        273–4, 279, 311, 325–6

Trigonella 135–6, 149
Trigonella foenum-graecum 240
Trogopterus xanthipes 26, 114, 224
Typha 224, 314
Typhonium giganteum 141

U

Uncaria 297

V

Vaccaria segetalis 27, 114, 139, 167,
        169
Vespa 114, 224, 273
Viola yedoensis 127, 134, 188,
        294

W

Wedelia chinensis 273
Wikstroemia indica 128
Withania somnifera 319

Z

Zanthoxylum 55, 325
Zanthoxylum bungeanum 56
Zaocys 270
Zaocys dhumnades 271
Zingiber officinale 26, 75, 210,
        326
Ziziphus jujuba 55, 75–6, 122–3, 243,
        249, 276, 325
Ziziphus spinosa 187, 295

Printed in the United States
By Bookmasters